Causes, Stages and Treatment of Ovarian Cancer

Causes, Stages and Treatment of Ovarian Cancer

Editor: Lester Price

FOSTER ACADEMICS

www.fosteracademics.com

www.fosteracademics.com

FOSTER ACADEMICS

Cataloging-in-Publication Data

Causes, stages and treatment of ovarian cancer / edited by Lester Price.
p. cm.
Includes bibliographical references and index.
ISBN 978-1-63242-531-7
1. Ovaries--Cancer. 2. Ovaries--Cancer--Prevention. 3. Ovaries--Cancer--Treatment.
I. Price, Lester.
RC280.O8 C38 2018
616.994 65--dc23

Foster Academics,
118-35 Queens Blvd., Suite 400,
Forest Hills, NY 11375, USA

ISBN 978-1-63242-531-7 (Hardback)

Printed and bound in China.

Contents

Preface

Ovarian cancer is caused when abnormal cells multiply and spread in an ovary. The main areas to which the cancer can spread are abdomen, liver, lungs, lymph nodes, bowel and bladder, etc. The treatments for this disease include chemotherapy and radiation therapy and sometimes the combination of both. This book presents researches and studies performed by experts across the globe on finding new and effective treatments of ovarian cancer. Researchers and students in this field will be assisted by this text.

This book is a result of research of several months to collate the most relevant data in the field.

When I was approached with the idea of this book and the proposal to edit it, I was overwhelmed. It gave me an opportunity to reach out to all those who share a common interest with me in this field. I had 3 main parameters for editing this text:

1. Accuracy - The data and information provided in this book should be up-to-date and valuable to the readers.

2. Structure - The data must be presented in a structured format for easy understanding and better grasping of the readers.

3. Universal Approach - This book not only targets students but also experts and innovators in the field, thus my aim was to present topics which are of use to all.

Thus, it took me a couple of months to finish the editing of this book.

I would like to make a special mention of my publisher who considered me worthy of this opportunity and also supported me throughout the editing process. I would also like to thank the editing team at the back-end who extended their help whenever required.

Editor

1

Discovery Analysis of TCGA Data Reveals Association between Germline Genotype and Survival in Ovarian Cancer Patients

Rosemary Braun[1,2*], Richard Finney[2], Chunhua Yan[2], Qing-Rong Chen[2], Ying Hu[2], Michael Edmonson[2], Daoud Meerzaman[2], Kenneth Buetow[3,2]

1 Robert H. Lurie Comprehensive Cancer Center, Northwestern University, Chicago, Illinois, United States of America, **2** Center for Biomedical Informatics and Information Technology, National Cancer Institute, National Institutes of Health, Bethesda, Maryland, United States of America, **3** Computational Science and Informatics Program, Complex Adaptive Systems Initiative, Arizona State University, Phoenix, Arizona, United States of America

Abstract

Background: Ovarian cancer remains a significant public health burden, with the highest mortality rate of all the gynecological cancers. This is attributable to the late stage at which the majority of ovarian cancers are diagnosed, coupled with the low and variable response of advanced tumors to standard chemotherapies. To date, clinically useful predictors of treatment response remain lacking. Identifying the genetic determinants of ovarian cancer survival and treatment response is crucial to the development of prognostic biomarkers and personalized therapies that may improve outcomes for the late-stage patients who comprise the majority of cases.

Methods: To identify constitutional genetic variations contributing to ovarian cancer mortality, we systematically investigated associations between germline polymorphisms and ovarian cancer survival using data from The Cancer Genome Atlas Project (TCGA). Using stage-stratified Cox proportional hazards regression, we examined >650,000 SNP loci for association with survival. We additionally examined whether the association of significant SNPs with survival was modified by somatic alterations.

Results: Germline polymorphisms at rs4934282 (AGAP11/C10orf116) and rs1857623 (DNAH14) were associated with stage-adjusted survival ($p = 1.12e\text{-}07$ and 1.80e-07, FDR $q = 1.2e\text{-}04$ and 2.4e-04, respectively). A third SNP, rs4869 (C10orf116), was additionally identified as significant in the exome sequencing data; it is in near-perfect LD with rs4934282. The associations with survival remained significant when somatic alterations.

Conclusions: Discovery analysis of TCGA data reveals germline genetic variations that may play a role in ovarian cancer survival even among late-stage cases. The significant loci are located near genes previously reported as having a possible relationship to platinum and taxol response. Because the variant alleles at the significant loci are common (frequencies for rs4934282 A/C alleles = 0.54/0.46, respectively; rs1857623 A/G alleles = 0.55/0.45, respectively) and germline variants can be assayed noninvasively, our findings provide potential targets for further exploration as prognostic biomarkers and individualized therapies.

Editor: Amanda Ewart Toland, Ohio State University Medical Center, United States of America

Funding: The authors are supported by the Intramural Research Program of the National Cancer Institute, United States National Institutes of Health, Bethesda, MD. There were no external funding sources for this study. The funders had no role in study design, data collection and analysis, decision to publish, or preparation of the manuscript.

Competing Interests: The authors have declared that no competing interests exist.

* E-mail: rbraun@northwestern.edu

Introduction

Ovarian cancer accounts for about three percent of all cancers in women and is the fifth leading cause of cancer-related death among women in the United States, with an age-adjusted incidence rate of 12.8 per 100,000 women per year and death rate of 8.6 per 100,000 women per year (2003–2007) [1]. Of the gynecological cancers, ovarian cancer has the highest mortality, with an overall five-year survival rate of 43.7% for white women and 34.9% for black women [1]. The poor survival statistics are attributable to the late stage at which ovarian cancers are diagnosed due to their asymptomatic nature: while stage I tumors have a 92.4% relative survival rate, they account only for 15% of ovarian cancer diagnoses; by contrast, stage III and IV cancers have survival rates of 34% and 18%, respectively, and together account for 65.4% of diagnoses [1]. Response to standard chemotherapy (platinum plus taxane) is highly variable [2,3], and tends to be poor for advanced cases [2]. Understanding the genetic determinants of ovarian cancer survival and response to treatment may improve these statistics, particularly for stage III and IV patients who comprise the majority of cases. In particular, identifying variations that predict response to chemotherapy allows for the possibility of administering alternate therapies that may improving outcomes.

Previous studies have examined the role of genetic variation in ovarian cancer susceptibility, progression, treatment response, and survival. It has been shown that BRCA1/2 germline mutations contribute to 10–15% of cases [4], and analysis of data from The Cancer Genome Atlas Project (TCGA [5]) has also shown that that BRCA1/2 germline mutation, somatic mutations and promoter methylation effect ovarian cancer survival [5]. Additionally, candidate gene studies have shown that polymorphisms in MDM2, along with TP53 status and SULF1, are associated with ovarian cancer survival [6–8]. Recently, Huang and coworkers reported a genetic variation is associated with carboplatin cytotoxicity in vitro and in vivo [3], a finding which may explain differential responsiveness to the standard platinum–based ovarian cancer therapy. The same authors later showed that the identified locus regulates miRNAs that contribute to platinum sensitivity, suggesting a mechanism of action [9].

To date, however, a clinically useful genomic marker of ovarian cancer survival remains elusive. The platinum–associated SNP investigated by Huang was not found to be significantly associated with survival in a validation cohort [3]. Likewise, Bolton and coworkers successfully identified several loci associated with ovarian cancer susceptibility, but those they initially found to be associated with survival failed to reach significance in the validation set [10], although it is hoped that future studies of this cohort will result in established associations with clinical outcome [10]. While tumor gene expression signatures predictive of treatment response and relapse have been reported (e.g., [11,12]), their clinical utility is limited by the cost, invasiveness, and variability inherent in evaluating tumor gene expression. Likewise, somatic copy number changes in certain genes have recently been reported to influence survival [13], but the utility of measuring CNV as a prognostic test is similarly limited.

The Cancer Genome Atlas Project (TCGA [5]) provides a collection of genomic and clinical data in which associations between genetics and survival can be thoroughly explored. Here, we carry out a genome-wide analysis to systematically investigate associations between *germline* genetic variation and overall survival in TCGA patients diagnosed with ovarian cancer (serous cystadenocarcinoma) [14]. The patients had an age and stage distribution typical of ovarian cancer, as shown in Table 1. Using the clinical and Affymetrix SNP6.0 ("SNP6") genotype data, we identified two single nucleotide polymorphism (SNP) loci at which the germline genotype is predictive of overall survival in ovarian cancer patients. The associations remain significant after adjusting for stage, and are associated with survival even amongst stage III patients. This suggests that constitutional genetic variation may play a role in treatment response and provides a potential avenue for a non-invasive prognostic biomarker test.

Results

Here, we report the association between germline SNPs and patient survival using TCGA ovarian cancer data. The filtered data comprised a total of 662,521 SNPs assayed in 489 clinically annotated ovarian cancer samples, with stage and age distributions as given in Table 1. Each of the 662,521 SNPs meeting the filtration criteria were tested for association with survival using Cox proportional hazards regression adjusted for stage using a non-additive model. Two SNPs, rs4934282 (A/C) in the gene AGAP11 (previously associated with C10orf116) and rs1857623 (A/G) upstream of DNAH14, showed a statistically significant univariate association with overall ovarian cancer survival, as summarized in Table 2. A *qq* plot of the *p*-values obtained is given in Figure 1. We additionally computed the per-allele hazard ratios for these SNPs using an additive model, obtaining HR = 0.599 ($p = 1.28e\text{-}08$) for the *C* allele at rs4934282 and HR = 1.425 ($p = 1.70e\text{-}05$) for the *G* allele at rs1857623. It should be noted that due to the small sample size, the power to detect a SNP with MAF = 0.45 (as these are) with $\alpha = 1e\text{-}06$ is 32% for HR = 0.6 and 3.5% for HR = 1.4; it is therefore likely that other SNPs with similar effect sizes may have been missed by chance in this analysis.

To illustrate the effect of rs4934282 (AGAP11/C10orf116) and rs1857623 (DNAH14) germline genotype on survival among patients with similar tumor stage, Kaplan-Meier plots for the 372 Stage III patients are given in Figures 2 and 3. Notably, the CC genotype at rs4934282 in AGAP11/C10orf116 confers a protective effect, nearly doubling the median survival time over the AA genotype group. Additionally, patients with homozygous CC at rs4934282 have a five-year survival rate of 45%, vs. 34% overall for Stage III patients [1].

To further investigate variation in the genomic regions surrounding these SNPs, we examined exome/capture sequencing data (for 375 patients with available germline data) in 100 Kbp windows centered about the two SNPs identified as significant in the SNP6 data, specifically chr10:88672456–88772455 and chr1:223081228–223181227. For ten samples with available whole-genome data, we were able to compare the intronic rs4934282 and rs1857623 Affymetrix SNP6.0 calls to those from the whole-genome sequencing, confirming the validity SNP6 calls. Of the 29 exome/capture SNPs tested (see Table 3) in the 375 samples, only rs4869 in C10orf116 remained significant after adjusting for the multiple hypotheses (FDR $q = 9.89e\text{-}03$). rs4869 is located ~2000b.p. upstream of rs4934282 and is in near-perfect linkage disequilibrium with rs4934282 (A/C at rs4934282 correlating with C/T at rs4869, respectively). rs4869 encodes a synonymous mutation in C10orf116 (Ile68Ile). We also investigated whether the variant alleles at any of these 29 loci led to deleterious nonsynonymous protein alterations; only five SNPs had mis-sense allelic variations, none of which were predicted to be deleterious (Table 4).

Finally, we used data derived from normal–paired tumor samples to assess whether the strong effect of germline genotype on survival was significantly mediated or moderated by tumor gene expression gain or loss of copy number in the tumor, or by loss of heterozygosity (see File S1) to test the hypothesis that the effect of germline genotype on ovarian cancer survival might be influenced by somatic events. We found no significant association of tumor gene expression, copy number variation, or loss of heterozygosity in these regions with survival (see File S1). Rather, the large effect of germline genotype at the loci on patient survival is independent of these somatic changes, and appears to suggest that constitutional genetic variation in these regions plays a role in treatment response.

Discussion

Recent studies have demonstrated that common genetic variants are associated with ovarian cancer risk [15,16]. However, it remains difficult to predict ovarian cancer survival independent of stage; current clinical findings show that tumor response and extreme drug resistance in vitro are not good predictors of ovarian cancer survival [17,18]. In our study, we comprehensively tested the SNPs assayed in the TCGA SNP6.0 data for association with survival, and additionally analyzed whole-genome and exome/capture SNPs in the genomic regions surrounding the significant

Table 1. Stage and age at diagnosis, organized by 5-year survival.

	Censored <5 yrs	Survival <5 yrs	Survival ≥ 5 yrs	All	p
N	187 (38%)	228 (47%)	74 (15%)	489	
Stage					1.3e-02
I	10	2	2	14	
II	11	6	8	25	
III	140	181	53	374	
IV	26	39	11	76	
Age	58.2 (49.6, 65.5)	59.9 (51.0, 68.1)	62.3 (54.7, 71.4)	59.1 (51.4, 69.1)	6.1e-02

Stage and age at diagnosis of samples, organized by 5-year survival. Median age is reported, with the first and third quartiles given in parentheses. p values for the univariate association between stage and survival and age and survival (logrank test) are also given.

SNP6.0 SNPs. We identified three SNPs in two genomic regions that had a statistically-significant association with survival. As shown in Table 2, the hazard ratios for homozygous minor alleles approached or exceeded two-fold in stage-stratified Cox proportional hazard models, and the per-allele effect sizes for these SNPs using a stage-stratified additive genotype model were HR = 0.599 and HR = 1.425 for rs4934282 *C* and rs1857623 *G*, respectively. Interestingly, none of the somatic variations we examined (tumor gene expression, copy number variation, and loss of heterozygosity) were associated either with the germline genotype at these loci or with survival, despite a plausible hypothesis that somatic changes in the tumor might have an effect on the genotype–survival association. Rather, these SNPs are strongly predictive of survival independent of somatic changes that had already occurred in the tumor (see File S1).

Two of the survival–associated SNPs are located within a 2200 bp region on chromosome 10 (rs4934282 at chr10:88732476 and rs4869 at chr10:88730312) and are in near–perfect LD in this data. This genomic region is associated with C10orf116 (chr10:88727949–88730672) and AGAP11 (chr10:88730498–88769960), which overlap; the biological significance of the variation probed by rs4934282 and rs4869 may be associated with either. AGAP11 is a member of the ankyrin repeat and GTPase domain Arf GTPase activating protein gene family [19]. C10orf116 (also referred to as APM2) is a protein of unknown function that is homologous to the medium chain of mammalian clathrin-associated protein complex and is involved in vesicular transport in yeast. The genomic region containing rs4934282 and rs4869 is shown in Figure 4.

While little prior evidence exists linking AGAP11 to cancer susceptibility, survival, or treatment response, some evidence exists for the role of C10orf116. C10orf116/APM2 expression has been implicated in other gynecological cancers; for instance, is has been shown to strongly differentiate between the BRCA1 associated breast tumor subclasses ESR1-positive and ESR1-negative [20] and is has been found to be downregulated in utering cancer in a number of studies [21]. More recently, C10orf116 has been shown to exhibit differential expression in different pathological grades of ovarian carcinoma [22] and in the response of breast cancer to chemotherapy [23,24].

More importantly, there exists from cell lines pointing to C10orf116 as a mediator of cisplatin resistance. Ovarian cancer has been treated with platinum compounds for many years [25,26], with cisplatin and carboplatin (which has a more acceptible toxicity profile) as a standard therapy for newly–diagnosed stage III ovarian cancers [26,27]. However, while many patients respond to initial treatment, the five-year survival rates remain poor (34% overall for stage III [1]). APM2 (C10orf116) has been shown to promote cisplatin resistance when overexpressed in HCT116 cell lines that were sensitive to chemotherapy and radiation [28], suggesting a possible mechanism by which rs4869 and rs4934282 influence survival. Silencing of APM2 by shRNA was shown to enhance the cytotoxic effects of cisplatin on tumor xenografts grown in CD-1 nude mice. Additionally, APM2 was found to be overexpressed in cisplatin resistant gastric cancer cells, but not in gastric cancer cells resistant to 5-FU or doxorubicin [29]. More recently, it was found that rs1649942, a SNP located ~5 Mb upstream of rs4934282/rs4869, had a modest association with carboplatin-induced cytotoxicity and the survival of ovarian cancer patients following carboplatin-based chemotherapy [3]. Although this SNP failed to reach significance in their phase 2 validation analysis (and likewise not significant in our study), it adds to the body of evidence implicating this genomic region in platinum sensitivity.

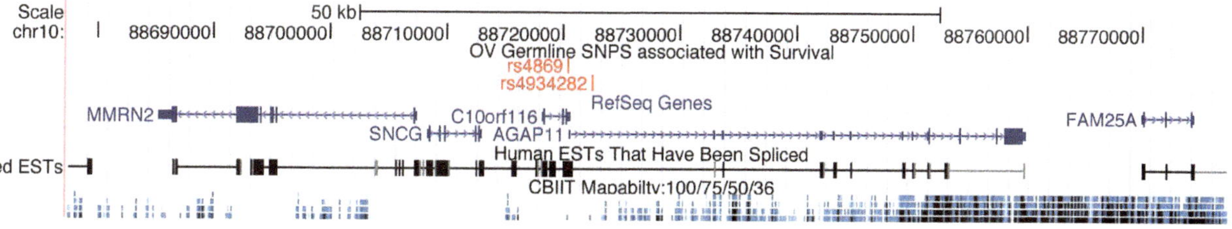

Figure 1. QQ plots. Quantile-quantile plot for observed p values for the likelihood ratio tests of the stage-adjusted Cox models versus the expected distribution of p values under independent null hypotheses. Points above the line indicate values that are more significant than expected; a large systematic deviation from this line would be indicative of population substructure driving the results. The two SNPs identified as significant, rs4934282 and rs1857623, lie well above the line and outside the small systematic deviation.

Table 2. Stage-adjusted survival.

rs4934282 (AGAP11/C10orf116, chr10:88732476)

	N (482)	HR	*p*	*q*	p_{perm}
AA	146	(ref)	(ref)	(ref)	(ref)
AC	231	0.686	8.0e-03	7.5e-01	8.4e-03
CC	105	0.355	3.6e-08	3.7e-03	<2e-06
Logrank			1.1e-07	1.2e-04	<2e-06

rs1857623 (DNAH14, chr1:223131228)

	N (486)	HR	*p*	*q*	p_{perm}
AA	151	(ref)	(ref)	(ref)	(ref)
AG	230	0.881	3.9e-01	9.8e-01	6.8e-01
GG	105	1.999	2.9e-05	4.5e-01	1.2e-04
Logrank			1.8e-07	2.4e-04	6.6e-05

rs4869 (C10orf116, chr10:88730312)

	N (304)	HR	*p*
TT	102	(ref)	(ref)
CT	152	1.763	2.6e-03
CC	108	2.132	1.3e-04
Logrank			3.4e-04

Significant survival associations after stratification by stage; rs4934282 and rs1857623 are from SNP6 data, rs4869 is from exome/capture data (29 SNPs tested). All tests of Schoefeld residuals had $p > 0.07$, meeting the proportional hazards assumption.

The third significant SNP, rs1857623, is found in an intergenic region on chromosome 1, 53 Kb upstream of DNAH14 and 136 Kb downstream from CNIH3. DNAH14 belongs to the dynein heavy chain family, a motor protein which attaches to microtubules and walks along cytoskeletal microtubules [30]. The mechanism by which variation in DNAH14 may impact survival is less clear. One possible avenue for future studies is its potential role in the context of taxol therapy: DNAH14 contains the microtubule-binding stalk of dynein motor (pfam12777 at Location:2910–3244 of reference protein NP_001364.1), and it has been demonstrated that taxol binds microtubules [28]. DNAH14 has also been found to be differentially regulated in response to taxane therapy in gastric cancers [31] and doxorubicin therapy in endometrial cells [32].

These findings suggest that consitutional genetic variations in these regions may play a role in ovarian cancer survival even among late-stage cases. However, it should be noted that the results presented here constitute a discovery-based analysis that did not include a validation cohort. As such, the findings may be spurious false positives, and require confirmation in follow-up studies. If validated, these SNPs may have important clinical potential as prognostic biomarkers since germline genotype can be assayed noninvasively and because the variant alleles at the significant loci are common (frequencies for rs4934282 A/C alleles = 0.54/0.46 respectively; rs1857623 A/G alleles = 0.55/0.45, respectvely; both comparable to allele frequencies for the Caucasian CEPH population in HapMap [33]). The significant loci are located in genes previously identified as having a possible relationship to chemotherapeutic response, suggesting that their association with survival may be due to their influence on treatment response. Our study suggests potential targets for prognositic tests and individualized therapies, and provides a basis for follow-up research.

Materials and Methods

Data

Data were collected by the TCGA project as described elsewhere [14]. Follow up times, vital status, tumor stage, and

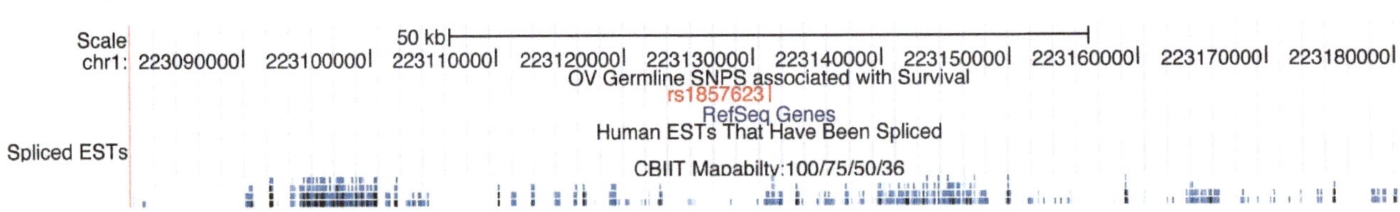

Figure 2. Survival of stage-III ovarian cancer patients by rs4934282 genotype. Kaplan-Meier survival plots for Stage III patients, stratified by germline genotype at rs4934282 (AGAP11): AA, black; AC, blue; CC, red. Confidence intervals are shown as a shaded region around each Kaplan-Meier curve. Censored observations are denoted with vertical ticks. The dashed horizontal and vertical lines mark 50% survival and five years (1825 days) respectively.

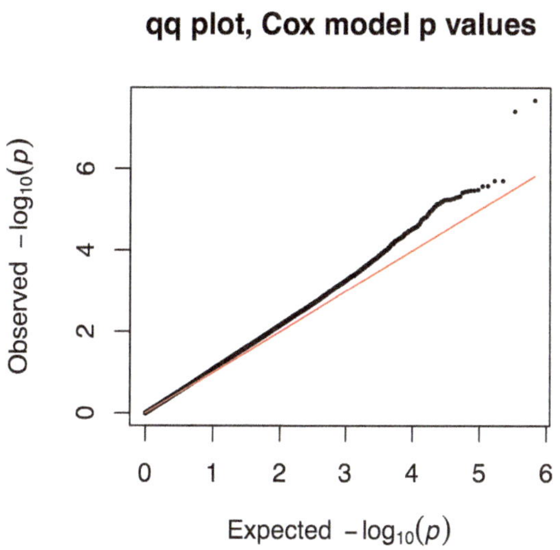

Figure 3. Survival of stage-III ovarian cancer patients by rs1857623 genotype. Kaplan-Meier survival plots for Stage III patients, stratified by germline genotype at rs1857623 (DNAH14): AA, black; AG, blue; GG, red. Confidence intervals are shown as a shaded region around each Kaplan-Meier curve. Censored observations are denoted with vertical ticks. The dashed horizontal and vertical lines mark 50% survival and five years (1825 days) respectively.

germline genotype data were obtained from the TCGA project [14] via the data portal on 06/03/2011.

SNP6 genotypes. Genotype calls for the 906,600 SNP probes assayed using the Affymetrix GenomeWide SNP6.0 platform and processed using Birdseed were obtained from TCGA. Samples that did not pass the TCGA quality control (per the TCGA copy number Sample Data Relationship Format file) were removed. A total of 496 ovarian serous cystadenocarcinoma patients had survival time and germline (either blood or tumor-adjacent normal) genotype data. Genotype calls were coded as 0, 1 or 2 according to the number of variant alleles and filtered according to a Birdseed confidence threshold of 0.05.

The genotype data were subject to additional quality control filtration criteria as follows. SNPs with call rates <0.95 or minor allele frequencies <0.05 were excluded, as were SNPs out of Hardy Weinberg equilibrium with $p<10^{-4}$. All samples with a call rate below 80% were excluded. Identity by state was computed using the R GenABEL package, and closely related samples with IBS >0.95 were removed. The SNP and sample filtration criteria were applied iteratively until all samples and SNPs met the stated thresholds. In total, 489 samples and 662,521 SNPs passed were kept in the analysis.

Tumor stage. Stage subcategories were coalesced for the purposes of this analysis into summary stage categories yielding four stage classifications (i.e., Stage IA, IB, IC were treated as Stage I, etc.). The number of samples in each stage category is given in Table 1.

Exome/capture data. Next generation exome/capture sequencing data were also retrieved for 375 patients with available germline data. The analysis was restricted to 100 Kbp windows centered about the two SNPs identified as significant in the SNP6 data, specifically chr10:88672456–88772455 and chr1:223081228–223181227. Graphical descriptions of these genomic regions are provided in Figures 5 and 6.

Binary Sequence Alignment/Map (BAM) files were downloaded from dbGAP, using for each sample the largest available normal BAM file. The "mpileup" and "bcftools" features of SAMtools [34] were used to generate the variant call information, with calling criteria as follows: if the coverage in a given sample for a given locus was less than the coverage threshold (see following paragraph), no call was made; otherwise, if non-reference allele frequency was less than 10%, the call was "homozygous reference;" if the non-reference frequency was greater than 90%, the call was "homozygous nonreference;" if it was between 10% and 90%, the call was "heterozygous."

To set the coverage threshold for the exome/capture data, we compared the exome/capture calls to the SNP6 germline genotype calls for 41 tag SNPs located in those regions. Treating the SNP6 calls as the gold standard for accuracy, we define the "mismatch rate" to be the number of calls for exome/capture and SNP6 data differ, divided by the total number of exome/capture calls made at that coverage depth. As coverage threshold is increased and the exome/capture data becomes more reliable, the mismatch rate decreases, but fewer exome/capture calls can be made. We varied the coverage threshold from 5 to 30, selecting the lowest coverage that yielded a mismatch rate smaller than 0.05. The optimum coverage was 9 (with a mismatch rate of 0.045).

We considered a locus to be informative (ie, having sufficient variation) if at least 20 germline samples had a heterozygous call at that coverage threshold; these criteria yield 29 total informative SNPs in the 100 Kbp regions surrounding rs4934282 and rs1857623, shown in Table 3, which we considered in the analysis.

Survival analysis

Survival analysis was carried out in R [35] using the "survival" package [36]. For each SNP represented in the data, Cox proportional hazards regression was used to model survival as a function of genotype. Because of the significant association of stage with survival, all models were stratified by stage. Genotype calls were treated as categorical variables with 0 as the referent group to avoid imposing linearity in the number of variant alleles. Each model yielded two hazard ratios per SNP (one for genotype = 1 with respect to genotype = 0 and another for genotype = 2 w.r.t. genotype = 0). The significance of the association was assessed using the logrank (Score) test [37]. A test of Schoenfeld residuals was used to check whether the proportional hazards assumption was met; only models with $p>0.05$ were considered valid. 639,510 SNPs tested met the proportional hazards assumption.

Because the large number of SNPs implies a vast number of hypotheses being tested, multiple testing adjustments were made to the p values. This was done in two ways. We report both the false discovery rate [38] (q) for the p values obtained for the parametric tests described above. In addition, we report permutation p_{perm} values obtained using 600,000 independent resamplings of the data. Permutation tests, while computationally intensive, are considered the strongest and most appropriate control of type-I error rates in genome-wide studies [39–41].

To investigate the existence and effect of any population stratification, the R package GenABEL [42] was used to examine population substructure. The genomic inflation factor was estimated to be $\lambda = 1.09$, indicating that population substructure, if present, should have no appreciable effect on the results. Using a randomly selected set of 12,000 independent (pairwise LD $r^2 < 0.01$) SNPs with MAF >0.3, population substructure was examined using principal component analysis. Pairwise plots of the first four components are provided in the File S2. We adjusted the models in two ways: using the first four PCs, and using cluster assignments identified from the PCA using R package mclust [43]. As expected based on $\lambda = 1.09$, we observed no appreciable changes in the Cox model results (data not shown). The results

Table 3. Cox model results for exome/capture loci.

					Alleles		N samples				AB		BB			
(lr)6–7 (lr)8–11 (lr)12–13 (lr)14–15 Source	rsID	Chr	Position	Gene	A	B	AA	AB	BB	tot	HR	p(HR)	HR	p(HR)	p.logRank	
NextGen	rs7074064	10	88673102	BMPR1A	T	C	220	115	29	364	0.94	6.97e-01	1.09	7.35e-01	8.46e-01	
NextGen	rs4447076	10	88686361	MMRN2	A	G	82	81	31	194	1.32	2.12e-01	0.92	8.02e-01	3.59e-01	
NextGen	rs34587013	10	88686602	MMRN2	C	G	287	40	2	329	1.09	7.15e-01			9.33e-01	
NextGen	rs4934281	10	88692330	MMRN2	G	C	1	25	269	295	1.61	6.51e-01	2.15	4.49e-01	4.77e-01	
NextGen	rs10887673	10	88692370	MMRN2	G	A	82	54	10	146	0.70	1.81e-01	0.88	7.96e-01	4.06e-01	
NextGen		10	88694221	MMRN2	G	T	289	20	0	309	1.40	2.86e-01			2.84e-01	
NextGen	rs3750822	10	88695286	MMRN2	T	G	63	21	2	86	0.53	8.97e-02			2.28e-01	
NextGen	rs4244973	10	88707120	MMRN2	T	A	5	31	291	327	1.27	7.08e-01	1.63	4.03e-01	4.45e-01	
NextGen	rs3750823	10	88707134	MMRN2	C	T	139	125	63	327	1.16	3.64e-01	1.07	7.52e-01	6.62e-01	
NextGen	rs1800373	10	88708416	SNCG	A	C	111	115	90	316	1.07	7.02e-01	0.95	8.17e-01	8.34e-01	
NextGen	rs760113	10	88709769	SNCG	C	G	159	72	9	240	0.97	8.73e-01	0.59	2.53e-01	5.13e-01	
NextGen	rs9864	10	88712378	SNCG	A	T	203	105	12	320	0.95	7.47e-01	0.50	1.28e-01	2.98e-01	
NextGen	rs62621086	10	88712453	SNCG	T	G	166	20	2	188	0.76	4.43e-01			4.53e-01	
NextGen	rs2279601	10	88720157	C10orf116	A	G	61	57	42	160	1.45	1.79e-01	1.76	5.66e-02	1.40e-01	
NextGen	rs4869	10	88720292	C10orf116	T	C	100	148	106	354	1.72	4.05e-03	2.06	2.75e-04	7.44e-04	*
NextGen	rs7960	10	88720354	C10orf116	C	T	75	99	38	212	1.23	3.26e-01	1.77	3.65e-02	1.08e-01	
SNP6.0	rs4934282	10	88732476	AGAP11	A	C	138	228	100	466	0.72	2.26e-02	0.37	3.12e-07	1.04e-06	*
NextGen		10	88748032	AGAP11	G	T	252	27	0	279	0.89	7.00e-01			6.99e-01	†
NextGen	rs1240370	10	88748297	AGAP11	T	C	97	118	38	253	1.08	6.85e-01	1.10	7.21e-01	8.99e-01	†
NextGen	rs1240371	10	88748466	AGAP11	C	G	12	26	12	50	2.12	3.22e-01	1.09	9.17e-01	4.62e-01	
NextGen	rs1240407	10	88753935	AGAP11	T	C	16	70	105	191	1.70	2.07e-01	2.17	5.95e-02	1.20e-01	†
NextGen	rs72644240	10	88754336	AGAP11	T	G	3	26	41	70	0.81	7.90e-01	1.01	9.88e-01	8.51e-01	†
NextGen		10	88757859	AGAP11	C	T	20	45	0	65	2.09	9.55e-02			8.85e-02	†
NextGen		10	88757910	AGAP11	G	T	33	34	8	75	1.24	5.75e-01	1.38	5.72e-01	7.87e-01	†
NextGen	rs36104328	10	88758019	AGAP11	A	G	175	58	4	237	0.83	3.92e-01			6.88e-01	†
NextGen	rs2641563	10	88758233	AGAP11	A	G	16	107	161	284	1.70	1.95e-01	2.17	5.26e-02	7.78e-02	
NextGen	rs2641562	10	88758403	AGAP11	A	G	86	119	52	257	1.23	3.08e-01	2.03	2.77e-03	8.99e-03	†
NextGen	rs1745901	10	88758637	AGAP11	C	T	21	124	181	326	1.78	9.58e-02	2.19	2.12e-02	4.38e-02	†
NextGen		1	223127807		C	T	29	25	0	54	1.40	4.69e-01			4.67e-01	
SNP6.0	rs1857623	1	223131228	DNAH14	A	G	145	220	104	469	0.88	3.91e-01	2.04	2.39e-05	1.06e-07	*
NextGen		1	223142168		A	G	19	34	0	53	1.16	7.34e-01			7.34e-01	

Cox model results for exome/capture loci, with significant SNP6.0 loci provided in context. Given are the sample numbers, hazard ratios and associated p values for each genotype, as well as the logrank p values for the Cox model.
*denotes significant SNPs;
†denotes non-specific regions in the exome/capture data that may reflect variation from another genomic region.

Table 4. SIFT and logRE predictions for missense SNPs.

					substitution		SIFT		logRE	
rsID	**Chr**	**Position**	**Gene**	**RefSeq**	**NT**	**AA**	**score**	**prediction**	**score**	**prediction**
rs3750823	10	88707134	MMRN2	NM_024756	c.G145A	p.G49S	0.15	borderline	0.27	neutral
rs4934281	10	88692330	MMRN2	NM_024756	c.C2191G	p.H731D	0.62	neutral	NA	NA
rs34587013	10	88686602	MMRN2	NM_024756	c.G2728C	p.V910L	0.91	neutral	NA	NA
rs9864	10	88712378	SNCG	NM_003087	c.A329T	p.E110V	0.15	borderline	0.36	neutral
rs2641563	10	88758233	AGAP11	NM_133447	c.A244G	p.I82V	1.00	neutral	NA	NA

SIFT and logRE predictions for missense SNPs. Shown are the location, gene, and RefSeq IDs for the SNPs, the nucleotide (NT) and amino acid (AA) substitutions, and the SIFT and logRE scores and predictions. SIFT scores are classified into predictions as follows: 0.00—0.05, probably damaging; 0.051—0.10, possibly damaging; 0.101—0.20, borderline; 0.201—1.00, neutral. logRE scores are classified into predictions as follows: 1—up, probably damaging; 0.7—0.99, possibly damaging; 0.5—0.69, borderline; 0.0—0.49, neutral.

presented here are therefore not adjusted for population substructure.

Sequencing data analysis

We compared the SNP6 genotypes at the significant loci (chr10:88722456 and chr1:223131228) to those from whole-genome sequencing data for 10 available samples; all 10 matched the SNP6 calls for the significant SNPs, supporting the SNP6 genotype calls.

For the two SNPs showing significant association with survival in the SNP6 data, we further investigated the surrounding genomic regions using combined whole-genome and exome/capture sequencing data. We investigated 29 SNPs in the the genomic regions surrounding rs4934282 and rs1857623 shown in Table 3 and chosen as described above. Stage-stratified Cox proportional hazards models were then constructed for the germline genotypes as described above. It should be noted neither rs4934282 nor rs1857623 were included due to insufficient exome/capture data (rs4934282

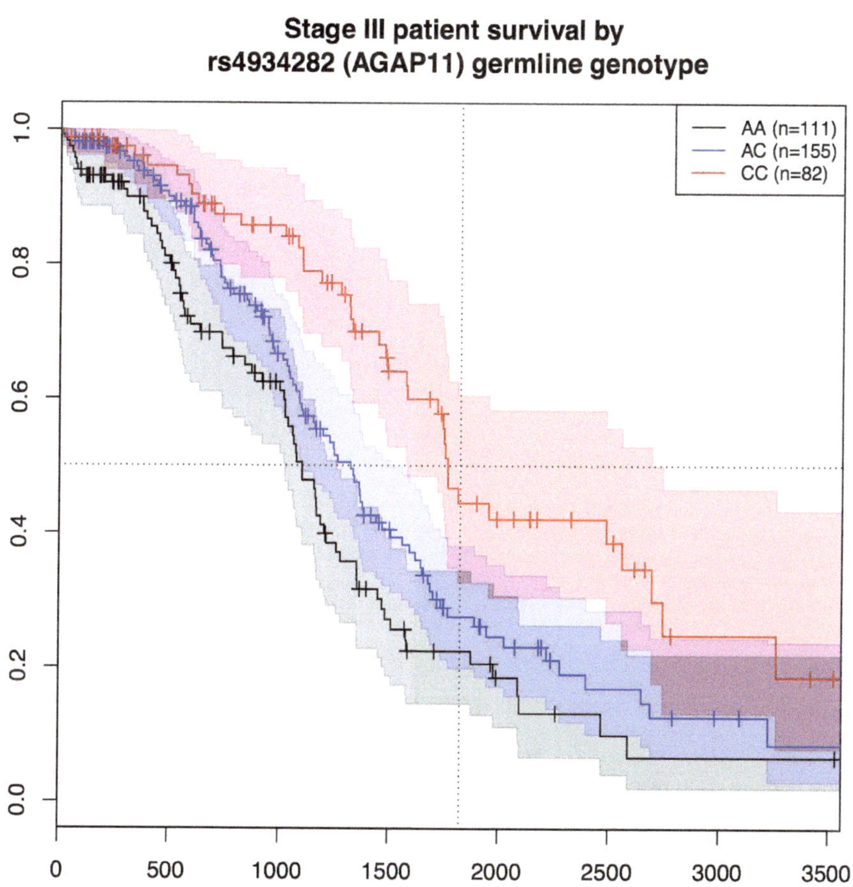

Figure 4. Genomic region containing rs4934282 and rs4869. Detailed description of the genomic region of chromosome 10 containing rs4934282 (second SNP from the right) and rs4869 (shown in green). Note the overlap between AGAP11 and C10orf116.

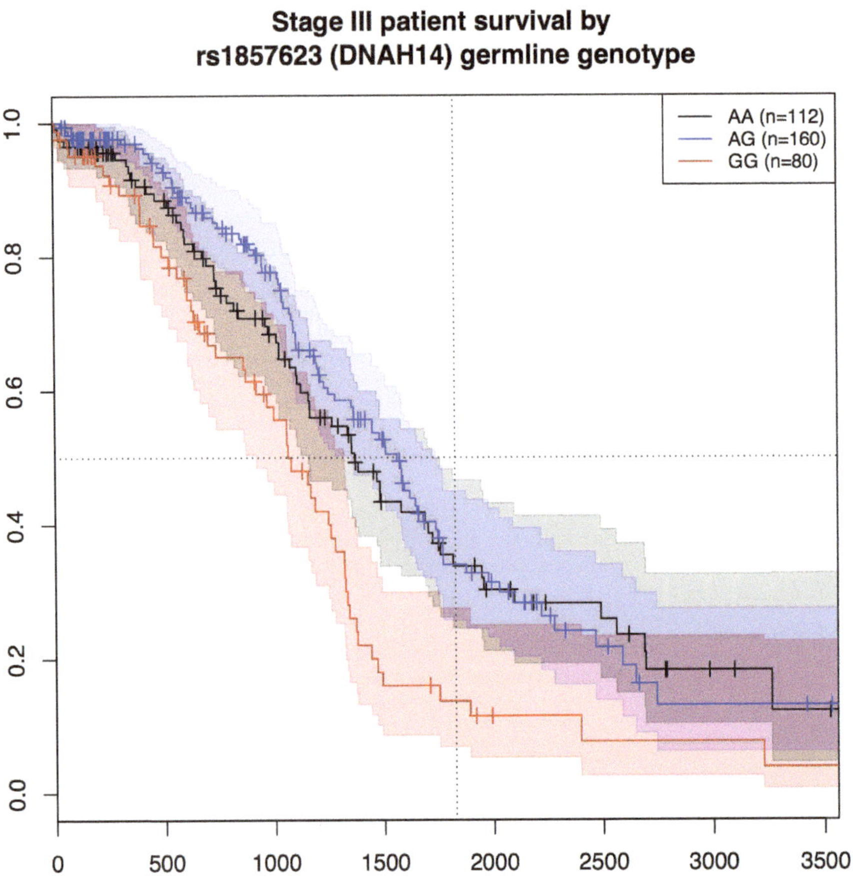

Figure 5. Genomic region surrounding rs4934282. Image from cgwb.nci.nih.gov of selected tracks for genome build NCBI36 (hg18) for the region surrounding two germline variations associated with survival in ovarian cancer in C10orf116/AGAP11 region on chromosome 10. The tracks are a custom track showing the SNPs rs4869 and rs4934282, RefSeq gene, mRNA, spliced ESTs and mapability.

is in an intronic region and hence not assayed in the exome/capture data; rs1857623 had no calls in the majority of samples).

It should be noted that not all the genomic regions contributing to these data have unique sequences. To assess this, we used the "mapability" criteria as implemented in CGWB [44]: for each

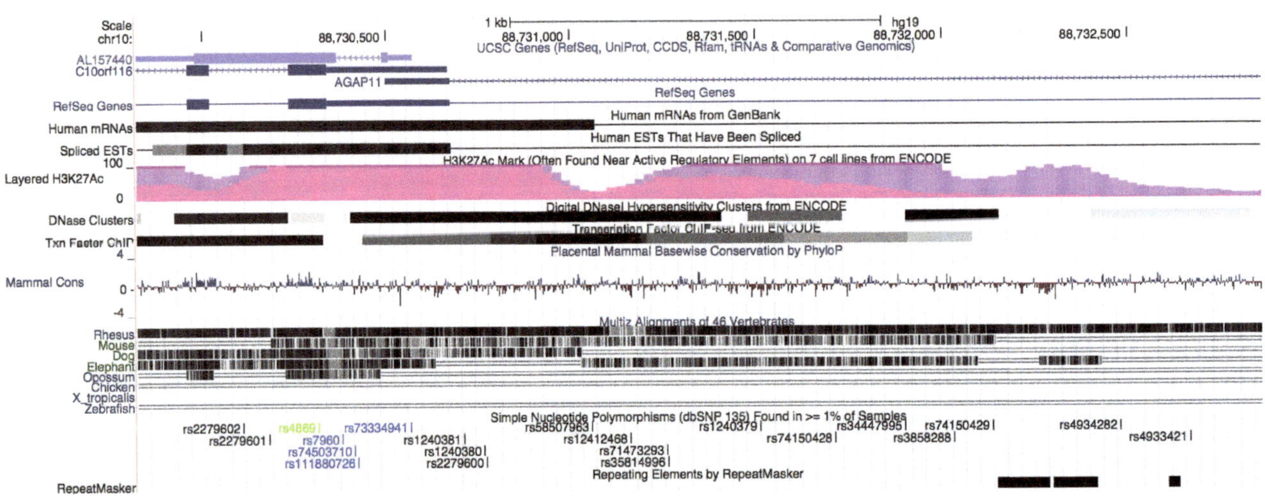

Figure 6. Genomic region surrounding rs1857623. Image from cgwb.nci.nih.gov of selected tracks for genome build NCBI36 (hg18) for the region surrounding a germline variation associated with survival in ovarian cancer upstream of DNAH14 on chromosome 1. The tracks are a custom track showing the SNP rs1857623, RefSeq gene, mRNA, spliced ESTs and mapability.

locus under consideration, we consider a sliding 75 base-pair window containing that locus and attempt to match it to other regions in the genome; the locus is flagged as unique if, for every position of the sliding window, the sequence only maps to the location of the window and no other genomic region. Loci for which some (or all) positions of the sliding window contain sequences that map to multiple genomic regions are flagged with a dagger in Table 3, denoting that the reads contributing to the calls at that locus may be nonspecific.

Prediction of amino-acid substitutions

We examined the SNPs in Table 3 for mis-sense substitutions using program ANNOVAR [45] and predicted their functional impact on protein sequences with logRE and SIFT. LogRE is the $\log_{10}$ of the ratio of HMMER E-values for the fit to a PFAM motif domain of two amino acid sequences that differ by an amino acid substitution. A logRE score whose absolute value is greater than or equal to 1 indicates that the amino acid alteration is likely to affect protein [46]. SIFT is a sequence homology-based tool that Sorts Intolerant From Tolerant amino acid substitutions and predicts deleterious amino acid substitutions. SIFT values ≤ 0.05 are predicted to be deleterious [47]. Of the SNPs considered above five mis-sense snps were identified: three in MMRN2 (rs3750823, rs4934281, rs34587013), one in SNCG (rs9864), and one in AGAP11 (rs2641563). However, there is no evidence that these amino acid changes have functional impact on the proteins (Table 4).

Analysis of somatic variations

To test the hypothesis that somatic changes might have an additive or moderating effect on the association between germline genotype and ovarian cancer survival, we used TCGA data derived from paired tumor samples to assess whether tumor gene expression, gain or loss of copy number in the tumor, or loss of heterozygosity were significantly associated with survival. A full description of the methods and results for this analysis is given in the File S1. None of these additional covariates were significant.

Supporting Information

File S1 Methods and results of analysis of somatic variations.

File S2 Methods and results of population substructure analysis.

Author Contributions

Conceived and designed the experiments: RB RF CY DM KB. Performed the experiments: RB RF CY QC. Analyzed the data: RB RF CY QC. Contributed reagents/materials/analysis tools: RB RF CY QC YH ME. Wrote the paper: RB RF CY DM KB.

References

1. Howlader N, Noone A, Krapcho M, Neyman N, Aminou R, et al. (2011) SEER cancer statistics review, 1975–2008. Bethesda, MD: National Cancer Institute.
2. Blackledge G, Lawton F, Redman C, Kelly K (1989) Response of patients in phase ii studies of chemotherapy in ovarian cancer: implications for patient treatment and the design of phase ii trials. British Journal of Cancer 59: 650.
3. Huang R, Johnatty S, Gamazon E, Im H, Ziliak D, et al. (2011) Platinum sensitivity-related germline polymorphism discovered via a cell-based approach and analysis of its association with outcome in ovarian cancer patients. Clinical Cancer Research.
4. Pal T, Permuth-Wey J, Betts JA, Krischer JP, Fiorica J, et al. (2005) BRCA1 and BRCA2 mutations account for a large proportion of ovarian carcinoma cases. Cancer 104: 2807–2816.
5. Bell D, Berchuck A, Birrer M, Chien J, Cramer DW, et al. (2011) Integrated genomic analyses of ovarian carcinoma. Nature 474: 609–615.
6. Han CH, Huang YJ, Lu KH, Liu Z, Mills GB, et al. (2011) Polymorphisms in the SULF1 gene are associated with early age of onset and survival of ovarian cancer. J Exp Clin Cancer Res 30: 5.
7. Bartel F, Jung J, Bohnke A, Gradhand E, Zeng K, et al. (2008) Both germ line and somatic genetics of the p53 pathway affect ovarian cancer incidence and survival. Clin Cancer Res 14: 89–96.
8. Marsh S, Paul J, King C, Gifford G, McLeod H, et al. (2007) Pharmacogenetic assessment of toxicity and outcome after platinum plus taxane chemotherapy in ovarian cancer: the scottish randomised trial in ovarian cancer. Journal of Clinical Oncology 25: 4528.
9. Ziliak D, Gamazon ER, Lacroix B, Kyung Im H, Wen Y, et al. (2012) Genetic Variation That Predicts Platinum Sensitivity Reveals the Role of miR-193b* in Chemotherapeutic Susceptibility. Mol Cancer Ther 11: 2054–2061.
10. Bolton KL, Ganda C, Berchuck A, Pharaoh PD, Gayther SA (2012) Role of common genetic variants in ovarian cancer susceptibility and outcome: progress to date from the Ovarian Cancer Association Consortium (OCAC). J Intern Med 271: 366–378.
11. Nikas J, Boylan K, Skubitz A, Low W (2011) Mathematical prognostic biomarker models for treatment response and survival in epithelial ovarian cancer. Cancer Informatics 10: 233–47.
12. Hartmann L, Lu K, Linette G, Cliby W, Kalli K, et al. (2005) Gene expression profiles predict early relapse in ovarian cancer after platinum-paclitaxel chemotherapy. Clinical Cancer Research 11: 2149.
13. Engler DA, Gupta S, Growdon WB, Drapkin RI, Nitta M, et al. (2012) Genome wide DNA copy number analysis of serous type ovarian carcinomas identifies genetic markers predictive of clinical outcome. PLoS ONE 7: e30996.
14. TCGA (2011) The results published here are in whole or part based upon data generated by The Cancer Genome Atlas Pilot Project established by the NCI and NHGRI. Information about TCGA and the investigators and institutions who constitute the TCGA research network can be found at http://cancergenome.nih.gov. (Data accessed 20 July 2011.).
15. Fasching P, Gayther S, Pearce L, Schildkraut J, Goode E, et al. (2009) Role of genetic polymorphisms and ovarian cancer susceptibility. Molecular Oncology 3: 171–181.
16. Bolton KL, Tyrer J, Song H, Ramus SJ, Notaridou M, et al. (2010) Common variants at 19p13 are associated with susceptibility to ovarian cancer. Nat Genet 42: 880–884.
17. Matsuo K, Bond V, Im D, Rosenshein N (2010) Prediction of chemotherapy response with platinum and taxane in the advanced stage of ovarian and uterine carcinosarcoma: a clinical implication of in vitro drug resistance assay. American Journal of Clinical Oncology 33: 358.
18. Rose P, Tian C, Bookman M (2010) Assessment of tumor response as a surrogate endpoint of survival in recurrent/platinum-resistant ovarian carcinoma: A gynecologic oncology group study. Gynecologic Oncology 117: 324–329.
19. Nie Z, Hirsch DS, Randazzo PA (2003) Arf and its many interactors. Curr Opin Cell Biol 15: 396–404.
20. Fernández-Ramires R, Solé X, De Cecco L, Llort G, Cazorla A, et al. (2009) Gene expression profiling integrated into network modelling reveals heterogeneity in the mechanisms of brca1 tumorigenesis. British Journal of Cancer 101: 1469–1480.
21. Arslan AA, Gold LI, Mittal K, Suen TC, Belitskaya-Levy I, et al. (2005) Gene expression studies provide clues to the pathogenesis of uterine leiomyoma: new evidence and a systematic review. Hum Reprod 20: 852–863.
22. Skubitz AP, Pambuccian SE, Argenta PA, Skubitz KM (2006) Differential gene expression identifies subgroups of ovarian carcinoma. Transl Res 148: 223–248.
23. Sano H, Wada S, Eguchi H, Osaki A, Saeki T, et al. (2012) Quantitative prediction of tumor response to neoadjuvant chemotherapy in breast cancer: novel marker genes and prediction model using the expression levels. Breast Cancer 19: 37–45.
24. Hernandez-Vargas H, Rodriguez-Pinilla SM, Julian-Tendero M, Sanchez-Rovira P, Cuevas C, et al. (2007) Gene expression profiling of breast cancer cells in response to gemcitabine: NF-kappaB pathway activation as a potential mechanism of resistance. Breast Cancer Res Treat 102: 157–172.
25. Prestayko A, d'Aoust J, Issell B, Crooke S (1979) Cisplatin (cis-diamminedichloroplatinum II). Cancer Treatment Reviews 6: 17–39.
26. Jakupec M, Galanski M, Keppler B (2003) Tumour-inhibiting platinum complexes—state of the art and future perspectives. Ergebnisse der Physiologie, Biologischen Chemie und Experimentellen Pharmakologie 146: 1–54.
27. Wang X (2010) Fresh platinum complexes with promising antitumor activity. Anti-Cancer Agents in Medicinal Chemistry 10: 396–411.
28. Alderson K, Holds JB, Anderson RL (1991) Botulinum-induced alteration of nerve-muscle interactions in the human orbicularis oculi following treatment for blepharospasm. Neurology 41: 1800–1805.
29. Kang H, Kim I, Park J, Shin Y, Ku J, et al. (2004) Identification of genes with differential expression in acquired drug-resistant gastric cancer cells using high-density oligonucleotide microarrays. Clinical Cancer Research 10: 272.

30. Pazour G, Agrin N, Walker B, Witman G (2006) Identification of predicted human outer dynein arm genes: candidates for primary ciliary dyskinesia genes. Journal of Medical Genetics 43: 62.
31. Chang H, Rha SY, Jeung HC, Jung JJ, Kim TS, et al. (2010) Identification of genes related to a synergistic effect of taxane and suberoylanilide hydroxamic acid combination treatment in gastric cancer cells. J Cancer Res Clin Oncol 136: 1901–1913.
32. Indermaur MD, Xiong Y, Kamath SG, Boren T, Hakam A, et al. (2010) Genomic-directed targeted therapy increases endometrial cancer cell sensitivity to doxorubicin. Am J Obstet Gynecol 203: 1–40.
33. The International HapMap Consortium (2003) The International HapMap Project. Nature 426: 789–796.
34. Li H, Handsaker B, Wysoker A, Fennell T, Ruan J, et al. (2009) The Sequence Alignment/Map format and SAMtools. Bioinformatics 25: 2078–2079.
35. R Development Core Team (2011) R: A Language and Environment for Statistical Computing. R Foundation for Statistical Computing, Vienna, Austria. ISBN 3-900051-07-0.
36. Therneau T, Lumley T (2011) survival: Survival analysis, including penalised likelihood. R package version 2.36-9.
37. Harrington D, Fleming T (1982) A class of rank test procedures for censored survival data. Biometrika 69: 553.
38. Benjamini Y, Hochberg Y (1995) Controlling the false discovery rate: a practical and powerful approach to multiple testing. Journal of the Royal Statistical Society Series B (Methodological) : 289–300.
39. Johnson RC, Nelson GW, Troyer JL, Lautenberger JA, Kessing BD, et al. (2010) Accounting for multiple comparisons in a genome-wide association study (GWAS). BMC Genomics 11: 724.
40. Cantor R, Lange K, Sinsheimer J (2010) Prioritizing gwas results: A review of statistical methods and recommendations for their application. The American Journal of Human Genetics 86: 6–22.
41. Han B, Kang H, Eskin E (2009) Rapid and accurate multiple testing correction and power estimation for millions of correlated markers. PLoS Genetics 5: e1000456.
42. Aulchenko Y, Ripke S, Isaacs A, Van Duijn C (2007) GenABEL: an R library for genome-wide association analysis.
43. Fraley C, Raftery A (2002) Model-based clustering, discriminant analysis, and density estimation. Journal of the American Statistical Association 97: 611–631.
44. Zhang J, Finney R, Rowe W, Edmonson M, Yang S, et al. (2007) Systematic analysis of genetic alterations in tumors using Cancer Genome WorkBench (CGWB). Genome research 17: 1111.
45. Wang K, Li M, Hakonarson H (2010) ANNOVAR: functional annotation of genetic variants from high-throughput sequencing data. Nucleic Acids Research 38: e164.
46. Clifford R, Edmonson M, Nguyen C, Buetow K (2004) Large-scale analysis of non-synonymous coding region single nucleotide polymorphisms. Bioinformatics 20: 1006.
47. Ng P, Henikoff S (2003) SIFT: Predicting amino acid changes that affect protein function. Nucleic Acids Research 31: 3812.

Resveratrol Inhibits Cisplatin-Induced Epithelial-to-Mesenchymal Transition in Ovarian Cancer Cell Lines

Sébastien Baribeau, Parvesh Chaudhry, Sophie Parent, Éric Asselin*

Research Group in Molecular Oncology and Endocrinology, Department of Medical Biology, Université du Québec à Trois-Rivières, Trois-Rivières, Québec, Canada

Abstract

Background: Many patients diagnosed with ovarian cancer experience recurrence and metastasis, two aspects that will often cause their demise. Epithelial-to-mesenchymal transition (EMT) is a key process involved in cancer progression. With increasing evidence linking Cisplatin and EMT, we wanted to identify a compound able to counter EMT progression when cancer cells are treated with Cisplatin.

Methodology/Principal Findings: Cell death was evaluated by cytometry with Annexin V/PI staining in A2780 and A2780CP cells. Ovarian cancer cell lines were treated with Cisplatin (24 h, 10 μM) and different concentrations of Resveratrol to evaluate its effect on Cisplatin-induced EMT using Western Blot and RT-PCR analysis. Morphological studies and wound healing assay to evaluate cell motility were performed using 72 h Cisplatin treatment with A2780 and A2780CP cells. Densitometry was done on Western Blot and PCR results, and statistical significance was determined using One-Way ANOVA followed by Tukey post-hoc test. Our results show that Cisplatin induced EMT-associated morphological changes in the A2780 ovarian cancer cell line and to a lesser extent in its Cisplatin-resistant counterpart A2780CP. Resveratrol caused cell death in A2780 and A2780CP cell lines in an apoptotic-independent manner. Resveratrol inhibited Cisplatin-induced Snail expression by reducing the Erk pathway activation, reverted morphological changes induced by Cisplatin and decreased cell migration.

Conclusions: These results indicate that Resveratrol has interesting potential to prevent Cisplatin-induced EMT in ovarian cancer cells. By increasing cell death, it also represents an inviting approach as adjuvant therapy to be used with chemotherapy. Using Erk pathway inhibitors could also prove helpful in ovarian cancer treatment to reduce the risk of metastasis.

Editor: Goli Samimi, Kinghorn Cancer Centre, Garvan Institute of Medical Research, Australia

Funding: This work has been supported by a grant from the Canadian Institutes for Health Research (MOP-66987). EA holds a Canadian Research Chair in Molecular-Gyneco-Oncology. The funders had no role in study design, data collection and analysis, decision to publish, or preparation of the manuscript.

Competing Interests: The authors have declared that no competing interests exist.

* E-mail: eric.asselin@uqtr.ca

Introduction

Ovarian cancer is the seventh most common cancer and the third most common amongst gynaecological cancers in canadian women. Ovarian cancer is also the gynaecological cancer with the highest mortality rate and a 5-year survival rate estimated to only 15–25% [1]. This can be explained by the fact that patients affected by ovarian cancer often already have a high-stage disease at the moment of diagnosis [2,3]. The usual treatment for ovarian cancer consists of surgical cytoreduction followed by platinum-based chemotherapy [4]. Despite initial response to the treatment, many patients will relapse and eventually be affected by metastases and ultimately meet their demise.

Epithelial-to-mesenchymal transition (EMT) is a physiological process that occurs during embryonic development and occasionally in adults, for example during wound healing [5]. EMT is a phenomenon during which cells will undergo a transition from an epithelial phenotype to a more motile and invasive mesenchymal phenotype, rendering them able to invade tissues and form metastases. The main hallmark of EMT is the loss of E-cadherin, a junction protein typically expressed in epithelial cells. In most cases, E-cadherin loss is mediated by transcriptional repressors, and mutations of the gene or the protein are not common events [6]. The most commonly involved repressors include Snail, Slug, and ZEB1 that directly bind to the E-cadherin promoter to repress its transcription [7,8]. Many factors are known to induce EMT, including cytokines such as TGF-β [9] or the MAPK-Erk pathway [10]. A recent study on ovarian cancer reported Cisplatin as an inducer of EMT [11].

Snail and Slug are transcription factors mainly known for their involvement in EMT where they repress the expression of epithelial markers, such as E-cadherin and Claudin-1, and increase the expression of mesenchymal markers, such as ZEB1 and MMP-9 [12–16]. They can also repress the expression and function of the tumor suppressor p53 and promote chemoresistance [17,18]. During EMT progression, it is believed that Snail will be the first factor to become active to initiate the transition whereas Slug would be expressed in later stages to allow the cells to retain their mesenchymal characteristics [19]. ZEB1 is another important promoter of EMT by repressing ZO-1 and E-cadherin [20], but can also be involved in increasing the proliferation rate of cells [21].

Resveratrol (trans-3,4′,5-trihydroxystilbene) is a natural compound produced in many plants including red grapes [22], and subsequently present in wine, known for its antioxidant and its protective effects on the cardiovascular system and against cancer in which it can inhibit multiple stages of the disease [23]. During the last years, these many effects placed Resveratrol in the spotlight of research.

In this study, we investigated the impact of Resveratrol on Cisplatin-induced EMT in ovarian cancer. We found that cells co-treated with Resveratrol and Cisplatin did not show the characteristic features of EMT, as Resveratrol treatment abrogated Cisplatin-induced Snail protein and mRNA expressions in a dose-dependent manner. This involved the Erk pathway, which was inhibited by Resveratrol and its involvement was confirmed via specific MEK1/2 inhibition with U0126. Resveratrol also blocked morphological changes in A2780 and A2780CP cells and decreased the migration ability of A2780 and A2780CP cells during a wound healing assay. Similar inhibition of migration was observed in OVCAR-3 and SKOV-3 cells. We also propose β-catenin as a marker of resistance to Cisplatin-induced apoptosis as it was cleaved only in Cisplatin-sensitive cell lines.

Methods

Reagents

Dulbecco's modified Eagle medium-F12 (DMEM-F12), and Bovine growth serum (BGS) were purchased from HyClone (South Logan, Utah). Gentamycin, Cisplatin, and Resveratrol were purchased from Sigma-Aldrich (St. Louis, MO). The MEK1/2 inhibitor and the Senescence β-galactosidase staining kit were purchased from Cell Signaling Technology (Danvers, MA). Dead cell apoptosis kit with annexin-V/PI, Trizol reagent and Moloney murine leukemia virus (M-MLV) reverse transcriptase were purchased from Invitrogen (Carlsbad, CA).

Cell culture and treatment

Human ovarian cancer cell lines A2780 and A2780CP (resistant to Cisplatin) cells were a kind gift from Dr G. Peter Raaphorst (Ottawa Regional Cancer Center, Ottawa, Canada) and were originally described in [24]. OVCAR-3 and SKOV-3 cell lines were purchased from the ATCC. A2780 and A2780CP cells were cultured in DMEM-F12 medium supplemented with 2% BGS. OVCAR-3 cells were cultured in RPMI-1640 medium and SKOV-3 cells were cultured in McCoy's medium both supplemented with 10% FBS. Gentamycin (50 μg/mL) was added to all culture media.

To study the impact of Resveratrol on Cisplatin-induced EMT, A2780 and A2780CP cells were co-treated with Resveratrol and 10 μM Cisplatin for 24 h. To study the impact of the Erk pathway on Cisplatin-induced EMT, ovarian cancer cell lines were pretreated with 20 μM U0126 for 1 h, then Cisplatin was added to the culture medium for 24 h at a final concentration of 10 μM. DMSO was used as control for U0126 and Resveratrol.

Detection of cell death by flow cytometry

A2780 and A2780CP cells were treated with Resveratrol and Cisplatin for 24 h. At harvest, cells were centrifuged at 500 rpm for 5 minutes, washed with PBS and then centrifuged 300 rpm for 5 minutes. Cell death was evaluated with Annexin-V-FITC and propidium iodide (PI) double staining using dead cell apoptosis kit according to the manufacturer's protocol. Fluorescence was read using a Cytomics FC 500 MPL flow cytometer (Beckman Coulter). Positive cells for Annexin-V and/or PI were considered as dead cells.

MTT assay

Proliferation of A2780 and A2780CP cells was evaluated by MTT assay. Cells were plated in duplicate in 96-well plates and left to adhere overnight. The following day, cells in growth phase were treated with 0–60 μM Resveratrol with or without 10 μM Cisplatin for 24 h in 100 μL culture medium. 4 h before the end of treatment, 10 μL of MTT solution was added to each well and plates were placed in the incubator. 4 h later, 100 μL solubilisation solution (10% SDS in 0.01 M HCl) was added to each well and plates were left in the incubator overnight. The following day, the absorbance was read at A_{595nm} with a Fluostar Optima plate reader.

Western Blot

Cells were harvested after 24 h Resveratrol-Cisplatin or U0126-Cisplatin treatment and washed twice with phosphate-buffered saline (PBS). Cells were then lysed in RIPA lysis buffer containing complete protease inhibitor cocktail (Roche Applied Science) and subjected to three freeze/thaw cycles at -20°C. Cells were then centrifuged and the supernatant was collected. Protein concentration was estimated using the BioRad DC Protein assay. Equal amount of proteins (20–40 μg) were then separated onto SDS-PAGE and transferred to nitrocellulose membranes (BioRad, Hercules, CA). Membranes were blocked in 5% non-fat skimmed milk in PBS-Tween 20 0.05% (PBS-T) for 1 h before incubation with primary antibody (diluted 1:1000 in PBS-T/milk) overnight at 4°C (all antibodies are from Cell Signaling Technology, Danvers, MA, except GAPDH from Abcam (Cambridge, MA)). Primary antibody targeting Snail was incubated 2 h at room temperature and HRP-conjugated-GAPDH was incubated 45 minutes at room temperature. After incubation, the membranes were washed four times in PBS-T before incubation with horseradish peroxidase conjugated secondary antibody (BioRad, Hercules, CA) diluted 1:3000 in PBS-T/milk. Membranes were washed four times in PBS-T and the antibodies were revealed using SuperSignal West Femto substrate (Thermo Scientific, Rockford, IL), as described by the manufacturer using UVP Bio Imaging System. GAPDH was used as loading control.

Cell morphology

Cells were grown in 6-well plates and then treated with 2.5 μM Cisplatin and/or 60 μM Resveratrol for 72 h in A2780 and A2780CP cells to allow enough time for EMT morphological changes to occur. After treatment, cells were washed with fresh medium to remove dead cells. Finally, cells were observed under a Carl Zeiss Axio observerZ1 microscope to determine their morphology and picture were taken in phase contrast microscopy using 20X magnification. Cells presenting mesenchymal characteristics, with a more fibroblast like morphology and cellular protusions, were considered as having undergone EMT.

Wound healing assay

To evaluate cell motility, cells were plated in 24-well plates and grown to confluency. A sterile tip was used to create a scratch in the cell layer. Cells were then treated with 2.5 μM Cisplatin and 60 μM Resveratrol and pictures were taken at appropriate times to evaluate wound closure. Wounds were evaluated using ImageJ software to measure the wound area at different time points. The percentage of wound closure was calculated as wound area at a given time compared to the initial wound surface. Pictures shown are representative of three independent experiments performed in duplicates.

Reverse Transcriptase PCR (RT-PCR)

Total RNA was extracted from treated cells using Trizol Reagent according to the manufacturer's instructions. 500 ng of RNA was reverse transcribed using M-MLV reverse transcriptase and oligo(dT) primers. The reverse-transcribed RNA was then amplified by PCR using specific primers. GAPDH was used as an internal control. Human Snail was amplified using the sense primer 5′-TCGGAAGCCTAACTACAGCGA-3′ and antisense primer 5′-AGATGAGCATTGGCAGCGAG-3′ (fragment length 140 bp). Human TCF8-ZEB1 was amplified using sense primer 5′-TTACACCTTTGCATACAGAACCC-3′ and antisense primer 5′-TTTACGATTACACCCAGACTGC-3′ (fragment length 100 bp). Human Vimentin was amplified using sense 5′-CGAAAACACCCTGCAATCTT-3′ and antisense primer 5′-CTGGATTTCCTCTTCGTGGA-3′ (fragment lenght 133 bp). GAPDH was amplified using sense 5′-GTCAGTGGTGGACCTGACCT-3′ and antisense primer 5′-GACTTGACAAAGTGGTCG-3′ (fragment length 139 bp). GAPDH was used as control.

Senescence-associated β-galactosidase staining

Cells were plated in 6-well plates and left to adhere overnight. The following day, cells were treated with 60 μM Resveratrol and 2.5 μM Cisplatin for 72 h. After the treatment, cells were washed to remove non-adherent cells and stained with the Senescence β-galactosidase staining kit according to the manufacturer's instructions. Cells were then counted under a light microscope to evaluate the percentage of senescent cells which appeared as blue cells.

Densitometry and Statistical analysis

Densitometric analysis was done on the Western Blot results and PCR pictures using Quantity One software (BioRad) to determine the abundance of proteins or amplified mRNA studied. In both cases, GAPDH was used as control. In wound healing assays, wound area was mesured using ImageJ software. Wound closure was evaluated by comparing the wound area at a given time to the initial wound area. Comparison between treatments was performed using GraphPad PRISM software version 5.00 (San Diego, CA) using one-way ANOVA analysis and the *post hoc* Tukey's test. Statistical significance was accepted when $p<0.05$. All experiments performed in this study were repeated three independent times.

Results

Resveratrol induces cell death in ovarian cancer cells

Treatment of A2780 and A2780CP ovarian cancer cells with Resveratrol increased cell death in a dose-dependent manner as shown by the proportion of PI-positive cells. The low proportion of Annexin-V staining in Resveratrol-treated samples but not in Cisplatin-treated samples suggests that Resveratrol might induce cell death through a different mechanism or occur faster than Cisplatin-induced cell death (Figure 1).

We investigated apoptosis and autophagy as potential cell death mechanisms. In A2780 cells, Cisplatin induced an increase in caspase-3 and PARP cleavage, indicating induction of cell death through apoptosis. By contrast, treatment of A2780 or A2780CP cells with Resveratrol did not affect the levels of cleaved caspase-3 despite the presence of dead cells, strengthening the possibility that a mechanism other than apoptosis is involved (Figure 2). We then decided to study autophagy induction by evaluating the expression levels of LC3B-II and Beclin-1, two proteins known for their involvement in autophagy progression. Resveratrol caused an increase in LC3B-II levels in both cell lines, supporting results from Opipari *et al.* showing autophagy as a potential mechanism responsible for Resveratrol-induced cell death [25]. In our model, we did not observe an increase in Beclin-1 levels, which is already expressed at relatively high levels in A2780 and A2780CP cell lines.

Resveratrol potentiates Cisplatin-induced decrease in cell proliferation

We next sought to evaluate the effect of Resveratrol on the proliferation of A2780 and A2780CP cell lines. As shown in Figure 3, low doses of Resveratrol (20–40 μM) slightly increases proliferation of both cell lines despite the cell death associated to this treatment. At the highest dose tested (60 μM) Resveratrol induced a slight decrease in proliferation in A2780 cells and almost no change in A2780CP cells. In Cisplatin-sensitive A2780 cells, Resveratrol potentiates the decrease in cell proliferation observed when Cisplatin is used as treatment suggesting a synergistic action between these two compounds. This was not observed in Cisplatin-resistant A2780CP cells but the highest Resveratrol dose did not increase proliferation when used in combination with Cisplatin.

Resveratrol inhibits Cisplatin-mediated EMT induction in ovarian cancer cell lines

To assess the impact of Resveratrol on Cisplatin-induced EMT, A2780 and A2780CP cells were co-treated with Resveratrol and Cisplatin. As expected, treating the cells with Cisplatin increased the protein levels of Snail, Vimentin and ZEB1, three of the main markers of EMT. Treating the cells with Cisplatin and Resveratrol decreased the expression levels of Snail, but did not show this effect on Vimentin and ZEB1 expression. By contrast, these two proteins were slightly increased when cells were exposed to Resveratrol alone (Figure 4A). The decrease in Snail levels in A2780 treated with Resveratrol and Cisplatin correlates with a decrease in Snail mRNA levels.However, this was not the case in A2780CP cells where no significant change was observed in Snail mRNA levels between samples treated with Cisplatin and those treated with both Cisplatin and Resveratrol, suggesting some post-translational mechanisms might also be involved in Snail downregulation in these cells (Figure 4B). ZEB1 and Vimentin mRNA levels remained mostly unaltered in cells treated with either Resveratrol, Cisplatin or both agents. In our cell model, we could not assess EMT progression based on downregulation of E-cadherin because A2780 and A2780CP cells do not express this protein.

Activation of the MAPK Erk is associated with Cisplatin-induced EMT

We next investigated the mechanism by which Resveratrol counters Cisplatin-induced Snail expression. The MAPK/Erk pathway is one of the possible mechanisms that can be involved in EMT induction in cells. In A2780 and A2780CP cells, Erk2 phosphorylation was increased in response to Cisplatin. The activation of this pathway was significantly inhibited by Resveratrol, corresponding to a decrease in Snail levels in A2780 and A2780CP cell lines (Figure 4). To further confirm the involvement of Erk in the increase of Snail levels in response to Cisplatin, we used U0126, a MEK1/2 specific inhibitor (Figure 5). Pretreatment of cells with this inhibitor significantly reduced the activation levels of Erk2 in A2780 and A2780CP cells, which also correlated with a significant decrease in Snail protein in both cell lines. Slight increases in the protein levels of Vimentin and ZEB1 were also observed (Figure 5A). Snail mRNA levels were decreased when both cells lines were treated with Cisplatin and U0126, suggesting

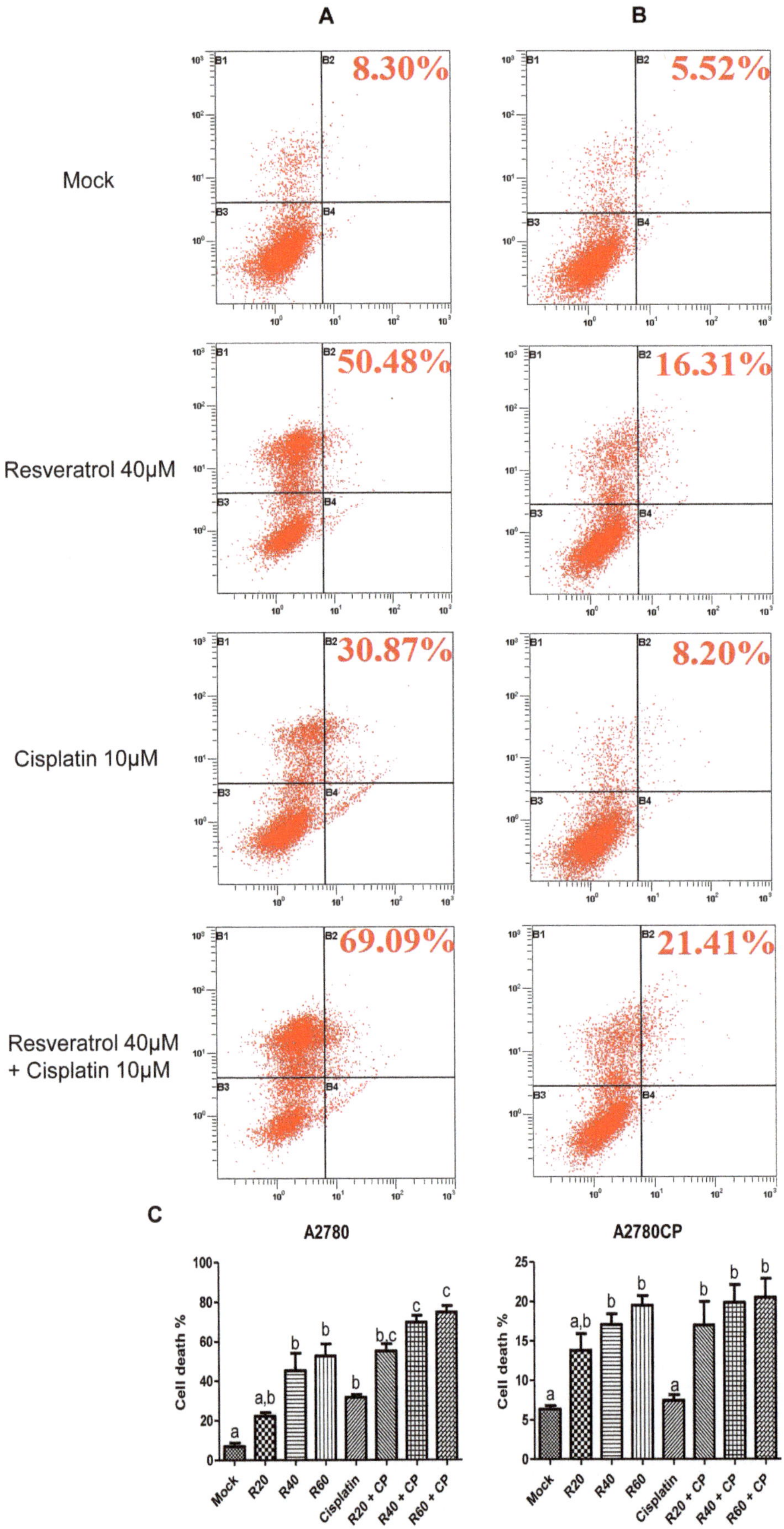
A
B
Mock
Resveratrol 40μM
Cisplatin 10μM
Resveratrol 40μM
+ Cisplatin 10μM
8.30%
5.52%
50.48%
16.31%
30.87%
8.20%
69.09%
21.41%
B1
B2
B3
B4
C
A2780
A2780CP
Cell death %
Mock
R20
R40
R60
Cisplatin
R20 + CP
R40 + CP
R60 + CP
a
a,b
b
b,c
c

Figure 1. Resveratrol induces cell death and potentiates Cisplatin cytotoxicity. Cell death levels were evaluated by flow cytometry with Annexin-V and PI staining in A2780 and A2780CP cells. Representative flow cytometry results are shown for A2780 (A) and A2780CP cells (B) treated with 10 μM Cisplatin and 40 μM Resveratrol. In the upper right corner, percentage of cell death is shown, corresponding to apoptotic and necrotic cell death. Annexin-V and PI negative cells (B3) are non-apoptotic. Annexin-V positive and PI negative cells (B4) are in the early stages of apoptosis. Annexin-V positive and PI positive cells (B2) are in late apoptosis. Annexin-V negative and PI positive cells (B1) are necrotic cells. Cell death percentage is shown in (C) for both cell lines treated with increasing doses of Resveratrol up to 60 μM with or without Cisplatin 10 μM. Results shown are representative of three independent experiments. In graphs, columns identified with different letters are significantly different ($p<0.05$). In graphs, mock: untreated cells, R20: Resveratrol 20 μM, R40: Resveratrol 40 μM, R60: Resveratrol 60 μM, CP: Cisplatin, R20CP: Resv. 20 μM + Cisplatin, R40CP: Resv. 40 μM + Cisplatin, R60CP: Resv. 60 μM + Cisplatin.

Cisplatin-induced Snail expression through the Erk pathway requires transcription of the Snail gene. ZEB1 and Vimentin mRNA levels did not show significant changes when A2780 and A2780CP cells were treated with Cisplatin and U0126 alone or in combination (Figure 5B). These results support Resveratrol-induced EMT inhibition through the Erk pathway.

Resveratrol blocks Cisplatin-induced morphological changes

In order to avoid excessive Cisplatin-induced cytotoxicity in A2780 cells, we decided to use 2.5 μM Cisplatin to assess morphological changes in A2780 and A2780CP cells for a 72 h treatment. Treatment of ovarian cancer cells with Cisplatin

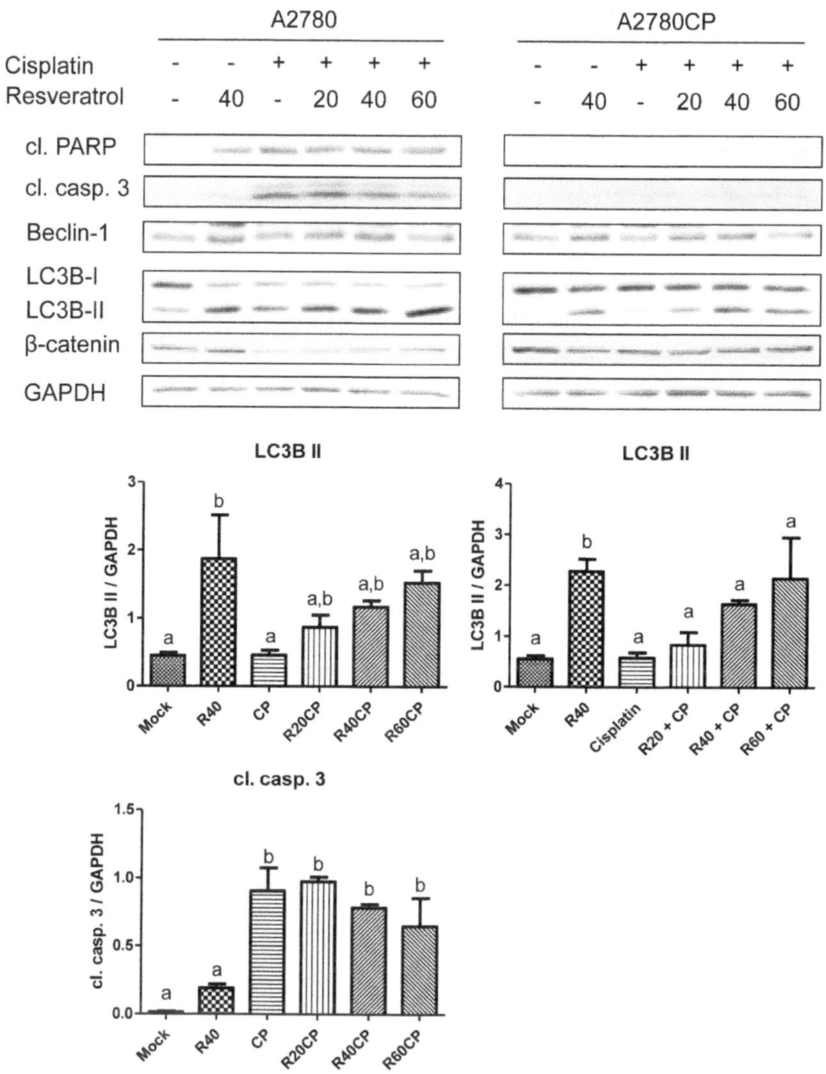

Figure 2. Resveratrol potentiates Cisplatin-induced cell death through autophagy. The mechanism of cell death was studied in A2780 and A2780CP cells in response to Cisplatin and Resveratrol. The absence of increase in cleaved PARP levels and caspase-3 cleavage when higher doses of Resveratrol are used suggests Resveratrol would induce cell death through a mechanism independent of apoptosis. The significant increase in LC3BII suggests Resveratrol could induce cell death through autophagy. Densitometry analysis is shown under Western Blot for each cell line. Results shown are representative of three independent experiments. In graphs, columns identified with different letters are significantly different ($p<0.05$). In graphs, mock: untreated cells, R40: Resveratrol 40 μM, CP: Cisplatin, R20CP: Resv. 20 μM + Cisplatin, R40CP: Resv. 40 μM + Cisplatin, R60CP: Resv. 60 μM + Cisplatin.

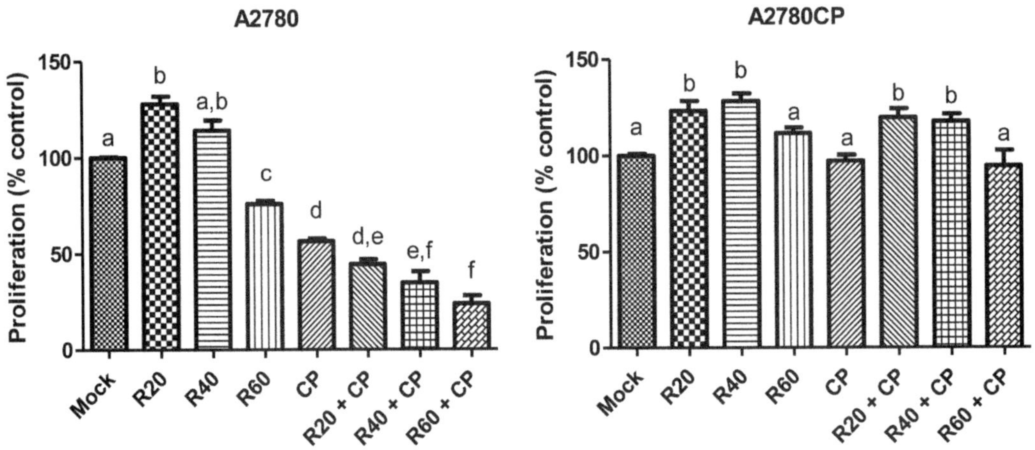

Figure 3. Resveratrol decreases proliferation of Cisplatin-sensitive A2780 cells but not Cisplatin-resistant A2780CP cells. MTT assay was performed to evaluate A2780 and A2780 cell lines proliferation in response to 10 μM Cisplatin and increasing doses up to 60 μM of Resveratrol. A2780 cells proliferation was increased by Resveratrol at 20 μM and decreased at 60 μM while all doses suggest an increase in proliferation in A2780CP cells. Resveratrol also potentiates Cisplatin decrease of proliferation in A2780 cells. Graph bars with different letters are statistically different ($p<0.05$). In graphs, mock: untreated cells, R20: Resveratrol 20 μM, R40: Resveratrol 40 μM, R60: Resveratrol 60 μM, CP: Cisplatin, R20CP: Resv. 20 μM + Cisplatin, R40CP: Resv. 40 μM + Cisplatin, R60CP: Resv. 60 μM + Cisplatin.

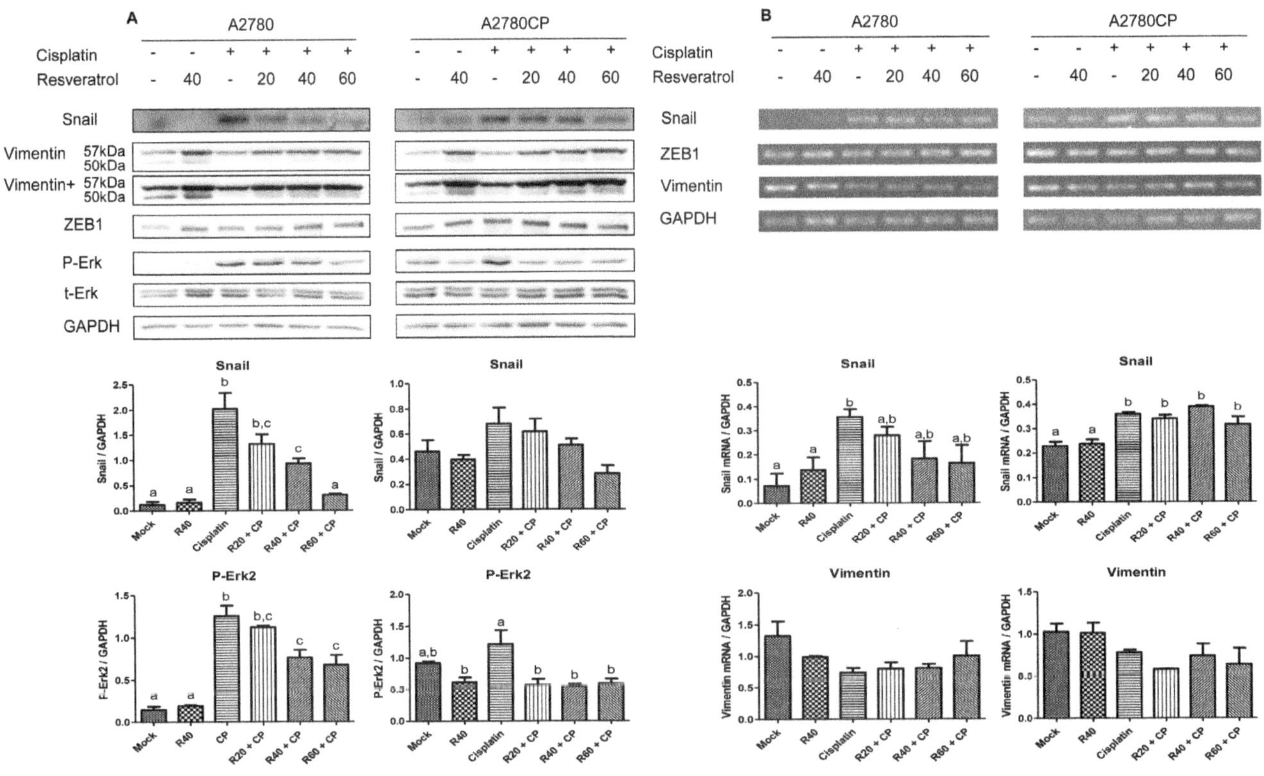

Figure 4. Resveratrol reduces Cisplatin-induced Snail expression. Western Blot analysis of EMT markers Snail, Vimentin and ZEB1 in A2780 and A2780CP (A) cells in response to 10 μm Cisplatin with or without increasing doses of Resveratrol. Densitometric analysis is shown under each cell line Western Blots. Resveratrol inhibits Cisplatin-induced Snail expression in a dose-dependent manner but slightly increases ZEB1 and Vimentin levels. The Resveratrol dose-dependent decrease in P-Erk2 levels suggests the involvement of the Erk pathway in Resveratrol-induced Snail downregulation. The EMT markers Snail, Vimentin and ZEB1 expression were analysed by RT-PCR in A2780 and A2780CP (B) cells treated with 10 μm Cisplatin with or without increasing doses of Resveratrol. Resveratrol or Cisplatin treatment had no effect on ZEB1 and Vimentin mRNA levels. Vimentin and ZEB1 densitometry is shown under each cell line. Snail mRNA expression was decreased only in A2780 cells, suggesting another mechanism could be involved in A2780CP cells. Images shown are representative of three independent experiments. In graphs, columns identified with different letters are significantly different ($p<0.05$). In graphs, mock: untreated cells, R40: Resveratrol 40 μM, CP: Cisplatin, R20CP: Resv. 20 μM + Cisplatin, R40CP: Resv. 40 μM + Cisplatin, R60CP: Resv. 60 μM + Cisplatin.

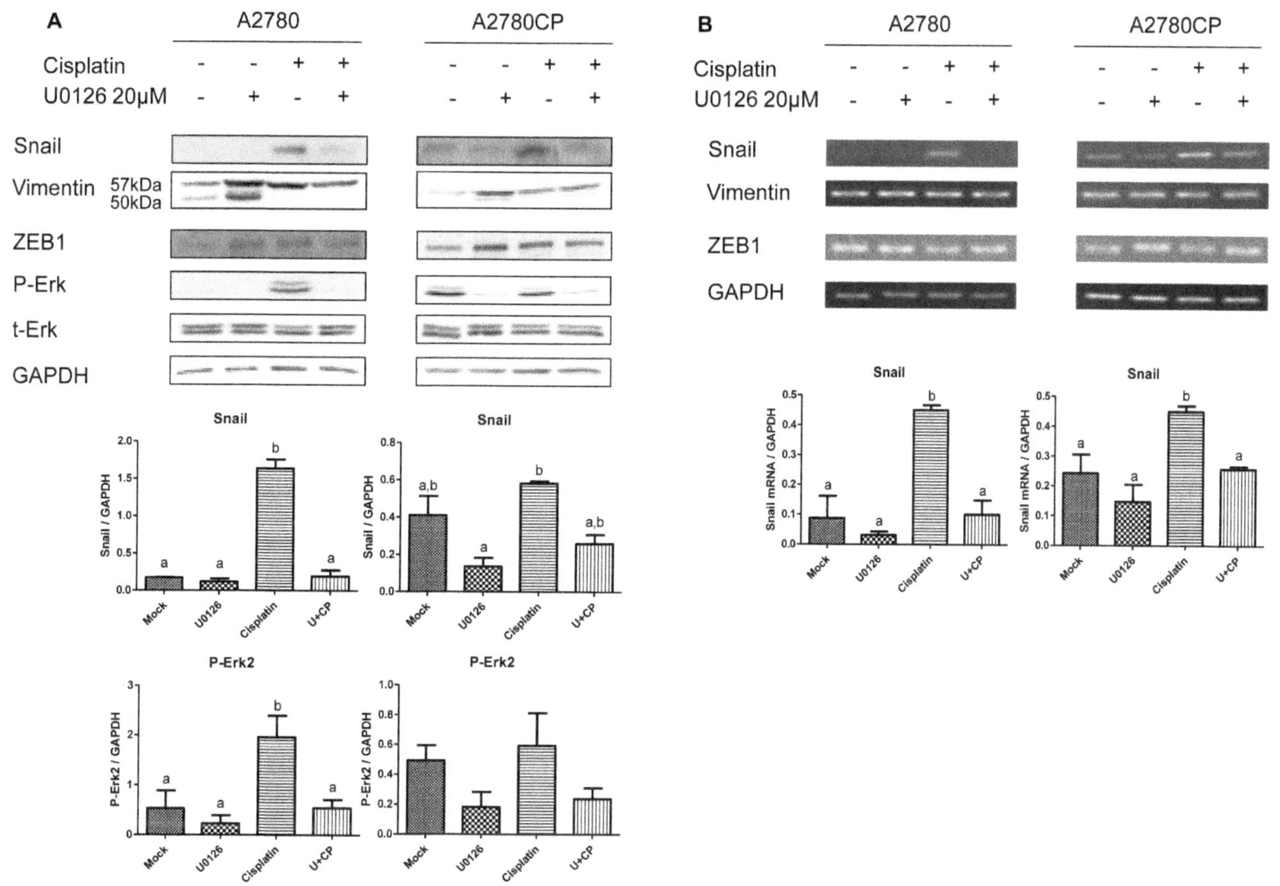

Figure 5. Erk inhibition abrogates Cisplatin-induced EMT in ovarian cancer cell lines. A2780 and A2780CP cell lines were pre-treated with U0126 to inhibit Erk activity and treated with Cisplatin for 24 h. Western Blot are shown in (A). Corresponding densitometry is shown under each cell line. Erk inhibition reduced Cisplatin-induced Snail expression but slightly increased ZEB1 and Vimentin expression in both cell lines. Corresponding PCR results are shown in (B). Snail mRNA decrease in U0126+Cisplatin treated samples suggests Snail regulation by Cisplatin involves gene transcription. Results shown are representative of three independent experiments. In graphs, columns identified with different letters are significantly different ($p<0.05$). In graphs, mock: untreated cells, CP: Cisplatine, U+CP: U0126+ Cisplatin.

induced morphological changes reminiscent of EMT as the cells lost their epithelial cobblestone-like morphology to acquire a more elongated fibroblast-like shape. Cellular protusions also appeared in Cisplatin-treated cells compared to control samples. Both A2780 and A2780CP cells showed these modifications indicating their progression through EMT. To test the effect of Resveratrol on this phenomenon, we used 60 μM, the concentration at which Snail downregulation was the most evident. Addition of Resveratrol to Cisplatin treatment blocked these morphological changes as the cells did not acquire any of the characteristic mesenchymal morphological features (Figure 6). It is also interesting to note that Resveratrol-treated cells became bigger and displayed an irregular appearance suggesting another cellular transformation, such as a senescence program, could be occurring [26].

Resveratrol induces senescence

We evaluated senescence induction in our cell lines after Cisplatin and Resveratrol treatment and observed a significant increase in Resveratrol-induced senescence in both cell lines after 72 h, with a more pronounced effect in A2780 cells (Figure 7). We also observed higher senescence levels in A2780 cells treated with Cisplatin and suggest that continuous exposure to Cisplatin might induce an oxidative stress leading to senescence in these Cisplatin-sensitive cells. Senescence induction in A2780 and A2780CP cells could be another mechanism involved in the inhibition of cisplatin-induced EMT by Resveratrol.

Resveratrol inhibits cell migration

Considering the morphological transformation occurring in A2780 and A2780CP cells, we next evaluated the migration ability of these cells with a wound healing assay. Cells were treated with 2.5 μM Cisplatin, to avoid excessive cytotoxicity in A2780 cells, and 60 μM Resveratrol. In both cell lines, 72 h were required for the wound to completely close up in untreated cells, suggesting that these cell lines don't have a very mobile phenotype. Resveratrol treatment clearly inhibited cell migration at every time point where wound closure was evaluated, reducing the wound closure to only 20–25% after 72 h for both cell lines whereas the control cells had almost completely closed the wounds (Figure 8A and 8B). Resveratrol's action would not be affected by Cisplatin in A2780CP cells where this agent exerted the same effect on the cells with or without Cisplatin.

Furthermore, we investigated the potential of Resveratrol to inhibit the migration ability of OVCAR-3 cells, an epithelial cell line expressing E-cadherin and without basal expression of ZEB1 or Vimentin which shows little migration potential, and SKOV-3 cells, a mesenchymal cell line showing basal expression of Vimentin and ZEB1 as well as a mesenchymal morphology and

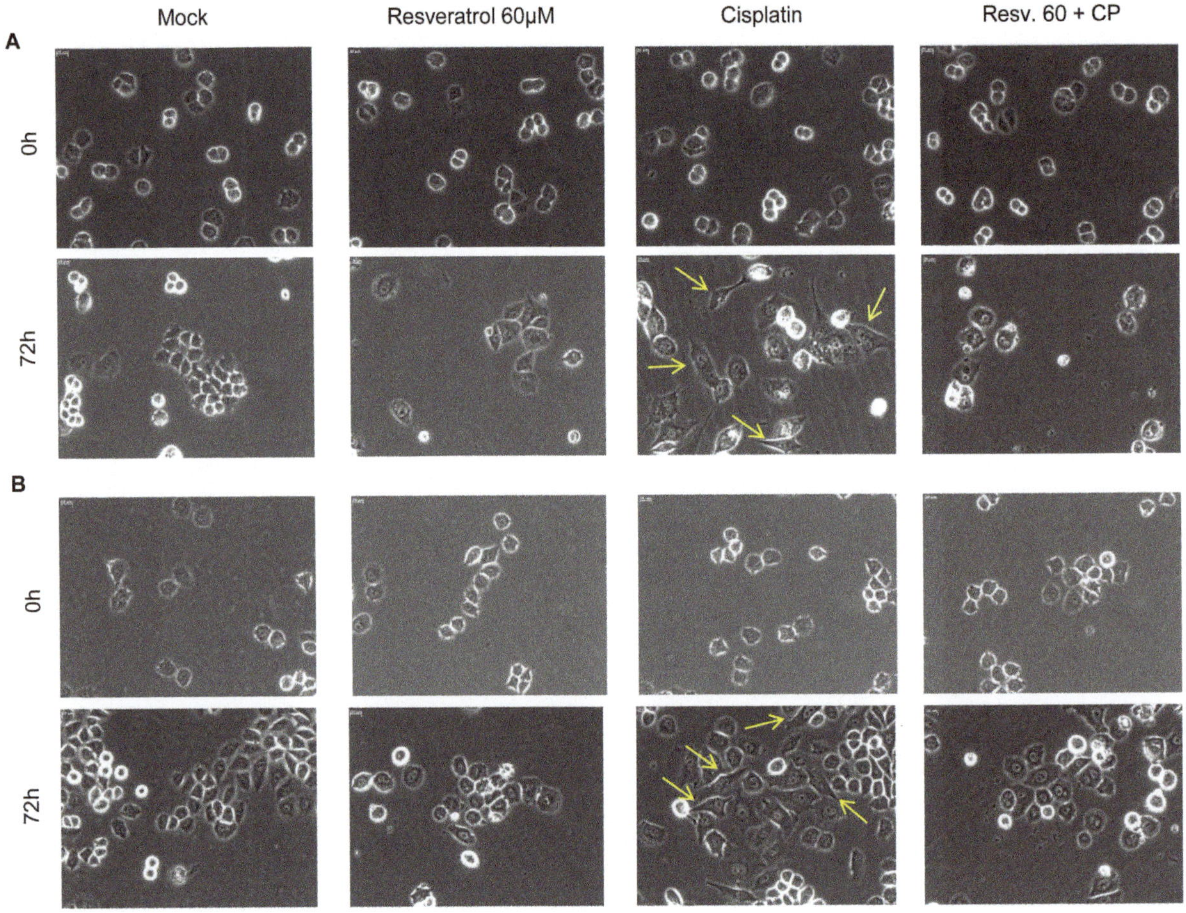

Figure 6. Resveratrol blocks EMT morphological changes induced by Cisplatin. A2780 (A) and A2780CP (B) cell lines were treated for 72 h with 2.5 μM Cisplatin with or without 60 μm Resveratrol to allow EMT morphological changes to become apparent. Cisplatin induced cellular morphological changes reminiscent of EMT in A2780 cells evident after 72 h, which were abrogated when Resveratrol was added to the treatment. Resveratrol exerted the same effect on A2780CP cells although the morphological changes induced by Cisplatin were less pronounced. Cells were observed under 20X magnification, scale bar in the upper left corner of the pictures represent 20 μm. Arrows indicate examples of cells having undergone an EMT. Images shown are representative of three independent experiments.

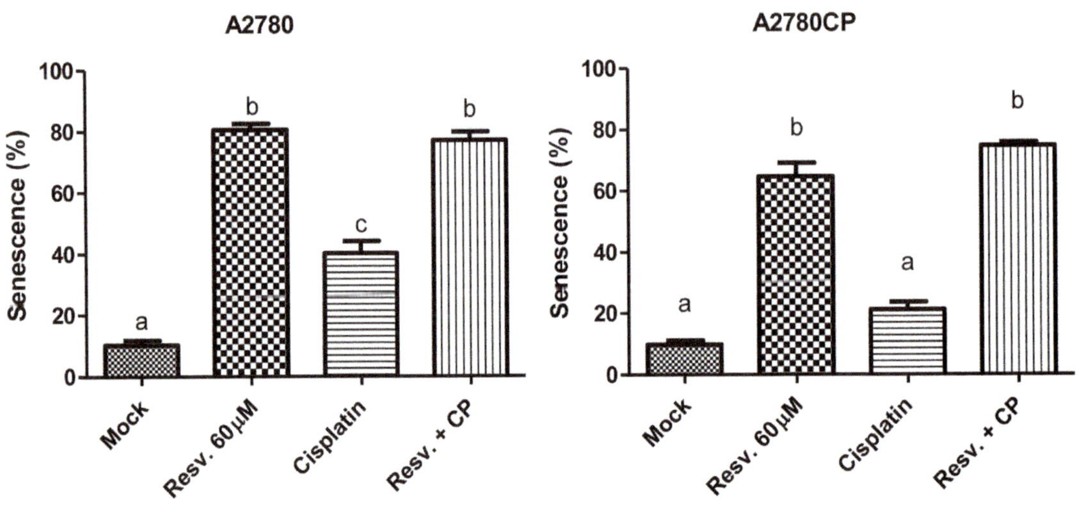

Figure 7. Resveratrol and Cisplatin induce senescence in ovarian cancer cell lines. Treatment of A2780 and A2780CP cells with Resveratrol significantly increased the proportion of senescent cells. Cisplatin induced a significant increase of senescence in A2780 cells. Cells were stained for β-galactosidase activity and counted under a light microscope to assess the percentage of senescent (blue) cells. In graphs, columns identified with different letters are significantly different ($p<0.05$). The analysis was performed with three independent experiments.

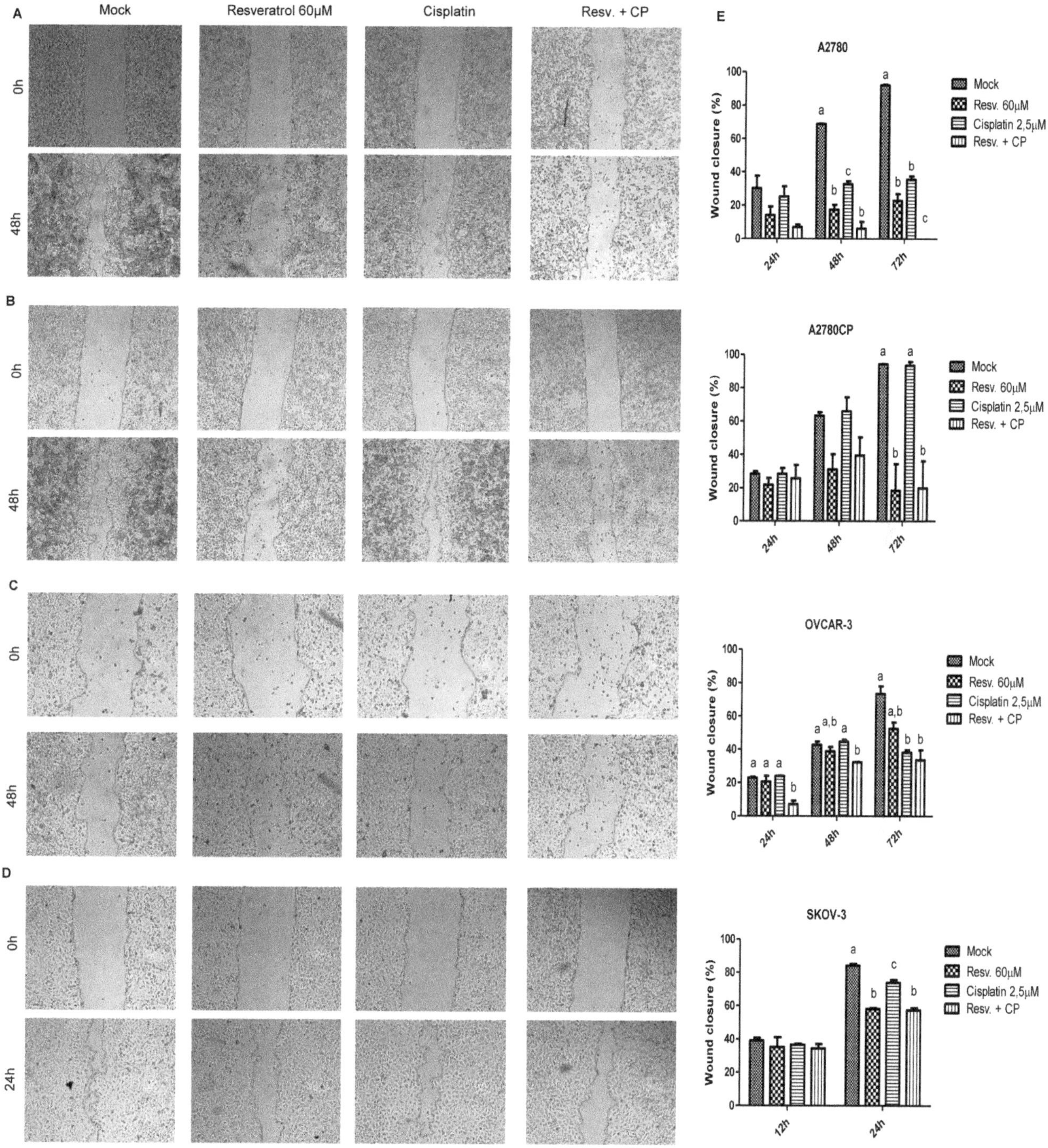

Figure 8. Wound healing capacity of ovarian cancer cell lines is impaired by Resveratrol. The migratory ability of A2780 (A), A2780CP (B), OVCAR-3 (C), and SKOV-3 (D) cells was evaluated by wound healing assay. A scratch was made with a sterile tip in a confluent layer of cells and wound closure was observed after 24, 48, and 72 h of Cisplatin and Resveratrol treatment for A2780, A2780CP, and OVCAR-3 cells, and 12 and 24 h for SKOV-3, corresponding to the moment where the wound was almost completely closed. In both cell lines, Resveratrol decreased the migration of the cells in the wound, preventing its closing after 72 h. Representative pictures are shown at t = 48 h. Graphical representation of wound closure after the different time points studied is shown in (E). Results shown are representative of three independent experiments performed in duplicates. In graphs, treatments are compared within each time point studied and columns identified with different letters are significantly different ($p < 0.05$).

high migration potential despite basal E-cadherin expression (Figure S1). Similar to A2780 and A2780CP cells, OVCAR-3 cells required at least 72 h to close the wound. In this cell line, Resveratrol significantly reduced the closure of the wound after 72 h and at every time point studied when used in combination with Cisplatin. In SKOV-3 cells, only 24 h were required to observe 80–85% wound closure and Resveratrol significantly decreased the migration of these cells when used alone or in combination with Cisplatin at this time point, indicating that this phytoalexin possesses the capacity to reduce the migration of cells that possess a high basal migration potential as well as cells with low migration potential (Figure 8C and 8D). Results observed in OVCAR-3 and SKOV-3 cells correlate with those observed in A2780 and A2780CP respectively, where sensitivity to cisplatin is also similar.

To address the possibility of an increase in the invasion potential of the cells, we performed a zymography assay in A2780. A2780CP, OVCAR-3 and SKOV-3 cells with Cisplatin and Resveratrol treatments. In all four cell lines, we only detected pro-MMPs at different levels, highest pro-MMP activity was observed in OVCAR-3 cells and lowest activity was observed in A2780 and A2780CP cells, which displayed almost no pro-MMP activity. We did not observe any active form of MMPs in this assay for any of the cell lines studied. Furthermore, Resveratrol and Cisplatin treatment, alone or in combination, did not affect pro-MMPs activity and did not induce active MMPs, suggesting that these treatment do not alter the invasion capacity of the cells (data not shown).

Discussion

Recently, Haslehurst *et al.* demonstrated an involvement for Snail and Slug, two of the main EMT activating transcription factors, in the chemoresistance of ovarian cancer [27]. Moreover, the demonstration that Cisplatin induces EMT [11] brings about a new challenge: how to fight back? Indeed, preventing EMT induction by Cisplatin shows an interesting potential to help patients overcome chemotherapy resistance and metastatic dissemination. In order to try to answer to this problem, we evaluated the impact of Resveratrol, a natural compound known for its wide array of beneficial effects [28], on Cisplatin-induced EMT in ovarian cancer.

First, we assessed cell death in response to Cisplatin and Resveratrol in A2780 and A2780CP cells. In A2780 cells, Resveratrol increased cell death when used as a single treatment and when used in combination with Cisplatin where it potentiated Cisplatin-induced cell death. By contrast, in Cisplatin-resistant A2780CP cells, Resveratrol induced cell death to a lesser extent compared to A2780 cells when used as a single treatment and failed to sensitise A2780CP cells to Cisplatin-induced death in our conditions where cell death remained the same as Resveratrol treatment alone. Our results suggest apoptosis is not responsible for Resveratrol-induced cell death as there is no increase in cleaved caspase-3. An alternative mechanism of cell death could be autophagy, which was previously shown to be involved in ovarian cancer cell death by Resveratrol [25]. We also show an increase in LC3B-II in both cell lines, suggesting cell death could be caused by this cellular process despite no increase in Beclin-1 levels, which could be due to the time point selected.

We suggest that β-catenin could be used as a marker to evaluate cancer sensitivity to Cisplatin. In our model, only the sensitive cell line (A2780) displayed β-catenin downregulation when treated with Cisplatin (Figure 2), consequent with a previous report demonstrating β-catenin cleavage by caspase-3 during apoptosis [29]. However, β-catenin could not be used as a marker for caspase-independent cell death mechanisms as its downregulation requires caspase-3 activation.

Despite an increase in cell death, Resveratrol increased cellular proliferation when used at low doses (20 and 40 μM) in our cell lines. We previously demonstrated that resveratrol can bind to the estrogen receptor α (ERα) in uterine cancer cells [30]. However, A2780 and A2780CP cell lines are ERα negative but we hypothesize that Resveratrol might bind to the estrogen receptor β (ERβ). This could also explain the synergistic action between Cisplatin and Resveratrol in A2780 cells since binding of Resveratrol to ERβ could increase gene transcription and then expose DNA to Cisplatin and increase its efficiency to induce cell death.

We confirmed results published earlier in a study on ovarian cancer reporting that Cisplatin increases EMT markers in ovarian cancer [11]. Cisplatin caused an increase in the protein levels of Snail, ZEB1 and Vimentin in both cell lines studied as soon as 24 h of treatment. Such a quick increase in Snail levels suggests that Cisplatin induces an EMT program even after a one-time/short-term treatment while TGF-β, a cytokine known for its ability to induce EMT, usually requires 72 h to achieve this process [31]. The increase in Snail levels was reverted by Resveratrol in a dose-dependent manner, which would involve the Erk pathway, as confirmed by MEK1/2 specific inhibition by U0126. However, Resveratrol and U0126 still increased Vimentin and ZEB1 levels.

Despite their lack of E-cadherin expression, A2780 and A2780CP cells represent an interesting model to study the induction of EMT since they possess many of the characteristics of epithelial cells such as an epithelial morphology that is altered by Cisplatin, thus allowing cells to gain a fibroblast-like mesenchymal morphology (Figure 6), and a low migration capacity in basal conditions (Figure 8). By contrast, SKOV-3 cells, which express basal E-cadherin levels, do not display an epithelial phenotype as they display fibroblast-like morphology (Figure S1) and possess an evident capacity to close a wound under basal conditions (Figure 8). Thus, we believe that A2780 and A2780CP cells, despite their defaults in their expression of some of the EMT markers, are an interesting model to study EMT induction by cisplatin as they display many epithelial characteristics. Other research groups also used A2780 cells as an epithelial model in their studies. Recently, Fangfang Du *et al.* demonstrated the potential involvement of EMT in the acquisition of paclitaxel resistance in A2780 cells [32].

Furthermore, Cisplatin-resistant A2780CP cells, which are less sensitive to Resveratrol-induced cell death, support that results observed in A2780 cells regarding EMT inhibition by Resveratrol are not due to excessive cell death and that Resveratrol possesses the potential to inhibit EMT in this cell model.

Another clue that Resveratrol inhibits Cisplatin-induced EMT came from the cellular morphology. Indeed, A2780 and A2780CP cells treated with Cisplatin alone displayed an evident morphology change from an epithelial cobblestone-like morphology to a more elongated morphology with cellular protusions reminiscent of cells having undergone EMT. However, cells treated with both Cisplatin and Resveratrol did not show such morphological modifications.

Recent studies in lung and colon cancer showed that Resveratrol induces senescence when used at doses in a range corresponding to the doses used in our study when treated for at least 10–12 days [33,34]. We were then interested in studying senescence induction by Resveratrol in A2780 and A2780CP cells. According to our results, Resveratrol induces a senescent phenotype in A2780 and A2780CP cells after 72 h of treatment in an interesting proportion of the cells. This phenomenon could also be a mechanism through which Resveratrol inhibits Cisplatin-induced EMT in A2780 and A2780CP cells since induction of senescence would inhibit the initiation of other cellular programs such as EMT and then block the effects of Cisplatin on these two ovarian cancer cell lines.

In wound healing assay, Resveratrol treatment displayed a marked decrease in cell migration in A2780 and A2780CP cells. This suggests that Resveratrol is able to inhibit migration, one of the main features acquired by cells undergoing EMT, and could then reduce metastatic potential of ovarian cancers. The decrease in migration observed for OVCAR-3 and SKOV-3 cells also holds potential for a wider application as Resveratrol also reduces the migration ability of another epithelial cell line, as well as a mesenchymal cell lines displaying a stronger migration capacity.

Recent studies using other cancer cell lines also support the role of Resveratrol in EMT inhibition. Vergara *et al.* demonstrated that Resveratrol inhibits EMT induction by EGF in MCF-7 breast cancer cell line via inhibition of the EGF-mediated Erk pathway activation [35]. A study from another group also supports the role of Resveratrol in inhibiting EMT induction in cancer cells in A549 lung cancer cells. In their study, the authors report that Resveratrol blocks TGF-β1 induced EMT and reduces the levels of EMT transcription factors Snail and Slug [36]. In our study, we suggest two mechanisms that can be responsible for EMT inhibition by Resveratrol (Figure 9). Resveratrol treatment reduced Cisplatin-mediated activation of the Erk pathway in A2780 and A2780CP cells, thus inhibiting Snail expression. Furthermore, Resveratrol significantly induced senescence in both cell lines, which could act as a dominant protection program in the cell to prevent the activation of other cellular differentiation pathways. In this regard, as a bonus to preventing EMT induction by Cisplatin, Resveratrol could alter cellular proliferation pathways and be a major determinant to prevent cancer progression.The fact that more than 90% of ovarian cancers are of epithelial origin [37] allows EMT to play a determinant role in ovarian cancer progression. Another important aspect of EMT is its possible involvement in the ability of cancer cells to resist to chemotherapeutic agents as well as acquire other important advantages such as resistance to anoikis and evasion from the immune system [38]. Combining these important consequences of EMT, it is clear that this phenomenon is a major factor involved in the high mortality rates associated with ovarian cancer. Considering this, finding new approaches to block EMT induction in cancer shows great promise to improve the outcome for patients. Our results suggest that Resveratrol might be an interesting compound to prevent cancer development or as an adjuvant molecule for cancer treatment once diagnosed.

However, bioavailability of Resveratrol might be a problem since it is quickly metabolised and it might be difficult to reach high local concentrations matching the doses used during *in vitro* studies [39]. To assess this problem it would be important to find alternate routes of administration, such as localised treatment or local injections, to improve Resveratrol's effect on cancer cells. In regard of our results, targeting the Erk pathway also shows interesting promise to decrease cancer progression towards metastasis and could reveal an important asset in the fight against cancer.

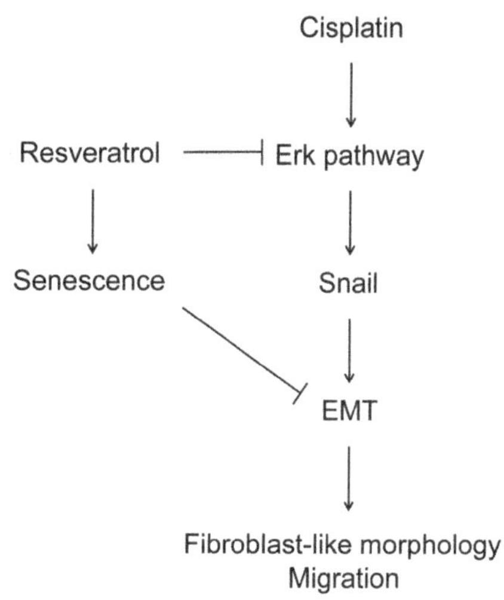

Figure 9. Involvement of Resveratrol in the inhibition of Cisplatin-induced EMT. Treatment of ovarian cancer cell lines with Cisplatin results in the activation of the Erk pathway and subsequent induction of Snail expression and induction of EMT. By contrast, Resveratrol prevents Cisplatin-mediated EMT induction by antagonizing the activation of the Erk pathway, thus preventing Snail levels increase and EMT induction. Furthermore, Resveratrol could also prevent Cisplatin-induced EMT through induction of a senescence program that would block the progression of other cellular differentiation programs like EMT.

Supporting Information

Figure S1 Epithelial and mesenchymal markers expressed in OVCAR-3 and SKOV-3 cells and their basal morphology. Expression of the epithelial marker (E-cadherin) and expression of the mesenchymal markers (ZEB1, Vimentin and Snail) was determined in OVCAR-3 and SKOV-3 cells treated or not with Cisplatin and Resveratrol (A). Basal morphology is shown for both cell lines under their corresponding protein expression profile (B). Despite its E-cadherin expression, SKOV-3 displays morphological characteristics of mesenchymal cells.

Acknowledgments

We are grateful to Valerie Leblanc for her technical assistance throughout the study.

Author Contributions

Conceived and designed the experiments: SB PC EA. Performed the experiments: SB PC SP. Analyzed the data: SB PC EA. Contributed reagents/materials/analysis tools: SB PC EA. Wrote the paper: SB EA.

References

1. Society CC (2011) Canadian Cancer Statistics.
2. Auersperg N, Wong AS, Choi KC, Kang SK, Leung PC (2001) Ovarian surface epithelium: biology, endocrinology, and pathology. Endocr Rev 22: 255–288.
3. Colombo PE, Fabbro M, Theillet C, Bibeau F, Rouanet P, et al. (2013) Sensitivity and resistance to treatment in the primary management of epithelial ovarian cancer. Crit Rev Oncol Hematol.
4. Kim A, Ueda Y, Naka T, Enomoto T (2012) Therapeutic strategies in epithelial ovarian cancer. J Exp Clin Cancer Res 31: 14.
5. Thiery JP (2002) Epithelial-mesenchymal transitions in tumour progression. Nat Rev Cancer 2: 442–454.
6. Lombaerts M, van Wezel T, Philippo K, Dierssen JW, Zimmerman RM, et al. (2006) E-cadherin transcriptional downregulation by promoter methylation but not mutation is related to epithelial-to-mesenchymal transition in breast cancer cell lines. Br J Cancer 94: 661–671.
7. Nieto MA (2002) The snail superfamily of zinc-finger transcription factors. Nat Rev Mol Cell Biol 3: 155–166.
8. Aigner K, Dampier B, Descovich L, Mikula M, Sultan A, et al. (2007) The transcription factor ZEB1 (deltaEF1) promotes tumour cell dedifferentiation by repressing master regulators of epithelial polarity. Oncogene 26: 6979–6988.
9. Bakin AV, Tomlinson AK, Bhowmick NA, Moses HL, Arteaga CL (2000) Phosphatidylinositol 3-kinase function is required for transforming growth factor beta-mediated epithelial to mesenchymal transition and cell migration. J Biol Chem 275: 36803–36810.
10. Cui W, Yazlovitskaya EM, Mayo MS, Pelling JC, Persons DL (2000) Cisplatin-induced response of c-jun N-terminal kinase 1 and extracellular signal–regulated protein kinases 1 and 2 in a series of cisplatin-resistant ovarian carcinoma cell lines. Mol Carcinog 29: 219–228.

11. Latifi A, Abubaker K, Castrechini N, Ward AC, Liongue C, et al. (2011) Cisplatin treatment of primary and metastatic epithelial ovarian carcinomas generates residual cells with mesenchymal stem cell-like profile. J Cell Biochem 112: 2850–2864.
12. Batlle E, Sancho E, Franci C, Dominguez D, Monfar M, et al. (2000) The transcription factor snail is a repressor of E-cadherin gene expression in epithelial tumour cells. Nat Cell Biol 2: 84–89.
13. Cano A, Perez-Moreno MA, Rodrigo I, Locascio A, Blanco MJ, et al. (2000) The transcription factor snail controls epithelial-mesenchymal transitions by repressing E-cadherin expression. Nat Cell Biol 2: 76–83.
14. Hajra KM, Chen DY, Fearon ER (2002) The SLUG zinc-finger protein represses E-cadherin in breast cancer. Cancer Res 62: 1613–1618.
15. Wels C, Joshi S, Koefinger P, Bergler H, Schaider H (2011) Transcriptional activation of ZEB1 by Slug leads to cooperative regulation of the epithelial-mesenchymal transition-like phenotype in melanoma. J Invest Dermatol 131: 1877–1885.
16. Kurrey NK, Amit K, Bapat SA (2005) Snail and Slug are major determinants of ovarian cancer invasiveness at the transcription level. Gynecol Oncol 97: 155–165.
17. Lee SH, Lee SJ, Jung YS, Xu Y, Kang HS, et al. (2009) Blocking of p53-Snail binding, promoted by oncogenic K-Ras, recovers p53 expression and function. Neoplasia 11: 22–31, 26p following 31.
18. Kurrey NK, Jalgaonkar SP, Joglekar AV, Ghanate AD, Chaskar PD, et al. (2009) Snail and slug mediate radioresistance and chemoresistance by antagonizing p53-mediated apoptosis and acquiring a stem-like phenotype in ovarian cancer cells. Stem Cells 27: 2059–2068.
19. Hotz B, Arndt M, Dullat S, Bhargava S, Buhr HJ, et al. (2007) Epithelial to mesenchymal transition: expression of the regulators snail, slug, and twist in pancreatic cancer. Clin Cancer Res 13: 4769–4776.
20. Eger A, Aigner K, Sonderegger S, Dampier B, Oehler S, et al. (2005) DeltaEF1 is a transcriptional repressor of E-cadherin and regulates epithelial plasticity in breast cancer cells. Oncogene 24: 2375–2385.
21. Hu F, Wang C, Du J, Sun W, Yan J, et al. (2010) DeltaEF1 promotes breast cancer cell proliferation through down-regulating p21 expression. Biochim Biophys Acta 1802: 301–312.
22. Cal C, Garban H, Jazirehi A, Yeh C, Mizutani Y, et al. (2003) Resveratrol and cancer: chemoprevention, apoptosis, and chemo-immunosensitizing activities. Curr Med Chem Anticancer Agents 3: 77–93.
23. Jang M, Cai L, Udeani GO, Slowing KV, Thomas CF, et al. (1997) Cancer chemopreventive activity of resveratrol, a natural product derived from grapes. Science 275: 218–220.
24. Louie KG, Behrens BC, Kinsella TJ, Hamilton TC, Grotzinger KR, et al. (1985) Radiation survival parameters of antineoplastic drug-sensitive and -resistant human ovarian cancer cell lines and their modification by buthionine sulfoximine. Cancer Res 45: 2110–2115.
25. Opipari AW Jr, Tan L, Boitano AE, Sorenson DR, Aurora A, et al. (2004) Resveratrol-induced autophagocytosis in ovarian cancer cells. Cancer Res 64: 696–703.
26. Chen QM, Tu VC, Catania J, Burton M, Toussaint O, et al. (2000) Involvement of Rb family proteins, focal adhesion proteins and protein synthesis in senescent morphogenesis induced by hydrogen peroxide. J Cell Sci 113 (Pt 22): 4087–4097.
27. Haslehurst AM, Koti M, Dharsee M, Nuin P, Evans K, et al. (2012) EMT transcription factors snail and slug directly contribute to cisplatin resistance in ovarian cancer. BMC Cancer 12: 91.
28. Catalgol B, Batirel S, Taga Y, Ozer NK (2012) Resveratrol: French paradox revisited. Front Pharmacol 3: 141.
29. Schmeiser K, Hammond EM, Roberts S, Grand RJ (1998) Specific cleavage of gamma catenin by caspases during apoptosis. FEBS Lett 433: 51–57.
30. Sexton E, Van Themsche C, Leblanc K, Parent S, Lemoine P, et al. (2006) Resveratrol interferes with AKT activity and triggers apoptosis in human uterine cancer cells. MolCancer 5: 45.
31. Xie L, Law BK, Chytil AM, Brown KA, Aakre ME, et al. (2004) Activation of the Erk pathway is required for TGF-beta1-induced EMT in vitro. Neoplasia 6: 603–610.
32. Du F, Wu X, Liu Y, Wang T, Qi X, et al. (2013) Acquisition of paclitaxel resistance via PI3Kdependent epithelialmesenchymal transition in A2780 human ovarian cancer cells. Oncol Rep.
33. Luo H, Yang A, Schulte BA, Wargovich MJ, Wang GY (2013) Resveratrol Induces Premature Senescence in Lung Cancer Cells via ROS-Mediated DNA Damage. PLoS One 8: e60065.
34. Heiss EH, Schilder YD, Dirsch VM (2007) Chronic treatment with resveratrol induces redox stress- and ataxia telangiectasia-mutated (ATM)-dependent senescence in p53-positive cancer cells. J Biol Chem 282: 26759–26766.
35. Vergara D, Valente CM, Tinelli A, Siciliano C, Lorusso V, et al. (2011) Resveratrol inhibits the epidermal growth factor-induced epithelial mesenchymal transition in MCF-7 cells. Cancer Lett 310: 1–8.
36. Wang H, Zhang H, Tang L, Chen H, Wu C, et al. (2013) Resveratrol inhibits TGF-beta1-induced epithelial-to-mesenchymal transition and suppresses lung cancer invasion and metastasis. Toxicology 303: 139–146.
37. Park SH, Cheung LW, Wong AS, Leung PC (2008) Estrogen regulates Snail and Slug in the down-regulation of E-cadherin and induces metastatic potential of ovarian cancer cells through estrogen receptor alpha. Mol Endocrinol 22: 2085–2098.
38. Tiwari N, Gheldof A, Tatari M, Christofori G (2012) EMT as the ultimate survival mechanism of cancer cells. Seminars in Cancer Biology 22: 194–207.
39. Gescher AJ, Steward WP (2003) Relationship between mechanisms, bioavailibility, and preclinical chemopreventive efficacy of resveratrol: a conundrum. Cancer Epidemiol Biomarkers Prev 12: 953–957.

3

Fibroblast Growth Factor 2 Induces E-Cadherin Down-Regulation via PI3K/Akt/mTOR and MAPK/ERK Signaling in Ovarian Cancer Cells

Man-Tat Lau, Wai-Kin So, Peter C. K. Leung*

Department of Obstetrics and Gynecology, Child and Family Research Institute, University of British Columbia, Vancouver, British Columbia, Canada

Abstract

Fibroblast growth factor 2 (FGF2) is produced by ovarian cancer cells and it has been suggested to play an important role in tumor progression. In this study, we report that FGF2 treatment down-regulated E-cadherin by up-regulating its transcriptional repressors, Slug and ZEB1, in human ovarian cancer cells. The pharmacological inhibition of phosphatidylinositol-3-kinase (PI3K), mammalian target of rapamycin (mTOR), and MEK suggests that both PI3K/Akt/mTOR and MAPK/ERK signaling are required for FGF2-induced E-cadherin down-regulation. Moreover, FGF2 up-regulated Slug and ZEB1 expression via the PI3K/Akt/mTOR and MAPK/ERK signaling pathways, respectively. Finally, FGF2-induced cell invasion was abolished by the inhibition of the PI3K/Akt/mTOR and MAPK/ERK pathways, and the forced expression of E-cadherin diminished the intrinsic invasiveness of ovarian cancer cells as well as the FGF2-induced cell invasion. This study demonstrates a novel mechanism in which FGF2 down-regulates E-cadherin expression through the activation of PI3K/Akt/mTOR and MAPK/ERK signaling, and the up-regulation of Slug and ZEB1 in human ovarian cancer cells.

Editor: Antimo Migliaccio, II Università di Napoli, Italy

Funding: This work was supported by an operating grant from the Canadian Institutes of Health Research to PCKL. The funders had no role in study design, data collection and analysis, decision to publish, or preparation of the manuscript.

Competing Interests: The authors have declared that no competing interests exist.

* E-mail: peter.leung@ubc.ca

Introduction

Epithelial ovarian cancer (EOC), which comprises 90% of all ovarian malignancies, is the most common and lethal form of gynecological cancer in developed countries [1], the death rate for this disease has not changed much in the last 50 years.

Fibroblast growth factor-2 (FGF2) mediates various cellular events, including proliferation, motility, and differentiation [2,3], and malignant ovarian tumors are common in patients with elevated FGF2 [4–6]. However, the role of FGF2 in ovarian cancer progression is still controversial. Ovarian tumors with high cytoplasmic FGF2 are associated with reduced tumor aggressiveness and increased survival rates compared with patients with low levels of FGF2 [7,8]. In contrast, previous *in vitro* studies and the gene expression profiling of advanced ovarian cancer suggest that FGF2 acts as an autocrine growth factor for ovarian cancer cell proliferation [9–11] and invasion [12]. Moreover, FGF2 regulates the expression of additional genes implicated in angiogenesis or metastasis, including metalloproteinases [13], vascular endothelial growth factor [14], and E-cadherin [13,15,16].

E-cadherin functions as a cell-cell adhesion protein and tumor suppressor that is silenced in many malignancies, and the loss of E-cadherin expression or function is a common event in tumor progression [17,18]. E-cadherin is known to suppress tumor cell invasion, and the re-expression of E-cadherin in E-cadherin-deficient carcinomas reverts cells to a less invasive, less aggressive phenotype [19–21], while the loss of E-cadherin is associated with ovarian cancer metastasis, peritoneal dissemination, and poor prognosis [22–26]. The loss of E-cadherin function can be achieved by the mutation of the E-cadherin gene [27], the hypermethylation of the E-cadherin promoter [28,29], and the transcriptional repression of E-cadherin [30–33]. Several transcription factors have been identified to suppress E-cadherin including Snail, Slug, Twist and ZEB1 via their interaction with the E-box binding site in the E-cadherin promoter [30,31,34–36].

Previous studies have demonstrated that FGF2 suppresses E-cadherin in various cell types [13,15,16]; however, the underlying mechanisms are still largely unknown. In the present study, we demonstrate that FGF2 reduces E-cadherin mRNA and protein levels in a time- and dose-dependent manner. Furthermore, increased Slug and ZEB1 expression via the activation of the PI3K/Akt/mTOR and the MAPK/ERK signaling pathways, respectively, potentially mediates the effects of FGF2 on E-cadherin. Finally, our results indicate that the down-regulation of E-cadherin-mediated FGF2 enhances the invasiveness in ovarian cancer cells.

Materials and Methods

Materials

FGF2 was purchased from Sigma-Aldrich (Ontario, Canada). Rapamycin, U0126 and wortmannin were purchased from Calbiochem (San Diego, CA). E-cadherin antibodies were purchased from BD Biosciences (San Jose, CA). Akt, phospho-Akt (Ser473), p44/42 MAPK (ERK), phospho-p44/42 MAPK (Thr202/Tyr204), p70S6K and phospho-p70S6K (Thr389) anti-

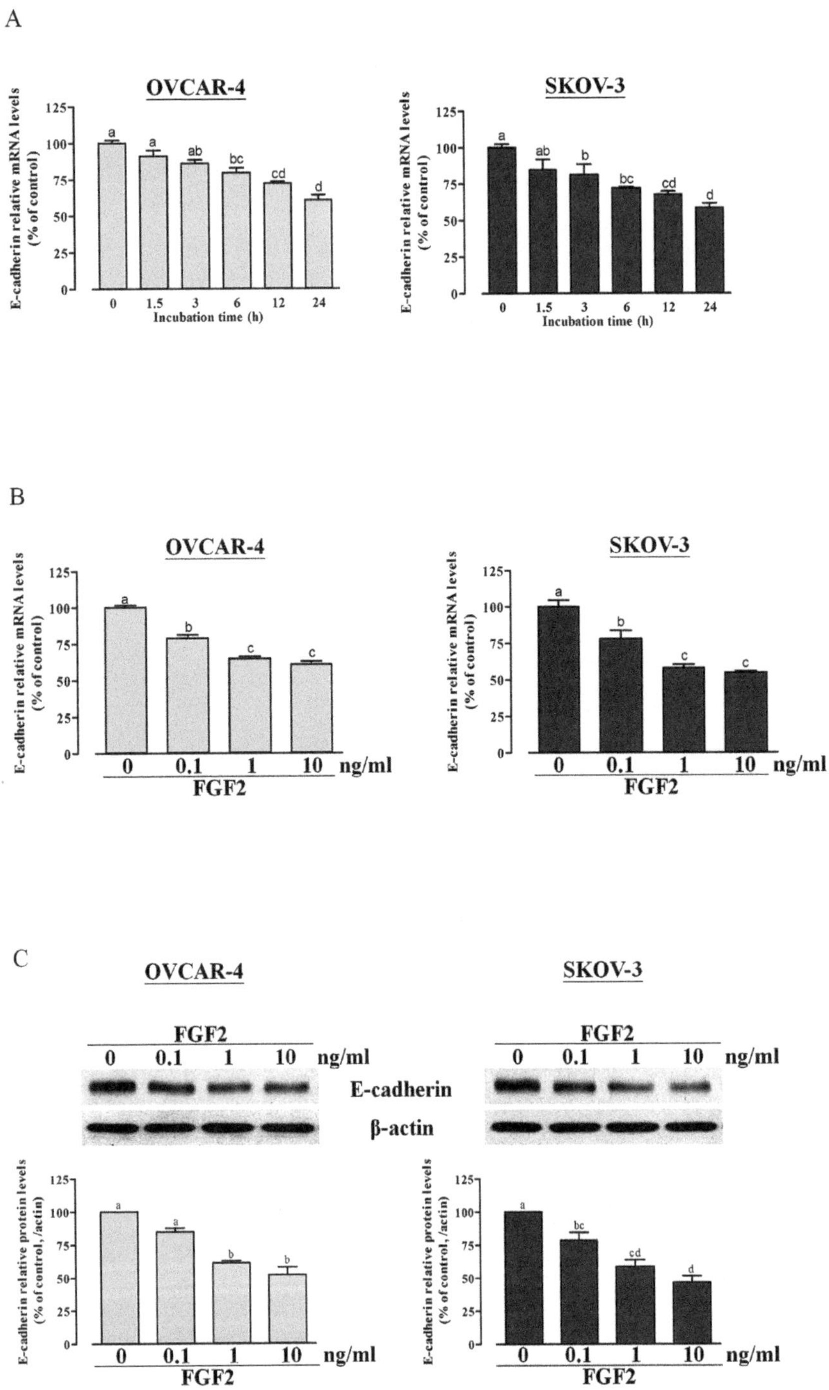

Figure 1. FGF2 suppresses E-cadherin mRNA and protein levels in OVCAR-4 and SKOV-3 cells. (A) OVCAR-4 and SKOV-3 cells were treated with 10 ng/ml FGF2 for 0 to 24 h as indicated, and then E-cadherin mRNA levels were analyzed by RT-qPCR. (B and C) OVCAR-4 and SKOV-3 cells were treated with different doses of FGF2 for 24 h after which E-cadherin mRNA levels (B) and protein levels (C) were analyzed by RT-qPCR and Western blotting, respectively. Results represent the mean ± SEM (n = 3; values without a common letter are significantly different, $P<0.05$). Data were analyzed by one-way ANOVA followed by Tukey's multiple comparison test.

bodies were purchased from Cell Signaling Technology, Inc. (Beverly, MA). The β-actin antibody was purchased from Santa Cruz Biotechnology (Santa Cruz, CA). Horseradish peroxidase-conjugated goat anti-rabbit IgG and goat anti-mouse IgG antibodies were purchased from Bio-Rad Laboratories (Hercules, CA).

Plasmid Constructs

The pcDNA-GFP (GFP) was generously provided by Dr. Alonzo H. Ross [37]. The pcDNA-Ecadherin-GFP (Ecad-GFP) was a kind gift from Dr. Jennifer L. Stow [38].

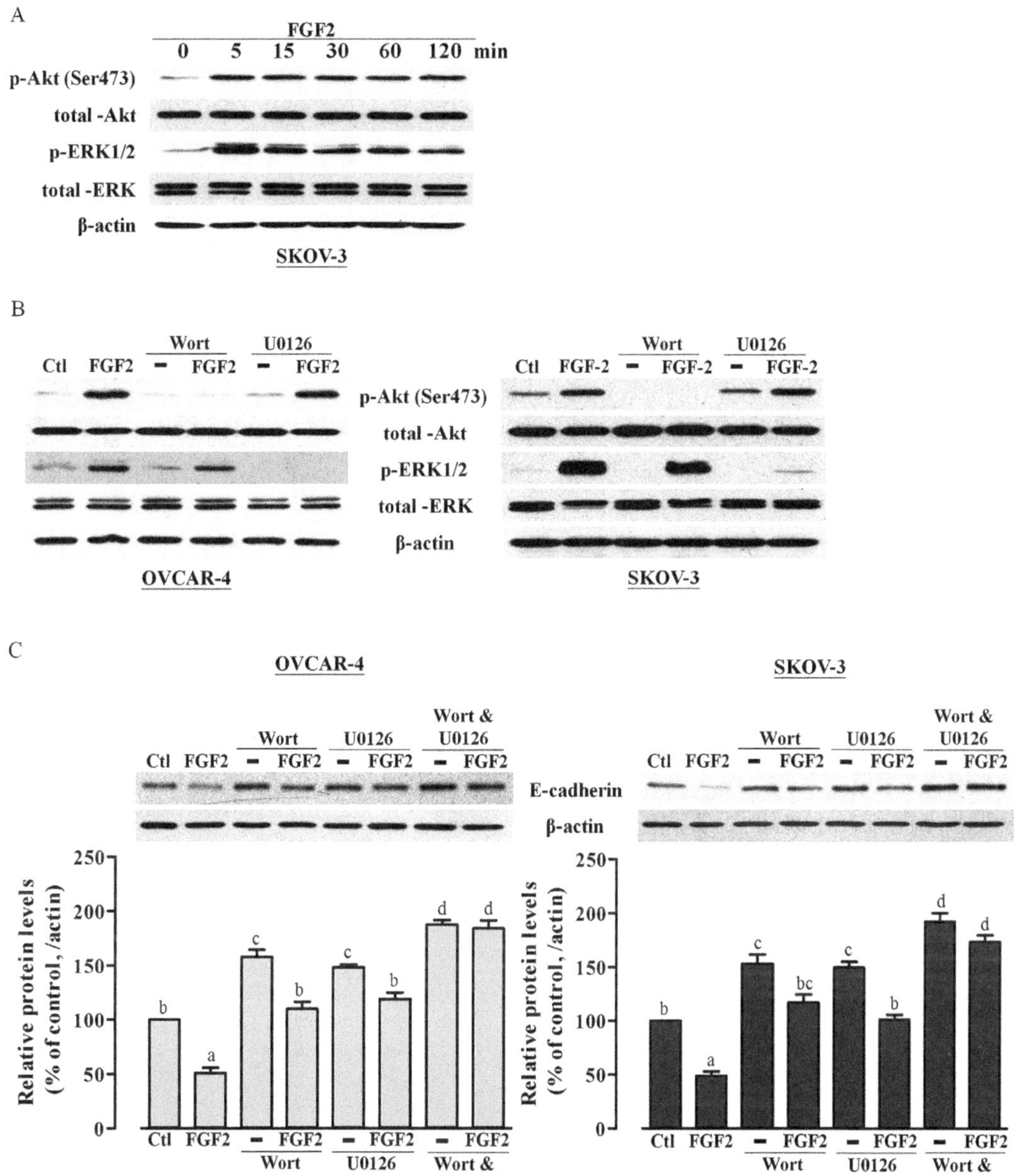

Figure 2. FGF2 suppresses E-cadherin expression via the PI3K/Akt and MAPK/ERK signaling pathways. (A) SKOV-3 cells were treated with 10 ng/ml FGF2 for 0 to 120 min as indicated. Phosphorylated and total Akt, phosphorylated and total ERK, and β-actin levels were analyzed by Western blot analysis. (B) OVCAR-4 and SKOV-3 cells were pretreated with wortmannin (1 μM) or U0126 (10 μM) for 30 min before the addition of FGF2 (10 ng/ml) for 30 min. Phosphorylated and total Akt, phosphorylated and total ERK protein levels were analyzed by Western blotting. The β-actin antibody was used as a control for equal loading. (C) OVCAR-4 and SKOV-3 cells were pretreated with wortmannin (1 μM) or U0126 (10 μM) alone or in the presence of 10 ng/ml FGF2 for 24 h, after which E-cadherin protein levels were analyzed by Western blotting. Results represent the mean ± SEM [(A) & (B) n = 3; (C) n = 6; values without a common letter are significantly different, $P<0.05$]. Data were analyzed by one-way ANOVA followed by Tukey's multiple comparison test.

Cell culture and transfections

Human ovarian cancer cell lines (OVCAR-4 and SKOV-3) were purchased from the American Type Culture Collection (ATCC, Manassas, VA), and their use was approved by the University of British Columbia Clinical Screening Committee for Research and Other Studies Involving Human Subjects. Cells were cultured in Medium 199:MCDB 105 (1:1; Sigma-Aldrich) containing 10% fetal bovine serum (FBS; Hyclone Laboratories Ltd., Logan, UT), 100 U/ml penicillin G and 100 μg/ml streptomycin (Life Technologies, Inc., Rockville, MD) in a humidified atmosphere of 5% CO_2 to 95% air at 37°C. The cells were passaged with 0.06% trypsin (1:250)/0.01% EDTA in Mg^{2+}/Ca^{2+} - free HBSS at confluence.

All transfections were carried out using Lipofectamine 2000 Reagent (Invitrogen, Burlington, ON, Canada) according to the manufacturer's protocol.

Reverse transcription quantitative real-time PCR (RT-qPCR)

Total RNA was prepared using TRIzol reagent (Invitrogen) according to the manufacturer's instructions. Single-stranded

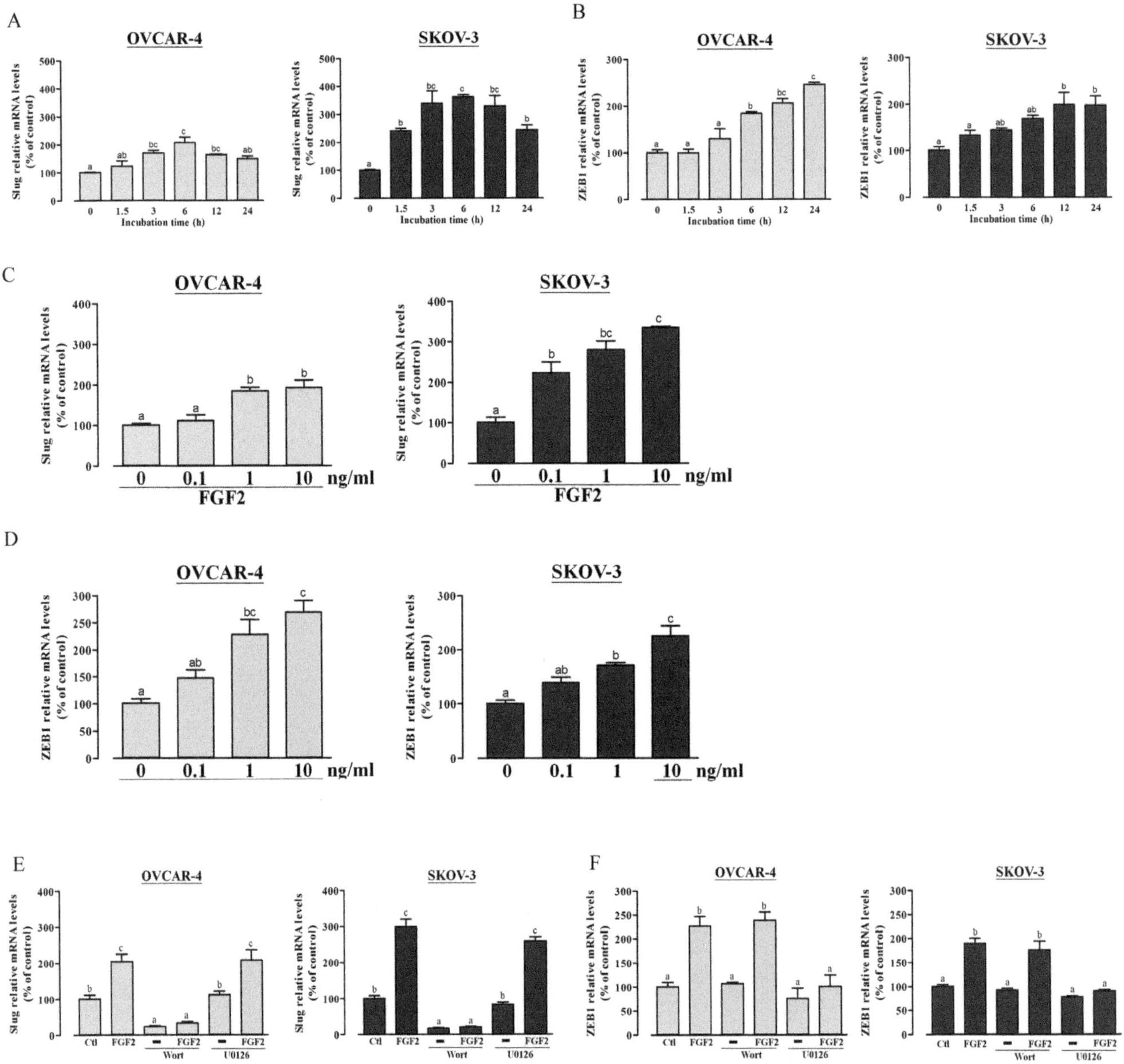

Figure 3. FGF2 increases Slug and ZEB1 mRNA levels in OVCAR-4 and SKOV-3 cells. (A and B) OVCAR-4 and SKOV-3 cells were treated with 10 ng/ml FGF2 for various times, and the mRNA levels of Slug (A) and ZEB1 (B) were analyzed by RT-qPCR. (C and D) OVCAR-4 and SKOV-3 cells were treated with different doses of FGF2 for 6 h (Slug; C) or 24 h (ZEB1; D), and mRNA levels were analyzed by RT-qPCR. (E and F) OVCAR-4 and SKOV-3 cells were pretreated with wortmannin (1 μM) or U0126 (10 μM) for 30 min prior to the addition of 10 ng/ml FGF2 for 6 h (E) and 24 h (F). Slug and ZEB1 mRNA levels were analyzed by RT-qPCR. Results represent the mean ± SEM (n = 3; values without a common letter are significantly different, $P<0.05$). Data were analyzed by one-way ANOVA followed by Tukey's multiple comparison test.

cDNA was synthesized from 2 μg total RNA according to the manufacturer's procedure (Amersham Biosciences, Quebec, Canada). The primers used for SYBR Green RT-qPCR were as follows: for human E-cadherin, sense, 5′-ACA GCC CCG CCT TAT GAT T-3′ and antisense, 5′-TCG GAA CCG CTT CCT TCA-3′; for Slug, sense, 5′-TTC GGA CCCACA CAT TAC CT-3′ and antisense, 5′-GCA GTG AGG GCA AGA AAA AG-3′ ; for ZEB1, sense, 5′-GCA CCT GAA GAG GAC CAG AG-3′ and antisense, 5′-TGC ATC TGG TGT TCC ATT TT-3′; and for GAPDH, sense, 5′-ATG GAA ATC CCA TCA CCA TCT T-3′ and antisense, 5′-CGC CCC ACT TGA TTT TGG -3′. RT-qPCR was performed using the Applied Biosystems 7300 Real-Time PCR System equipped with a 96-well optical reaction plate. Relative quantification of mRNA levels was performed using the comparative Cq method ($\Delta\Delta$Cq method) with GAPDH as the reference gene.

Western blot analysis

Cells were harvested in lysis buffer [50 mM Tris (pH 7.5), 150 mM NaCl, 1% NP40, 0.5% sodium deoxycholate, 1 mM EDTA, 0.1% SDS] containing protease inhibitor cocktail (Sigma-Aldrich), and protein concentrations were determined using the DC Protein Assay (Bio-Rad Laboratories, Inc., Hercules, CA). Protein (40 μg) was electrophoresed on 7.5% SDS-polyacrylamide gels, transferred to nitrocellulose mem-

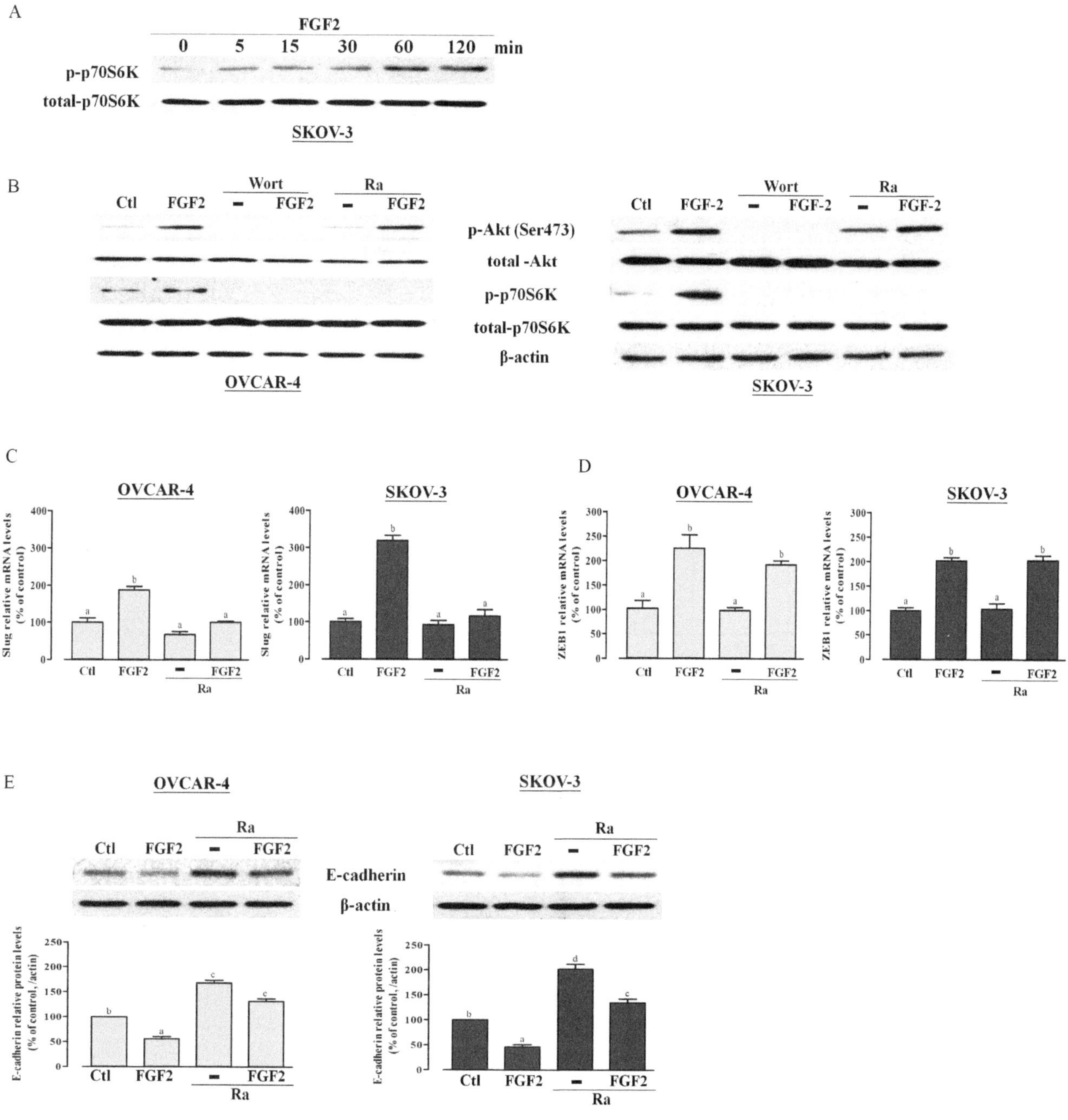

Figure 4. FGF2 suppresses E-cadherin expression via the PI3K/Akt/mTOR signaling pathway. (A) SKOV-3 cells were treated with 10 ng/ml FGF2 for 0 to 120 min as indicated. Phosphorylated and total p70S6K levels were analyzed by Western blot analysis. (B) OVCAR-4 and SKOV-3 cells were pretreated with wortmannin (1 μM) or rapamycin (20 nM) for 30 min prior to the addition of 10 ng/ml FGF2 for 30 min. Phospho-Akt and Akt, along with phospho-p70S6K and p70S6K protein levels were analyzed by Western blotting. The β-actin antibody was used as a control for equal loading. (C and D) OVCAR-4 and SKOV-3 cells were pretreated with rapamycin (20 nM) for 30 min prior to addition of 10 ng/ml FGF2 for 6 h (C) and 24 h (D). Slug and ZEB1 mRNA levels were analyzed by RT-qPCR. (E) OVCAR-4 and SKOV-3 cells were pretreated with rapamycin (20 nM) for 30 min prior to addition of 10 ng/ml FGF2 for 24 h, after which E-cadherin protein levels were analyzed by Western blotting. Results represent the mean ± SEM [(A)–(D) n = 3; (E) n = 6; values without a common letter are significantly different, $P<0.05$). Data were analyzed by one-way ANOVA followed by Tukey's multiple comparison test.

branes (Amersham Bioscience), and incubated with specific primary antibodies at 4°C overnight. After washing, the membranes were incubated with horseradish peroxidase-conjugated secondary antibodies for 1 h and were visualized with enhanced chemiluminescent substrate (Thermo Fisher Scientific Inc, Waltham, MA).

Invasion assay

Twenty-four-well transwell inserts with an 8-μm pore coated with 1 mg/ml Matrigel (50 μl/well; BD sciences, Mississauga, ON, Canada) were used to assess cell invasion. Trypsinized cells (1×10^5) in 0.1% FBS medium, with or without FGF2, were seeded

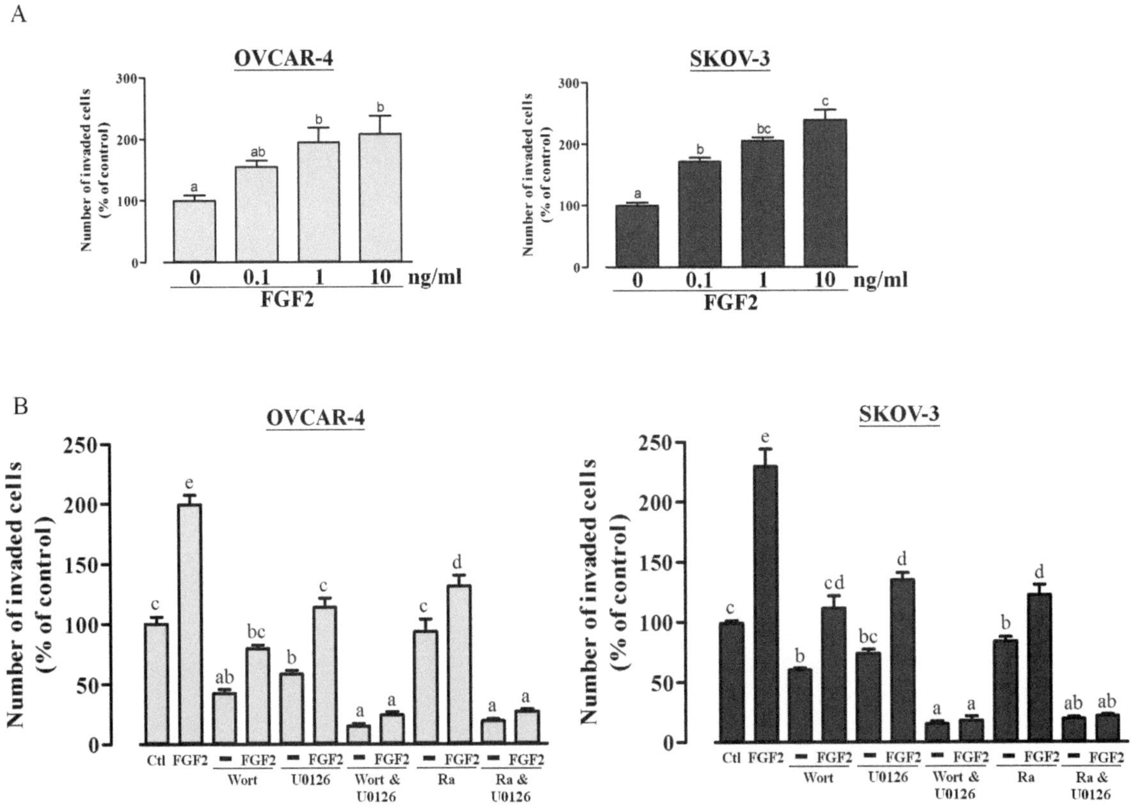

Figure 5. FGF2 induces ovarian cancer cell invasion via the PI3K/Akt/mTOR and MAPK/ERK signaling pathways. (A) Ovarian cancer cells were seeded in Matrigel-coated transwell inserts and treated with different doses of FGF2 for 24 h. (B) Cells were pre-treated with wortmannin (1 μM), rapamycin (20 nM) or U0126 (10 μM) for 30 min and seeded in Matrigel-coated transwell inserts and cultured with 10 ng/ml FGF2 for 24 h. Results represent the mean ± SEM [(A) n = 3; (B) n = 6; values without a common letter are significantly different, $P<0.05$]. Data were analyzed by one-way ANOVA followed by Tukey's multiple comparison test.

in triplicate in the upper chamber. 1% FBS medium was placed in the lower wells. The chambers were incubated for 24 h at 37°C in a 5% CO_2 atmosphere. Cells that did not penetrate the filter were wiped off, and invaded cells on the lower surface of the filter were fixed with ice-cold methanol and stained with 0.5% crystal violet. Results are presented as the mean number of invaded cells of five fields (at 100× magnification) ± SEM from three independent experiments.

Data analysis

All values are expressed as mean ± SEM from three to six independent experiments. Data were analyzed by a one-way ANOVA followed by Tukey's *post hoc* test using GraphPad Prism 5 (GraphPad Software, San Diego, CA). $P<0.05$ was considered statistically significant.

Results

Effect of FGF2 on E-cadherin expression in ovarian cancer cells

As a first step toward analyzing the role of FGF2 in ovarian cancer progression, we investigated the effect of FGF2 on E-cadherin expression in OVCAR-4 and SKOV-3 cells. Our results showed that treatment with FGF2 down-regulated E-cadherin mRNA levels in both a time- (Fig 1A) and dose-dependent manner (Fig 1B). Similarly, Western blot analysis showed that treatment with FGF2 down-regulated E-cadherin protein levels in a dose-dependent manner in ovarian cancer cells (Fig 1C).

FGF2-induces E-cadherin down-regulation via the PI3K/Akt and MAPK/ERK pathways

It is well documented that the PI3K/Akt and MAPK/ERK pathways are frequently amplified and serve as survival pathways in ovarian carcinomas [39]. In addition, FGF2 is known to activate the PI3K/Akt and MAPK/ERK pathways [40,41] and, has been reported to regulate E-cadherin down-regulation [42,43]. Therefore, we analyzed whether these two pathways were involved in the suppression of E-cadherin expression by FGF2. We first examined the phosphorylation status of Akt and ERK upon treatment with 10 ng/ml FGF2 at 5, 15, 30, 60, and 120 minutes post-treatment and found that FGF2 treatment induced the phosphorylation of Akt (Ser473) and ERK (Thr202/Tyr204) in a time-dependent manner in SKOV-3 cells (Fig 2A). To determine whether these two pathways were involved in the suppression of E-cadherin expression by FGF2, we used two pharmacological inhibitors, wortmannin and U0126, to specifically block the PI3K/Akt and MAPK/ERK pathways, respectively, in SKOV-3 cells and OVCAR-4 (Fig 2B), respectively. As shown in Fig. 2C, the PI3K and ERK inhibitors significantly increased basal E-cadherin expression and markedly diminished, but did not completely abolish, FGF2-induced suppression of E-cadherin expression, which demonstrated the involvement of the PI3K/Akt and

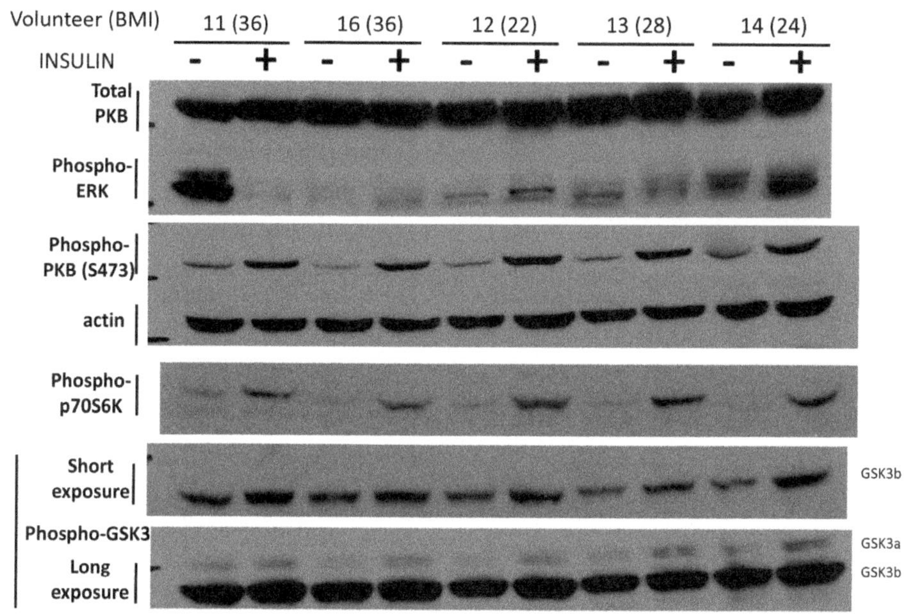

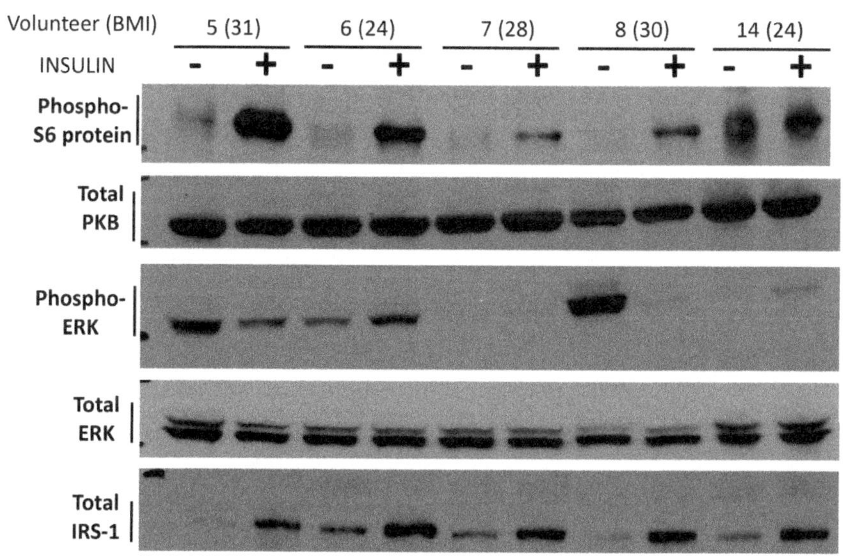

Figure 6. The loss of E-cadherin mediates FGF2-induced invasion. (A) SKOV-3 cells were transient transfected with the pcDNA-GFP (GFP) or human E-cadherin expression plasmids (Ecad-GFP) for 48 h. After transfection, cells were treated with 10 ng/ml FGF2 for 24 h and subjected to immunoblotting for E-cadherin and β-actin. (B) After 48 h of transfection, the trypsinized cells were seeded in Matrigel-coated transwell inserts, and cultured with 10ng/ml FGF2 for 24 h. Results represent the mean ± SEM (n = 6; values without a common letter are significantly different, $P<0.05$). Data were analyzed by one-way ANOVA followed by Tukey's multiple comparison test.

MAPK/ERK pathways in the FGF2-mediated down-regulation of E-cadherin expression in ovarian cancer cells.

FGF2 differentially up-regulates Slug and ZEB1 expression via the PI3K/Akt and MAPK/ERK pathways, respectively

To investigate whether FGF2 down-regulates E-cadherin expression by modulating the transcriptional regulation of E-cadherin, we used RT-qPCR to examine the mRNA levels of the E-cadherin transcriptional repressors Snail, Slug, Twist and ZEB1. Treatment with FGF2 significantly increased Slug and ZEB1 mRNA levels in a time- (Fig 3A and 3B) and dose-dependent manner (Fig 3C and 3D) but had no significant influence on Snail and Twist mRNA levels (data not shown). To determine whether the PI3K/Akt and MAPK/ERK signaling pathways are involved in FGF2-induced increases in Slug and ZEB1 mRNA, cells were treated with PI3K inhibitor (wortmannin) or MEK inhibitor (U0126) in the presence or absence of FGF2. Interestingly, wortmannin significantly suppressed the basal Slug mRNA level and totally abolished the effects of FGF2 on Slug mRNA levels (Fig 3E), whereas FGF2-enhanced ZEB1 mRNA levels were not affected (Fig 3F). On the other hand, U0126 treatment totally abolished the effects of FGF2 on ZEB1 mRNA levels (Fig 3F), the drug had no effect on Slug mRNA levels (Fig 3E).

FGF2-induced E-cadherin down-regulation via the PI3K/Akt/mTOR pathway

Next, we investigated the role of the mTOR pathway in FGF2-induced E-cadherin down-regulation, because mTOR is a pathway downstream of PI3K/Akt signaling that has been shown to be involved in E-cadherin down-regulation [44]. As shown, treatment with FGF2 induced the activation of mTOR signaling in a time-dependent manner in SKOV-3 cells, as indicated by phosphorylation of the mTOR downstream molecule, p70S6K (Fig 4A). To determine whether the PI3K/Akt/mTOR signaling pathway was involved in the regulation of E-cadherin levels by FGF2, we used the mTOR-specific inhibitor rapamycin to block the mTOR pathway in SKOV-3 cells and OVCAR-4 (Fig 4B). Similar to wortmannin, rapamycin totally abolished the FGF2-induced elevation of Slug mRNA (Fig 4C), whereas rapamycin showed no effect on ZEB1 mRNA levels (Fig 4D). Moreover, rapamycin treatment significantly increased the protein levels of E-cadherin and markedly diminished the suppressive effect of FGF2 on E-cadherin protein levels (Fig 4E), indicating that the PI3K/Akt/mTOR pathway is involved in FGF2-induced E-cadherin suppression in ovarian cancer cells.

Activation of the PI3K/Akt/mTOR and MAPK/ERK signaling pathways are critical for FGF2-induced cell invasion

Several lines of evidence indicate that FGF2 plays an important role in the invasive properties of human cancer cells [45,46]. Thus, we examined the effect of FGF2 on cell invasion in ovarian cancer cells using Matrigel-coated Transwell invasion assays. OVCAR-4 and SKOV-3 cells were treated with increasing concentrations of FGF2, resulted in a dose-dependent stimulation of invasion (Fig 5A). The involvement of the PI3K/Akt/mTOR and MAPK/ERK signaling pathways in FGF2-stimulated cell invasion were also evaluated. Our results showed that FGF2-induced cell invasion was markedly diminished, but not totally, by treatment with wortmannin, rapamycin or U0126 alone (Fig 5B), while combined inhibition of the PI3K/Akt/mTOR and MAPK/ERK signaling pathways totally abolished FGF2-induced cell invasion (Fig 5B). Taken together, these results indicate that the MAPK/ERK and PI3K/Akt/mTOR pathways are involved in FGF2-induced ovarian cancer cell invasion.

Down-regulation of E-cadherin mediates FGF2-stimulated ovarian cancer cell invasion

Next, we asked whether down-regulation of E-cadherin mediated the FGF2-induced cell invasion. SKOV-3 cells were transiently transfected with wild-type human E-cadherin expression plasmid for 48 h and then were treated with FGF2 for further 24 h (Fig 6A). FGF2 treatment reduced E-cadherin protein levels in cells transfected with empty vector, whereas no effect was detected in cells overexpressing E-cadherin (Fig 6A). Overexpression of E-cadherin decreased basal invasiveness and abolished the ability of FGF2 to induce ovarian cancer cell invasion (Fig 6B), implicating that E-cadherin plays an essential role in FGF-stimulated ovarian cancer cell invasion.

Discussion

FGF2, which is a member of the FGF family, normally presents in plasma at a concentration less than 10 pg/ml, and elevated levels (up to 6 ng/ml) can be found in ascetic fluid from ovarian cancer patients [4]. Clinical studies have shown a high levels of FGF2 and its mRNA in advanced primary ovarian cancers when compared to normal ovaries [6]. Also, several studies have shown increased plasma levels of FGF2 in ovarian cancer patients [4,47,48]. The elevated levels of FGF2 and its receptors present in ovarian malignant tumors suggest that FGF2 plays an important role in ovarian tumor progression [9]. Several *in vitro* studies and the gene expression profiling studies in advanced ovarian cancer reveal that FGF2 functions as an autocrine growth factor for ovarian cancer cell proliferation [9–11], and invasion [12]. Moreover, FGF2 regulates expression of various genes implicated in angiogenesis or metastasis [13–15,49], suggesting the FGF2 signaling may be a potential therapeutic target. However, the role of FGF2 in ovarian tumor progression remains to be elucidated. The present study shows that FGF2 induced the down-regulation of E-cadherin expression, which is involved in FGF2-induced ovarian cancer cell invasion. In addition, our studies suggest that FGF2 exerts its effects in human ovarian cancer cells via the activation of the PI3K/Akt/mTOR and MAPK/ERK signaling pathways and the subsequent increased expression of Slug and ZEB1.

FGF2 plays a fundamental role in various biological activities, including cell proliferation, migration, and differentiation [2,3]. FGF2 has also been described as an angiogenic factor [50] and more recently has been shown to contribute to the development of peritioneal metastasis [51]. Dysregulated FGF signaling is common in many cancers including ovarian cancer [4–6,52], suggesting that this signaling can promote tumor development and progression. FGF2 has been reported to modulate E-cadherin expression in a variety of cell types. However, its role on E-cadherin expression seems to be cell type specific. In pancreatic adenocarcinoma, FGF-1 and FGF2 have been shown to up-regulate E-cadherin expression [53]. In contrast, the down-regulation of E-cadherin expression with FGF2 treatment has been observed in tubular epithelial cells and NBT-II carcinoma cells, resulting in increased cell migration and invasion [13,15]. Also, FGF2 has been shown to down-regulate E-cadherin

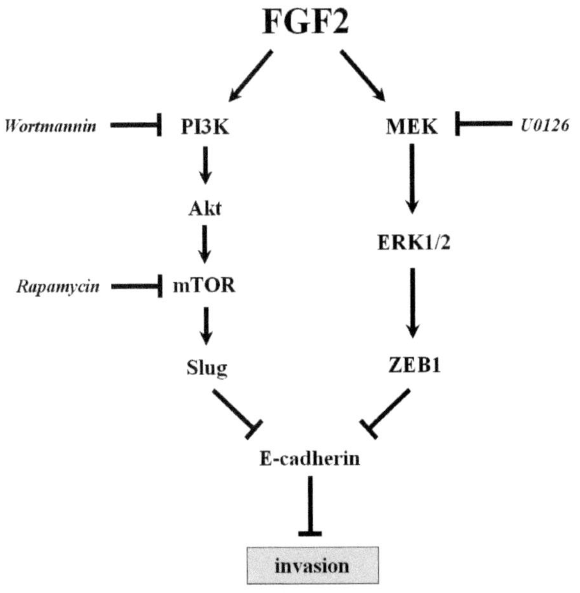

Figure 7. Proposed model illustrating how FGF2 suppressed E-cadherin may contribute to ovarian cancer cell invasion.

expression in human umbilical vein endothelial cells via the JNK signaling pathway [16]. The current data support a crucial role for FGF2 in the down-regulation of E-cadherin in ovarian carcinoma cells via the PI3K/Akt/mTOR and MAPK/ERK signaling pathways. The binding of FGF2 to its receptors leads to the activation of downstream signaling pathways such as PI3K/Akt and MAPK/ERK [40,41]. Emerging evidence suggests that these pathways are involved in the regulation of E-cadherin [42,43]. Moreover, the aberrant inhibition of the mTOR pathway, which is downstream of PI3K/Akt signaling blocked FGF2-induced E-cadherin down-regulation and cell invasion. These results are consistent with our previous study demonstrating a requirement for mTOR signaling in insulin-like growrh factor 1-induced E-cadherin down-regulation in ovarian cancer cells [54]. Taken together, our results indicate that the FGF2-dependent PI3K/Akt/mTOR and MAPK/ERK activation is involved in FGF2-induced E-cadherin down-regulation and cell invasion in ovarian cancer cells.

The loss of E-cadherin gene expression is mainly due to an overexpression of transcriptional repressors including Snail, Slug and ZEB1 [34–36]. Indeed, elevated Slug and ZEB1 mRNA levels have been found in ovarian carcinoma [55,56]. Moreover, a previous study demonstrated that the overexpression of Slug in SKOV-3 cells results in the down-regulation of E-cadherin, enhanced motility and invasiveness [57]. However, much less is known about the regulation of these transcriptional repressors. Slug expression can be regulated by PI3K/Akt signaling, which can also be activated by FGF treatment [40,41,43,45]. Consistent with these results, the inhibition of PI3K/Akt signaling by wortmannin reduced the basal and abolished FGF2-induced Slug levels expression, suggesting that this pathway is critical for Slug expression. The activation of PI3K/Akt signaling has been demonstrated to stimulate Slug expression via GSK-3β/β-catenin signaling and to subsequently down-regulate E-cadherin in uterine carcinosarcomas and normal hepatocytes [43,58]. It is well known that PI3K/Akt signaling induces nuclear β-catenin accumulation through the inhibition of GSK3β [59,60]. In addition, the inhibition of mTOR signaling by rapamycin blocks increased β-catenin translocation into the nucleus in human pancreatic β-cells [61]. FGF2 may activate PI3K/Akt signaling and its downstream GSK3β and mTOR pathways to induce β-catenin-dependent transcription including that of Slug. Further studies are required to elucidate the precise mechanism of the elevation of Slug levels by the mTOR pathway. Notably, E-cadherin protein levels were clearly increased by rapamycin, while basal Slug mRNA levels were not affected. Thus, our results suggest that the mTOR signaling pathway also modulates the E-cadherin levels in Slug-independent manner. Interestingly, treatment with the MEK inhibitor U0126 only blocked FGF2-induced ZEB1 expression, but did not inhibit FGF2-induced Slug expression. Our data suggest that MAPK/ERK is an upstream factor of ZEB1 activation in ovarian cancer cells *in vitro*. FGF2 has been shown to activate the MAPK/ERK pathway in various cancer cells [62,63], and we show in OVCAR-4 and SKOV-3 cells that ZEB1 expression is MAPK/ERK-dependent. These results are consistent with a previous study demonstrating a requirement for MAPK/ERK signaling in IGF-1-induced ZEB1 expression in prostate cancer cells [42]. Furthermore, a recent study demonstrated that ERK2, but not ERK1, reduced E-cadherin levels via Fra1-mediated ZEB1/2 in a nontransformed human mammary epithelial cell line, MCF-10A cells [64]. Taken together, our findings indicate that FGF2 differentially regulates Slug and ZEB1 expression via the PI3K/Akt/mTOR and MAPK/ERK signaling pathways in human ovarian cancer cells.

The biological significance of E-cadherin reduction in ovarian cancer invasiveness was demonstrated by the fact that overexpression of E-cadherin blocked FGF2-induced cell invasion *in vitro*. Evidence indicates that the loss of E-cadherin is associated with ovarian cancer metastasis, peritoneal dissemination and poor patient survival [22–26], suggesting that E-cadherin functions as a suppressor of tumor invasiveness. Indeed, silencing E-cadherin by siRNA enhances ovarian cancer cell invasion via an up-regulation of the α5-integrin [24]. We have also found that E-cadherin knockdown by RNA interference increases the PI3K/Akt signaling pathway [65], which, in turns, mediates E-cadherin-depletion-induced invasion in ovarian cancer cells (Lau *et al.*, unpublished). Moreover, the overexpression of a dominant-negative E-cadherin mutant in ovarian carcinoma cells results in increased mesenchymal cell migration [66]. Our results demonstrate that FGF2 enhances cell invasiveness by down-regulating E-cadherin and that E-cadherin overexpression inhibits basal invasiveness and abolishes FGF2-induced invasion. The PI3K/Akt and MAPK/ERK signaling pathways are involved in FGF2-induced cell invasion [45,46]. Furthermore, additional mechanisms such as the elevation of protease activity/secretion, the modulation of actin cytoskeleton, and increased motility have also been described [12,46,67]. Whereas loss of E-cadherin has been shown to stimulate MMP-mediated invasion in prostate cancer and bronchial tumor cells [68,69]. Taken together, these results demonstrate that E-cadherin acts as a crucial suppressor of ovarian cancer invasiveness, and along with other described mechanisms, the loss of E-cadherin plays an important role in FGF2-induced cell invasion.

In summary, our results show that FGF2 down-regulates E-cadherin expression, most likely through the transcriptional suppression of Slug and ZEB1, which are concomitantly expressed by the activation of the PI3K/Akt/mTOR and MAPK/ERK pathways. In addition, the present study suggests that the down-regulation of E-cadherin mediates FGF2-induced ovarian cancer cell invasion (Fig 7). Inhibition of either PI3K/Akt/mTOR or MAPK/ERK signaling results in partially blocked the FGF2-induced E-cadherin down-regulation and cell invasion. Thus, these findings indicate that the design of combined treatments targeting FGF2-related signaling cascades may have relevant implications in the prevention and treatment of this malignancy.

Acknowledgments

We thank Dr. Alonzo H. Ross (University of Massachusetts Medical School, Massachusetts), Dr. Jennifer L. Stow (University of Queensland, Brisbane, Queensland, Australia) for kindly and generously giving us the constructs.

PCKL is recipient of a Distinguished Scientist Award from the Child and Family Research Institute.

Author Contributions

Conceived and designed the experiments: M-TL. Performed the experiments: M-TL W-KS. Analyzed the data: M-TL W-KS. Contributed reagents/materials/analysis tools: PCKL. Wrote the paper: M-TL W-KS PCKL.

References

1. Jemal A, Murray T, Ward E, Samuels A, Tiwari RC, et al. (2005) Cancer statistics, 2005. CA Cancer J Clin 55: 10–30.

2. Bottcher RT, Niehrs C (2005) Fibroblast growth factor signaling during early vertebrate development. Endocr Rev 26: 63–77

3. Chalkiadaki G, Nikitovic D, Berdiaki A, Sifaki M, Krasagakis K, et al. (2009) Fibroblast growth factor-2 modulates melanoma adhesion and migration through a syndecan-4-dependent mechanism. Int J Biochem Cell Biol 41: 1323–1331
4. Barton DP, Cai A, Wendt K, Young M, Gamero A, et al. (1997) Angiogenic protein expression in advanced epithelial ovarian cancer. Clin Cancer Res 3: 1579–1586.
5. Davidson B, Goldberg I, Gotlieb WH, Kopolovic J, Ben-Baruch G, et al. (2002) The prognostic value of metalloproteinases and angiogenic factors in ovarian carcinoma. Mol Cell Endocrinol 187: 39–45.
6. Fujimoto J, Ichigo S, Hori M, Hirose R, Sakaguchi H, et al. (1997) Expression of basic fibroblast growth factor and its mRNA in advanced ovarian cancers. Eur J Gynaecol Oncol 18: 349–352.
7. Secord AA, Darcy KM, Hutson A, Lee PS, Havrilesky LJ, et al. (2007) Co-expression of angiogenic markers and associations with prognosis in advanced epithelial ovarian cancer: a Gynecologic Oncology Group study. Gynecol Oncol 106: 221–232.
8. Obermair A, Speiser P, Reisenberger K, Ullrich R, Czerwenka K, et al. (1998) Influence of intratumoral basic fibroblast growth factor concentration on survival in ovarian cancer patients. Cancer Lett 130: 69–76.
9. Crickard K, Gross JL, Crickard U, Yoonessi M, Lele S, et al. (1994) Basic fibroblast growth factor and receptor expression in human ovarian cancer. Gynecol Oncol 55: 277–284.
10. De Cecco L, Marchionni L, Gariboldi M, Reid JF, Lagonigro MS, et al. (2004) Gene expression profiling of advanced ovarian cancer: characterization of a molecular signature involving fibroblast growth factor 2. Oncogene 23: 8171–8183.
11. Di Blasio AM, Cremonesi L, Vigano P, Ferrari M, Gospodarowicz D, et al. (1993) Basic fibroblast growth factor and its receptor messenger ribonucleic acids are expressed in human ovarian epithelial neoplasms. Am J Obstet Gynecol 169: 1517–1523.
12. Li T, Jiang S (2010) Effect of bFGF on invasion of ovarian cancer cells through the regulation of Ets-1 and urokinase-type plasminogen activator. Pharm Biol 48: 161–165.
13. Strutz F, Zeisberg M, Ziyadeh FN, Yang CQ, Kalluri R, et al. (2002) Role of basic fibroblast growth factor-2 in epithelial-mesenchymal transformation. Kidney Int 61: 1714–1728.
14. Giavazzi R, Sennino B, Coltrini D, Garofalo A, Dossi R, et al. (2003) Distinct role of fibroblast growth factor-2 and vascular endothelial growth factor on tumor growth and angiogenesis. Am J Pathol 162: 1913–1926.
15. Billottet C, Elkhatib N, Thiery JP, Jouanneau J (2004) Targets of fibroblast growth factor 1 (FGF-1) and FGF-2 signaling involved in the invasive and tumorigenic behavior of carcinoma cells. Mol Biol Cell 15: 4725–4734.
16. Wu JC, Yan HC, Chen WT, Chen WH, Wang CJ, et al. (2008) JNK signaling pathway is required for bFGF-mediated surface cadherin downregulation on HUVEC. Exp Cell Res 314: 421–429.
17. Nollet F, Berx G, van Roy F (1999) The role of the E-cadherin/catenin adhesion complex in the development and progression of cancer. Mol Cell Biol Res Commun 2: 77–85.
18. Yap AS (1998) The morphogenetic role of cadherin cell adhesion molecules in human cancer: a thematic review. Cancer Invest 16: 252–261.
19. Gottardi CJ, Wong E, Gumbiner BM (2001) E-cadherin suppresses cellular transformation by inhibiting beta-catenin signaling in an adhesion-independent manner. J Cell Biol 153: 1049–1060.
20. St Croix B, Sheehan C, Rak JW, Florenes VA, Slingerland JM, et al. (1998) E-Cadherin-dependent growth suppression is mediated by the cyclin-dependent kinase inhibitor p27(KIP1). J Cell Biol 142: 557–571.
21. Yanagisawa M, Anastasiadis PZ (2006) p120 catenin is essential for mesenchymal cadherin-mediated regulation of cell motility and invasiveness. J Cell Biol 174: 1087–1096.
22. Daraï E, Scoazec JY, Walker-Combrouze F, Mlika-Cabanne N, Feldmann G, et al. (1997) Expression of cadherins in benign, borderline, and malignant ovarian epithelial tumors: a clinicopathologic study of 60 cases. Hum Pathol 28: 922–928.
23. Hudson LG, Zeineldin R, Stack MS (2008) Phenotypic plasticity of neoplastic ovarian epithelium: unique cadherin profiles in tumor progression. Clin Exp Metastasis 25: 643–655.
24. Sawada K, Mitra AK, Radjabi AR, Bhaskar V, Kistner EO, et al. (2008) Loss of E-cadherin promotes ovarian cancer metastasis via alpha 5-integrin, which is a therapeutic target. Cancer Res 68: 2329–2339.
25. Veatch AL, Carson LF, Ramakrishnan S (1994) Differential expression of the cell-cell adhesion molecule E-cadherin in ascites and solid human ovarian tumor cells. Int J Cancer 58: 393–399.
26. Yuecheng Y, Hongmei L, Xiaoyan X (2006) Clinical evaluation of E-cadherin expression and its regulation mechanism in epithelial ovarian cancer. Clin Exp Metastasis 23: 65–74.
27. Hajra KM, Fearon ER (2002) Cadherin and catenin alterations in human cancer. Genes Chromosomes Cancer 34: 255-268.
28. Graff JR, Herman JG, Lapidus RG, Chopra H, Xu R, et al. (1995) E-cadherin expression is silenced by DNA hypermethylation in human breast and prostate carcinomas. Cancer Res 55: 5195–5199.
29. Hennig G, Behrens J, Truss M, Frisch S, Reichmann E, et al. (1995) Progression of carcinoma cells is associated with alterations in chromatin structure and factor binding at the E-cadherin promoter in vivo. Oncogene 11: 475–484.
30. Batlle E, Sancho E, Franci C, Dominguez D, Monfar M, et al. (2000) The transcription factor snail is a repressor of E-cadherin gene expression in epithelial tumour cells. Nat Cell Biol 2: 84–89.
31. Cano A, Perez-Moreno MA, Rodrigo I, Locascio A, Blanco MJ, et al. (2000) The transcription factor snail controls epithelial-mesenchymal transitions by repressing E-cadherin expression. Nat Cell Biol 2: 76–83.
32. Comijn J, Berx G, Vermassen P, Verschueren K, van Grunsven L, et al. (2001) The two-handed E box binding zinc finger protein SIP1 downregulates E-cadherin and induces invasion. Mol Cell 7: 1267–1278.
33. Hajra KM, Chen DY, Fearon ER (2002) The SLUG zinc-finger protein represses E-cadherin in breast cancer. Cancer Res 62: 1613–1618.
34. Bolos V, Peinado H, Perez-Moreno MA, Fraga MF, Esteller M, et al. (2003) The transcription factor Slug represses E-cadherin expression and induces epithelial to mesenchymal transitions: a comparison with Snail and E47 repressors. J Cell Sci 116: 499–511.
35. Grooteclaes ML, Frisch SM (2000) Evidence for a function of CtBP in epithelial gene regulation and anoikis. Oncogene 19: 3823–3828.
36. Peinado H, Olmeda D, Cano A (2007) Snail, Zeb and bHLH factors in tumour progression: an alliance against the epithelial phenotype? Nat Rev Cancer 7: 415–428.
37. Liu F, Wagner S, Campbell RB, Nickerson JA, Schiffer CA, et al. (2005) PTEN enters the nucleus by diffusion. J Cell Biochem 96: 221–234.
38. Miranda KC, Khromykh T, Christy P, Le TL, Gottardi CJ, et al. (2001) A dileucine motif targets E-cadherin to the basolateral cell surface in Madin-Darby canine kidney and LLC-PK1 epithelial cells. J Biol Chem 276: 22565–22572.
39. Nicosia SV, Bai W, Cheng JQ, Coppola D, Kruk PA (2003) Oncogenic pathways implicated in ovarian epithelial cancer. Hematol Oncol Clin North Am 17: 927–943.
40. Eswarakumar VP, Lax I, Schlessinger J (2005) Cellular signaling by fibroblast growth factor receptors. Cytokine Growth Factor Rev 16: 139–149.
41. Schlessinger J (2004) Common and distinct elements in cellular signaling via EGF and FGF receptors. Science 306: 1506–1507.
42. Graham TR, Zhau HE, Odero-Marah VA, Osunkoya AO, Kimbro KS, et al. (2008) Insulin-like growth factor-I-dependent up-regulation of ZEB1 drives epithelial-to-mesenchymal transition in human prostate cancer cells. Cancer Res 68: 2479–2488.
43. Saegusa M, Hashimura M, Kuwata T, Okayasu I (2009) Requirement of the Akt/beta-catenin pathway for uterine carcinosarcoma genesis, modulating E-cadherin expression through the transactivation of slug. Am J Pathol 174: 2107–2115.
44. van der Poel HG (2004) Mammalian target of rapamycin and 3-phosphatidylinositol 3-kinase pathway inhibition enhances growth inhibition of transforming growth factor-beta1 in prostate cancer cells. J Urol 172: 1333–1337.
45. Blair KJ, Kiang A, Wang-Rodriguez J, Yu MA, Doherty JK, et al. (2010) EGF and bFGF Promote Invasion That Is Modulated by PI3/Akt Kinase and Erk in Vestibular Schwannoma. Otol Neurotol 32:308–14
46. Kamura S, Matsumoto Y, Fukushi JI, Fujiwara T, Iida K, et al. (2010) Basic fibroblast growth factor in the bone microenvironment enhances cell motility and invasion of Ewing's sarcoma family of tumours by activating the FGFR1-PI3K-Rac1 pathway. Br J Cancer 103: 370–381.
47. Dirix LY, Vermeulen PB, Pawinski A, Prove A, Benoy I, et al. (1997) Elevated levels of the angiogenic cytokines basic fibroblast growth factor and vascular endothelial growth factor in sera of cancer patients. Br J Cancer 76: 238–243.
48. Salgado R, Benoy I, Vermeulen P, van Dam P, Van Mark E, et al. (2004) Circulating basic fibroblast growth factor is partly derived from the tumour in patients with colon, cervical and ovarian cancer. Angiogenesis 7: 29–32.
49. Wu JC, Yan HC, Chen WT, Chen WH, Wang CJ, et al. (2008) JNK signaling pathway is required for bFGF-mediated surface cadherin downregulation on HUVEC. Exp Cell Res 314: 421–429.
50. Werner S, Grose R (2003) Regulation of wound healing by growth factors and cytokines. Physiol Rev 83: 835–870.
51. Sako A, Kitayama J, Yamaguchi H, Kaisaki S, Suzuki H, et al. (2003) Vascular endothelial growth factor synthesis by human omental mesothelial cells is augmented by fibroblast growth factor-2: possible role of mesothelial cell on the development of peritoneal metastasis. J Surg Res 115: 113–120.
52. Turner N, Grose R (2010) Fibroblast growth factor signalling: from development to cancer. Nat Rev Cancer 10: 116–129.
53. El-Hariry I, Pignatelli M, Lemoine NR (2001) FGF-1 and FGF-2 modulate the E-cadherin/catenin system in pancreatic adenocarcinoma cell lines. Br J Cancer 84: 1656–1663.
54. Lau MT, Leung PC (2012) The PI3K/Akt/mTOR signaling pathway mediates insulin-like growth factor 1-induced E-cadherin down-regulation and cell proliferation in ovarian cancer cells. Cancer Lett 326: 191–198.
55. Elloul S, Silins I, Trope CG, Benshushan A, Davidson B, et al. (2006) Expression of E-cadherin transcriptional regulators in ovarian carcinoma. Virchows Arch 449: 520–528.
56. Elloul S, Vaksman O, Stavnes HT, Trope CG, Davidson B, et al. (2010) Mesenchymal-to-epithelial transition determinants as characteristics of ovarian carcinoma effusions. Clin Exp Metastasis 27: 161–172.
57. Kurrey NK, K A, Bapat SA (2005) Snail and Slug are major determinants of ovarian cancer invasiveness at the transcription level. Gynecol Oncol 97: 155–165.

58. Wu J, Ru NY, Zhang Y, Li Y, Wei D, et al. (2011) HAb18G/CD147 promotes epithelial-mesenchymal transition through TGF-beta signaling and is transcriptionally regulated by Slug. Oncogene 30:4410–27
59. Cross DA, Alessi DR, Cohen P, Andjelkovich M, Hemmings BA (1995) Inhibition of glycogen synthase kinase-3 by insulin mediated by protein kinase B. Nature 378: 785–789.
60. Li DM, Sun H (1998) PTEN/MMAC1/TEP1 suppresses the tumorigenicity and induces G1 cell cycle arrest in human glioblastoma cells. Proc Natl Acad Sci U S A 95: 15406–15411.
61. Liu H, Remedi MS, Pappan KL, Kwon G, Rohatgi N, et al. (2009) Glycogen synthase kinase-3 and mammalian target of rapamycin pathways contribute to DNA synthesis, cell cycle progression, and proliferation in human islets. Diabetes 58: 663–672.
62. Wesley UV, McGroarty M, Homoyouni A (2005) Dipeptidyl peptidase inhibits malignant phenotype of prostate cancer cells by blocking basic fibroblast growth factor signaling pathway. Cancer Res 65: 1325–1334.
63. Hatziapostolou M, Polytarchou C, Katsoris P, Courty J, Papadimitriou E (2006) Heparin affin regulatory peptide/pleiotrophin mediates fibroblast growth factor 2 stimulatory effects on human prostate cancer cells. J Biol Chem 281: 32217–32226.
64. Shin S, Dimitri CA, Yoon SO, Dowdle W, Blenis J (2010) ERK2 but not ERK1 induces epithelial-to-mesenchymal transformation via DEF motif-dependent signaling events. Mol Cell 38: 114–127.
65. Lau MT, Klausen C, Leung PC (2011) E-cadherin inhibits tumor cell growth by suppressing PI3K/Akt signaling via beta-catenin-Egr1-mediated PTEN expression. Oncogene 30: 2753–66
66. Wu C, Cipollone J, Maines-Bandiera S, Tan C, Karsan A, et al. (2008) The morphogenic function of E-cadherin-mediated adherens junctions in epithelial ovarian carcinoma formation and progression. Differentiation 76: 193–205.
67. Lee JG, Kay EP (2006) Cross-talk among Rho GTPases acting downstream of PI 3-kinase induces mesenchymal transformation of corneal endothelial cells mediated by FGF-2. Invest Ophthalmol Vis Sci 47: 2358–2368.
68. Luo J, Lubaroff DM, Hendrix MJ (1999) Suppression of prostate cancer invasive potential and matrix metalloproteinase activity by E-cadherin transfection. Cancer Res 59: 3552–3556.
69. Nawrocki-Raby B, Gilles C, Polette M, Martinella-Catusse C, Bonnet N, et al. (2003) E-Cadherin mediates MMP down-regulation in highly invasive bronchial tumor cells. Am J Pathol 163: 653–661.

4

Ovarian Cancer Spheroid Cells with Stem Cell-Like Properties Contribute to Tumor Generation, Metastasis and Chemotherapy Resistance through Hypoxia-Resistant Metabolism

Jianqun Liao[1,4], Feng Qian[2,3], Nana Tchabo[9], Paulette Mhawech-Fauceglia[7], Amy Beck[3], Zikun Qian[3], Xinhui Wang[8], Wendy J. Huss[5,6], Shashikant B. Lele[1], Carl D. Morrison[7], Kunle Odunsi[1,2,3]*

1 Departments of Gynecologic Oncology, Roswell Park Cancer Institute, Buffalo, New York, United States of America, **2** Immunology; Roswell Park Cancer Institute, Buffalo, New York, United States of America, **3** Center for Immunotherapy; Roswell Park Cancer Institute, Buffalo, New York, United States of America, **4** Surgical Oncology, Roswell Park Cancer Institute, Buffalo, New York, United States of America, **5** Urology Oncology, Roswell Park Cancer Institute, Buffalo, New York, United States of America, **6** Pharmacology & Therapeutics, Roswell Park Cancer Institute, Buffalo, New York, United States of America, **7** Pathology, Roswell Park Cancer Institute, Buffalo, New York, United States of America, **8** Surgical Oncology, Massachusetts General Hospital, Harvard Medical School, Boston, United States of America, **9** Atlantic Health System Morristown/Overlook Medical Centers, Women's Cancer Center, Morristown and Summit, New Jersey, United States of America

Abstract

Cells with sphere forming capacity, spheroid cells, are present in the malignant ascites of patients with epithelial ovarian cancer (EOC) and represent a significant impediment to efficacious treatment due to their putative role in progression, metastasis and chemotherapy resistance. The exact mechanisms that underlie EOC metastasis and drug resistance are not clear. Understanding the biology of sphere forming cells may contribute to the identification of novel therapeutic opportunities for metastatic EOC. Here we generated spheroid cells from human ovarian cancer cell lines and primary ovarian cancer. Xenoengraftment of as few as 2000 dissociated spheroid cells into immune-deficient mice allowed full recapitulation of the original tumor, whereas $>10^5$ parent tumor cells remained non-tumorigenic. The spheroid cells were found to be enriched for cells with cancer stem cell-like characteristics such as upregulation of stem cell genes, self-renewal, high proliferative and differentiation potential, and high aldehyde dehydrogenase (ALDH) activity. Furthermore, spheroid cells were more aggressive in growth, migration, invasion, scratch recovery, clonogenic survival, anchorage-independent growth, and more resistant to chemotherapy *in vitro*. ^{13}C-glucose metabolic studies revealed that spheroid cells route glucose predominantly to anaerobic glycolysis and pentose cycle to the detriment of re-routing glucose for anabolic purposes. These metabolic properties of sphere forming cells appear to confer increased resistance to apoptosis and contribute to more aggressive tumor growth. Collectively, we demonstrated that spheroid cells with cancer stem cell-like characteristics contributed to tumor generation, progression and chemotherapy resistance. This study provides insight into the relationship between tumor dissemination and metabolic attributes of human cancer stem cells and has clinical implications for cancer therapy.

Editor: Sandra Orsulic, Cedars-Sinai Medical Center, United States of America

Funding: This work was supported in part by Cancer Research Institute Ovarian Cancer Working Group Grant, Cancer Vaccine Collaborative Grant of the Cancer Research Institute and Ludwig Institute for Cancer Research, Anna-Maria Kellen Clinical Investigator Award of the Cancer Research Institute (to KO), Roswell Park Cancer Institute Alliance Foundation, NIH P30 CA016056; NIH R01CA158318-01A1 and RPCI-UPCI Ovarian Cancer SPORE P50CA159981-01A1. The funders had no role in study design, data collection and analysis, decision to publish, or preparation of the manuscript.

Competing Interests: The authors have declared that no competing interests exist.

* E-mail: kunle.odunsi@roswellpark.org

Introduction

Epithelial ovarian cancer (EOC) is the leading cause of death from gynecologic malignancies. There are more than 23,000 cases annually in the United States, and 14,000 women can be expected to die from the disease [1]. Despite modest improvements in response rates, progression-free and median survival using adjuvant platinum and taxane chemotherapy following cytoreductive surgery, overall survival rates for patients with advanced EOC and ovarian-like malignancies (primary peritoneal) remain disappointing [2]. This has been attributed to several reasons. First, in contrast to most other solid tumors, more than 75% of EOC patients present with advanced stage disease (FIGO III or IV). Secondly, although most patients initially respond to platinum and paclitaxel chemotherapy including complete responses, the relapse rate is approximately 85%. Within 2 years of cytoreductive surgery and systemic chemotherapy, tumors usually recur and once relapse occurs, curative therapy is difficult. Therefore, it is imperative to understand the mechanism(s) of EOC metastasis and chemotherapy resistance in order to improve clinical outcomes in this disease.

The primary mode of distant metastasis in EOC involves the shedding of cells from the primary tumor, into the abdominal cavity, followed by implantation on the mesothelial lining of the peritoneum [3,4]. Currently, there are data to demonstrate that "sphere forming cells" or "spheroids" are commonly found in ascites and are capable of tumorigenesis *in vivo*, have a reduced response to chemotherapeutic drugs *in vitro*, and may play an important role in metastatic disease [5–9]. Because metabolic changes may confer an advantage on the ability of cancer cells to survive, proliferate, and invade [10–12], we hypothesized that sphere forming cells are likely to exhibit metabolic attributes that promote their ability to survive and metastasize. In present study, we generated spheroid cells from EOC cell lines and from patients with primary ovarian cancer. Our *in vivo* and *in vitro* biologic studies suggested that these sphere forming cells are enriched in cancer stem-like cells (CSCL) that critically contribute to ovarian cancer tumorigenesis, metastasis and chemotherapy resistance. We then utilized isotope-based dynamic metabolic profiling [13,14], to simultaneously assess the substrate flux within and among major metabolic pathways of macromolecule synthesis and energy production under various physiologic conditions. We found that spheroid cells increase anaerobic glycolysis and pentose cycle and decrease re-routing of glucose for anabolic purposes. This study provides insights into the relationship between tumor dissemination and metabolic attributes of ovarian CSCL cells, and has clinical implications for cancer therapy.

Materials and Methods

Isolation of Tumor Cells from Human Ovarian Cancer

Tumor specimens and ascitic fluid were obtained from patients undergoing tumor debulking surgery for epithelial ovarian cancer (EOC) at Roswell Park Cancer Institute (RPCI), Buffalo, NY. All specimens were collected under an approved protocol CIC 02–15 from the Institutional Review Board at RPCI, and informed written consent was obtained from each patient. Tumor cells from ascites were obtained from centrifuged cell pellets of ascitic fluid. The pellets were washed twice in PBS, placed on Ficoll-Hypaque density gradients and centrifuged again to harvest tumor cells. To obtain tumor cells from solid tumor tissue, tumor specimens were finely minced in cell culture medium and single cell suspensions were washed twice in PBS followed by Ficoll-Hypaque purification.

Cell Culture

Primary EOC cell lines were established from solid tumor and ascites by culturing cells in 13 different conditions [15,16] from 30 EOC patients over a period of 2 years. Spheroid cells were generated from new EOC cell lines and from an established ovarian cancer cell line, OV2774, which were obtained from Sloan Kettering Institute, New York, NY (courtesy of Lloyd J. Old, Ludwig Institute for Cancer Research, NY), by the method as described [17] with modifications by resuspending 8×10^4 cells with serum-free DMEM/F12 supplemented with 10 ng/mL human recombinant epidermal growth factor (EGF; Invitrogen), 10 ng/mL basic fibroblast growth factor (bFGF; Invitrogen), and N2 supplement-A (Stemcell Technologies Inc) in Ultra Low Attachment 6-well plates (Corning) and subsequent organization into spheres.

In vivo Xenograft Experiments

All animal studies adhered to protocols approved by the Institutional Animal Care and Use Committee of RPCI. Dissociated spheroid or parent tumor cells were counted, resuspended in 50 µL 1:1 RPMI/Matrigel (BD Biosciences), and injected subcutaneous (s.c.) into the right legs of 3- to 4-wk-old female SCID mice (C.B-igh-1blcrTac-Prkdcscid/Ros) provided by RPCI Animal Facility (originated from Taconic Farms, Hudson, NY). Engrafted mice were inspected biweekly for tumor appearance by visual observation and palpation, and tumor latencies were determined. Mice were sacrificed by cervical dislocation at a tumor diameter of 1 cm or at 6 months post-transplantation. Xenograft tumors were resected, fixed in 10% neutral, buffered formalin, and embedded in paraffin for sectioning (5 µm) on a rotary microtome, followed by slide mounting, H&E staining, and histologic assessment by a pathologist for tumor type, grade, and stage. To determine xenograft recapitulation of the parental tumor phenotype, the same process was performed on human tumors. To evaluate formation of ovarian tumors in their native environment, SCID mice were injected intraperitoneal (i.p.) with various amounts of spheroid-derived cells or their parent tumors, monitored biweekly for weight change and ascites formation, and euthanized upon excessive abdominal distention or palpable tumor growth.

Stem Cell Marker Gene Expression Profiling

Signosis's Human stem cell marker cDNA plate array was used to examine stem cell related gene expression on spheroid cells and parent cells according to the manufacturer's protocol. Briefly, total RNA isolated from cells by Tri Reagent (Molecular Research Center, Inc.) was reverse transcribed into cDNA, which was hybridized with gene-specific oligonucleotide pre-coated in individual wells. The expression level of genes was detected by chemiluminescent signals by a plate reader.

Quantitative PCR

Total RNA was exacted from spheroid or non-spheroid cells using Qiagen's RNeasy Mini Kit per manufacture's procedure and reverse transcribed into cDNA by iScript cDNA Synthesis Kit from Bio-Rad. Quantitative real-time PCR was performed using Bio-Rad's iQ SYBR Green Supermix per company's protocols in a iCycler iQ system also from Bio-Rad. Real-time PCR primer sequences are shown in Table 1. Thermal cycling was performed by an initial denaturing step at 95°C for 3 min followed by 40 cycles of denaturation at 95°C for 10 sec, then 60°C for 1 min for annealing and data collection. Melt-curve analysis was performed immediately after the amplification protocol under the following conditions: 80 cycles of 0.5°C increments (10 sec each) beginning at 57.5°C (data collection step). Each experiment was performed in triplicate, with normalization to the ribosomal protein L4 (RPL4) gene as an internal control and target gene expression level was calculated by $\Delta\Delta C_t$ method using Bio-Rad's iQ5 quantitative PCR analysis software.

ALDH Activity Analysis

The ALDEFLUOR kit (StemCell Technologies, Vacouver, Canada) uses a fluorescent substrate which accumulates within cells after oxidized by ALDH enzyme. Cells in a concentration of 2×10^5/ml were stained by 5 µl ALDEFLUOR reagent at 37°C for 45 min. In each experiment, a sample of cells was stained under identical conditions with specific ALDH inhibitor diethylaminobenzaldehyde (DEAB) as negative control for setting up flow cytometry gate. The BioVision ALDH Activity Assay kit (BioVision) quantifies ALDH enzymatic activity by absorbance reading at 450 nm. Acetaldehyde is oxidized by ALDH generating NADH which then reduces a colorless probe to a colored product. Spheroid cells or parental cells (1×10^6) were lysed by 200 µl ALDH Assay Buffer and 10 µl of the cell lysate were used for the assay. OD450s were read at 10 min and 1 hr intervals and ALDH activities were calculated according to manufacturer's protocol. All tests were done in duplicate.

Table 1. Quantitate real time PCR primers used in this study.

	Type	Sequence
Notch1		
ACC# NM_017617.3	Forward	GGGACCAACTGTGACATCAA
	Reverse	GTAGCCACTGGTCATGTCTTT
CD34		
ACC# NM_001773.2	Forward	TAGCCTGTCACCTGGAAATG
	Reverse	TGCCTTGATGTCACTTAGGATAG
Cdcp1		
ACC# AF468010.1	Forward	AAGGACACAGACATTCCCTTAC
	Reverse	GTCTCAGTGCCCTGCTTTAT
Nanog		
ACC# NM_024865.2	Forward	TCCTGAACCTCAGCTACAAAC
	Reverse	GCGTCACACCATTGCTATTC
Myc		
ACC# NM_002467.4	Forward	CTTCTCTGAAAGGCTCTCCTTG
	Reverse	GTCGAGGTCATAGTTCCTGTTG
RPL4		
ACC# AK294113.1	Forward	GGCTACAAGAAGACCAAGGAA
	Reverse	CTCATTCGCTGAGAGGCATAG

Proliferation Assay

Parental and spheroid EOC cells were cultured in complete medium (CM, 10%FBS+RPMI) or unsupplemented RPMI for 24 h. Then the same amounts of cells were seeded in tissue culture plate with CM, half of the medium was changed every 3 days and cell growth was detected by CellTiter-Glo Luminescent Cell Viability Assay as described [18] (Promega Corp). The proliferation assays were done in triplicate.

Migration Assay

Parental and spheroid EOC cells were treated with unsupplemented RPMI for 24 h. In a transwell plate, 2×10^5/well cells were put into insert with 0.2%BSA-RPMI medium, the chamber has no cells except RPMI medium with 2.5% FBS. After culture for 1, 2, and 3 days, the numbers of cells that passed through membrane as well as cells fall into chamber were calculated under microscope after 10% formaldehyde fixing for 20 min followed by 0.1% crystal blue staining for another 20 min both at room temperature (RT). All tests were done in duplicate.

Wound Healing (Scratch) Assay

Parental and spheroid EOC cells were cultured in CM for 24 h. Then cells were seeded into 6-well plates to 80–90% confluence and the cell monolayer was scratched in a straight line with a 200 µl pipette tip to create a "scratch". Debris was removed with PBS and then the culture was re-fed with fresh medium. Images were taken at 0 and 24 hr after the scratch to calculate the cell migration rate.

Invasion Assay

Parental and spheroid EOC cells were treated with RPMI only medium for 24 h. In a transwell plate, 40000/well cells were put into insert which is coated with matrigel in 0.2%BSA-RPMI medium, the chamber has no cells except RPMI medium with 5% FBS. After culture for 1, 2, and 3 days, inserts were collected and the surface of membranes were cleaned, cells in matrigel were fixed by 10% formaldehyde for 20 min RT and the numbers of cells that invaded into matrigel were determined after staining with 0.1% crystal blue 20 min RT. All experiments were done in duplicate.

Anchorage-independent Growth Assay

Five hundred cells were seeded in triplicate in 6-well plates containing a top layer of 0.3% soft agar and a 0.5% agar base in DMEM, 10% FBS. Twenty-four hours later, the average number of cells seeded per field was determined by counting cells in 5 different fields under the light microscope. Colonies formed (>0.1 mm in diameter) after 3 weeks of growth in soft agar were counted; 10 different fields were quantified per well and the average number of colonies per field was calculated. The AIG (anchorage-independent growth) index was expressed relative to the number of cells seeded.

Chemotherapy Resistance Assay

Spheres were dissociated by trypsinization and pipetting and cells were seeded at 5,000 cells per well (96-well plates; Corning) in 200 µL CM medium. All cells were treated for 24 h with 0 to 6 µg/mL Cisplatin (BD Biosciences) or 0 to 18 µg/mL Paclitaxel (Sigma; n = 5 per drug dose). Relative cell numbers were determined by CellTiter-Glo Luminescent Cell Viability Assay [18]. Dose-response experiments were performed in duplicate. Percentage cell survival is expressed relative to untreated control. Spheroid cell drug cytotoxicities were compared after 48-h treatment with Cisplatin (4 µg/mL). After drug treatments, cells were incubated for 8 days in drug-free CM medium and cell colonies were examined under microscopy.

Clonogenic Survival Assay

Cells were treated with various amounts of Cisplatin for 24 h. After removing the drug, cells were washed with PBS, harvested and 300 of surviving cells/well were re-fed with CM medium in 6-well plate. 10–14 days later, colonies were stained with 0.1% crystal violet and counted.

Immunohistochemistry

Tumor specimens were fixed with buffered formalin and embedded in paraffin. Sections (5 µm) were placed on glass slides, heated at 60°C for 20 min, and then deparaffinized with xylene and ethanol. For antigen retrieval, tumor specimens mounted on glass slides were immersed in preheated antigen retrieval solution (DAKO high pH solution; DAKO, Carpinteria, CA) for 20 min and allowed to cool for 20 min at room temperature. After the inactivation of endogenous peroxidase, purified specific monoclonal antibody CA125 (Ov 185:1, Novocastra) (1:200 dilution) and CK7 (Dako) (1:20 dilution or 75 µg/ml) were then added, and incubated overnight at 4°C. The primary antibody was detected with a biotinylated anti-mouse IgG (DAKO). Diaminobenzidine tetrahydrochloride was then added for development for 10 min, followed by counterstaining with hematoxylin solution.

Biochemical Analyses

The use of [U-$^{13}C_6$] glucose tracer in combination with mass spectrometry allows the evaluation of metabolic flux through the main pathways facilitating energy production and biosynthetic metabolism of the cell. Normal ovarian cells (RPNLOv78) were kindly provided by Dr. T Pejovic [19]. The cells were cultured in 1:1 mixture of RPMI and DMEM (glucose-free) +10% FBS +10 ug/ml Insulin +10 ng/ml EGF+0.1% Gentamicin+

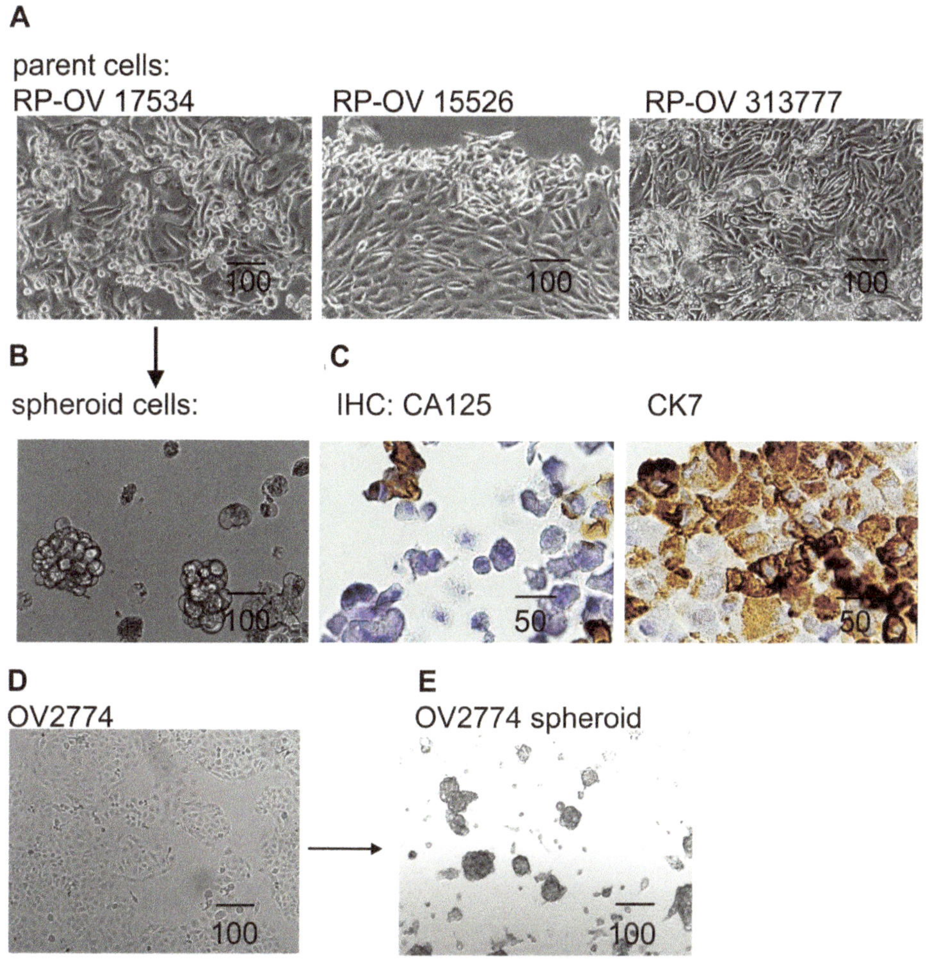

Figure 1. Spheroid cells were generated from primary and established EOC cells. (A) Three primary cell lines generated from EOC patients show epithelial cells morphology. (B) One of primary EOC cell line generated 3-D independent, self-renewing spheroid cells under stem-cell selection media. (C) Primary cell lines express ovarian carcinoma marker CA-125 and epithelial marker CK-7, as shown by IHC for RP-OV17534. (D) EOC cell line OV2774 is able to generate OV2774 spheroid cells (E). All scale bar unit in this figure and following figures are in μm.

[U-$^{13}C_6$]glucose (180 mg/ml). Parent cells (RP-OV17534) were cultured in RPMI (glucose-free) +10%FBS+[U-$^{13}C_6$]glucose (180 mg/ml). RP-OV17534 spheroid cells were cultured in DMEM/F12 (glucose-free) +N2 Supplement-A +EGF 10 ng/ml +bFGF 10 ng/ml+[U-$^{13}C_6$]glucose (180 mg/ml). After 24 hrs of the incubation, cells were centrifuged (1,500 rpm for 5 minutes) and incubation medium and cell pellets were obtained. Glucose and lactate incubation medium concentrations were determined as previously described [20]. Lactate from the cell culture media was extracted by ethyl acetate after acidification with HCl. Lactate was derivatized to its propylamide-heptafluorobutyric form and the m/z 330 and 331 (carbons 2–3 of lactate, chemical ionization) was monitored for the detection of *m2* (^{13}C double-labeled lactate) and *m3* (triple-labeled lactate) for the estimation of pentose cycle activity versus anaerobic glycolysis [21]. Glutamate was separated from the medium using ion-exchange chromatography [22]. Glutamate was converted to its *n*-trifluoroacetyl-*n*-butyl derivative and the ion clusters m/z 198 (carbons 2–5 of glutamate, electron impact ionization) were monitored. $^{13}CO_2$ release was measured by a Finnegan Delta-S ion ratio mass spectroscope and was used to estimate glucose carbon utilization through oxidation by the cell lines [23]. Mass spectral analyses were carried out by three independent automatic injections by the sampler and accepted only if the standard sample deviation was <1% of the normalized peak intensity.

Data Analysis and Statistical Methods

Statistical analyses were done using the parametric unpaired, two-tailed independent sample t test with 99% confidence intervals.

Results

Generation of Spheroid Cells from Primary Ovarian Cancer Specimens and Established EOC Cell Lines

Stable cell lines were established successfully from 3 of 30 (10%) cultures initiated from primary EOC specimens over a period of 2 years. RP-OV15526 was derived from solid tumor while RP-OV17534 and RP-OV313777 were derived from EOC ascites. These cells have been cultured *in vitro* for 465, 312, and 125 days with 68, 65, and 17 passages, respectively. All lines were from late-stage (IIIC or IV) ovarian serous adenocarcinoma cancer patients. Confluent monolayer of primary human EOC cells depicted typical epithelial cobblestone morphology with 3-dimensional growing upwards in cell-condensed areas (**Fig. 1A**). Examination

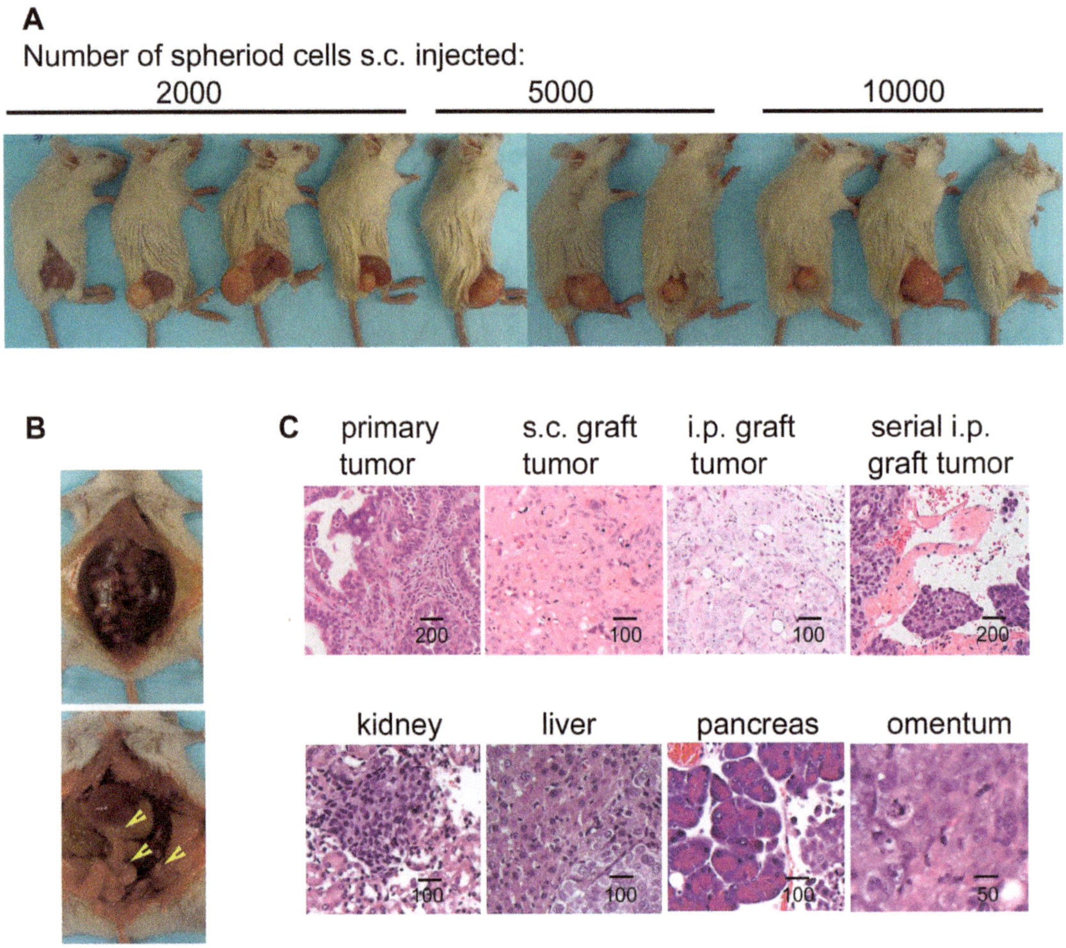

Figure 2. RP-OV17534 Spheroid cells generated tumors in immune-deficient mice. (A) Different amount of spheroid cells s.c. injected into SCID mice formed tumors. (B) Spheroid cells i.p. injected into SCID mice formed bloody ascites and tumors in different organs as indicated by arrows. (C) Representative H&E staining sections (upper panel) shows RP-OV17534 primary tumor, subcutaneous graft tumor from spheroids, intraperitoneal graft tumor from spheroids, and serial intraperitoneal graft tumor from SCID mouse ascites. Histological analysis (lower panel) shows frequent metastasis of tumor cells into various organs of spheroid cells recipients.

of epithelial markers CK-7 and CA-125 further confirmed the epithelial nature of these primary cell lines (**Fig. 1C**). In order to generate spheroid cells, ovarian cancer cell line OV2774 or primary EOC cells were enzymatically dissociated and inoculated on ultra-low attachment culture plates in serum-free medium with EGF, bFGF, and N2 supplement-A. In this culture condition some cells died from serum starvation, while others were forced into suspension and formed aggregates. Three weeks after plating, some aggregates compacted into spheres which could not be dissociated by pipetting. Some of the spheres also aggregated to form sphere clusters. Floating spheres and clusters were dissociated by pipetting, and replated twice a week, with the resulting cells generating secondary spheres, appearing as distinct prototypical spheroids (**Figs. 1B, 1E**), similar to those found in patient ascites [5,6]. Using this approach, we obtained sustainable spheroids from established cell line OV2774 (**Figs. 1D and 1E**) and primary EOC cells RP-OV17534 (**Figs. 1A and 1B**) under stem-selective conditions. We have cultured the OV2774 and RP-OV17534 cells as spheroids for 6 months, demonstrating the self-renewing ability of the spheroid cells.

Spheroid Cells Tumorigenicity and Metastasis in Immune-deficient Mice

Next, we investigated the tumorigenicity of sphere-forming cells. We examined whether exponentially smaller numbers (compared with parental cancer cells) were capable of tumorigenesis, as previously shown for other epithelial cancer initiating cells (CICs) [24–28]. Spheroid cells or corresponding parental bulk tumor cells were injected s.c. into right legs of SCID mice. With injections of only 2,000 cells per mouse, spheroid cells were tumorigenic in 4 of 4 SCID mice for RP-OV17534 spheroid cells and 2 of 2 for OV2774 spheroid cells, as evidenced by palpable tumors at the injection site (**Fig. 2A; Table 2**). The median tumor latency time in this cohort was 31 to 90 days for RP-OV17534 spheroid and 50 to 57 for OV2774 spheroid, similar to or less than CICs of other malignancies [24–27]. Correspondingly, injections of 5,000 and 10,000 RP-OV17534 spheroid cells were also tumorigenic in three of three mice with shorter tumor latencies (**Fig. 2A; Table 2**). Without non-adherent spheroid selection, bulk tumor cells failed to form tumors even at 40,000 cells for RP-OV17534 engraftment (**Table 2**). All subcutaneous xenograft tumors derived from spheroid cells were categorized as serous adenocarcinomas of moderate/poor differentiation (grade 2/grade 3), similar to the

Table 2. In vivo tumorigenicity of ovarian cancer spheroid cells.

Cell type	*Injection cell type*	*Injection site*	*Cell dose*[a]	*Tumor formation*[b]	*Latency*[c] *days*
Primary	Spheroid	S.c.	2000	4/4	31/38/42/90
EOC		S.c.	5000	3/3	40/52/54
RP-OV		S.c.	10000	3/3	31/37/38
17534	Parental	S.c.	5000	0/2	–
		S.c.	10000	0/2	–
		S.c.	40000	0/2	–
	Spheroid	I.p.	10000	4/4	75/80/80/84
		I.p.	20000	3/3	59/63/63
		I.p.	40000	3/3	54/54/63
	Parental	I.p.	20000	0/2	–
		I.p.	40000	0/2	–
		I.p.	60000	0/2	–
		I.p.	80000	0/3	–
		I.p.	1.7×10^7	1/1	92
		I.p.	2×10^7	3/3	105
EOC cell	Spheroid	S.c.	2000	2/2	50/57
line	Parental	S.c.	2000	1/2	57
OV2774	Spheroid	I.p.	5000	1/1	126
		I.p.	15000	1/1	85
		I.p.	20000	1/1	126
		I.p.	300000	1/1	79
	Parental	I.p.	20000	0/1	–
		I.p.	40000	0/1	–
			1.2×10^7	1/1	50
			2×10^7	1/1	38

[a]Number of cells per injection.
[b]Number of tumors formed per number of injection.
[c]The time from injection to the first appearance of a palpable tumor or ascites.
S.c.: subcutaneous; I.p.: intraperitoneal.

parental primary patient tumors (H&E stained sections; **Fig. 2C**). No architectural/cytologic differences were observed between primary and graft tumors.

A major limitation of studies of CICs is engraftment into non-native microenvironments [29,30]. To establish that CICs faithfully recapitulate the well-established progression of ovarian cancer in its native setting, the experiments were conducted with intra-peritoneal (i.p.) injections. The i.p. injection of only 10,000 cells per mouse of RP-OV17534 spheroid cells resulted in development of bloody ascites in 4 of 4 SCID mice (**Fig. 2B; Table 2**), with tumor latencies of 75 to 84 days, similar to or less than CICs of other malignancies [17]. Correspondingly, i.p. injections of 20,000 and 40,000 spheroid cells were also tumorigenic in three of three mice with shorter tumor latencies (**Table 2**). Without non-adherent spheroid selection, bulk tumor cells failed to form bloody ascites and tumors even at 80,000 cells per injection, whereas one of one and 3 of 3 mice i.p. injected respectively with 1.7×10^7 and 2×10^7 parental primary EOC cells were tumorigenic, albeit with extended latency (92–105 days; **Table 2**). I.p. injection of sphere-forming cells resulted in development of bloody ascites and peritoneal metastasis to the omentum, liver, colon, stomach, and kidney (**Fig. 2B**), and intraperitoneal tumor histology similar to both subcutaneous xenograft and primary patient tumors (**Fig. 2C**). Consistent with the results for RP-OV17534, we also observed higher tumorigenicity of OV2774 spheroid cells compared to their parent cells, in similar i.p. engraftment animal experiments using OV2774 derived cells (**Table 2**).

Another essential criterion for CICs is their ability to serially propagate tumors in consecutively engrafted animals [31]. To examine this definitive stemness characteristic, serial engraftments of xenografts were performed. 2×10^4 of spheroid cells were i.p. injected into SCID mice and ascites developed as expected in 3 out of 3 mice in approximately 60 days. Transplantation of 8×10^4, 1×10^5, and 5×10^5 such ascites cells into SCID mice resulted in ascites and tumors, with a latency significantly shorter than the parental patient tumor cells (66/63/49 days respectively for passage 2 xenografts versus no tumor development for parent tumor cells of 8×10^4 transplantation in 0 out of 3 SCID mice). The pathology of the omental mass was similar to that of s.c. tumors (**Fig. 2C**). These results indicate that sphere-forming cells are more tumorigenic than their parental tumor cells, demonstrating that a highly tumorigenic subpopulation of cells are present within the sphere-forming cells, and may reside within ovarian neoplasms. Since RP-OV17534 spheroid cells and OV2774 spheroid cells demonstrated similar characteristics, the following results are shown for RP-OV17534 derived cells with similar observations for OV2774 cells.

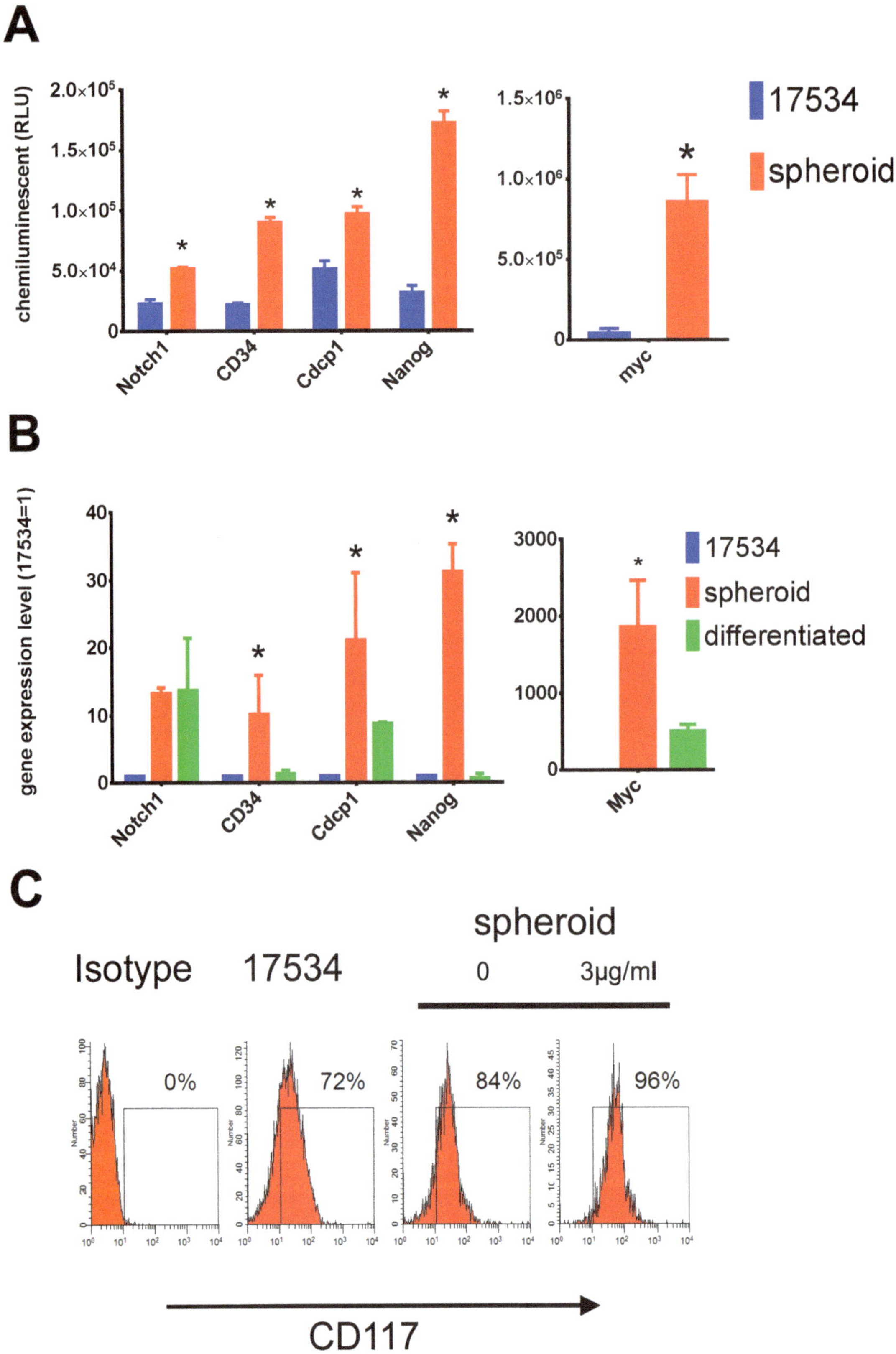

Figure 3. Spheroid cells overexpressed stem cell genes. (A) Total RNA isolated from spheroid cells and parent cells were examined for their gene expression by a human stem cell markers cDNA array and stem cell-genes showed higher expression levels in spheroid cells to non-spheroid cells. (B) The overexpression levels of Notch1, Nanog, Cdcp1, CD34, and Myc in spheroid cells compared to non-spheroid cells were confirmed by quantitative real-time PCR. These stem cell-genes' expression were lost or down-regulated when spheroid cells were differentiated by culturing in CM without growth factors for 14 days. Expression levels are represented as fold changes compared to these of non-spheroid cells. (C) FACS examination

of CD117 expression on spheroid cells and parent cells showing high CD117 expression in spheroid cells. Some spheroid cells were treated with Cisplatin for 24 hrs before surface staining by CD117 Abs. Error bars: SD, N = 3. *: $p<0.05$.

Ovarian Tumor Sphere-forming Cells Express Stem Cell Genes

To examine the expression of gene specific to embryonic stem cells, total RNA from spheroid cells and parent cells were analyzed by a Human Stem Cell Marker cDNA Plate Array. Among 32 genes tested, spheroid cells upregulated Notch1, Nanog, Cdcp1, CD34, and Myc expression (**Fig. 3A**). Each of these genes is essential for developmental processes (embryogenesis, neurogenesis, stem cell expansion, and hematopoiesis [32–34]). These results were confirmed by quantitative real-time PCR data. The expression levels of Notch1, Nanog, Cdcp1, CD34, and Myc in spheroid cells were approximately 10 to 2000 fold higher than that of non-spheroid cells detected by real-time PCR (**Fig. 3B**, red bar). When spheroid cells were cultured in CM without growth factors, a differentiating condition, floating cells adhered and grew into epithelial cells. Next we compared the same sets of gene expression level by real-time PCR in spheroid cells, culturing in either stem cell-selective or differentiating conditions for 14 days. Expression of CD34 and Nanog were approximately 1 fold of that of non-spheroid cells, Cdcp1 and Myc decreased to 9 and 500 fold, respectively. Notch1 expression level in spheroid cells stayed at 12 fold of that of non-spheroid cells after culturing in CM for 14 days (**Fig. 3B**, green bar). Stem cell factor receptor CD117 (c-kit) has been reported in previous studies on ovarian cancer tumor progenitors [17,35]. Therefore, we examined CD117 expression by FACS in these spheroid cells. Consistent with previous reports, we also detected CD117 up-regulation in spheroid cells compared with parent cells. Since a large number of spheroid cells killed by chemotherapy drugs were differentiated non-stem cells, whereas stem-like cells survived (see below), we found that CD117 expression further increased in spheroid cells after cisplatin treatment for 24 hrs (**Fig. 3C**). These data indicate that spheroid cells from ovarian cancer overexpress stem cell genes under stem cell-selective conditions and lose or decrease these gene expressions under differentiation conditions.

Increased ALDH Activity in Spheroid Cells

ALDH plays a vital role in cellular detoxification. Recent studies show that increased ALDH activity leads to several types of malignancies, serves as a cancer stem cell marker and correlated with poor prognosis [36–39]. Our ALDEFLUOR assay showed more $ALDH^+$ cells in spheroid cells in the absence of ALDH inhibitor DEAB (**Fig. 4A**). The increased ALDH function in spheroid cells was confirmed by an ALDH activity colorimetric assay, showing significant enhanced activity in spheroid cells (**Fig. 4B**).

Spheroid Cells have High Proliferation and Migration Potential than their Parental Cells

The relationship of spheroid formation and cell growth potential was examined in a kinetic cell proliferation assay. Increased cell proliferation was demonstrated in spheroid cells compared with parent cells. More cells appeared at day 6 and continued increasing to day 17 (**Fig. 5A**). Since all cell cultures were maintained at identical growth conditions in the same culture milieu, their varying growth kinetics could be attributed to cell intrinsic mechanisms.

Cell motility is one of the factors that contribute to tumor cell invasion [40]. To detect the migration kinetics of spheroids versus non-spheroid cells, parental and spheroid EOC cells were studied in a migration assay. Very few parental cells migrated while significant amount of spheroid cells passed through transwell membrane. The difference started to show on day 2 and continued on day 3 (**Fig. 5B**). The observation that spheroid cells migrated quicker than their parental cells was further confirmed by a wound healing assay. As shown in **Figure 5C**, more spheroid cells migrated into the scratch than parental cells. The data also suggest spheroid cells may utilize different wound healing pathways.

Ovarian Tumor Spheroid Cells Showed Invasion Abilities and Anchorage-independent Growth

To study the relationship between spheroid formation and cell invasion, spheroid cells and parental cells were tested in an

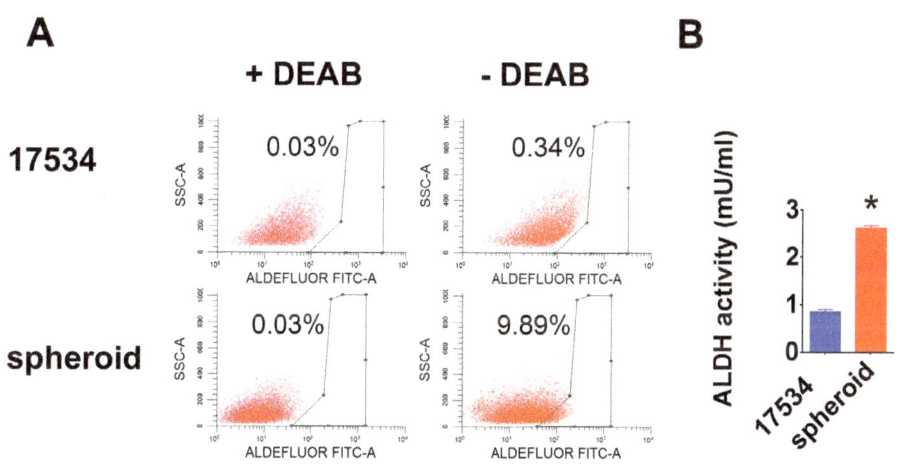

Figure 4. Increased ALDH activity in spheroid cells. (A) The ALDEFLOUR kit labels the population with a high ALDH enzymatic activity in spheroid cells. An aliquot of each sample of cells was treated with ALDH inhibitor DEAB as negative control for setting FACS gate. (B) The BioVision ALDH colorimetric assay detected enhanced ALDH activity in spheroid cell lysate. Error bars: SD, N = 2. *: $p<0.05$.

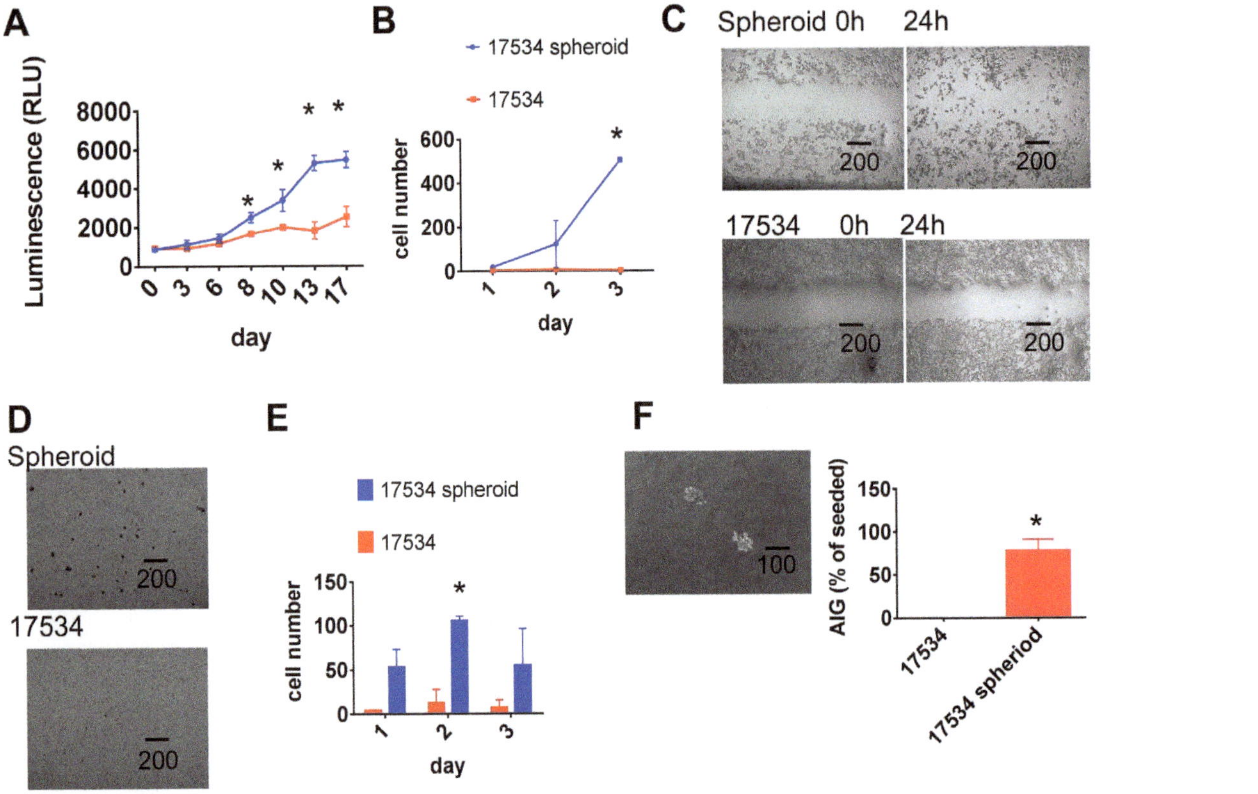

Figure 5. Spheroid cells show a more aggressive growth pattern. (A) Spheroid cells had higher proliferation potential than their parent cells. Both spheroid cells and parental cells were cultured in CM for 24 h, then 5000/well cells were cultured in CM in 96 well plates. Half of media was changed every 3 days. Cell proliferations were detected from day 0 to day 17 by CellTiter-Glo Luminescent Cell Viability Assay. (B) Spheroid cells had higher migration ability than parent cells. Parental and spheroid EOC cells were treated with RPMI only medium for 24 hrs. In a transwell plate, 2×10^5/well cells were put into insert with 0.2%BSA-RPMI medium, the lower chamber contains no cells except RPMI medium with 2.5% FBS. After culture for 1, 2, and 3 days, the numbers of cells that passed through membrane as well as cells fall into chamber were calculated under microscope. (C) Spheroid cells recovered 'scratch' made by 200-μL pipette tip after 24 hours more efficient than their parent cells. Experiments were repeated three times with similar results. (D) More spheroid cells invaded into matrigel than parent cells as shown by microscopy. Spheroid cells and parental cells were treated with serum-free medium RPMI for 24 h. In a transwell plate, 40000/well of cells were put into insert coated with matrigel with 0.2% BSA, while the chamber had only media with 5% FBS, after culture for 1, 2, and 3 days, The number of cells invading into matrigel were counted after 0.1% crystal blue staining. (E) Invasion tests were done in duplicate and average and SD were shown. *,$p<0.01$. (F) Spheroid cells formed colonies in top agar detected in anchorage-independent growth assay (AIG) as shown under microscopy. 500 cells were seeded in 6 well plates containing a top layer of 0.3% soft agar and 0.5% agar base in DMEM, 10% FBS. 24 hrs later, the number of cells seeded was determined by counting cells under the light microscope. After 3 weeks of growth in soft agar, the number of colonies (Colonies >5 cells) were counted; 10 different fields were quantified per well and the average number of colonies per field was calculated. The AIG index was expressed relative to the number of cells seeded. More than 70% of seeded spheroid cells formed colonies while none of seeded parent cells formed colonies. Experiments were repeated twice with similar results. *,$p<0.01$. Error bars: SD.

invasion assay. In this assay, cells need to break down matrigel while in migration assay cells just moved through a membrane. The invasion assay mimics the *in vivo* situation more closely. As shown in **Figure 5D**, very few parent cells invaded into matrigel while significantly more spheroid cells invaded into matrigel after 3 days of culture. Spheroid cells had higher invasion ability than their parental cells detected on day 1, 2, and 3 (**Fig. 5E**). Since spheroid cells show increased proliferation ability after 6 days of culture in proliferation assay, it is unlikely that the superior invasion ability of spheroid cells is merely due to their higher proliferation property. This *in vitro* invasion potential is consistent with the observed *in vivo* spheroid cells tumorigenicity as shown in **Fig. 2**. To further confirm the aggressive properties of spheroid cells, we next investigated their tumorigenic potential using the anchorage-independent growth (AIG) assay. **Fig. 5F** shows that parent cells could not form colony in soft agar while spheroid cells produced significant numbers of colonies, providing additional evidence for the increased tumorigenic attributes of spheroid cells.

Spheroid Cells are Resistant to Conventional Chemotherapies

To determine whether spheroid cells possess a cancer stem cell chemoresistant phenotype, spheroid cells and parent cells were treated in the same serum-free culture medium for 24 h. After which, 5000/well of cells was treated by various amounts of Cisplatin in CM. Numbers of cells were determined by CellTiter-Glo Luminescent Cell Viability Assay at different time points. More spheroid cells were killed by Cisplatin at concentrations above 4 μg/mL on day2 while only few non-spheroid cells were dead at the same concentrations, suggesting that spheroid cells are initially more sensitive to Cisplatin than non-spheroid cells due to their proliferation potential (**Fig. 6A**). However, when cells treated with Cisplatin for 48 h were washed and cultured in CM for another 8 days, spheroid cells formed more colonies than non-spheroid cells (**Fig. 6B**). These results suggested that a large number of spheroid cells killed by Cisplatin are differentiated

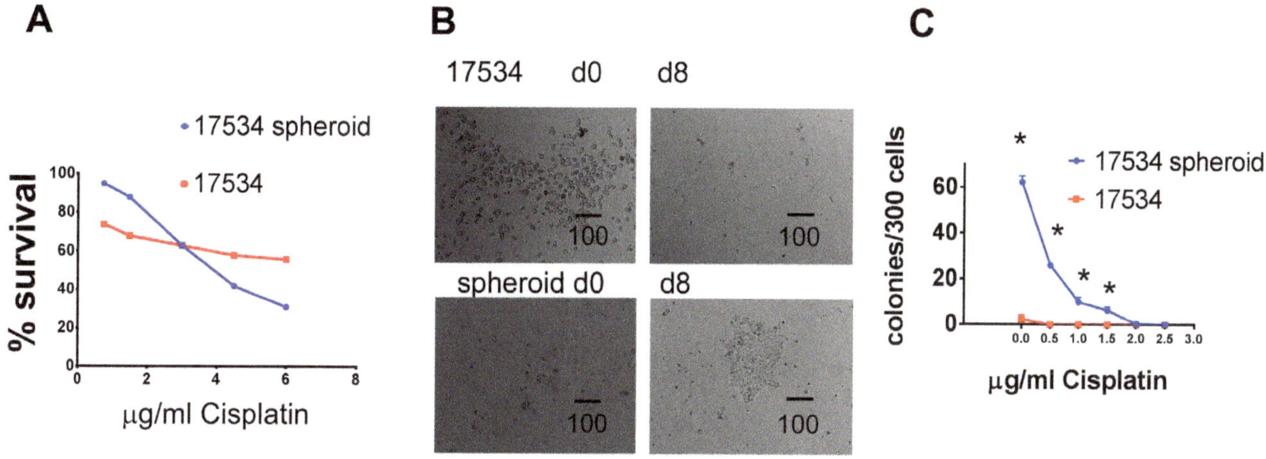

Figure 6. Spheroid cells are resistant to chemotherapy *in vitro*. (A) More spheroid cells were killed by Cisplatin than parent cells. The same numbers of spheroid and parent cells were cultured in CM with indicated amount of Cisplatin for 2 days and numbers of cells from different time points were determined. (B) More parent cells survived after Cisplatin treatment for 48 h (Left). However, 8 days later, only spheroid cells were growing while parent cells disappeared (Right). (C) Spheroid and parent cells were treated with indicated amount of Cisplatin for 24 h, washed, and 300 of survived cells/well were cultured in CM for another 10 days, cell colonies were shown after crystal violet staining. The same clonogenic survival assays were repeated twice with similar results. Colonies formed (>5 cells) after 10 days of growth were counted and average and SD were shown. *,$p<0.05$.

non-stem cells while the small number of cells that survived the chemotherapy treatment are resistant stem-like cells with more proliferative potential compared to non-spheroid cells once chemotherapy treatment was removed. To confirm this hypothesis, we investigated clonogenecity of residual cells after Cisplatin treatment. Spheroid cells and parent cells were treated with increasing concentration of Cisplatin for 24 hr, washed and 300/well of treated cells were cultured in 6-well-plate for another 10 days, the numbers of colonies (>5 cells) were counted under microscopy. Untreated spheroid cells generated many colonies while parent cells formed significantly less colonies, consistent with our chemotherapy survival assays. As the Cisplatin concentration increased, the number of colonies decreased. However, spheroid cells still formed significantly more colonies than parent cells after Cisplatin treatment (**Fig. 6C**).

Metabolism Studies Reveal Spheroid Cells' Resistance to Oxygen Deprivation

Cancer cells adopt an alternative metabolic pathway and increase their glycolytic activity through a process called the Warburg effect [41]. The Warburg effect is necessary for cancer cells to resist oxidative stress and to adapt to hypoxic conditions [42]. Since glycolysis could play an essential role in tumorigenesis during both the immortalization and transformation steps [43], we investigated the dynamic metabolic flux of spheroid cells. Lactate secreted into cell culture medium can be used to measure label incorporation into the three-carbon metabolite pool. Direct [U-$^{13}C_6$] glucose catabolism through glycolysis results in m3 lactate, whereas passage through the oxidative and nonoxidative branches of the pentose phosphate pathway of glucose results in m2 lactate. As expected, the majority of lactate is produced via glycolysis in all tumor cell cultures (**Fig. 7A**). Spheroid cells showed significant increase in oxidizing glucose directly in the pentose cycle (**Fig. 7B**). Metabolism flux comparison between Glucose-6-P Dehydrogenase (G6PDH) and glycolysis revealed increased pentose cycle flux and NADPH production in spheroid cells, indicating increased acetate use for *de novo* fatty acid synthesis instead of complete oxidation in spheroid cell cultures (**Fig. 7C**). The ^{13}C label enrichment of lactate from glucose in spheroid cells showed a more than two fold increase compared with their parent cells (**Fig. 7D**). The ^{13}C isotopomer distribution showed a significant increase in anaerobic glycolysis and defective aerobic glucose metabolism in spheroid cells. This is indicative and important marker of decreased tricarboxylic acid (TCA) cycle flux and energy production via complete glucose/substrate oxidation. TCA cycle anaplerotic flux was measured using the equilibrium between glutamate and α-ketoglutarate. The large increase in glutamate labeling in two carbon positions with ^{13}C indicated a defective TCA cycle and limited turnover of ketoglutarate into succinate and fumarate (**Fig. 7E**). This indicates a complex-II defect in spheroid cell cultures. Consistently, ^{13}C-labeled carbon dioxide release from glucose was significantly decreased in spheroid cells (**Fig. 7F**), which also indicated that spheroid cells have defects in complete glucose oxidation in the TCA cycle. ^{13}C-gultamate and acetyl-CoA are the transported products of the citrate shuttle from mitochondria to the cytosol for *de novo* fatty acid synthesis, fatty acid chain elongation and glutamate recycling. Glutamate labeling in the cytosol is similar to that of malonyl-CoA and fatty acids up to palmitate (C:16) via substrate sharing through the citrate shuttle. ^{13}C-acetate incorporation from substrate into fatty acids and rate of new fatty acid synthesis, which corresponds with the fraction of newly synthesized glutamate, was measured by glutamate labeling in the cytosol. The fraction of newly synthesized fatty acid increased significantly in spheroid cells (**Fig. 7G**), and ^{13}C enrichment of acetate for fatty acid synthesis also showed significant increase (**Fig. 7H**). Spheroid cells had significant increase in malonyl-CoA synthesis and fatty acid *de novo* synthesis and breakdown via peroxisomal beta oxidation. The large increase of glucose derived acetate used for malonyl-CoA synthesis also indicated severe defect in TCA cycle energy production and turnover. The main energy production and biosynthetic metabolism pathways for both spheroid cells and parent cells are summarized in Figure **7I**.

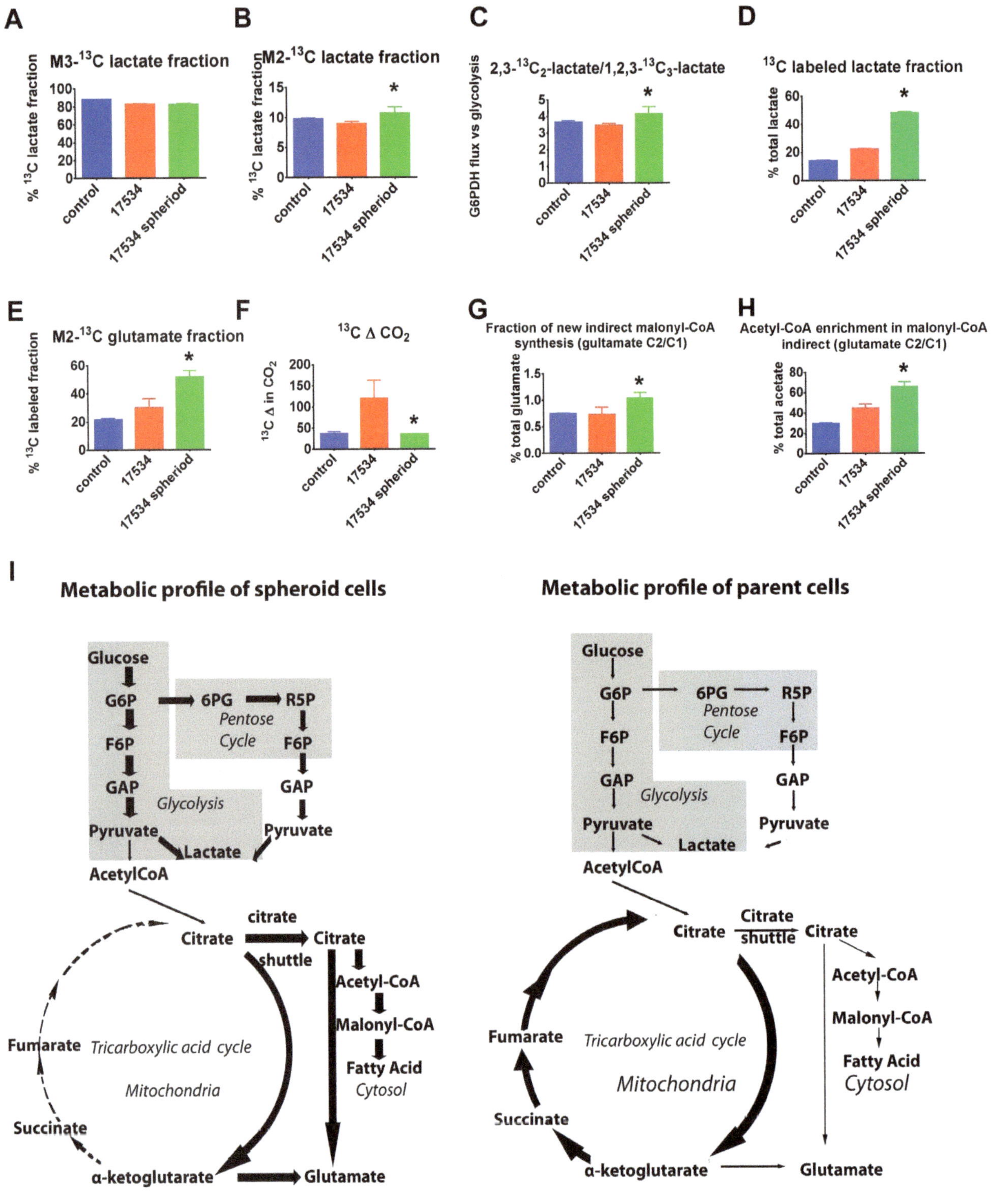

Figure 7. Spheroid cells show a hypoxia-resistant metabolism profile. Metabolic profiles of a normal ovarian cell line RPNLOv78 as control, EOC cells RP-OV17534, and spheroid RP-OV17534 cells cultures in the presence of [U-$^{13}C_6$]glucose for 24 hrs (n = 3) showing (A) percentages of m3-^{13}C lactate derived directed from glycolysis; (B) percentages of m2-^{13}C lactate derived from pentose cycle; (C) ratio of m2 to m3 lactate; (D) percentage of ^{13}C-labeled lactate of total lactate; (E) percentages of ^{13}C-double-labeled glutamate in total ^{13}C-labeled glutamate; (F) $^{13}CO_2$ release from [U-$^{13}C_6$]glucose; (G) The fraction of newly synthesized palmitate and the ^{13}C enrichment of acetyl units (H). Error bars: SD; *,$p<0.01$, compared with parental EOC cells. (I) EOC spheroid cells show increased anaerobic glycolysis, increased direct glucose oxidation in the pentose cycle, but low TCA cycle carbon flux, low anaplerotic flux, and *de novo* fatty acid synthesis. In contrast, parent EOC cells show increased TCA cycle and high anaplerotic flux. G6P, glucose-6-P; F6P, fructose-6-P; GAP, glyceraldehyde-3-P; 6PG, 6-P-gluconate; R5P, ribulose-5-P. Various thickness of lines represent different strengths of metabolic flux.

Discussion

There are both single cells and spheroid cells in EOC tumors and ascites [44,45]. Previous research in ovarian cancer has focused mainly on the metastatic behavior of single cells. Currently, there is data to demonstrate that spheroids are capable of tumorigenesis *in vivo*, and have a reduced response to chemotherapeutic drugs *in vitro* [46–48]. In order to study EOC pathogenesis, we cultured EOC primary cells under stem cell-selective conditions and generated anchorage-independent, self-renewing spheroids morphologically similar to spheroids isolated from patient ascites [5,6]. These spheroid cells expressed numerous stem cell markers and were sustainable indefinitely under stem cell-selecting conditions. The spheroid cells had shorter doubling time than their parental cells and showed additional attributes that are distinct from their parent cells. Strikingly, as few as 2000 spheroid cells from primary tumor cells engrafted into immune-deficient mice and allowed full recapitulation of the original tumor, whereas $>10^5$ parent tumor cells remained non-tumorigenic. These spheroid cells also could serially propagate tumors of identical phenotypes *in vivo*. In order to address concerns regarding engraftment into non-native microenvironment [29,30], we i.p. injected EOC spheroid cells into SCID mice which resulted in a pathology essentially identical to the human malignancy, with formation of bloody ascites and extensive peritoneal dissemination. Although there is a long history of transplanting human tumor cells into immune-deficient mice, the strong host resistance in these mice allowed only the most aggressive tumors and cell lines to be engrafted. Our *in vivo* engraftment experiments not only indicated that spheroid cells are highly tumorigenic but also that EOC is hierarchically organized so that only a subset of cells-cancer stem cells- possess the potential to initiate and sustain tumor growth.

Cell motility is one of the factors that contribute to tumor cell invasion. Indeed, spheroid cells showed higher migration ability than their parent cells both in migration and wound healing assays. Importantly, spheroid cells had higher invasion ability than parent cells in invasion assays. They also showed 3-D growth in anchorage-independent growth assays. These results are consistent with previous reports [5,7,49,50] indicating that spheroids could adhere to, migrate on and infiltrate into other monolayer cells. In addition, our data demonstrated that aggressive properties of spheroid cells enriched with cancer stem cells contributes to ovarian cancer pathogenesis.

Contrary to previous reports that spheroid cells are more resistant to chemotherapy drugs [5–8], we demonstrated that spheroid cells were initially more sensitive than parent cells to cisplatin and paclitaxel treatment (**Fig. 6** and data not shown). However, our clonogenic survival assay indicated that more spheroid cells survived after 24 hrs of cisplatin treatment, compared with parent cells. This may be because spheroid cells proliferate faster than parent cells in CM, and therefore more dividing spheroid cells were killed by drug than their parent cells. However, after drug removal, the surviving spheroid cells recovered faster than parent cells. These two lines of evidence suggested that a large fraction of spheroid cells killed by cisplatin are more differentiated non-stem cells, while the small fraction of spheroid cells that survived chemotherapy are cancer stem cells. The stemness properties of these surviving spheroid cells was demonstrated by their ability to generate more tumor colonies than the large numbers of parent cells that survived from cisplatin treatment. These results may explain why current chemotherapeutic regimens are unable to achieve sustained remission in ovarian cancer patients, despite frequently producing a complete response at the time of first line treatment.

It has been shown that cancer cells use more glucose compared to normal cells and accumulate extracellular lactate even in normoxic conditions, a feature called Warburg effect [51,52]. In addition, recent reports have shown that human pluripotent stem cells rely mostly on glycolysis to meet their energy demands [53,54]. Using stable ^{13}C-glucose isotope, we demonstrated that spheroid cells have a significant increase in glycolysis flux compared to their parent cells (**Fig. 7**). This pattern of glycolytic flux is similar to what has been observed for pluripotent stem cells [53]. The very different patterns of substrate utilization likely explain their aggressiveness and resistance to chemotherapies. Our results indicate that spheroid cells mainly route glucose to anaerobic glycolysis. This direct oxidation of glucose through anaerobic glycolysis is in accord with recent publications suggesting that CSCs may have even more active glycolytic activity compared to the bulk of general cancer cells [55–58]. In addition, we demonstrated that the amount of glucose utilized in the pentose phosphate pathway is far greater than that oxidized through the TCA cycle by spheroid cells. Since the oxidative branch of the pentose cycle is an efficient means for producing cytoplasmic NADPH and high NADPH production would be necessary for increased fatty acid synthesis, a NADPH dependent process, our data shows that synthesis of fatty acids are indeed increased in spheroid cells. Since hypoxia is associated with the formation and maintenance of cancer stem cells [59], our metabolic data suggest that ovarian CSCs are likely to survive in severely hypoxic microenvironments. These spheroid cell metabolic attributes may confer the increased chemoresistance observed in this study. On the contrary, parent cells display increased use of anabolic pathways to the detriment of anaerobic glycolysis and are likely to be more vulnerable to chemotherapy.

Acknowledgments

We thank SiDMAP LLC for assistance with some experiments.

Author Contributions

Conceived and designed the experiments: JL FQ NT XW WJH SBL KO. Performed the experiments: JL NT AB ZQ. Analyzed the data: JL FQ NT AB ZQ PMF KO. Contributed reagents/materials/analysis tools: CDM. Wrote the paper: JL FQ KO. These authors contributed equally to the study: JL FQ.

References

1. Jemal A, Siegel R, Ward E, Hao Y, Xu J, et al. (2009) Cancer statistics, 2009. CA Cancer J Clin 59: 225–249.
2. Armstrong D (2010) Update on treatment options for newly diagnosed ovarian cancer. Clin Adv Hematol Oncol 8: 675–678.
3. Colombo N, Van Gorp T, Parma G, Amant F, Gatta G, et al. (2006) Ovarian cancer. Crit Rev Oncol Hematol 60: 159–179.
4. Cannistra SA (2004) Cancer of the ovary. N Engl J Med 351: 2519–2529.
5. Burleson KM, Boente MP, Pambuccian SE, Skubitz AP (2006) Disaggregation and invasion of ovarian carcinoma ascites spheroids. J Transl Med 4: 6.
6. L'Esperance S, Bachvarova M, Tetu B, Mes-Masson AM, Bachvarov D (2008) Global gene expression analysis of early response to chemotherapy treatment in ovarian cancer spheroids. BMC Genomics 9: 99.
7. Shield K, Riley C, Quinn MA, Rice GE, Ackland ML, et al. (2007) Alpha2beta1 integrin affects metastatic potential of ovarian carcinoma spheroids by supporting disaggregation and proteolysis. J Carcinog 6: 11.
8. Zietarska M, Maugard CM, Filali-Mouhim A, Alam-Fahmy M, Tonin PN, et al. (2007) Molecular description of a 3D in vitro model for the study of epithelial ovarian cancer (EOC). Mol Carcinog 46: 872–885.

9. Shield K, Ackland ML, Ahmed N, Rice GE (2009) Multicellular spheroids in ovarian cancer metastases: Biology and pathology. Gynecol Oncol 113: 143–148.
10. Boros LG, Lapis K, Szende B, Tomoskozi-Farkas R, Balogh A, et al. (2001) Wheat germ extract decreases glucose uptake and RNA ribose formation but increases fatty acid synthesis in MIA pancreatic adenocarcinoma cells. Pancreas 23: 141–147.
11. Boros LG, Lee PW, Brandes JL, Cascante M, Muscarella P, et al. (1998) Nonoxidative pentose phosphate pathways and their direct role in ribose synthesis in tumors: is cancer a disease of cellular glucose metabolism? Med Hypotheses 50: 55–59.
12. Dang CV, Semenza GL (1999) Oncogenic alterations of metabolism. Trends Biochem Sci 24: 68–72.
13. Boros LG, Cascante M, Lee WN (2002) Metabolic profiling of cell growth and death in cancer: applications in drug discovery. Drug Discov Today 7: 364–372.
14. Raamsdonk LM, Teusink B, Broadhurst D, Zhang N, Hayes A, et al. (2001) A functional genomics strategy that uses metabolome data to reveal the phenotype of silent mutations. Nat Biotechnol 19: 45–50.
15. Bertozzi CC, Chang CY, Jairaj S, Shan X, Huang J, et al. (2006) Multiple initial culture conditions enhance the establishment of cell lines from primary ovarian cancer specimens. In Vitro Cell Dev Biol Anim 42: 58–62.
16. Shepherd TG, Theriault BL, Campbell EJ, Nachtigal MW (2006) Primary culture of ovarian surface epithelial cells and ascites-derived ovarian cancer cells from patients. Nat Protoc 1: 2643–2649.
17. Zhang S, Balch C, Chan MW, Lai HC, Matei D, et al. (2008) Identification and characterization of ovarian cancer-initiating cells from primary human tumors. Cancer Res 68: 4311–4320.
18. Crouch SP, Kozlowski R, Slater KJ, Fletcher J (1993) The use of ATP bioluminescence as a measure of cell proliferation and cytotoxicity. J Immunol Methods 160: 81–88.
19. Pejovic T, Pande NT, Mori M, Mhawech-Fauceglia P, Harrington C, et al. (2009) Expression profiling of the ovarian surface kinome reveals candidate genes for early neoplastic changes. Transl Oncol 2: 341–349.
20. Vizan P, Boros LG, Figueras A, Capella G, Mangues R, et al. (2005) K-ras codon-specific mutations produce distinctive metabolic phenotypes in NIH3T3 mice [corrected] fibroblasts. Cancer Res 65: 5512–5515.
21. Lee WN, Boros LG, Puigjaner J, Bassilian S, Lim S, et al. (1998) Mass isotopomer study of the nonoxidative pathways of the pentose cycle with [1,2–13C2]glucose. Am J Physiol 274: E843–851.
22. Katz J, Lee WN, Wals PA, Bergner EA (1989) Studies of glycogen synthesis and the Krebs cycle by mass isotopomer analysis with [U-13C]glucose in rats. J Biol Chem 264: 12994–13004.
23. Kasho VN, Cheng S, Jensen DM, Ajie H, Lee WN, et al. (1996) Feasibility of analysing [13C]urea breath tests for Helicobacter pylori by gas chromatography-mass spectrometry in the selected ion monitoring mode. Aliment Pharmacol Ther 10: 985–995.
24. Al-Hajj M, Wicha MS, Benito-Hernandez A, Morrison SJ, Clarke MF (2003) Prospective identification of tumorigenic breast cancer cells. Proc Natl Acad Sci U S A 100: 3983–3988.
25. Collins AT, Berry PA, Hyde C, Stower MJ, Maitland NJ (2005) Prospective identification of tumorigenic prostate cancer stem cells. Cancer Res 65: 10946–10951.
26. Dalerba P, Dylla SJ, Park IK, Liu R, Wang X, et al. (2007) Phenotypic characterization of human colorectal cancer stem cells. Proc Natl Acad Sci U S A 104: 10158–10163.
27. Li C, Heidt DG, Dalerba P, Burant CF, Zhang L, et al. (2007) Identification of pancreatic cancer stem cells. Cancer Res 67: 1030–1037.
28. Patrawala L, Calhoun T, Schneider-Broussard R, Li H, Bhatia B, et al. (2006) Highly purified CD44+ prostate cancer cells from xenograft human tumors are enriched in tumorigenic and metastatic progenitor cells. Oncogene 25: 1696–1708.
29. Hill RP, Perris R (2007) "Destemming" cancer stem cells. J Natl Cancer Inst 99: 1435–1440.
30. Kelly PN, Dakic A, Adams JM, Nutt SL, Strasser A (2007) Tumor growth need not be driven by rare cancer stem cells. Science 317: 337.
31. Clarke MF, Dick JE, Dirks PB, Eaves CJ, Jamieson CH, et al. (2006) Cancer stem cells–perspectives on current status and future directions: AACR Workshop on cancer stem cells. Cancer Res 66: 9339–9344.
32. Loh YH, Wu Q, Chew JL, Vega VB, Zhang W, et al. (2006) The Oct4 and Nanog transcription network regulates pluripotency in mouse embryonic stem cells. Nat Genet 38: 431–440.
33. Mohle R, Kanz L (2007) Hematopoietic growth factors for hematopoietic stem cell mobilization and expansion. Semin Hematol 44: 193–202.
34. Wiese C, Rolletschek A, Kania G, Blyszczuk P, Tarasov KV, et al. (2004) Nestin expression–a property of multi-lineage progenitor cells? Cell Mol Life Sci 61: 2510–2522.
35. Bapat SA, Mali AM, Koppikar CB, Kurrey NK (2005) Stem and progenitor-like cells contribute to the aggressive behavior of human epithelial ovarian cancer. Cancer Res 65: 3025–3029.
36. Ginestier C, Hur MH, Charafe-Jauffret E, Monville F, Dutcher J, et al. (2007) ALDH1 is a marker of normal and malignant human mammary stem cells and a predictor of poor clinical outcome. Cell Stem Cell 1: 555–567.
37. Carpentino JE, Hynes MJ, Appelman HD, Zheng T, Steindler DA, et al. (2009) Aldehyde dehydrogenase-expressing colon stem cells contribute to tumorigenesis in the transition from colitis to cancer. Cancer Res 69: 8208–8215.
38. van den Hoogen C, van der Horst G, Cheung H, Buijs JT, Lippitt JM, et al. (2010) High aldehyde dehydrogenase activity identifies tumor-initiating and metastasis-initiating cells in human prostate cancer. Cancer Res 70: 5163–5173.
39. Charafe-Jauffret E, Ginestier C, Bertucci F, Cabaud O, Wicinski J, et al. (2013) ALDH1-positive cancer stem cells predict engraftment of primary breast tumors and are governed by a common stem cell program. Cancer Res.
40. Puiffe ML, Le Page C, Filali-Mouhim A, Zietarska M, Ouellet V, et al. (2007) Characterization of ovarian cancer ascites on cell invasion, proliferation, spheroid formation, and gene expression in an in vitro model of epithelial ovarian cancer. Neoplasia 9: 820–829.
41. Warburg O (1956) On the origin of cancer cells. Science 123: 309–314.
42. Lyssiotis CA, Vander-Heiden MG, Munoz-Pinedo C, Emerling BM (2012) Emerging concepts: linking hypoxic signaling and cancer metabolism. Cell Death Dis 3: e303.
43. Kondoh H (2008) Cellular life span and the Warburg effect. Exp Cell Res 314: 1923–1928.
44. Naora H, Montell DJ (2005) Ovarian cancer metastasis: integrating insights from disparate model organisms. Nat Rev Cancer 5: 355–366.
45. Allen HJ, Porter C, Gamarra M, Piver MS, Johnson EA (1987) Isolation and morphologic characterization of human ovarian carcinoma cell clusters present in effusions. Exp Cell Biol 55: 194–208.
46. Aaberg-Jessen C, Norregaard A, Christensen K, Pedersen CB, Andersen C, et al. (2013) Invasion of primary glioma- and cell line-derived spheroids implanted into corticostriatal slice cultures. Int J Clin Exp Pathol 6: 546–560.
47. Luca AC, Mersch S, Deenen R, Schmidt S, Messner I, et al. (2013) Impact of the 3D Microenvironment on Phenotype, Gene Expression, and EGFR Inhibition of Colorectal Cancer Cell Lines. PLoS One 8: e59689.
48. Vang S, Wu HT, Fischer A, Miller DH, Maclaughlan S, et al. (2013) Identification of Ovarian Cancer Metastatic miRNAs. PLoS One 8: e58226.
49. Burleson KM, Hansen LK, Skubitz AP (2004) Ovarian carcinoma spheroids disaggregate on type I collagen and invade live human mesothelial cell monolayers. Clin Exp Metastasis 21: 685–697.
50. Burleson KM, Casey RC, Skubitz KM, Pambuccian SE, Oegema TR Jr, et al. (2004) Ovarian carcinoma ascites spheroids adhere to extracellular matrix components and mesothelial cell monolayers. Gynecol Oncol 93: 170–181.
51. Chiaradonna F, Moresco RM, Airoldi C, Gaglio D, Palorini R, et al. (2012) From cancer metabolism to new biomarkers and drug targets. Biotechnol Adv 30: 30–51.
52. Ward PS, Thompson CB (2012) Metabolic reprogramming: a cancer hallmark even warburg did not anticipate. Cancer Cell 21: 297–308.
53. Chen CT, Hsu SH, Wei YH (2010) Upregulation of mitochondrial function and antioxidant defense in the differentiation of stem cells. Biochim Biophys Acta 1800: 257–263.
54. Prigione A, Fauler B, Lurz R, Lehrach H, Adjaye J (2010) The senescence-related mitochondrial/oxidative stress pathway is repressed in human induced pluripotent stem cells. Stem Cells 28: 721–733.
55. Zhou Y, Zhou Y, Shingu T, Feng L, Chen Z, et al. (2011) Metabolic alterations in highly tumorigenic glioblastoma cells: preference for hypoxia and high dependency on glycolysis. J Biol Chem 286: 32843–32853.
56. Yuan S, Wang F, Chen G, Zhang H, Feng L, et al. (2013) Effective elimination of cancer stem cells by a novel drug combination strategy. Stem Cells 31: 23–34.
57. Nakano A, Tsuji D, Miki H, Cui Q, El Sayed SM, et al. (2011) Glycolysis inhibition inactivates ABC transporters to restore drug sensitivity in malignant cells. PLoS One 6: e27222.
58. Liu PP, Liao J, Tang ZJ, Wu WJ, Yang J, et al. (2013) Metabolic regulation of cancer cell side population by glucose through activation of the Akt pathway. Cell Death Differ.
59. Keith B, Simon MC (2007) Hypoxia-inducible factors, stem cells, and cancer. Cell 129: 465–472.

5

MiR-26a Promotes Ovarian Cancer Proliferation and Tumorigenesis

Wenjing Shen[1]*, Min Song[2]*, Jie Liu[3], Guangrong Qiu[4], Tianren Li[1], Yanjie Hu[1], Hongbo Liu[5]

1 Department of Gynecology, The First Affiliated Hospital of China Medical University, Shenyang, China, **2** Department of Pathology, The First Affiliated Hospital and College of Basic Medical Sciences, China Medical University, Institute of Pathology and Pathophysiology, Shenyang, China, **3** Experimental Technology Center, China Medical University, Shenyang, China, **4** Department of Medical Genetics, China Medical University, Shenyang, China, **5** Department of Health Statistics, School of Public Health, China Medical University, Shenyang, China

Abstract

MicroRNAs (miRNAs) important for posttranscriptional gene expression are involved in the initiation and progression of human cancer. In this study, we reported that *miR-26a* was over-expressed in human EOC specimens and the expression level of extracellular *miR-26a* in plasma can distinguish patients from healthy controls in EOC. Ectopic expression of *miR-26a* in ovarian cancer (OC) cells increased cell proliferation and clonal formation. This growth promoting effect of OC cell growth was mediated by *miR-26a* inhibition of the posttranscription of ER-α. Furthermore, inhibition of *miR-26a* suppressed the tumor formation generated by injecting OC cells in nude mice. Our results suggest that aberrantly expressed *miR-26a* may contribute to OC development.

Editor: Jin Q. Cheng, H. Lee Moffitt Cancer Center & Research Institute, United States of America

Funding: This work was sponsored by grants from the Project No. 30571836 from the NNSF(National Natural Science Foundation) of China. In addition, the work presented is part of projects with Project No.L2010681 financially supported by Science Foundation of the Education Department of Liaoning Province of China, and Project No.201202259 financially supported by Science Foundation of Science and Technology Bureau of Liaoning Province of China. Author Min Song contributed to experimental conceiving and design, guidance and discussion of the project, so she is the co-correspondence author of this paper. All the other funders had no role in study design, data collection and analysis, decision to publish, or preparation of the manuscript.

Competing Interests: The authors have declared that no competing interests exist.

* E-mail: wenjing0326@163.com (WS); songmin6@sohu.com (MS)

Introduction

OC is the fifth most common cancer in women and the leading cause of cancer deaths from gynecological malignancy in western countries [1]. In 2012, there are 22,280 new cases and 15,500 deaths from OC in the United States according to the national cancer statistics. EOC accounts for 85%–90% of ovarian cancer. Unfortunately, the overall prognosis is poor and the molecular events that lead to the development of this disease are still little-known.

MiRNAs represent a large family of endogenous noncoding RNAs and posttranscriptionally regulate gene expression [2]. Recent studies have revealed critical functions of miRNAs in essential processes, including proliferation, differentiation and cell death [3]. Altered expression or mutation of miRNAs has been reported in cancer, such as lung cancer, breast cancer, leukemia and other carcinomas [4]. In lung cancer cells, over-expression of *let-7* inhibited their growth by targeting Ras [5,6]. Furthermore, *miR-21* directly targets the tumor suppressor PTEN in hepatocellular cancer [7]. Moreover, several studies showed that miRNAs can function either as tumor suppressors (as is the case for the *miR-15a-miR-16-1* cluster [8]) or oncogenes (as is the case for *miR-21* [9]).

Genome-wide miRNA expression profiling showed *miR-26a* dysregulation in diverse cancers[10]. In this study, we found that *miR-26a* is over-expressed in human EOC. We demonstrate that inhibition of *miR-26a* decreased proliferation of human EOC cells, and suppressed growth of EOC cells in nude mice. In addition, ERα was down-regulated by *miR-26a* in EOC cells. Furthermore, we found that extracellular *miR-26a* levels in plasma can distinguish patients from healthy controls in EOC. Our study suggests that aberrant expression of *miR-26a* is critical for the development of human EOC and measurement of circulating *miR-26a* may be a good approach to EOC diagnosis.

Materials and Methods

Patients

Clinical specimens (including tissue and plasma samples) were collected from patients registered at The First Affiliated Hospital of China Medical University (Shenyang, China). The patients's information is summarized in Table 1, Table S1 and Table S2.

Materials

Antibody against ERα was from Santa Cruz (Santa Cruz, CA, USA), antibody against α-tubulin from Sigma (St Louis, MO, USA). All other reagents were from Sigma. Anti-miR-26a and nonsense of anti-miR were from GenePharma (Shanghai, PR China). Cel-miR-39 mimics were from IBS (Shanghai, PR China).

Quantative RT-PCR (qRT-PCR, Quantitative Reverse Transcriptase-polymerase Chain Reaction)

Total RNA isolated from clinical specimens or cells using Trizol Reagent (Invitrogen, Carlsbad, CA, USA) were reverse-transcribed into cDNA according to the previous report [11]. Isolation of RNA from plasma and quantification of miRNA were carried

Table 1. clinicopathologic data of ovarian cancer patients.

Total number	26
Pathological tumor stage	
I	3
II	4
III	17
IV	2
Grade	
G1	10
G2	9
G3	7
Histological type	
Serous cystadenocarcinoma	15
Mucinous cystadenocarcinoma	5
Endometrioid carcinoma	3
Clear cell carcinoma	3

out as described in [12]. In brief, 25 fmol of Cel-miR-39 mimics was added to 400 ul plasma. Real-time PCR was carried out using SYBR green PCR master mix (TaKaRa, Otus, Shiga, Japan). Amplification and detection were performed using ABI Prism 7700 system (Applied Biosystems, Foster City, CA, USA) according to the manufacturer's instructions. Cel-miR-39 was taken as reference gene for plasma samples. Primers used were listed in Table S3.

Cell Culture

The human OC cell lines, SKOV-3, ES2 (Cellbank, Shanghai, PR China) were maintained in McCoy's 5a supplemented with 10% (v/v) fetal calf serum (Invitrogen, Carlsbad, CA, USA). These cells were incubated at 37°C with 5% CO_2.

Vector Construction

Full-length human *miR-26a* was amplified from human genomic DNA and cloned into the pcDNA3.1 at KpnI and XhoI sites according to the previous report [13] and [14]. The human wild-type ERα was generated by PCR from cDNA and the PCR products were inserted into pcDNA3.1 as described in [15].

Cell Growth Assay

Cell growth was estimated by determination of the cell number and the colony formation. The cells were transfected with *miR-26a* or anti-miR-*26a* using FuGene HD (Roche, Indianapolis, IN) according to the manufacturer's protocol. After culture for 24 hours the cells were seeded at an initial density of 1×10^5 per 35 mm-dish. The cells were then harvested at the indicated times and the numbers were counted using the COULTERTM (Beckman, Fullerton, CA, USA).

Cells transfected with *miR-26a* were seeded into 96 well plates at a concentration of 2.5×10^3 cells, and measured after 48 h using a WST-1 assay (Boster, Wuhan, PR China), performed according to the manufacturer's protocol.

A total of 500 cells transfected with *miR-26a* or empty vector (Ctrl) were seeded in 35 mm dishes separately in triplicate. Three weeks later, the colonies were fixed with 4% paraformaldehyde, permeated with 20% methanol and stained with crystal violet. The stained cells were eluted by 10% glacial acetic acid and the

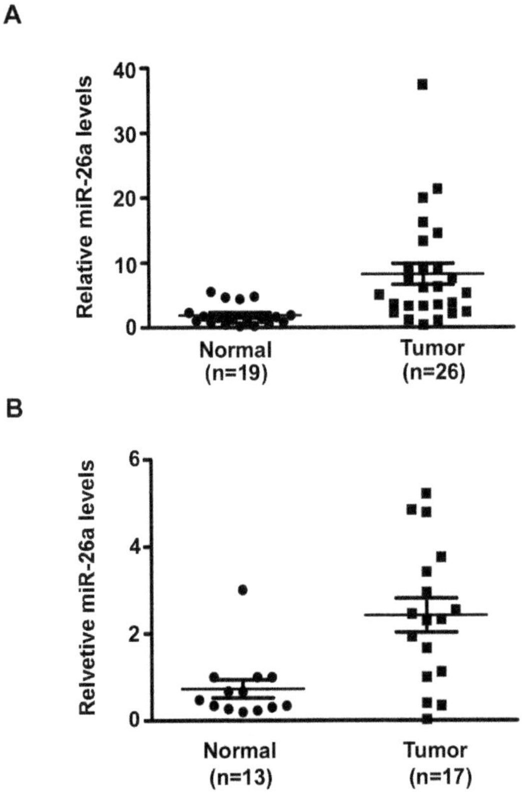

Figure 1. The expression of *miR-26a* was increased in EOC patients. (A)Quantitative analysis of the expression levels of *miR-26a* in EOC samples normalized to those of 18s rRNA by qRT-PCR. Data for each dot were mean value of one sample repeated in three independent experiments (normal, n = 19; tumor, n = 26). **P<0.01 vs Normal. (B)Quantitative analysis of the expression levels of plasma *miR-26a* by qRT-PCR. Data for each dot were mean value of one sample repeated in three independent experiments (normal, n = 13; tumor, n = 17).

OD595 values were measured by spectrophotometer as the indicator of cell number.

Luciferase Reporter Assay

1.5×10^5 SKOV3 stable cells in 35 mm dishes were co-transfected with pGL3-ERα-WT (1 μg) or pGL3-ERα-Mut (1 μg) and pRL-TK (1 μg) using.

FuGENE® HD Transfection Reagent(Roche, Diagnostics Corp., Indianapolis, IN) following the manufacturer's protocol. Forty-eight hours after transfection, luciferase activity was measured using a dual luciferase reporter assay system (Promega) and normalized to Renilla luciferase activity.

Western Blotting

Proteins were separated on SDS–8%PAGE, transferred to PVDF membranes (Amersham, Buckinghamshire, UK) and probed with primary antibodies and secondary antibodies conjugated with horseradish peroxidase. The protein bands were visualized by the Amersham ECL system and scanned. Their densities were determined by ImageQuant 5.2 software (Amersham).

In vivo Tumorigenesis

SKOV3 cells transfected with *miR-26a* or anti-miR-*26a* separately. Each nude mouse was subcutaneously injected with

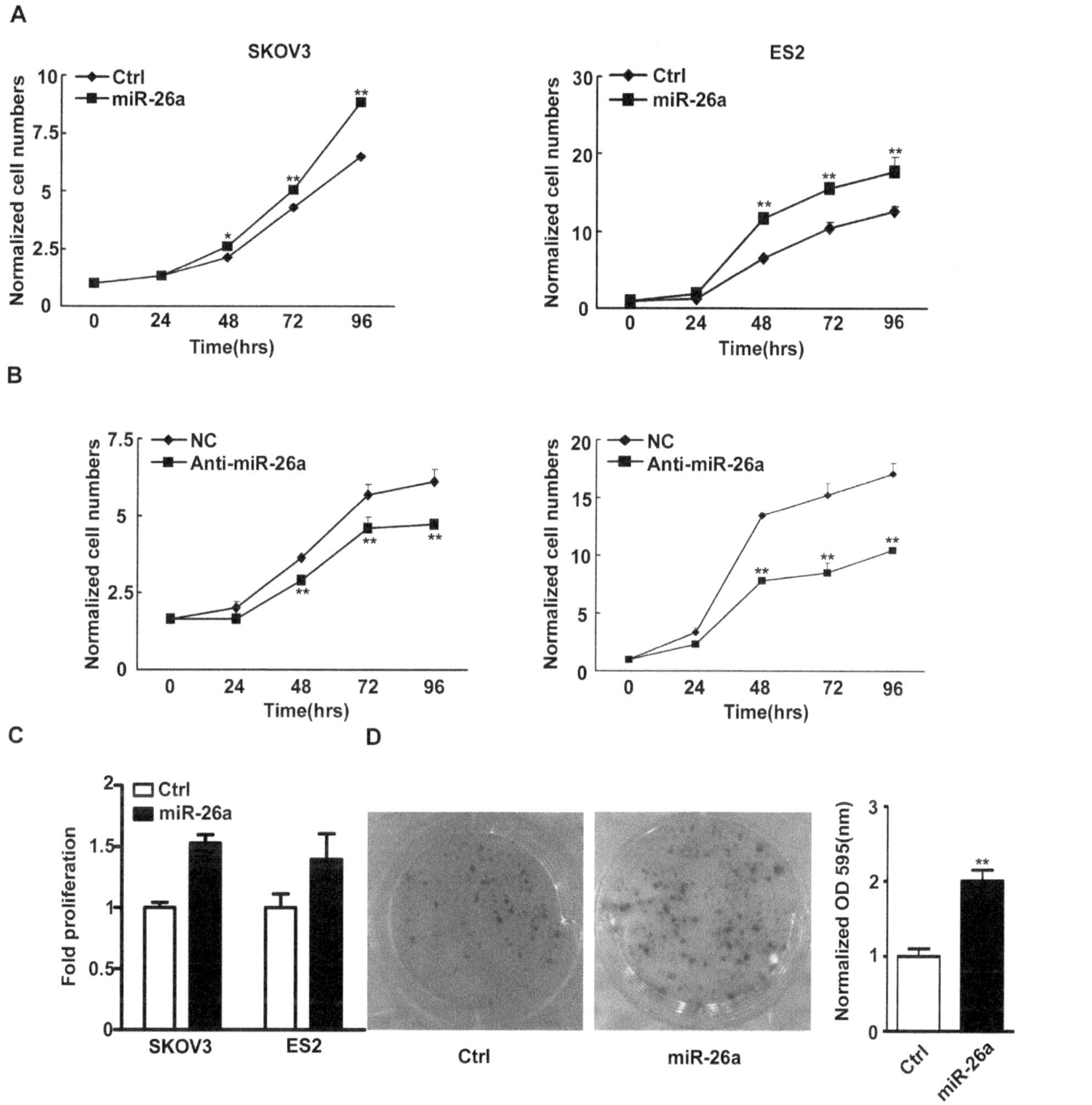

Figure 2. *MiR-26a* promoted EOC cell growth. Growth curves of SKOV3 (A) or ES2 (B) cells transfected with *miR-26a* (left panel) or anti-miR-26a (right panel). Cell numbers were normalized to those in 0 hr. Data were mean±s.e. of three independent experiments in triplicate. $*p<0.05$, $**p<0.01$ vs empty vector (Ctrl) or negative control (NC). (C) Cell proliferation transfected with *miR-26a* was measured by a WST-1 assay. Data were mean±s.e. of three independent experiments in triplicate. $**p<0.01$ vs empty vector (Ctrl) (D) Quantification of the colonies formed by Ctrl or *miR-26a* transfected cells. Data were mean±s.e. of three independent experiments. $**P<0.01$ vs Ctrl.

2×10^6 transfected SKOV3 cells. Thirty or thirty-five days after injection the mice were killed and the tumors were taken. The longest and shortest diameter of the tumor was noted as d1 and d2. The tumor volume was calculated using the equation: $V = d1 \times d2 \times d2/2$. Tumor weight was then measured.

Statistics

Multiple comparisons were assessed by SPSS statistical software for statistical analysis. Wilcoxon Test and Krusikal Wallis H Test were used in statistical analysis of patient samples. Other comparisons between groups for statistical significance were performed with Student's t test and analysis of variance (ANOVA). Results were considered significant difference at $*P<0.05$; $**P<0.01$.

Ethics Statement

The research meets all requirements for the ethics of experiment. Clinical specimens were collected with consent of patients and healthy volunteers and approval of Medical Research Ethics Committee of the First Affiliated Hospital of China Medical

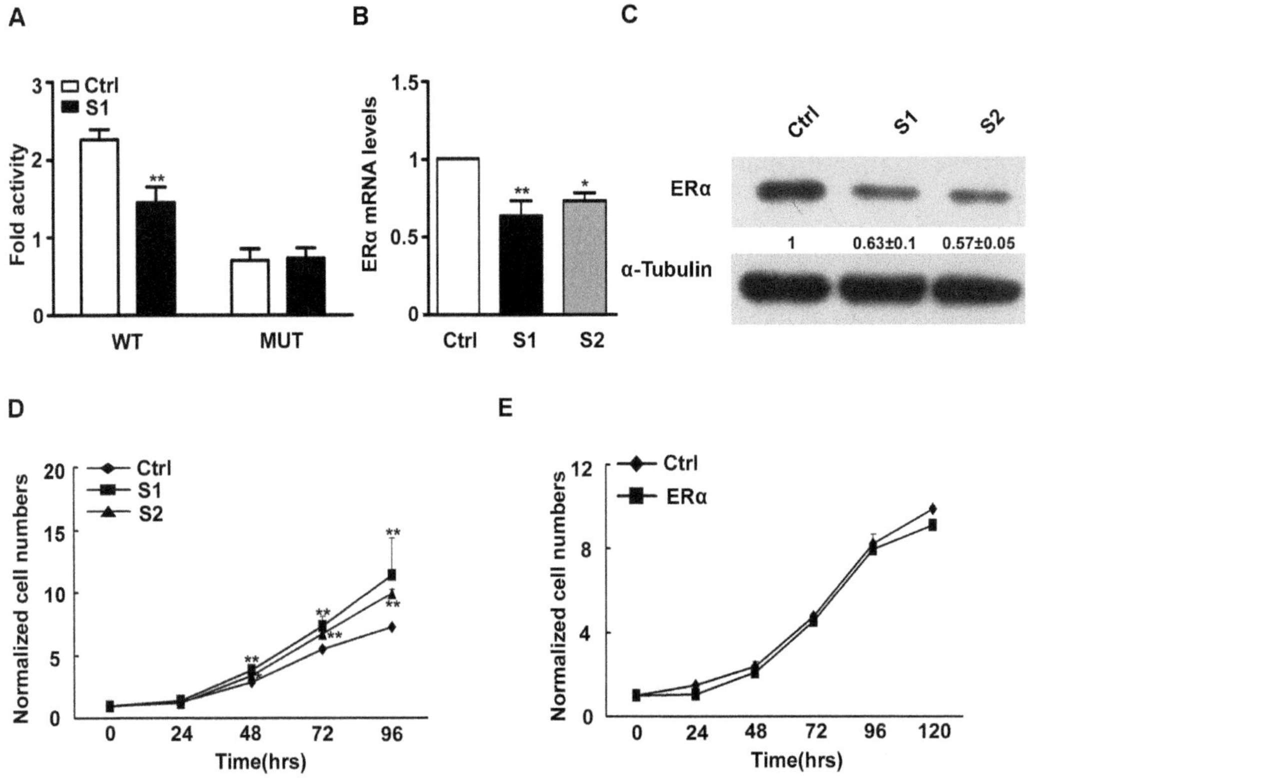

Figure 3. ERα was a target of *miR-26a*. (A) Stable 1 cells (S1) were transfected with pGL3-ERα-WT (WT) reporter vector or pGL3-ERα-Mut (MUT). Data were mean±s.e. of three independent experiments. **P<0.01 vs control cells (Ctrl). (B) Quantitative analysis of the expression levels of ERα in Stable1 (S1), Stable2 (S2) and control (Ctrl) cells were determined and normalized to GAPDH mRNA levels. *p<0.05,**P<0.01 vs Ctrl. (C) Western-blot analysis of total cell lysates extracted from indicated stable cells using the indicated antibodies. Data was representative of three independent experiments and quantitation normalized with the Ctrl. Tubulin served as a loading control. (D) The growth curves of S1, S2 and Ctrl cells. Data were mean±s.e. of three independent experiments in triplicate. *p<0.05, **P<0.01 vs Ctrl. (E) Over-expression of ERα decreased the growth of S1 cells after transfection. Cell numbers were normalized to Ctrl cells. Data were mean±s.e. of three independent experiments in triplicate.

University. All participants have provided their written informed consent to participate in this study. All procedures involving animals were approved by the Institutional Animal Care and Use Committee of China Medical University.

Results

Increased Expression of miR-26a in Specimens and Plasma in Human EOC

It has been observed that the expression level of *miR-26a* was decreased or increased in human malignancies, such as breast carcinoma [16], nasopharyngeal carcinoma [17,18], and glioblastoma [19], indicating a complicated role of *miR-26a* in progression of the malignancies. To investigate the possible role of *miR-26a* in EOC development, we first examined the expression of *miR-26a* in specimens and plasma in EOC by SYBR-Green stem-loop qRT-PCR [20]. We examined the expression of *miR-26a* in 26 tumor samples and 19 normal ovaries. As shown in Figure 1A, the expression levels of *miR-26a* in tumor samples were much higher than those in normal ovary samples. Similarly, the concentrations of *miR-26a* were higher in plasma from EOC patients (n = 17) than in that from healthy controls (n = 13) (Figure 1B). Together, these results provide us initial evidence that *miR-26a* may play a role in the development of human EOC.

Over-expressing miR-26a Promoted EOC Cell Growth and Inhibiting miR-26a Suppressed EOC Cell Proliferation

We next examined whether *miR-26a* affects EOC cell growth using SKOV3 and ES2 cells as models. As shown in Figure 2A, the growth ability of SKOV3 and ES2 cells was increased by over-expression of *miR-26a*. On the contrary, the proliferation of the cells transfected with anti-miR-26a was markedly decreased compared with that of the cells transfected with nonsense (Figure 2B). WST-1 assay showed similar results in cell proliferation (Figure 2C). These results suggest that *miR-26a* indeed affected EOC cell growth.

The notion was further tested in the clonal formation assay. The number and size of the colonies formed were markedly increased in *miR-26a* transfected cells (Figure 2D). Together, these results suggest that *miR-26a* was indeed involved in the regulation of EOC cell growth.

ERα was a Target Gene of miR-26a in EOC Cells

We then investigated the mechanisms by which *miR-26a* promote EOC cell proliferation. In patients with hepatocellular carcinoma, the expression of *miR-26a* was higher in women than in men [21]. Moreover, *miR-26a* regulated liver tumor cell growth by targeting ERα [22]. As shown in Figure 3A, the luciferase activity of pGL3-ERα-WT in SKOV3-stable1 cells (S1) was much lower than in control cells. The luciferase activity of pGL3-ERα-Mut was rescued in Stable1 cells. We next examined whether *miR-*

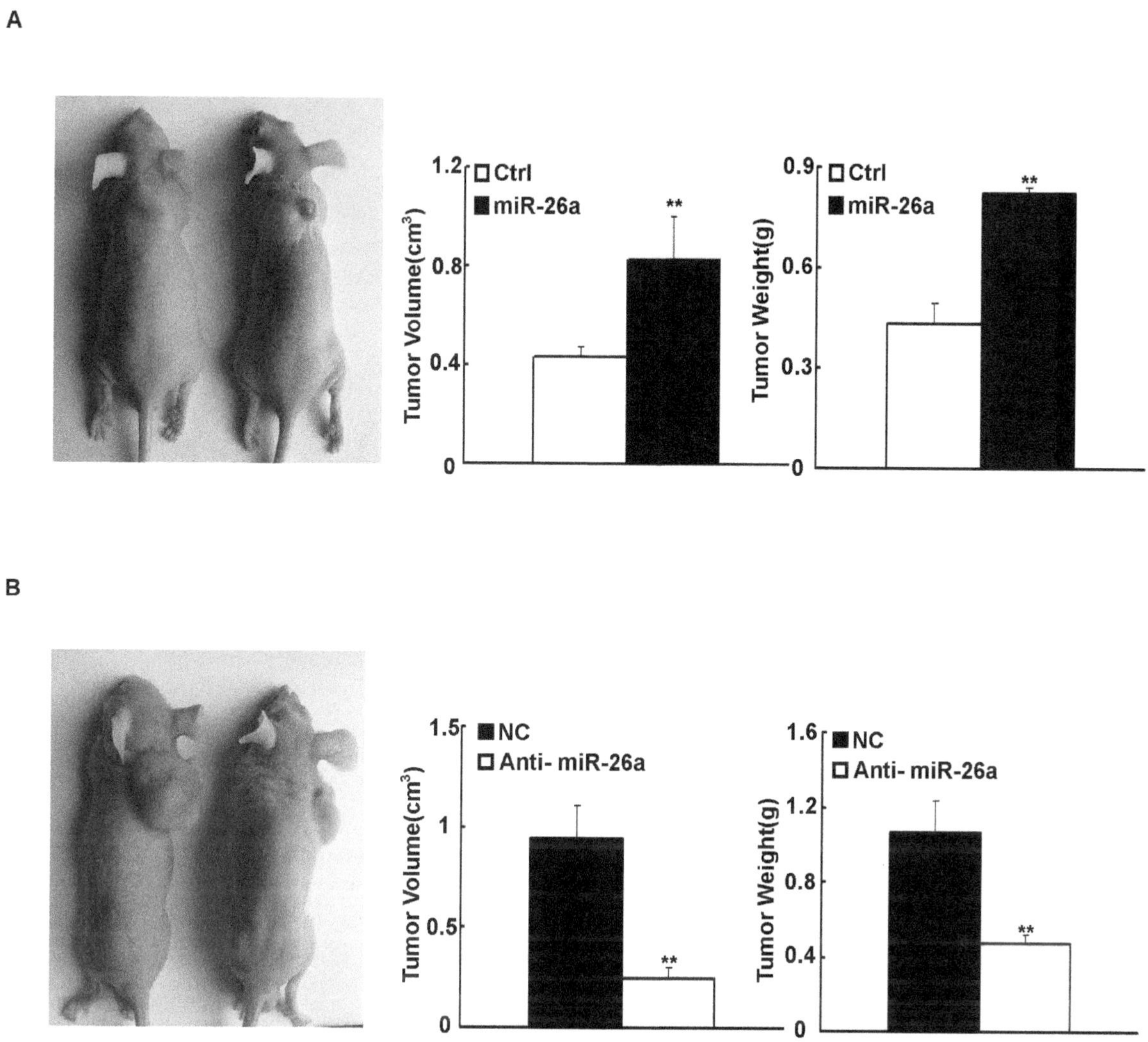

Figure 4. *MiR-26a* promoted the development of tumor in nude mice. Tumor formation generated by the SKOV3 cells. (A) transfected with *miR-26a* or anti-miR-26a(B) Nude mice were subcutaneously injected with 2×10^6 transfected cells. Representative images, measurement of the final volume and weight of the tumors formed. The tumor sizes were measured and calculated in Materials and methods. Data were mean±s.d. of 4–6 mice. **P<0.01 vs empty vector or nonsense.

26a could regulate endogenous ERα expression in EOC cells. Compared with control, endogenous ERα mRNA levels (Figure 3B) and protein levels (Figure 3C) were down-regulated when cells were transfected with *miR-26a*.

MiR-26a Controlled the Proliferation of EOC Cells through ERα

Given the fact that *miR-26a* was involved in proliferation of EOC cells and ERα was a target of *miR-26a*, we next tested whether over-expression of ERα could rescue promotion of proliferation by *miR-26a* in EOC cells. Moreover, stable expression of *miR-26a* in two SKOV3 cell clones (S1 or S2) increased the growth of the cells about 1.58 or 1.37 fold, respectively (Figure 3D). QRT-PCR analysis showed that *miR-26a* expression level was greatly increased in S1 and S2 cells (Figure S1). As shown in Figure 3E, whereas growth of S1 cells transfected with ERα, were not different from that of control cells. These results indicate that *miR-26a* controlled proliferation of EOC cells through regulation of ERα expression.

MiR-26a Promoted the Development of Tumor in Nude Mice

To provide direct evidence that *miR-26a* was responsible for EOC development, SKOV3 cells transfected with either *miR-26a* or anti-miR-26a were injected into the flank of nude mice as described. A week after implantation, xenografted tumors could be seen. After thirty or thirty-five days, all nude mice were killed and the tumors were taken out and weighed. At the macroscopic observation, the differences in tumor size and volume among the two groups were indicated. The tumor volume generated from empty vector was 0.435±0.042 (cm^3, P<0.01), that in *miR-26a* group was 0.829±0.172 (cm^3, P<0.01) (Figure 4A), that in negative control group was 0.941±0.163 (cm^3, P<0.01), and that in anti-miR-26a was 0.248±0.05 (cm^3, P<0.01) (Figure 4B). The average weight of the tumor generated from empty vector was 0.433±0.07, whereas the average weight of the tumor generated from *miR-26a* was 0.821±0.02 (gram, P<0.01). The average weight of the tumor generated from nonsense was 1.062±0.169, whereas the average weight of the tumor generated from anti-miR-26a was 0.473±0.05 (gram, P<0.01), respectively. The results mentioned above suggest that *miR-26a* was critical for the development of EOC *in vivo*.

Discussion

In this study, we have shown that expression level of *miR-26a* was greatly increased in human EOC samples, and blood-based *miR-26a* level can distinguish patients from healthy controls in EOC. Our results also displayed that expression level of *miR-26a* affected EOC cell growth in culture. Moreover, ERα was a target for *miR-26a* in EOC cells. Furthermore, expression level of *miR-26a* affected tumor formation in nude mice. Therefore, our results are consistent with an idea that *miR-26a* is critical for the development of human EOC.

MicroRNAs are known to regulate the expression of genes involved in several biological processes such as development, proliferation, apoptosis and stress response [23]. Recent studies showed a direct link between miRNAs and human cancers [4,24,25,26]. MiRNAs can be oncogenic miRNA (oncomirs) or tumor suppressor relevant to cancer. As previously shown, loss of oncogenic *miR-21*, acting to repress RHOB expression, is associated with an elevation of RHOB in hepatocellular carcinoma and breast cancer cells [13]. The importance of other miRNAs, such as *let-7*, *miR-16*, *miR-126* and *miR-125b* has also been demonstrated [27]. Recent microarray profile data shows *miR-26a* dysregulation in diverse cancer [4]. In liver cancer, *miR-26a* protects normal liver tissue from hepatocellular carcinoma-promoting inflammation[21], and appears to antagonize human breast cancer [16] and rhabdomyosarcoma [28]. On the contrary, *miR-26a* facilitates glioblastoma formation as an oncogene [19]. Our results obtained from gain-of-function and loss-of-function approaches indicated that *miR-26a* promoted proliferation and inhibition of *miR-26a* suppressed EOC cell proliferation.

In ovarian cancer, ERα expression has been studied to correlate to chlinico-pathological parameters and prognosis [29,30]. Previous study showed that it did not reveal any correlations with histologic type of tumors and ovarian cancer grading [30]. Univariate survival analysis revealed that patients with positive-ERα status had a significant better progression-free survival compared with the patients with no expression[31]. In our results, the expression of *miR-26a* in specimens and plasma in EOC were much higher than those in normal ovary samples, and *miR-26a* promote EOC cell proliferation by targeting ERα. It means that *miR-26a* might be an important factor in the survival of ovarian cancer.

Circulating biomarkers are used to diagnostic disease, monitor therapeutic effect and predict recurrence in clinical applications. The discovery of circulating miRNAs in cancer patients indicates their potential application as powerful biomarkers in cancer diagnostics[32]. Recent studies revealed that cancer-related miRNAs could stably detectable in plasma and serum which originate from cancer tissues [4,33]. Our results investigate the possibility of *miR-26a* applied as a biomarker in clinical setting through examining the expression of *miR-26a* in plasma of EOC patients.

In conclusion, inhibition of *miR-26a* decreased EOC cell growth in culture and in nude mice. *MiR-26a* affected proliferation of EOC cells by targeting ERα. An important implication of current study is that *miR-26a* might be a potential target for therapeutic intervention to human EOC.

Supporting Information

Figure S1 *MiR-26a* expression level was greatly increased in S1 and S2 cells. QRT-PCR determined the expression levels of *miR-26a* in S1 and S2 cells. Data were mean±s.e. of three independent experiments in triplicate. $^{**}P<0.01$ vs Ctrl.

Table S1 clinicopathologic data and *miR-26a* expression level of control.

Table S2 clinicopathologic data and *miR-26a* expression level of ovarian cancer patients.

Table S3 Primers used in Quantative RT-PCR.

Author Contributions

Conceived and designed the experiments: WS MS. Performed the experiments: WS MS JL GQ TL YH HL. Analyzed the data: WS MS HL. Contributed reagents/materials/analysis tools: WS MS JL GQ TL YH HL. Wrote the paper: WS.

References

1. Hoskins WJ (1995) Prospective on ovarian cancer: why prevent? J Cell Biochem Suppl 23: 189–199.
2. Filipowicz W, Bhattacharyya SN, Sonenberg N (2008) Mechanisms of post-transcriptional regulation by microRNAs: are the answers in sight? Nat Rev Genet 9: 102–114.
3. Hwang HW, Mendell JT (2006) MicroRNAs in cell proliferation, cell death, and tumorigenesis. Br J Cancer 94: 776–780.
4. Calin GA, Croce CM (2006) MicroRNA signatures in human cancers. Nat Rev Cancer 6: 857–866.
5. Takamizawa J, Konishi H, Yanagisawa K, Tomida S, Osada H, et al. (2004) Reduced expression of the let-7 microRNAs in human lung cancers in association with shortened postoperative survival. Cancer Res 64: 3753–3756.
6. Johnson SM, Grosshans H, Shingara J, Byrom M, Jarvis R, et al. (2005) RAS is regulated by the let-7 microRNA family. Cell 120: 635–647.
7. Meng F, Henson R, Wehbe-Janek H, Ghoshal K, Jacob ST, et al. (2007) MicroRNA-21 regulates expression of the PTEN tumor suppressor gene in human hepatocellular cancer. Gastroenterology 133: 647–658.
8. Bonci D, Coppola V, Musumeci M, Addario A, Giuffrida R, et al. (2008) The miR-15a-miR-16-1 cluster controls prostate cancer by targeting multiple oncogenic activities. Nat Med 14: 1271–1277.
9. Medina PP, Nolde M, Slack FJ (2010) OncomiR addiction in an in vivo model of microRNA-21-induced pre-B-cell lymphoma. Nature 467: 86–90.
10. Zhang L, Volinia S, Bonome T, Calin GA, Greshock J, et al. (2008) Genomic and epigenetic alterations deregulate microRNA expression in human epithelial ovarian cancer. Proc Natl Acad Sci U S A 105: 7004–7009.
11. Chen C, Ridzon DA, Broomer AJ, Zhou Z, Lee DH, et al. (2005) Real-time quantification of microRNAs by stem-loop RT-PCR. Nucleic Acids Res 33: e179.
12. Mitchell PS, Parkin RK, Kroh EM, Fritz BR, Wyman SK, et al. (2008) Circulating microRNAs as stable blood-based markers for cancer detection. Proc Natl Acad Sci U S A 105: 10513–10518.
13. Chang TC, Yu D, Lee YS, Wentzel EA, Arking DE, et al. (2008) Widespread microRNA repression by Myc contributes to tumorigenesis. Nat Genet 40: 43–50.
14. Mohamed JS, Lopez MA, Boriek AM (2010) Mechanical stretch up-regulates microRNA-26a and induces human airway smooth muscle hypertrophy by suppressing glycogen synthase kinase-3beta. J Biol Chem 285: 29336–29347.
15. Bake S, Ma L, Sohrabji F (2008) Estrogen receptor-alpha overexpression suppresses 17beta-estradiol-mediated vascular endothelial growth factor expression and activation of survival kinases. Endocrinology 149: 3881–3889.
16. Zhang B, Liu XX, He JR, Zhou CX, Guo M, et al. (2011) Pathologically decreased miR-26a antagonizes apoptosis and facilitates carcinogenesis by targeting MTDH and EZH2 in breast cancer. Carcinogenesis 32: 2–9.
17. Baffa R, Fassan M, Volinia S, O'Hara B, Liu CG, et al. (2009) MicroRNA expression profiling of human metastatic cancers identifies cancer gene targets. J Pathol 219: 214–221.
18. Lu J, He ML, Wang L, Chen Y, Liu X, et al. (2011) MiR-26a inhibits cell growth and tumorigenesis of nasopharyngeal carcinoma through repression of EZH2. Cancer Res 71: 225–233.

19. Huse JT, Brennan C, Hambardzumyan D, Wee B, Pena J, et al. (2009) The PTEN-regulating microRNA miR-26a is amplified in high-grade glioma and facilitates gliomagenesis in vivo. Genes Dev 23: 1327–1337.
20. Feng J, Wang K, Liu X, Chen S, Chen J (2009) The quantification of tomato microRNAs response to viral infection by stem-loop real-time RT-PCR. Gene 437: 14–21.
21. Ji J, Shi J, Budhu A, Yu Z, Forgues M, et al. (2009) MicroRNA expression, survival, and response to interferon in liver cancer. N Engl J Med 361: 1437–1447.
22. Chen L, Zheng J, Zhang Y, Yang L, Wang J, et al. (2011) Tumor-specific expression of microRNA-26a suppresses human hepatocellular carcinoma growth via cyclin-dependent and -independent pathways. Mol Ther 19: 1521–1528.
23. He L, Hannon GJ (2004) MicroRNAs: small RNAs with a big role in gene regulation. Nat Rev Genet 5: 522–531.
24. Calin GA, Dumitru CD, Shimizu M, Bichi R, Zupo S, et al. (2002) Frequent deletions and down-regulation of micro- RNA genes miR15 and miR16 at 13q14 in chronic lymphocytic leukemia. Proc Natl Acad Sci U S A 99: 15524–15529.
25. Michael MZ, SM OC, van Holst Pellekaan NG, Young GP, James RJ (2003) Reduced accumulation of specific microRNAs in colorectal neoplasia. Mol Cancer Res 1: 882–891.
26. Garofalo M, Croce CM (2011) microRNAs: Master regulators as potential therapeutics in cancer. Annu Rev Pharmacol Toxicol 51: 25–43.
27. Fujii YR (2009) Oncoviruses and Pathogenic MicroRNAs in Humans. Open Virol J 3: 37–51.
28. Ciarapica R, Russo G, Verginelli F, Raimondi L, Donfrancesco A, et al. (2009) Deregulated expression of miR-26a and Ezh2 in rhabdomyosarcoma. Cell Cycle 8: 172–175.
29. Cunat S, Hoffmann P, Pujol P (2004) Estrogens and epithelial ovarian cancer. Gynecol Oncol 94: 25–32.
30. Hecht JL, Kotsopoulos J, Hankinson SE, Tworoger SS (2009) Relationship between epidemiologic risk factors and hormone receptor expression in ovarian cancer: results from the Nurses' Health Study. Cancer Epidemiol Biomarkers Prev 18: 1624–1630.
31. Halon A, Materna V, Drag-Zalesinska M, Nowak-Markwitz E, Gansukh T, et al. (2011) Estrogen receptor alpha expression in ovarian cancer predicts longer overall survival. Pathol Oncol Res 17: 511–518.
32. Ma R, Jiang T, Kang X (2012) Circulating microRNAs in cancer: origin, function and application. J Exp Clin Cancer Res 31: 38.
33. Chen X, Ba Y, Ma L, Cai X, Yin Y, et al. (2008) Characterization of microRNAs in serum: a novel class of biomarkers for diagnosis of cancer and other diseases. Cell Res 18: 997–1006.

6

Molecular Profiling of Multiple Human Cancers Defines an Inflammatory Cancer-Associated Molecular Pattern and Uncovers KPNA2 as a Uniform Poor Prognostic Cancer Marker

Saleh M. Rachidi[1,2], Tingting Qin[3], Shaoli Sun[4], W. Jim Zheng[3,5], Zihai Li[1,2]*

1 Department of Microbiology and Immunology, South Carolina Clinical and Translational Research Institute (SCTR), Medical University of South Carolina, Charleston, South Carolina, United States of America, **2** Hollings Cancer Center, South Carolina Clinical and Translational Research Institute (SCTR), Medical University of South Carolina, Charleston, South Carolina, United States of America, **3** Division of Bioinformatics, Department of Biochemistry and Molecular Biology, South Carolina Clinical and Translational Research Institute (SCTR), Medical University of South Carolina, Charleston, South Carolina, United States of America, **4** Department of Pathology and Laboratory Medicine, South Carolina Clinical and Translational Research Institute (SCTR), Medical University of South Carolina, Charleston, South Carolina, United States of America, **5** Computational Biology Core Facility, South Carolina Clinical and Translational Research Institute (SCTR), Medical University of South Carolina, Charleston, South Carolina, United States of America

Abstract

Background: Immune evasion is one of the recognized hallmarks of cancer. Inflammatory responses to cancer can also contribute directly to oncogenesis. Since the immune system is hardwired to protect the host, there is a possibility that cancers, regardless of their histological origins, endow themselves with a common and shared inflammatory cancer-associated molecular pattern (iCAMP) to promote oncoinflammation. However, the definition of iCAMP has not been conceptually and experimentally investigated.

Methods and Findings: Genome-wide cDNA expression data was analyzed for 221 normal and 324 cancer specimens from 7 cancer types: breast, prostate, lung, colon, gastric, oral and pancreatic. A total of 96 inflammatory genes with consistent dysregulation were identified, including 44 up-regulated and 52 down-regulated genes. Protein expression was confirmed by immunohistochemistry for some of these genes. The iCAMP contains proteins whose roles in cancer have been implicated and others which are yet to be appreciated. The clinical significance of many iCAMP genes was confirmed in multiple independent cohorts of colon and ovarian cancer patients. In both cases, better prognosis correlated strongly with high *CXCL13* and low level of *GREM1, LOX, TNFAIP6, CD36*, and *EDNRA*. An "Inflammatory Gene Integrated Score" was further developed from the combination of 18 iCAMP genes in ovarian cancer, which predicted overall survival. Noticeably, as a selective nuclear import protein whose immuno-regulatory function just begins to emerge, karyopherin alpha 2 (KPNA2) is uniformly up-regulated across cancer types. For the first time, the cancer-specific up-regulation of KPNA2 and its clinical significance were verified by tissue microarray analysis in colon and head-neck cancers.

Conclusion: This work defines an inflammatory signature shared by seven epithelial cancer types and KPNA2 as a consistently up-regulated protein in cancer. Identification of iCAMP may not only serve as a novel biomarker for prognostication and individualized treatment of cancer, but also have significant biological implications.

Editor: Matthew L. Anderson, Baylor College of Medicine, United States of America

Funding: This research was partly supported by pilot projects from National Institutes of Health/National Center for Research Resources (NIH/NCRR) grants P20 RR017696-05 and P20 RR017677; National Institute of General Medical Sciences (NIH/NIGMS) R01GM063265-09S1; PhRMA Foundation Research Starter Grant (to W.J.Z); T.Q. was supported by PhRMA Foundation Research Starter Grant, NIH/NCRR 5P20RR017677-10, NIH/NIGMS R01GM063265-09S1 and T32GM074934 07. Z.L. is supported by NIH grants. The funders had no role in study design, data collection and analysis, decision to publish, or preparation of the manuscript.

Competing Interests: The authors have declared that no competing interests exist.

* E-mail: zihai@musc.edu

Introduction

The relationship between cancer and inflammation was observed as early as the 19th century, when Ronald Virchow described tumor-infiltrating leukocytes. However, it was not until the past two decades that the inflammatory microenvironment has been recognized as a key component in carcinogenesis, being involved in cancer initiation, promotion and metastasis [1]. Chronic infections are established etiological factors for many human cancers [2]. Similarly, chronic inflammation such as inflammatory bowel disease and chronic hepatitis increases the risk for colorectal and hepatocellular carcinomas, respectively. In most cases, immune-surveillance is thought to eliminate tumorigenic foci [3]. However, cancer-initiating cells reprogram immune cells to create a tumor-friendly microenvironment, thereby evading antitumor immunity. In addition, cancer can educate both the

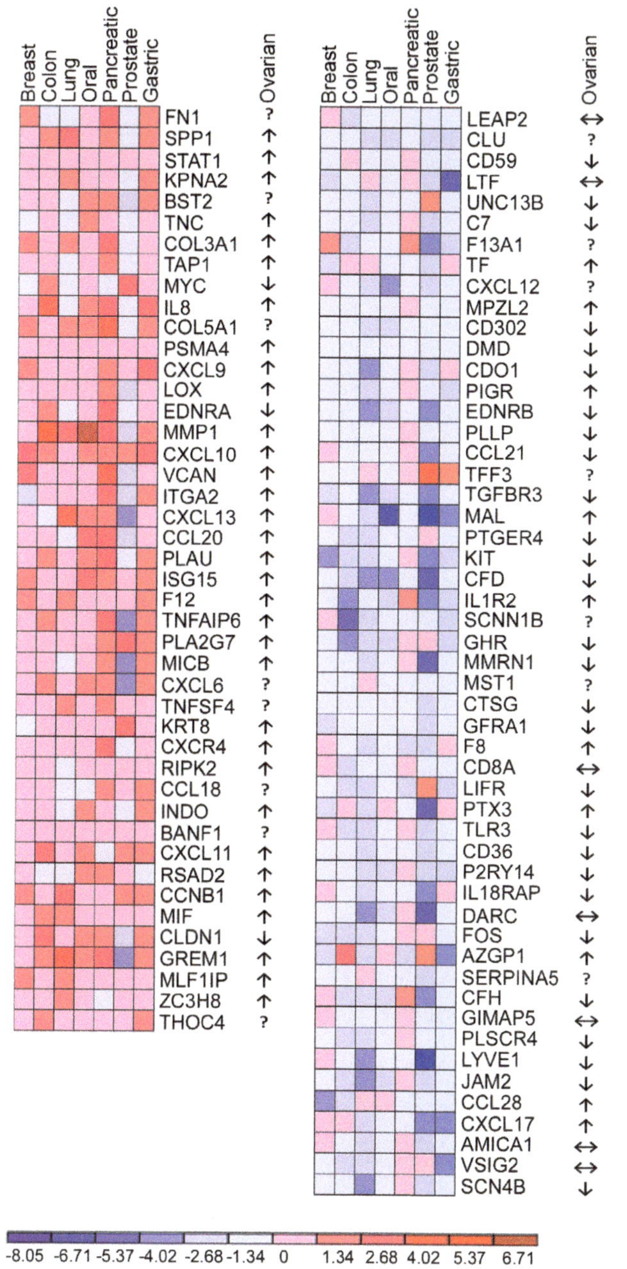

Figure 1. Heat map of dysregulated inflammatory genes. Heat map showing the 44 up-regulated and 52 down-regulated genes across the seven cancer types, in addition to the direction of dysregulation in ovarian cancer. ↑, up-regulated. ↓, down-regulated. ↔, unchanged.

innate and adaptive arms of the immune system through myeloid-derived suppressor cells [4], regulatory T cells [5] and other mediators, to promote growth and invasion.

The role of inflammation in carcinogenesis begins with tumor initiation, through multiple mechanisms such as genotoxic stress via reactive oxygen species, induction of activation-induced cytidine deaminase (AID) [6], TNF-α-induced entry of β-catenin into the nucleus [7] and others. Beyond initiation, cytokines activate pro-tumorigenic transcription factors such as STAT3 and NF-κB in existing cancer cells [8]. Inflammatory cells also dampen antitumor immunity through molecules such as indoleamine-2,3-dioxygenase and arginase 1, which interfere with the function of T lymphocytes [4]. Epithelial-mesenchymal transition is also favored by cytokines such as TGF-β, promoting distal metastasis [9].

"Onco-inflammation" therefore contributes to the different cancer hallmarks, including cell proliferation, angiogenesis and escape from apoptosis. However, despite this elaborate cross-talk between cancer cells and the inflammatory microenvironment, the approach to uncover critical players in this interaction has so far been sporadic and non-comprehensive. In this study, we hypothesize that a common inflammatory pattern exists among different cancer types, constituting a signature profile termed as iCAMP. We performed a comprehensive analysis of gene expression across 7 common epithelial cancer types. A robust oncoinflammatory profile was identified, demonstrating independent and strong predictive values in clinical outcomes of multiple cancers. This approach has also led to the discovery and validation of KPNA2 as the single most consistently up-regulated protein in cancer.

Methods

Ethics Statement

Access to patient samples and anonymous analysis of data was approved by the Institutional Review Board for Human Research at the Medical University of South Carolina.

Datasets

This analysis included gene expression profiles from 7 types of cancer. One dataset was included for each cancer type, resulting in a total of 7 datasets. The cancers included in this study are: breast,

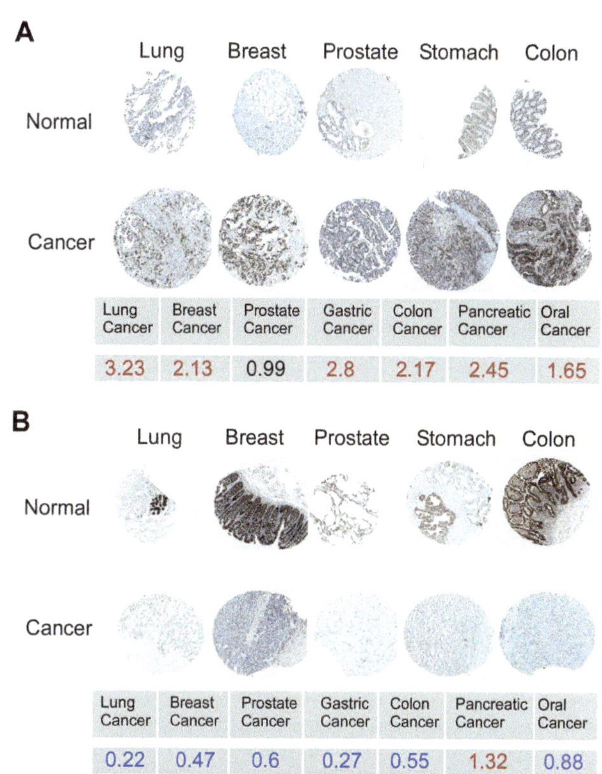

Figure 2. Expression of KPNA2 and PIGR in multiple cancer types. An example of an up-regulated gene (KPNA2) (A) and a down-regulated gene (PIGR) (B) in 5 cancer types on the protein level. Numbers correspond to average fold changes of the mRNA levels across all 7 cancer types in the current study.

colon, lung, oral, prostate, pancreatic and gastric cancers [10,11,12,13,14,15,16]. Datasets were obtained from Gene Expression Omnibus (GEO) Datasets, an NCBI public database. Each of the datasets included microarray mRNA expression data from cancer and normal tissue (Table S1). All of the datasets used [HG-U133_Plus_2] Affymetrix Human Genome U133 Plus 2.0 Array platform for quantification of gene expression levels.

CDEP analysis on seven GEO datasets

The seven epithelial cancer types were investigated to identify genes showing consistent differential expression using the recently developed Consistent Differential Expression Pattern (CDEP) method [17]. The raw microarray data comparing gene expression between normal and cancer cells was downloaded from NCBI's GEO database (http://www.ncbi.nlm.nih.gov/gds/) (Table S1). After excluding 10 adenoma samples in the colon dataset, 545 samples were studied, of which 324 were from cancer tissue and 221 were normal. The expression values of the replicate samples in the pancreatic cancer dataset were averaged. The raw datasets were pre-processed individually. For each dataset, gene expression values were adjusted and normalized by the GCRMA approach implemented in R [18]. The false discovery rate (FDR) of each gene on each normalized dataset was calculated using permutation method implemented by the "RankProd" package in R [19]. Each gene in each dataset was then associated with a raw FDR, $F_{gi}^{up}(F_{gi}^{down})$ for being up/down-regulated [17]. For genes not present in the platform of a dataset, the median FDR value of that dataset was assigned [17].

CDEP meta-analysis was then applied to the raw FDRs of the seven datasets. For each dataset, the false positive rate is defined as the probability of a non-up-regulated gene being falsely called as over-expressed (or a non-down-regulated gene being falsely called as repressed). The number of genes being up-regulated, down-regulated, and non-differentially expressed for each dataset was estimated by a Beta mixture model implemented in WinBUGS [20]. Based on this rate and using independent Bernoulli distributions, we calculated the likelihood of a gene to be falsely identified as over/under-expressed among the seven datasets for each FDR threshold l. The procedure was evaluated by estimating the false discovery rate (FDR_g) observing the above expected log likelihood, i.e. the proportion of false positives among the genes identified to be consistently differentially expressed. The "null log likelihood" was computed by permuting the $F_{gi}^{up}(F_{gi}^{down})$values relative to the genes within each dataset, and then performing the same above procedures to calculate the expected value of the "null log likelihood" in each permutation b for every gene, using $FDR_g = 0.05$ as a cutoff.

Database for Annotation, Visualization and Integrated Discovery (DAVID)

After identifying the differentially expressed genes across the 7 cancer types, the set of up-regulated and down-regulated genes was entered into DAVID database (http://david.abcc.ncifcrf.gov/), and those with gene annotations related to inflammation and/or immune response were selected for further analysis.

Human Protein Atlas (HPAT)

Six of the seven cancer types and their corresponding normal tissue were investigated for the protein expression level of all of the immune-related genes by HPAT (www.proteinatlas.org).

Oncomine Cancer Database

Oncomine database (www.oncomine.org) was used to identify the clinical significance of the immune-related genes and their ability to predict patient survival and disease recurrence. X-tile software [21] was used to determine the optimal cut-off points for separating low risk from high risk patients.

Inflammatory Gene Integrated Score (IGIS)

IGIS for each ovarian cancer patient is the summation of the risk value of 18 iCAMP genes with independent prognostic significance demonstrated by the training dataset [22]. These genes are *CCL28, CXL12, EDNRRB, GFRA1, GREM1, IL8, JAM2, LOX, MAL, MIF, MPZL2, PIGR, PTGER4, RSAD2, SERPINA5, TFF3, TNFAIP6 and TNFSF4.* The predictive value of IGIS was tested using an independent TCGA ovarian cancer dataset, based on cut-off values pre-determined by the training dataset [22]. For a given patient, the value of a gene conferring poor prognosis is its relative risk (RR), whereas the value of a gene whose expression in that patient predicts better prognosis was set as zero. As an example, if a patient A falls in the high risk group for genes 1 and 2 but in the low risk group for gene 3, this patient's IGIS will be the summation of Relative Risk for gene 1 and Relative Risk for gene 2, since the value of gene 3 is zero.

Ingenuity Pathway Analysis (IPA)

Using the Ingenuity Pathway Analysis tool (www.ingenuity.com), inflammatory genes were mapped into multiple networks, each showing over-expressed and under-expressed ones.

Tissue Microarrays

Tissue microarrays (TMAs) for colon cancer and head-neck cancer specimens contained formalin-fixed, paraffin embedded tissues. Colon cancer TMAs were developed from patient specimens obtained at the Medical University of South Carolina (MUSC), Charleston, SC, USA. Our study was approved by the Institutional Review Board. The colon cancer cohort consisted of tumors from 55 patients and adjacent normal tissue from 50 of them, along with 15 lymph node metastatic samples. Each of the normal and cancer specimens was at least in duplicate. Clinical and demographic information including age, sex, histologic type, grade, tumor (T) and lymph node (N) stages, overall and recurrence-free survival were obtained from the Cancer Registry of the Hollings Cancer Center at the Medical University of South Carolina. The head-neck cancer TMA was obtained from US Biomax, which contained 60 head-neck squamous cell carcinomas and normal specimens from 9 independent patients.

Immunohistochemistry (IHC)

5-μm sections were cut from the TMA blocks. KPNA2 staining was performed using a rabbit polyclonal antibody specific to human KPNA2 (Abcam, Cat # 84440) at 1:500 dilution. Slides were baked for 1 hour at 60°C and de-paraffinized. After antigen retrieval using citrate buffer (pH = 6.0), endogenous peroxidase was quenched using 3% H_2O_2 in dH_2O for 5 minutes and non-specific binding was blocked by 2% normal goat serum for 3 hours at room temperature. Samples were incubated with anti-KPNA2 antibody at 4°C for 16 hours, followed by secondary antibody (Vectastain ABC Kit, PK-4001) and development using DAB substrate (Vector Labs SK-4100). Staining showed absolute specificity to the nucleus without discernible off-target signal. KPNA2 quantification was performed by a surgical pathologist (S.S.) who was blinded to the patient's clinical parameters. Quantification included nuclear staining intensity (1: faint;

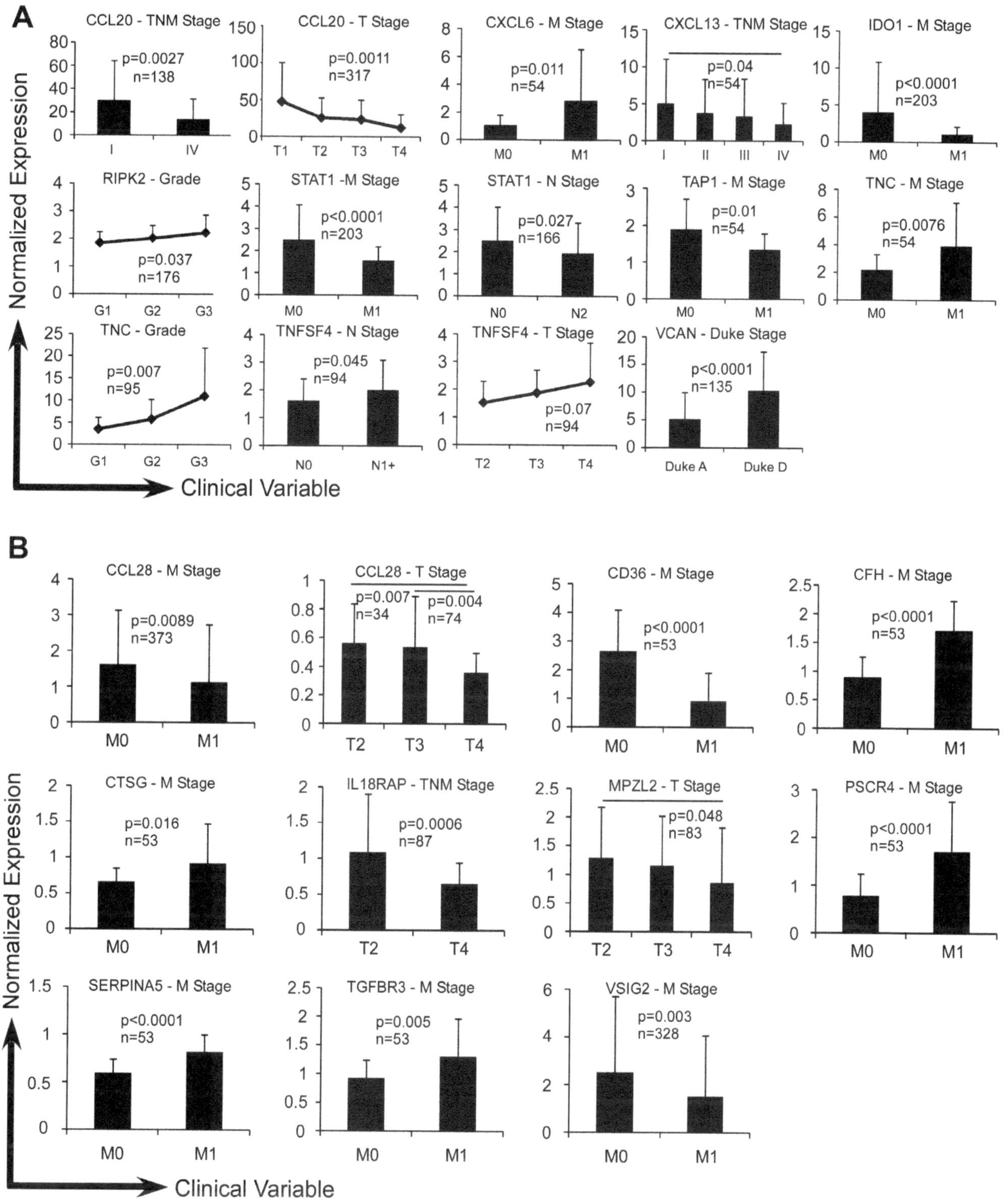

Figure 3. Up-regulated (A) and down-regulated (B) genes with clinical correlations in colon cancer. Four independent studies were analyzed for the expression of indicated genes and their clinical significance. The vertical axis represents the normalized expression intensity of each gene relative to the median intensity of the entire gene probes. Error bars represent standard deviation. Genes are listed in alphabetical order.

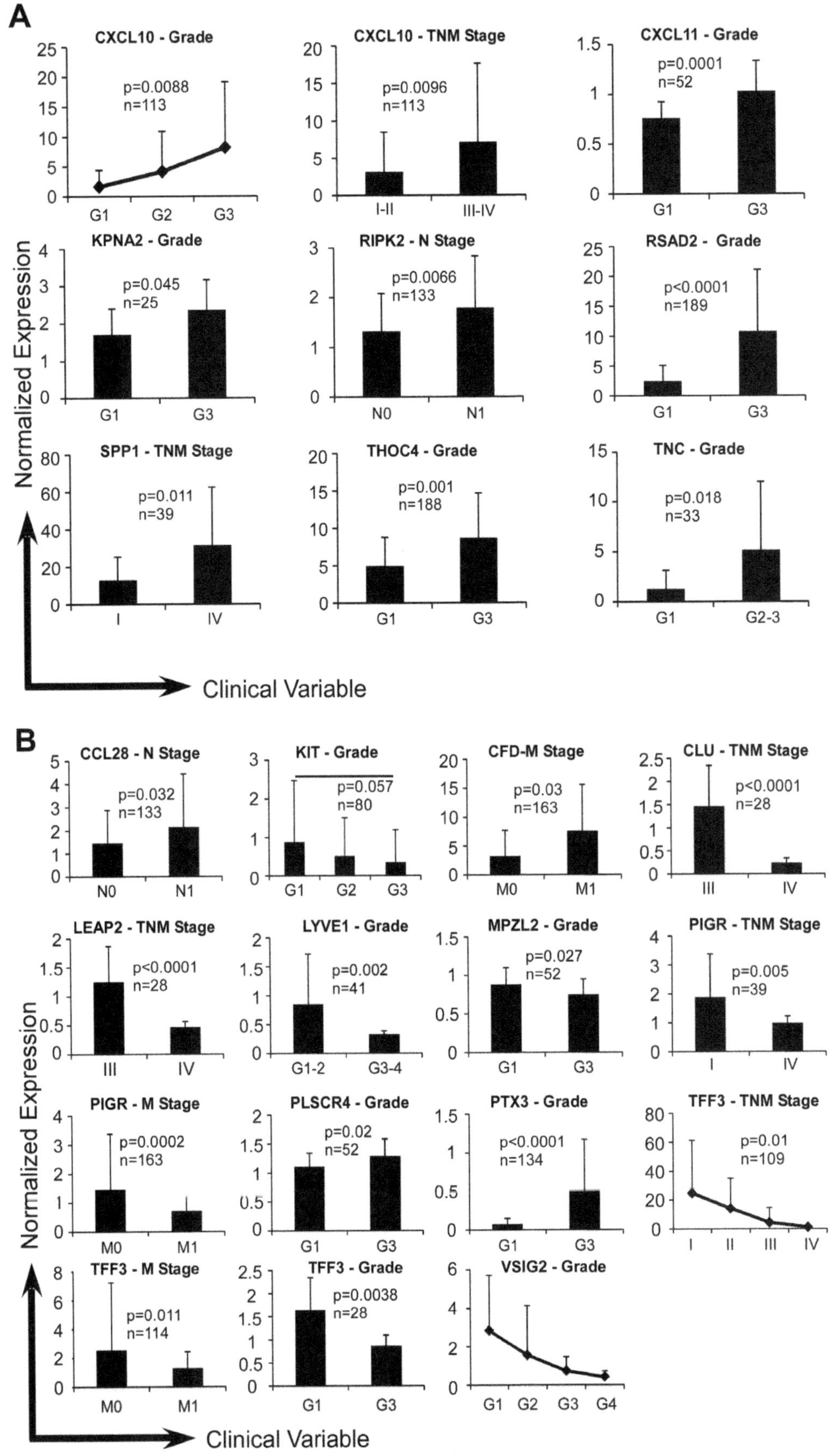
A
CXCL10 - Grade
p=0.0088
n=113
CXCL10 - TNM Stage
p=0.0096
n=113
CXCL11 - Grade
p=0.0001
n=52
KPNA2 - Grade
p=0.045
n=25
RIPK2 - N Stage
p=0.0066
n=133
RSAD2 - Grade
p<0.0001
n=189
SPP1 - TNM Stage
p=0.011
n=39
THOC4 - Grade
p=0.001
n=188
TNC - Grade
p=0.018
n=33
Normalized Expression
Clinical Variable
B
CCL28 - N Stage
p=0.032
n=133
KIT - Grade
p=0.057
n=80
CFD-M Stage
p=0.03
n=163
CLU - TNM Stage
p<0.0001
n=28
LEAP2 - TNM Stage
p<0.0001
n=28
LYVE1 - Grade
p=0.002
n=41
MPZL2 - Grade
p=0.027
n=52
PIGR - TNM Stage
p=0.005
n=39
PIGR - M Stage
p=0.0002
n=163
PLSCR4 - Grade
p=0.02
n=52
PTX3 - Grade
p<0.0001
n=134
TFF3 - TNM Stage
p=0.01
n=109
TFF3 - M Stage
p=0.011
n=114
TFF3 - Grade
p=0.0038
n=28
VSIG2 - Grade
Normalized Expression
Clinical Variable

Figure 4. Up-regulated (A) and down-regulated (B) genes with clinical correlations in ovarian cancer. Same as in Figure 3 except that five independent studies of ovarian cancer were analyzed for the expression of indicated genes and their clinical value.

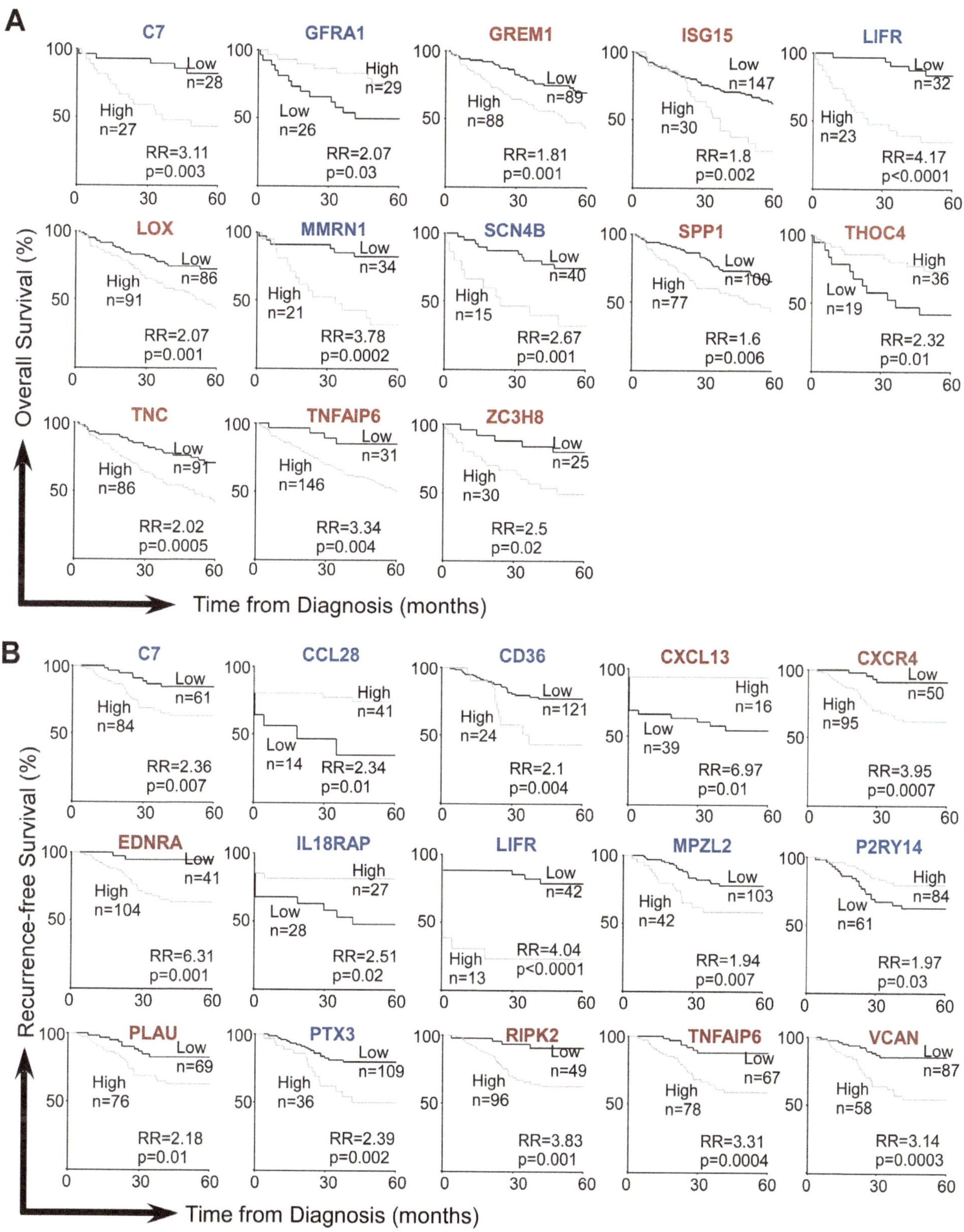

Figure 5. Inflammatory genes predicting overall (A) and recurrence-free (B) survivals in colon cancer. Two datasets from Smith *et al.* [37] were examined for the indicated genes. High, patients with high gene expression. Low, patients with low gene expression. RR, relative risk. Genes are listed in alphabetical order. Red: Elevated iCAMP gene, Blue: Repressed iCAMP gene.

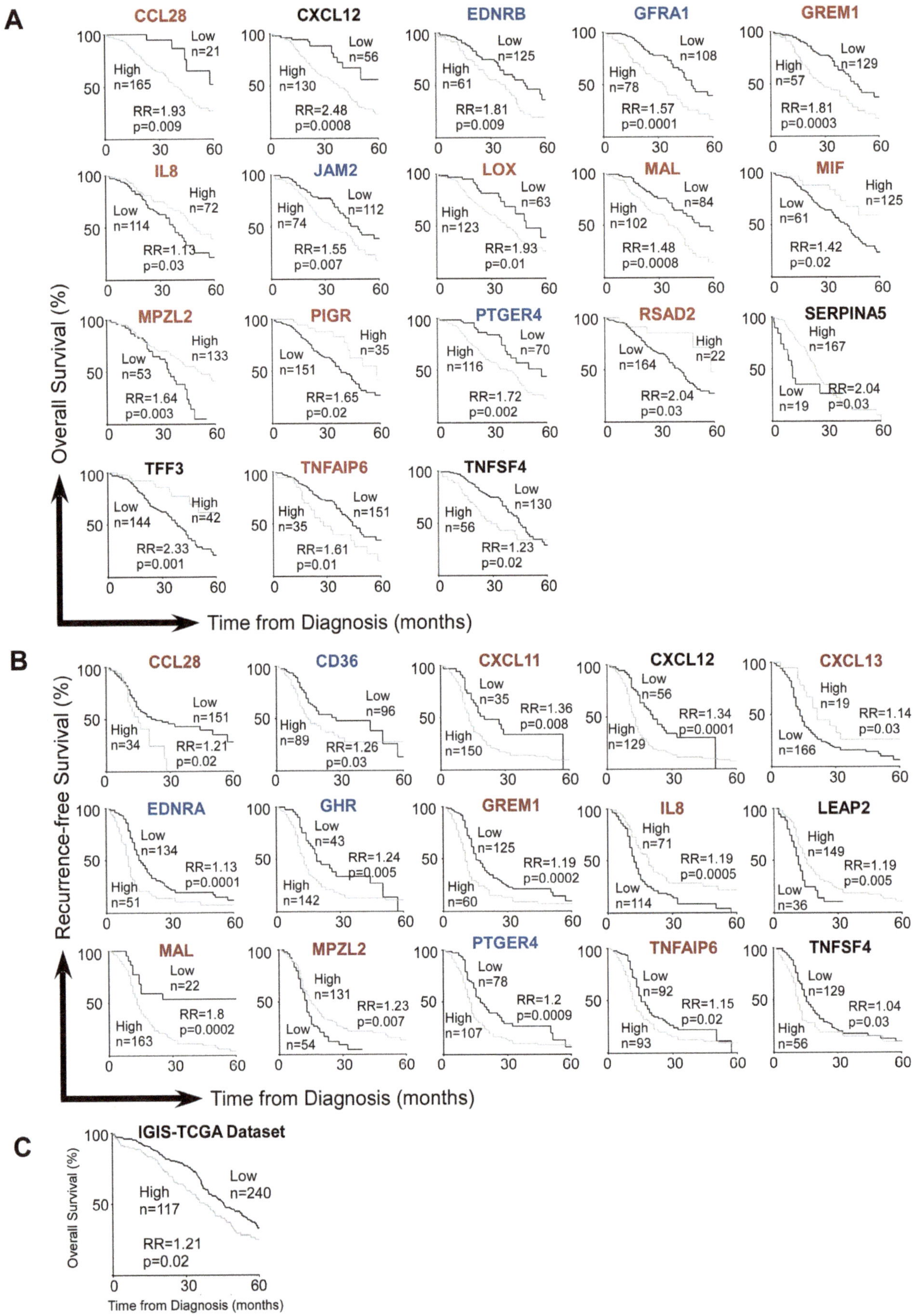
A
Overall Survival (%)
Time from Diagnosis (months)
CCL28 Low n=21 High n=165 RR=1.93 p=0.009
CXCL12 Low n=56 High n=130 RR=2.48 p=0.0008
EDNRB Low n=125 High n=61 RR=1.81 p=0.009
GFRA1 Low n=108 High n=78 RR=1.57 p=0.0001
GREM1 Low n=129 High n=57 RR=1.81 p=0.0003
IL8 High n=72 Low n=114 RR=1.13 p=0.03
JAM2 Low n=112 High n=74 RR=1.55 p=0.007
LOX Low n=63 High n=123 RR=1.93 p=0.01
MAL Low n=84 High n=102 RR=1.48 p=0.0008
MIF High n=125 Low n=61 RR=1.42 p=0.02
MPZL2 High n=133 Low n=53 RR=1.64 p=0.003
PIGR High n=35 Low n=151 RR=1.65 p=0.02
PTGER4 Low n=70 High n=116 RR=1.72 p=0.002
RSAD2 High n=22 Low n=164 RR=2.04 p=0.03
SERPINA5 High n=167 Low n=19 RR=2.04 p=0.03
TFF3 High n=42 Low n=144 RR=2.33 p=0.001
TNFAIP6 Low n=151 High n=35 RR=1.61 p=0.01
TNFSF4 Low n=130 High n=56 RR=1.23 p=0.02
B
Recurrence-free Survival (%)
Time from Diagnosis (months)
CCL28 Low n=151 High n=34 RR=1.21 p=0.02
CD36 Low n=96 High n=89 RR=1.26 p=0.03
CXCL11 Low n=35 High n=150 RR=1.36 p=0.008
CXCL12 Low n=56 High n=129 RR=1.34 p=0.0001
CXCL13 High n=19 Low n=166 RR=1.14 p=0.03
EDNRA Low n=134 High n=51 RR=1.13 p=0.0001
GHR Low n=43 High n=142 RR=1.24 p=0.005
GREM1 Low n=125 High n=60 RR=1.19 p=0.0002
IL8 High n=71 Low n=114 RR=1.19 p=0.0005
LEAP2 High n=149 Low n=36 RR=1.19 p=0.005
MAL Low n=22 High n=163 RR=1.8 p=0.0002
MPZL2 High n=131 Low n=54 RR=1.23 p=0.007
PTGER4 Low n=78 High n=107 RR=1.2 p=0.0009
TNFAIP6 Low n=92 High n=93 RR=1.15 p=0.02
TNFSF4 Low n=129 High n=56 RR=1.04 p=0.03
C
IGIS-TCGA Dataset
Overall Survival (%)
Low n=240 High n=117 RR=1.21 p=0.02
Time from Diagnosis (months)

Figure 6. Inflammatory genes predicting patient prognosis in stage IIIC ovarian cancer. A. Overall survival. B. Recurrence-free survival. C. IGIS predicts overall survival in TCGA dataset. Raw gene expression data was obtained from Tothill *et al.* [22] for (A) and (B), and from TCGA for (C). Red: Elevated in ovarian cancer, Blue: Repressed in ovarian cancer, Black: Unchanged or unknown. IGIS score was calculated based on all the 18 genes indicated in (A).

2: moderate; 3: strong but less intense than 4; and 4: intense) and percentage of positive nuclei over all tumor cells in one TMA core.

Results

Data-mining workflow and identification of consistently differentially expressed genes in seven human cancer types

Raw data from 7 datasets (Table S1) was first obtained from Gene Expression Omnibus (GEO). Each dataset corresponds to one cancer type: breast, colon, lung, oral, pancreatic, prostate and gastric cancers. These datasets include expression microarray profiles from cancer tissues and corresponding normal tissues. After determining dysregulated genes in each cancer type, the Consistent Differential Expression Pattern (CDEP) methodology was implemented to identify differentially expressed genes across the seven datasets. 911 genes were up-regulated and 618 genes were down-regulated. Using DAVID, these genes were then functionally classified and the immune-related genes were identified (Figure S2, Table S2). To further improve the signal-to-noise ratio, genes which showed a fold change (FC) <2 in five or more cancer types were excluded. This resulted in a robust inflammatory profile, termed iCAMP, of 44 up-regulated and 52 down-regulated genes at the mRNA level (Figure 1). The protein expression of iCAMP was verified by IHC in 6 cancer types: breast, colon, lung, pancreatic, prostate and gastric by mining the Human Protein Atlas (Table S3, Figure S5). The clinical significance of iCAMP was determined by using Oncomine database. Finally, the Ingenuity Pathway Analysis tool was used to pinpoint the function of iCAMP in cancer-associated inflammation.

Identification of immune-related genes

Among the up-regulated genes in iCAMP, those involved in the positive regulation of lymphocyte apoptosis were significantly enriched by 11.2 folds. Small chemokines of the CXC family, such as *CXCL9*, *CXCL10* and *CXCL11* were enriched by 9.5 folds (Figure S2A). Additionally, tumors were also enriched with genes in other immunological categories such as host-virus interaction and response to wounding (Figure S2A). Down-regulated genes were highly enriched for complement components in the alternative pathway (9.9 folds), T-cell-associated genes such as CD8α, granzyme A and mal, T cell differentiation proteins (7.3 folds) and genes involved in regulating NK cell function such as lectin-like receptor subfamily K, member 1 (*KLRK1*) (Figure S2B).

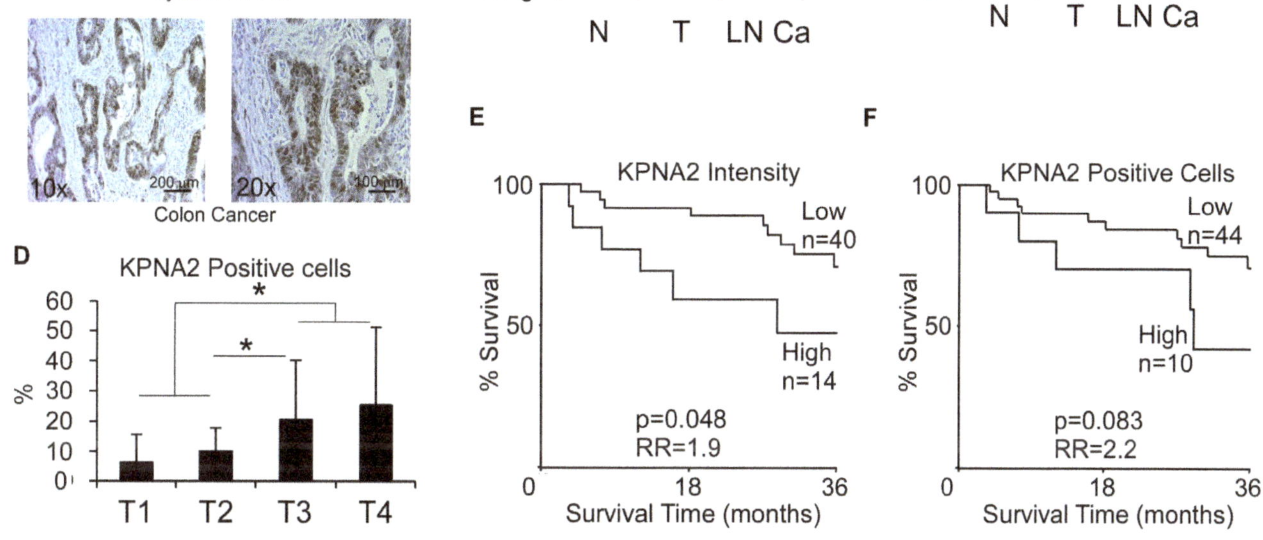

Figure 7. Correlation of KPNA2 expression with colon cancer stage and survival. A. Representative images of KPNA2 immunohistochemical staining from normal and malignant colon tissues. **B.** Quantification of KPNA2 staining intensity in normal tissues (N, n = 50), primary tumor (T, n = 55) and lymph node metastasis (LN Ca, n = 15). *p<0.0001. **C.** Frequency of KPNA2 positive cells. *p<0.0001. **D.** The percentage of KPNA2-positive cells correlates with T stage. *p<0.05. **E.** Kaplan-Meier curve showing the overall survival of colon cancer patients with different KPNA2 expression.

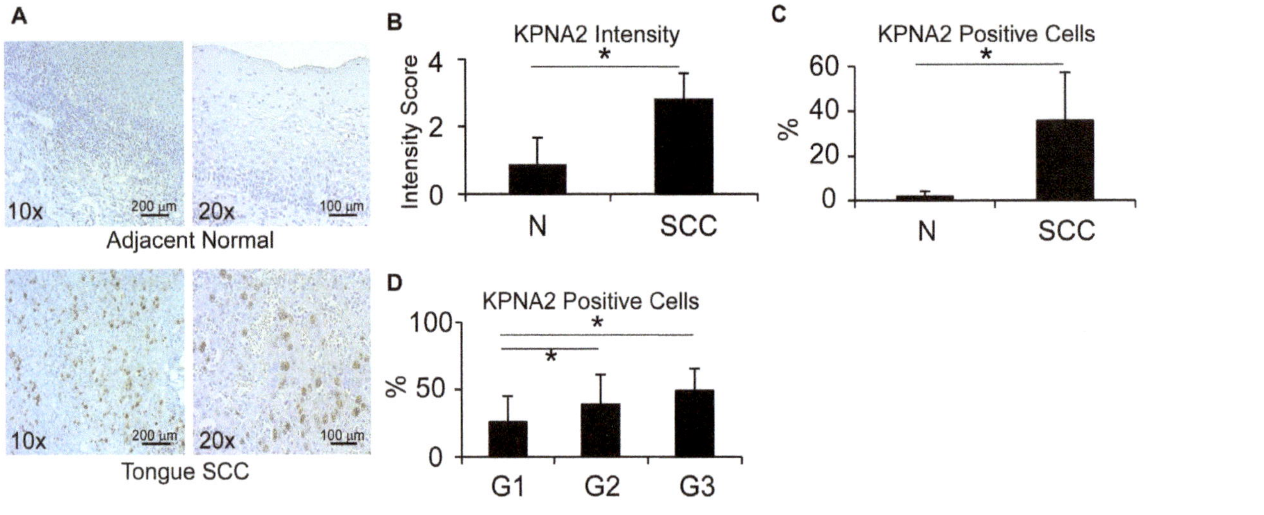

Figure 8. Preferential expression of KPNA2 in head-neck SCC. A. Representative images of KPNA2 immunohistochemical staining from normal and malignant tongue tissues. **B.** KPNA2 staining intensity in primary tumor and adjacent normal tissue *p<0.0001. **C.** Frequency of KPNA2 positive cells in primary tumor and adjacent normal tissue (2%). *p<0.0001. **D.** Correlation between KPNA2 expression and tumor grade. *p<0.05.

The functions of many iCAMP genes are yet to be understood. For example, KPNA2 was shown to be upregulated across a broad-spectrum of cancer types (Figure 1) [23,24,25,26,27]. It is unclear, however, if the possible tumor-promoting activity of KPNA2 is due to its function as a nuclear transporter for selective immunoregulatory proteins such as STAT1 [28] and interferon-γ-induced transcription factor IRF-1 [29].

Expression of iCAMP at the protein level

To examine the protein expression pattern of the iCAMP genes, we took advantage of the publically available protein expression database, HPAT. Genes which did not show differential expression by IHC were not excluded due to the limited sensitivity of this method. Using IHC as a filtering step would expand the false negative observations, limiting the power of this study. However, it was informative to define which genes showed protein changes in what cancer types as this has direct implications on the choice of genes for further functional analyses. For example, KPNA2 was found to be increased in all cancer types except pancreatic cancer (Figure 2). On the other hand, polymeric immunoglobulin receptor (PIGR), a protein involved in the trans-epithelial transport of immunoglobulins, is consistently down-regulated in cancer cells (Figure 2). Altogether, protein expression data is available for 34 up-regulated and 38 down-regulated genes (total = 72) of the 96 genes (Table S3, Figure S5). Of the 34 up-regulated genes at the mRNA level, 13 were also up-regulated by IHC in at least 3 of 6 cancer types studied. As for the transcriptionally down-regulated genes (38 were examined for protein expression), 20 showed down-regulation by IHC in ≥3 of the same 6 cancer types.

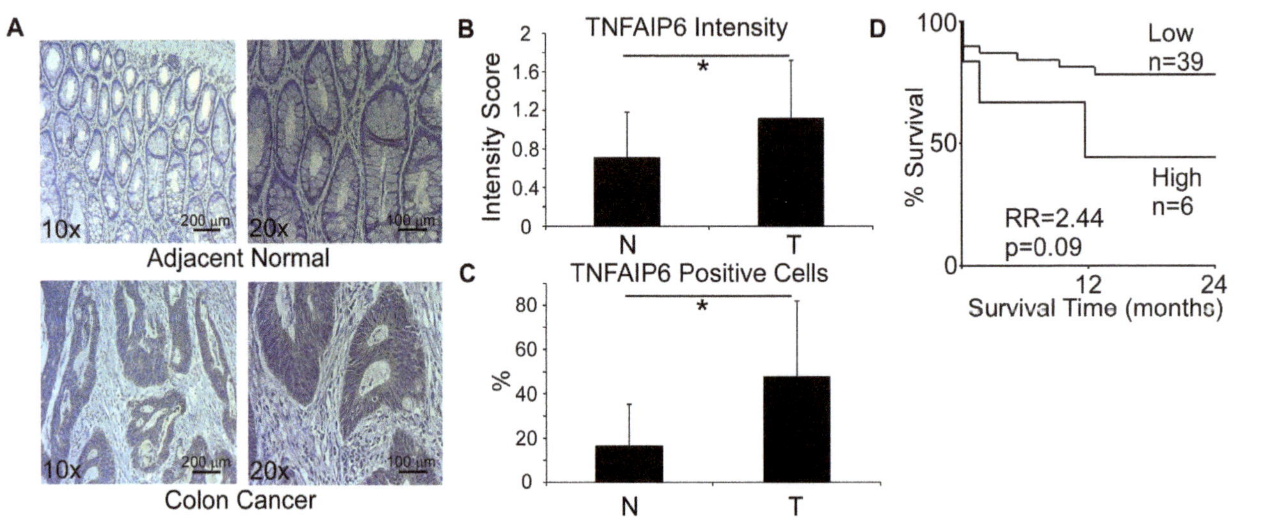

Figure 9. Elevation of TNFAIP6 in colon cancer. A. Representative images of TNFAIP6 immunohistochemical staining from normal and malignant colon tissues. **B.** TNFAIP6 staining intensity in primary colon tumor (n = 55) and adjacent normal tissue (n = 50). *p<0.001. **C.** Frequency of TNFAIP6 positive cells in primary tumor (n = 55) and adjacent normal tissue (n = 50). *p<0.0001. **D.** Kaplan-Meier curve showing recurrence-free survival of colon cancer patients with different TNFAIP6 expression, based on the percentage of positive cells.

Table 1. Selected iCAMP genes consistently elevated or repressed in cancer and their clinical significance.

Elevated Genes	Background Information	Current Findings
EDNRA	Up-regulated in colon cancer [63]	Higher levels confer worse survival in colon and ovarian cancers
SPP1	Elevated in multiple types of carcinoma [64]	Elevated with higher stages of ovarian cancer – Predicts worse overall survival in colon cancer
KPNA2	Correlates with worse disease and survival [24,26,65]	Up-regulated in several cancer types – Correlates with poor prognosis in ovarian, head/neck and colon cancer
BST2	Poorly studied in the context of cancer	Elevated in gastric, pancreatic, oral, breast, colon and lung cancers by mRNA and/or IHC.
TNC	Elevated in multiple cancers – Induces focal adhesion [66]	Over-expression confers poorer survival in colon cancer.
TNFAIP6	Induces the stability of the ECM and promote cell migration – Elevated mRNA in peripheral blood of colon cancer patients [43]	Up-regulated in metastatic ovarian cancer – Elevated with higher T stage – Predicts worse survival in ovarian and colon cancers
TNFSF4	Dendritic cell co-stimulatory molecule	Confers worse survival in ovarian cancer – Positively correlates with grade, nodal stage and tumor size in colon cancer
LOX	Hypoxia-induced mediator of metastasis – Recruits CD11b+ cells to metastatic niche facilitating malignant cell seeding [67]	Up-regulated in 6 of 7 cancer types – Higher levels confer worse survival in colon and ovarian cancers
VCAN	Upregulated in tumors of the breast, ovary, colon and prostate – Confers poor prognosis in endometrial cancer patients [68]	Higher levels predict worse survival in colon and ovarian cancers
Repressed Genes	**Background Information**	**Current Findings**
LEAP2	Expressed in gastro-intestinal epithelial tissue – Upregulated in response to *Salmonella enterica* and TLR ligands – Role in tumorigenesis unknown [69,70]	Down-regulated in multiple cancer types – Lower expression predicts worse survival in ovarian cancer
MPZL2	Cellular localization and homology to myelin suggest its involvement in cellular attachment – Unclear roles in cancer	Decreased in higher grade ovarian cancer – Lower with higher stage colon cancer – Lower expression predicts worse survival in ovarian cancer – Lower expression predicts worse survival in colon cancer
PIGR	Decreased in non-small cell lung cancer [71,72] – Elevation predicts earlier recurrence of human hepatoma – Promotes metastasis in mouse models [73]	Down-regulated with higher stage ovarian cancer – Lower expression predicts worse survival in ovarian cancer
LIFR	IL6 type cytokine receptor – Suppressed in colorectal and liver cancers [74,75]	Down-regulated on the mRNA level in 6 of the 7 cancers and on the protein level in all 7 cancer types
PTX3	A glycoprotein secreted by antigen presenting cells, endothelial cells and fibroblasts in response to inflammatory stimuli [76]	Lower expression predicts better survival in colon cancer – Lower expression in grade 1 compared to grade 3 ovarian cancer
SERPINA5	Inhibitor of urokinase-type plasminogen activator (UPA) – Downregulation in advanced-stage ovarian cancer [77]	Lower expression confers worse survival in ovarian cancer – Higher in patients with metastatic disease
CCL28	Secreted by ovarian cancer cells in response to hypoxia to mediate Treg recruitment – Higher expression predicts worse survival in ovarian cancer [78]	Increased CCL28 in ovarian cancer with nodal metastasis – Higher levels predict worse overall and recurrence-free survival – Consistently repressed in other cancer including colon, breast, prostate, gastric and pancreatic cancers – lower expression in colon cancer predicts worse survival

Clinical significance of iCAMP genes

We next chose to use ovarian cancer to study the significance of iCAMP genes based on two considerations. First, most of ovarian malignancies are of epithelial origin which is histologically similar to the seven cancer types from which the gene profile was defined. Second, ovarian cancer was not used to generate the iCAMP genes. The predictive value of these genes in ovarian cancer would validate the utility of our gene discovery approach. As a control, the clinical predictive values of these genes were also examined in colon cancer. To determine the direction of dysregulation of each gene in ovarian cancer, we mined 5 published datasets [30,31,32,33,34] and one additional dataset from The Cancer Genome Atlas (TCGA) (Table S4), which collectively contain 35 normal and 878 cancer samples. Based on the number of datasets showing dysregulation in each direction, each gene was labeled as elevated, unchanged or repressed in ovarian cancer (Figure 1). A gene is determined to be elevated if 1) at least 1 dataset shows up-regulation ($p<0.05$) and none of the other datasets shows down-regulation, or 2) at least 3 datasets show up-regulation and not more than one dataset shows down-regulation ($p<0.05$). The inverse applies to repressed genes. Based on that, 33 of the 44 up-regulated genes were also elevated in ovarian cancer, 3 were repressed and 8 could not be determined. Among the 52 down-regulated genes, 28 were also repressed in ovarian cancer, 7 were unchanged, 10 were elevated and 7 were undetermined (Figure 1). Thus, at least 61 out of 96 iCAMP genes were concordantly dysregulated in ovarian cancer.

Colon [35,36,37] and ovarian cancer datasets [22,30,38,39,40] from Oncomine, as well as TCGA colon cancer dataset, were then analyzed for clinical significance of expression level of individual iCAMP gene. A number of genes such as *CCL20*, *CD36* and *IL18RAP* individually showed significant correlations with clinical variables in colon cancer such as tumor stage (T1 to T4), lymph node status (N0 to N2), metastasis (M0 or M1), pathological grade

(G1 to G4) and Duke stage (A to D) (Figures 3A and 3B). In ovarian cancer, all of the up-regulated genes were increased with more advanced stage (*CXCL10*, *RIPK2* and *SPP1*) or higher pathological grade (*CXCL11*, *KPNA2*, *RSAD2*, *THOC4* and *TNC*) (Figure 4A). As for the down-regulated iCAMP genes, more advanced stages conferred higher expression of some genes (*CCL28* and *CFD*) and lower expression of others (*CLU*, *LEAP2*, *PIGR* and *TFF3*) (Figure 4B).

We next determined if iCAMP gene expression level predicts survival, based on raw microarray data for colon cancer [37] and ovarian cancer [22]. Genes which showed different expression levels between survivors and non-survivors at one, three and/or five years were tested by Kaplan-Meier analysis (Figures 5 and 6). In colon cancer, better overall survival was predicted with higher levels of GFRA1 and THOC4, and lower levels of C7, GREM1, ISG15, LIFR, LOX, MMRN1, SCN4B, SPP1, TNC, TNFAIP6 and ZC3H8 (Figure 5A). The dysregulated expression of many iCAMP genes also has significant predictive value for cancer recurrence (Figure 5B).

In stage IIIC ovarian cancer, improved overall survival was associated with higher mRNA levels of IL8, MIF, MPZL2, PIGR, RSAD2, SERPINA5 and TFF3, but lower levels of CCL28, CXCL12, EDNRB, GFRA1, GREM1, JAM2, LOX, MAL, PTGER4, TNFAIP6 and TNFSF4 (Figure 6A). The dysegulation of many of these genes also predicts recurrence-free survival (Figure 6B).

Interestingly, lower expression of a number of genes (GREM1, LOX, TNFAIP6, CD36, and EDNRA) predicted better prognosis in both ovarian and colon cancers. On the other hand, CXCL13 elevation predicted better prognosis in both diseases (Figures 5 and 6).

To determine the prognostic value of iCAMP genes as a group, an inflammatory gene integrated score (IGIS) was devised for ovarian cancer (Figures 6C). IGIS included 18 genes which independently showed significant predictability ($p<0.05$) by Kaplan-Meier analysis. This score takes into consideration the number of genes within which the patient falls in the high risk group, as well as the risk each of these genes confers. The robustness of IGIS was validated using the independent ovarian cancer TCGA dataset. Based on cutoff values pre-determined from the initial training dataset above [22], stage IIIC patients from the TCGA dataset were categorized as either high or low risk for each gene. Then, for each gene where a TCGA patient shows poor prognosis, relative risk (RR pre-determined by the training dataset) of that gene was added to the patients IGIS score. The TCGA patients eventually were distributed with different IGIS scores based on expression levels of all 18 IGIS genes. We found that IGIS indeed predicted overall survival (RR = 1.21, $p = 0.02$) (Figures 6C).

Clinical significance of KPNA2 in colon adenocarcinoma and head-neck squamous cell carcinomas

We next focused on KPNA2 in colon adenocarcinoma and head/neck squamous cell carcinoma, since KPNA2 overexpression has not been reported in these two cancer types. KPNA2 is a nuclear/cytoplasmic protein involved in the import of select cytoplasmic proteins into the nucleus. It binds to the nuclear localization sequence (NLS) of its cargo protein and to karyopherin β1, and the whole protein complex translocates across the nuclear envelope through the nuclear pore complex (NPC) [41]. Among KPNA2 clients is the interferon-γ-induced transcription factor IRF-1 [29] and STAT1 [28], both of which are involved in host immune response.

We examined the KPNA2 expression with immunohistrochemistry using our in-house tumor microarray which contains 55 primary colon cancer specimens, 15 lymph node metastases and 50 corresponding adjacent normal tissues from patients of various disease stages. We found a drastic increase in KPNA2 expression in primary and lymph node metastatic colon tumors compared to adjacent normal tissues (Figures 7A, 7B and 7C). KPNA2 expression also correlated with the tumor (T) stage, where the percentage of positive cells increased from T1 through T4 (T1: 6.4%, T2: 10%, T3: 20.6% and T4: 25.4%) (Figure 7D). Given that most of the patients were in the T2 ($n = 11$) and T3 ($n = 31$) categories, we found significant difference in KPNA2 expression between T2 and T3 ($p = 0.017$). The difference was also significant between combined T1–T2 and T3–T4 stages ($p = 0.003$) (Figure 7D). More importantly, patients with KPNA2 intensity score ≥3 displayed worse overall survival than those with KPNA2 intensity ≤2 (Relative risk = 1.9, $p = 0.048$) (Figure 7E).

Similar to colon cancer, oral and laryngeal squamous cell carcinomas displayed elevated levels of KPNA2 compared to independent mouth and larynx normal tissues (Figure 8A, 8B and 8C). Although KPNA2 showed no correlation with the disease stage, it was higher in each of grade 2 (39.2% positive cells) and grade 3 (49% positive cells) carcinomas compared to grade 1 (26.3%). (p(G1 vs. G2) = 0.03 and p(G1 vs. G3) = 0.002) (Figure 8D).

TNFAIP6 is overexpressed in colon adenocarcinoma

Tumor necrosis factor alpha-induced protein 6 (TNFAIP6) is a secreted glycoprotein expressed by epithelial cells and leukocytes under normal and inflammatory conditions. Its anti-inflammatory function is well established in different inflammatory conditions such as osteoarthritis, and it is detectable in serum samples from patients with autoimmune disorders [42]. Recently, transcriptional profiling of blood from colorectal patients and normal controls by qRT-PCR identified TNFAIP6 as a biomarker for colorectal cancer [43]. This study shows that TNFAIP6 mRNA is elevated in peripheral blood cells of colorectal cancer patients. Here, we investigated the protein levels of TNFAIP6 in colon cancer cells and adjacent normal epithelium. Immunohistochemical staining of 55 colon cancer specimens and 50 adjacent normal tissues revealed an increased expression in cancer on a per cell basis, as well as an increase in the frequency of TNFAIP6-expressing cells (Figures 9A, B and C). TNFAIP6 protein levels did not predict overall patient survival (data not shown). As for disease recurrence, we found a trend towards worse recurrence-free survival in highly expressing patients (Figure 9D), without reaching statistical significance (RR = 2.44, $p = 0.09$).

Discussion

This study was designed to conceptually and experimentally address a novel hypothesis that cancers, irrespective of their etiology, harbor shared iCAMPs to evade immune surveillance and to highjack host immunity for promoting onco-inflammatory growth and metastasis. An unbiased and comprehensive data-mining strategy was undertaken to address this hypothesis and to mine common molecular expression patterns in a large number of patients from many independent studies to ensure the consistency of our findings. The expression of selective genes was confirmed by tissue microarrays. Although the biological significance of our finding awaits further studies, it is clear that the iCAMP not only exists but also shows significant clinical relevance. The core iCAMP gene set reproduces many well-established genes that are aberrantly expressed in cancer tissue, such as VCAN and KPNA2.

It also uncovers a number of new consistently dysregulated genes that have not been studied in the context of anti-cancer immunity, such as BST2, LEAP2, TNFAIP6, TNFSF4 and KPNA2 (Table 1).

The existence of iCAMP highlighted the importance of "onco-inflammation" as one of the common drivers for oncogenesis [44]. The consistent dysregulation of these genes across cancers of different histological origins suggests similar set of "rules" all cancers have to follow in order to sabotage the host immune response and engage it in growth and invasion. Remarkably, these iCAMP genes can potentially be harnessed as biomarkers for cancer aggressiveness, as we found striking predictability of these genes for disease recurrence and patient survival in a number of cancers. The fact that these molecules show consistent aberrant expression and prognostic significance also suggests that they could potentially be therapeutic targets for multiple cancers.

Data-mining is helpful not only in identifying biomarkers and potential therapeutic targets, but also to uncover the underlying biology of human cancer. As an example, molecular profiling of colon cancer revealed higher levels of T cell homing and adhesion molecules to confer more favorable prognosis [45]. In our study, the iCAMP gene set is enriched for genes in positive regulation of lymphocyte apoptosis, which could be a defense mechanism for cancer cells to decrease the pressure of anti-tumor immunity. CXC chemokines are also enriched among the over-expressed genes. These chemokines have been reported to play different roles, ranging from recruiting inflammatory cells to aid cancer invasion to dampening the positive signaling in antitumor immunity.

As for down-regulated genes, they were mostly enriched for immune effector molecules such as granzyme A, Mal and NKG2D (Figure S2B). In fact, NKG2D, which confers activation and anti-tumor immunity in T cells and NK cells, was shown to be shut down in esophageal cancer [46]. Moreover, ligands of this receptor were down-regulated in colorectal cancer [47], which provides a mechanism for evading immune-surveillance. Similarly, granzyme A is part of the cytotoxic T cell and eosinophil arsenal for tumoricidal activity [48]. Mal, which was first described in myelin and lymphocytes was later reported to function in apical transport in epithelial cells, thus, its disruption could lead to disorganized polarity [49]. This protein was down-regulated in multiple types of cancer, including breast and head and neck cancers [49,50].

The concept of iCAMP is analogous to pathogen-associated molecular patterns (PAMPs) that was postulated more than two decades ago [51]. Importantly, not all up/down-regulated genes contribute to the invasiveness of the cancers studied. The tumor microenvironment consists of a complex interaction among cancer, stromal, endothelial, and immune cells. Any given change in gene expression could be an active process initiated by cancer cells and eventually promote invasiveness, or alternatively, be a reaction by other cells of the immune system. This is best illustrated by some up-regulated genes whose elevation predicts better prognosis, and down-regulated genes whose repression correlates with longer survival.

Among the genes that drew our attention was KPNA2, which was increased in expression in 6 of 7 cancer types at the mRNA and the protein levels, with limited expression in normal epithelia. KPNA2 is an embryonic antigen, shown to be expressed in mouse embryonic stem cells [52] and normal human testis [53,54], and emerges again in a variety of epithelial [23,24,25,26,27,55,56] and non-epithelial [57,58] cancers. Despite the exceptional correlation of this gene with cancer behavior across multiple cancer types, its function in shaping tumor behavior remains unclear. One study showed KPNA2 to promote invasive phenotypes of human breast cancer cells *in vitro* [59], but the mechanism underlying this observation was not investigated. In a cell-free system, KPNA2 was reported to interact with OCT4, a transcription factor involved in maintaining pluripotency and self-renewal in embryonic stem cells [54]. Could KPNA2 expression lead to a significant activity in cancer cells to produce oncogenic inflammatory mediators? This is possible, particularly since KPNA2 does not seem to be a general nuclear importer. The selective transport of some key immunologically important transcription factors such as STAT1 and IRF1 by KPNA2 raises a strong possibility of underlying immunological properties of KPNA2. Thus, the potential dual roles of KPNA2 to regulate inflammation as well as stemness of cells suggests that it could serve as a critical link between chronic inflammation and oncogenesis. This speculation warrants further studies.

Since iCAMP represents a list of multiple gene products, an integrated score or index shall be expected to predict the clinical behavior of cancers, which indeed was proven to be the case for both colon and ovarian cancers. This predictive value of iCAMP as a biomarker awaits further investigation in prospective studies, much like the MamaPrint® [60] and Oncotype DX® [61] in optimizing personalized medical practice. Given the inflammatory function of iCAMP genes, the integrated score could prove effective in identifying high risk patients who would benefit from immunotherapy. In this regard, significant efforts are already undertaken to implement the immune score into the staging of cancer, in conjunction with the tumor (T), lymph node infiltration (N) and distal metastasis (M) parameters [62].

Supporting Information

Figure S1 Methodology followed to identify the inflammatory cancer-associated molecular pattern (iCAMP).

Figure S2 Enrichment of inflammatory gene ontologies within the cancer-associated molecular pattern. (A) Up-regulated genes, (B) Down-regulated genes. Using DAVID database, all differentially expressed genes were assigned gene ontology terms based on their known functions in the literature. Immune-related gene ontologies are presented here. The horizontal axis represents the enrichment fold: The proportion of a given functional class within our list relative to its proportion in the whole human genome.

Figure S3 Distribution of the dysregulated genes in different cellular compartments. Obtained from WebGestalt gene set analysis toolkit. (http://bioinfo.vanderbilt.edu/webgestalt/).

Figure S4 Distribution of dysregulated genes, their functional classes and previously established interactions. Each line represents a direct interaction corroborated by at least one evidence from the literature. Obtained from Ingenuity Pathway Analysis (www.ingenuity.com).

Figure S5 Immunohistochemical stains of selected genes on representative specimens from the Human Protein Atlas (HPAT). Up-regulated Genes. A: FN1, STAT1, BST2; B: TNC, COL3A1, ISG15; C: PLA2G7, KRT8, CXCL11. **Down-regulated Genes.** D: UNC13B, C7, CDO1; E: TGFBR3, PITGR4, IL1R2; F: SCNN1B, MST1, LIFR; G: PTX3, AZGP1, GIMAP5; H: VSIG2.

Table S1 GEO datasets. Summary of the GEO datasets from which differentially expressed genes were identified. HG-

U133_Plus_2] Affymetrix Human Genome U133 Plus 2.0 platform was used in all datasets.

Table S2 Immune-related genes and their corresponding mRNA ratios (cancer:normal). Shaded genes are those presented in figure 1. These genes have a Fold Change (FC)>2 in 3–7 cancer types, in addition to some genes whose FC values are slightly less than 2 in more than 3 cancer types.

Table S3 Protein expression of iCAMP genes. Protein expression changes (Interpreted from the Human Protein Atlas immunohistochemical stains) of the up-regulated and down-regulated genes which showed mRNA differential expression with a fold change FC>2 in 3–7 cancer types. ↑, elevated. ↓, repressed. ↔, no change. NA, Not available.

Table S4 The number of Oncomine datasets showing elevation or repression of each gene in ovarian cancer. U, up. D, down. X, no change.

Acknowledgments

We thank Ms. Kiwana Gibbs and the Tissue Biorepository at MUSC for their assistance in acquiring samples and collecting information for colon cancer patients.

Author Contributions

Conceived and designed the experiments: SMR WJZ ZL. Performed the experiments: SMR TQ. Analyzed the data: SMR ZL. Contributed reagents/materials/analysis tools: SS ZL. Wrote the paper: SMR ZL.

References

1. Grivennikov SI, Greten FR, Karin M (2010) Immunity, inflammation, and cancer. Cell 140: 883–899.
2. Goldstein MG, Li Z (2009) Heat-shock proteins in infection-mediated inflammation-induced tumorigenesis. J Hematol Oncol 2: 5.
3. Schreiber RD, Old LJ, Smyth MJ (2011) Cancer immunoediting: integrating immunity's roles in cancer suppression and promotion. Science 331: 1565–1570.
4. Gabrilovich DI, Nagaraj S (2009) Myeloid-derived suppressor cells as regulators of the immune system. Nat Rev Immunol 9: 162–174.
5. Zou W (2006) Regulatory T cells, tumour immunity and immunotherapy. Nat Rev Immunol 6: 295–307.
6. Okazaki IM, Kotani A, Honjo T (2007) Role of AID in tumorigenesis. Adv Immunol 94: 245–273.
7. Oguma K, Oshima H, Aoki M, Uchio R, Naka K, et al. (2008) Activated macrophages promote Wnt signalling through tumour necrosis factor-alpha in gastric tumour cells. EMBO J 27: 1671–1681.
8. Grivennikov SI, Karin M (2010) Dangerous liaisons: STAT3 and NF-kappaB collaboration and crosstalk in cancer. Cytokine Growth Factor Rev 21: 11–19.
9. Yang J, Weinberg RA (2008) Epithelial-mesenchymal transition: at the crossroads of development and tumor metastasis. Dev Cell 14: 818–829.
10. Turashvili G, Bouchal J, Baumforth K, Wei W, Dziechciarkova M, et al. (2007) Novel markers for differentiation of lobular and ductal invasive breast carcinomas by laser microdissection and microarray analysis. BMC Cancer 7: 55.
11. Skrzypczak M, Goryca K, Rubel T, Paziewska A, Mikula M, et al. (2010) Modeling oncogenic signaling in colon tumors by multidirectional analyses of microarray data directed for maximization of analytical reliability. PLoS One 5.
12. D'Errico M, de Rinaldis E, Blasi MF, Viti V, Falchetti M, et al. (2009) Genome-wide expression profile of sporadic gastric cancers with microsatellite instability. Eur J Cancer 45: 461–469.
13. Hou J, Aerts J, den Hamer B, van Ijcken W, den Bakker M, et al. (2010) Gene expression-based classification of non-small cell lung carcinomas and survival prediction. PLoS One 5: e10312.
14. Ye H, Yu T, Temam S, Ziober BL, Wang J, et al. (2008) Transcriptomic dissection of tongue squamous cell carcinoma. BMC Genomics 9: 69.
15. Badea L, Herlea V, Dima SO, Dumitrascu T, Popescu I (2008) Combined gene expression analysis of whole-tissue and microdissected pancreatic ductal adenocarcinoma identifies genes specifically overexpressed in tumor epithelia. Hepatogastroenterology 55: 2016–2027.
16. Wang Y, Xia XQ, Jia Z, Sawyers A, Yao H, et al. (2010) In silico estimates of tissue components in surgical samples based on expression profiling data. Cancer Res 70: 6448–6455.
17. Tsoi LC, Qin T, Slate EH, Zheng WJ (2011) Consistent Differential Expression Pattern (CDEP) on microarray to identify genes related to metastatic behavior. BMC Bioinformatics 12: 438.
18. Gentleman R, Irizarry RA, Martinez-Murillo F, Spencer F, Wu Z (2004) A Model-Based Background Adjustment for Oligonucleotide Expression Arrays. Journal of the American Statistical Association 99: 909–917.
19. Hong F, Breitling R, McEntee CW, Wittner BS, Nemhauser JL, et al. (2006) RankProd: a bioconductor package for detecting differentially expressed genes in meta-analysis. Bioinformatics 22: 2825–2827.
20. Lunn D, Spiegelhalter D, Thomas A, Best N (2009) The BUGS project: Evolution, critique and future directions. Stat Med 28: 3049–3067.
21. Camp RL, Dolled-Filhart M, Rimm DL (2004) X-tile: a new bio-informatics tool for biomarker assessment and outcome-based cut-point optimization. Clin Cancer Res 10: 7252–7259.
22. Tothill RW, Tinker AV, George J, Brown R, Fox SB, et al. (2008) Novel molecular subtypes of serous and endometrioid ovarian cancer linked to clinical outcome. Clin Cancer Res 14: 5198–5208.
23. Dankof A, Fritzsche FR, Dahl E, Pahl S, Wild P, et al. (2007) KPNA2 protein expression in invasive breast carcinoma and matched peritumoral ductal carcinoma in situ. Virchows Arch 451: 877–881.
24. Mortezavi A, Hermanns T, Seifert HH, Baumgartner MK, Provenzano M, et al. (2011) KPNA2 expression is an independent adverse predictor of biochemical recurrence after radical prostatectomy. Clin Cancer Res 17: 1111–1121.
25. Sakai M, Sohda M, Miyazaki T, Suzuki S, Sano A, et al. (2010) Significance of karyopherin-{alpha} 2 (KPNA2) expression in esophageal squamous cell carcinoma. Anticancer Res 30: 851–856.
26. Zheng M, Tang L, Huang L, Ding H, Liao WT, et al. (2010) Overexpression of karyopherin-2 in epithelial ovarian cancer and correlation with poor prognosis. Obstet Gynecol 116: 884–891.
27. Gousias K, Becker AJ, Simon M, Niehusmann P (2012) Nuclear karyopherin a2: a novel biomarker for infiltrative astrocytomas. J Neurooncol 109: 545–553.
28. Frieman M, Yount B, Heise M, Kopecky-Bromberg SA, Palese P, et al. (2007) Severe acute respiratory syndrome coronavirus ORF6 antagonizes STAT1 function by sequestering nuclear import factors on the rough endoplasmic reticulum/Golgi membrane. J Virol 81: 9812–9824.
29. Umegaki N, Tamai K, Nakano H, Moritsugu R, Yamazaki T, et al. (2007) Differential regulation of karyopherin alpha 2 expression by TGF-beta1 and IFN-gamma in normal human epidermal keratinocytes: evident contribution of KPNA2 for nuclear translocation of IRF-1. J Invest Dermatol 127: 1456–1464.
30. Hendrix ND, Wu R, Kuick R, Schwartz DR, Fearon ER, et al. (2006) Fibroblast growth factor 9 has oncogenic activity and is a downstream target of Wnt signaling in ovarian endometrioid adenocarcinomas. Cancer Res 66: 1354–1362.
31. Lu KH, Patterson AP, Wang L, Marquez RT, Atkinson EN, et al. (2004) Selection of potential markers for epithelial ovarian cancer with gene expression arrays and recursive descent partition analysis. Clin Cancer Res 10: 3291–3300.
32. Welsh JB, Zarrinkar PP, Sapinoso LM, Kern SG, Behling CA, et al. (2001) Analysis of gene expression profiles in normal and neoplastic ovarian tissue samples identifies candidate molecular markers of epithelial ovarian cancer. Proc Natl Acad Sci U S A 98: 1176–1181.
33. Bonome T, Levine DA, Shih J, Randonovich M, Pise-Masison CA, et al. (2008) A gene signature predicting for survival in suboptimally debulked patients with ovarian cancer. Cancer Res 68: 5478–5486.
34. Adib TR, Henderson S, Perrett C, Hewitt D, Bourmpoulia D, et al. (2004) Predicting biomarkers for ovarian cancer using gene-expression microarrays. Br J Cancer 90: 686–692.
35. Kaiser S, Park YK, Franklin JL, Halberg RB, Yu M, et al. (2007) Transcriptional recapitulation and subversion of embryonic colon development by mouse colon tumor models and human colon cancer. Genome Biol 8: R131.
36. Ki DH, Jeung HC, Park CH, Kang SH, Lee GY, et al. (2007) Whole genome analysis for liver metastasis gene signatures in colorectal cancer. Int J Cancer 121: 2005–2012.
37. Smith JJ, Deane NG, Wu F, Merchant NB, Zhang B, et al. (2010) Experimentally derived metastasis gene expression profile predicts recurrence and death in patients with colon cancer. Gastroenterology 138: 958–968.
38. Schwartz DR, Kardia SL, Shedden KA, Kuick R, Michailidis G, et al. (2002) Gene expression in ovarian cancer reflects both morphology and biological behavior, distinguishing clear cell from other poor-prognosis ovarian carcinomas. Cancer Res 62: 4722–4729.
39. Sieben NL, Oosting J, Flanagan AM, Prat J, Roemen GM, et al. (2005) Differential gene expression in ovarian tumors reveals Dusp 4 and Serpina 5 as key regulators for benign behavior of serous borderline tumors. J Clin Oncol 23: 7257–7264.
40. Schaner ME, Ross DT, Ciaravino G, Sorlie T, Troyanskaya O, et al. (2003) Gene expression patterns in ovarian carcinomas. Mol Biol Cell 14: 4376–4386.

41. Moroianu J, Hijikata M, Blobel G, Radu A (1995) Mammalian karyopherin alpha 1 beta and alpha 2 beta heterodimers: alpha 1 or alpha 2 subunit binds nuclear localization signal and beta subunit interacts with peptide repeat-containing nucleoporins. Proc Natl Acad Sci U S A 92: 6532–6536.
42. Wisniewski HG, Vilcek J (1997) TSG-6: an IL-1/TNF-inducible protein with anti-inflammatory activity. Cytokine Growth Factor Rev 8: 143–156.
43. Marshall KW, Mohr S, Khettabi FE, Nossova N, Chao S, et al. (2010) A blood-based biomarker panel for stratifying current risk for colorectal cancer. Int J Cancer 126: 1177–1186.
44. Hanahan D, Weinberg RA (2011) Hallmarks of cancer: the next generation. Cell 144: 646–674.
45. Mlecnik B, Tosolini M, Charoentong P, Kirilovsky A, Bindea G, et al. (2010) Biomolecular network reconstruction identifies T-cell homing factors associated with survival in colorectal cancer. Gastroenterology 138: 1429–1440.
46. Osaki T, Saito H, Fukumoto Y, Yamada Y, Fukuda K, et al. (2009) Inverse correlation between NKG2D expression on CD8+ T cells and the frequency of CD4+CD25+ regulatory T cells in patients with esophageal cancer. Dis Esophagus 22: 49–54.
47. Sers C, Kuner R, Falk CS, Lund P, Sueltmann H, et al. (2009) Down-regulation of HLA Class I and NKG2D ligands through a concerted action of MAPK and DNA methyltransferases in colorectal cancer cells. Int J Cancer 125: 1626–1639.
48. Legrand F, Driss V, Delbeke M, Loiseau S, Hermann E, et al. (2010) Human eosinophils exert TNF-alpha and granzyme A-mediated tumoricidal activity toward colon carcinoma cells. J Immunol 185: 7443–7451.
49. Horne HN, Lee PS, Murphy SK, Alonso MA, Olson JA Jr, et al. (2009) Inactivation of the MAL gene in breast cancer is a common event that predicts benefit from adjuvant chemotherapy. Mol Cancer Res 7: 199–209.
50. Beder LB, Gunduz M, Hotomi M, Fujihara K, Shimada J, et al. (2009) T-lymphocyte maturation-associated protein gene as a candidate metastasis suppressor for head and neck squamous cell carcinomas. Cancer Sci 100: 873–880.
51. Janeway CA Jr (1989) Approaching the asymptote? Evolution and revolution in immunology. Cold Spring Harb Symp Quant Biol 54: 1–13.
52. Young JC, Major AT, Miyamoto Y, Loveland KL, Jans DA (2011) Distinct effects of importin alpha2 and alpha4 on Oct3/4 localization and expression in mouse embryonic stem cells. FASEB J 25: 3958–3965.
53. Ly-Huynh JD, Lieu KG, Major AT, Whiley PA, Holt JE, et al. (2011) Importin alpha2-interacting proteins with nuclear roles during mammalian spermatogenesis. Biol Reprod 85: 1191–1202.
54. Li X, Sun L, Jin Y (2008) Identification of karyopherin-alpha 2 as an Oct4 associated protein. J Genet Genomics 35: 723–728.
55. Jensen JB, Munksgaard PP, Sorensen CM, Fristrup N, Birkenkamp-Demtroder K, et al. (2011) High expression of karyopherin-alpha2 defines poor prognosis in non-muscle-invasive bladder cancer and in patients with invasive bladder cancer undergoing radical cystectomy. Eur Urol 59: 841–848.
56. Wang CI, Wang CL, Wang CW, Chen CD, Wu CC, et al. (2011) Importin subunit alpha-2 is identified as a potential biomarker for non-small cell lung cancer by integration of the cancer cell secretome and tissue transcriptome. Int J Cancer 128: 2364–2372.
57. He L, Ding H, Wang JH, Zhou Y, Li L, et al. (2012) Overexpression of karyopherin 2 in human ovarian malignant germ cell tumor correlates with poor prognosis. PLoS One 7: e42992.
58. Winnepenninckx V, Lazar V, Michiels S, Dessen P, Stas M, et al. (2006) Gene expression profiling of primary cutaneous melanoma and clinical outcome. J Natl Cancer Inst 98: 472–482.
59. Noetzel E, Rose M, Bornemann J, Gajewski M, Knuchel R, et al. (2012) Nuclear transport receptor karyopherin-alpha2 promotes malignant breast cancer phenotypes in vitro. Oncogene 31: 2101–2114.
60. Cardoso F, Van't Veer L, Rutgers E, Loi S, Mook S, et al. (2008) Clinical application of the 70-gene profile: the MINDACT trial. J Clin Oncol 26: 729–735.
61. Paik S, Shak S, Tang G, Kim C, Baker J, et al. (2004) A multigene assay to predict recurrence of tamoxifen-treated, node-negative breast cancer. N Engl J Med 351: 2817–2826.
62. Galon J, Franck P, Marincola FM, Angell HK, Thurin M, et al. (2012) Cancer classification using the Immunoscore: a worldwide task force. J Transl Med 10: 205.
63. Hoosein MM, Dashwood MR, Dawas K, Ali HM, Grant K, et al. (2007) Altered endothelin receptor subtypes in colorectal cancer. Eur J Gastroenterol Hepatol 19: 775–782.
64. Brown LF, Papadopoulos-Sergiou A, Berse B, Manseau EJ, Tognazzi K, et al. (1994) Osteopontin expression and distribution in human carcinomas. Am J Pathol 145: 610–623.
65. Noetzel E, Rose M, Bornemann J, Gajewski M, Knuchel R, et al. (2011) Nuclear transport receptor karyopherin-alpha2 promotes malignant breast cancer phenotypes in vitro. Oncogene.
66. Lange K, Kammerer M, Hegi ME, Grotegut S, Dittmann A, et al. (2007) Endothelin receptor type B counteracts tenascin-C-induced endothelin receptor type A-dependent focal adhesion and actin stress fiber disorganization. Cancer Res 67: 6163–6173.
67. Erler JT, Bennewith KL, Cox TR, Lang G, Bird D, et al. (2009) Hypoxia-induced lysyl oxidase is a critical mediator of bone marrow cell recruitment to form the premetastatic niche. Cancer Cell 15: 35–44.
68. Kodama J, Hasengaowa, Kusumoto T, Seki N, Matsuo T, et al. (2007) Prognostic significance of stromal versican expression in human endometrial cancer. Ann Oncol 18: 269–274.
69. Townes CL, Michailidis G, Nile CJ, Hall J (2004) Induction of cationic chicken liver-expressed antimicrobial peptide 2 in response to Salmonella enterica infection. Infect Immun 72: 6987–6993.
70. Howard A, Townes C, Milona P, Nile CJ, Michailidis G, et al. (2010) Expression and functional analyses of liver expressed antimicrobial peptide-2 (LEAP-2) variant forms in human tissues. Cell Immunol 261: 128–133.
71. Khattar NH, Lele SM, Kaetzel CS (2005) Down-regulation of the polymeric immunoglobulin receptor in non-small cell lung carcinoma: correlation with dysregulated expression of the transcription factors USF and AP2. J Biomed Sci 12: 65–77.
72. Ocak S, Pedchenko TV, Chen H, Harris FT, Qian J, et al. (2011) Loss of polymeric immunoglobulin receptor expression is associated with lung tumorigenesis. Eur Respir J.
73. Ai J, Tang Q, Wu Y, Xu Y, Feng T, et al. (2011) The role of polymeric immunoglobulin receptor in inflammation-induced tumor metastasis of human hepatocellular carcinoma. J Natl Cancer Inst 103: 1696–1712.
74. Cho YG, Chang X, Park IS, Yamashita K, Shao C, et al. (2011) Promoter methylation of leukemia inhibitory factor receptor gene in colorectal carcinoma. Int J Oncol 39: 337–344.
75. Okamura Y, Nomoto S, Kanda M, Li Q, Nishikawa Y, et al. (2010) Leukemia inhibitory factor receptor (LIFR) is detected as a novel suppressor gene of hepatocellular carcinoma using double-combination array. Cancer Lett 289: 170–177.
76. Garlanda C, Bottazzi B, Bastone A, Mantovani A (2005) Pentraxins at the crossroads between innate immunity, inflammation, matrix deposition, and female fertility. Annu Rev Immunol 23: 337–366.
77. Bijsmans IT, Smits KM, de Graeff P, Wisman GB, van der Zee AG, et al. (2011) Loss of SerpinA5 protein expression is associated with advanced-stage serous ovarian tumors. Mod Pathol 24: 463–470.
78. Facciabene A, Peng X, Hagemann IS, Balint K, Barchetti A, et al. (2011) Tumour hypoxia promotes tolerance and angiogenesis via CCL28 and T(reg) cells. Nature 475: 226–230.

7

Inhibition of HDAC1 and DNMT1 Modulate RGS10 Expression and Decrease Ovarian Cancer Chemoresistance

Ercan Cacan[1], Mourad W. Ali[2], Nathaniel H. Boyd[1], Shelley B. Hooks[2], Susanna F. Greer[1]*

1 Division of Cellular Biology and Immunology, Center for Inflammation, Immunity and Infection, Department of Biology, Georgia State University, Atlanta, Georgia, United States of America, **2** Department of Pharmaceutical and Biomedical Sciences, University of Georgia, Athens, Georgia, United States of America

Abstract

RGS10 is an important regulator of cell survival and chemoresistance in ovarian cancer. We recently showed that RGS10 transcript expression is suppressed during acquired chemoresistance in ovarian cancer. The suppression of RGS10 is due to DNA hypermethylation and histone deacetylation, two important mechanisms that contribute to silencing of tumor suppressor genes during cancer progression. Here, we fully investigate the molecular mechanisms of epigenetic silencing of RGS10 expression in chemoresistant A2780-AD ovarian cancer cells. We identify two important epigenetic regulators, HDAC1 and DNMT1, that exhibit aberrant association with RGS10 promoters in chemoresistant ovarian cancer cells. Knockdown of HDAC1 or DNMT1 expression, and pharmacological inhibition of DNMT or HDAC enzymatic activity, significantly increases RGS10 expression and cisplatin-mediated cell death. Finally, DNMT1 knock down also decreases HDAC1 binding to the RGS10 promoter in chemoresistant cells, suggesting HDAC1 recruitment to RGS10 promoters requires DNMT1 activity. Our results suggest that HDAC1 and DNMT1 contribute to the suppression of RGS10 during acquired chemoresistance and support inhibition of HDAC1 and DNMT1 as an adjuvant therapeutic approach to overcome ovarian cancer chemoresistance.

Editor: Malú G. Tansey, Emory University, United States of America

Funding: Research was supported by grant # RSG-09-067-01-LB from the American Cancer Society. The funder had no role in study design, data collection and analysis, decision to publish, or preparation of the manuscript.

Competing Interests: The authors have declared that no competing interests exist.

* E-mail: sgreer@gsu.edu

Introduction

Ovarian cancer is one of the deadliest gynecological cancers, with a 60% mortality rate in patients and a 5-year survival rate of lower than 30% in advanced stage disease [1]. The high mortality rate is due in large part to the development of resistance to chemotherapeutic drugs [2,3]. Thus, understanding the molecular and genetic mechanisms that drive the development of acquired chemoresistance will enable us to improve current therapeutic agents for ovarian cancer treatment. G-protein coupled receptors (GPCRs) initiate multiple oncogenic signaling pathways in cancer cells by activating their associated G-proteins [4,5]. Activation of GPCRs by growth factors such as Lysophosphatidic acid (LPA) triggers survival signaling pathways that drive resistance to chemotherapeutic drugs such as cisplatin and taxane [6]. GPCR activation of G-proteins is opposed by the activity of regulator of G-protein signaling (RGS) proteins. RGS proteins inhibit G-protein signaling pathways by directly binding to the activated Gα subunit of G-proteins to accelerate hydrolysis of GTP into GDP, which returns G-proteins to an inactive state [7–10]. Relevant to our studies, recent reports indicate that RGS proteins inhibit breast, lung, prostate, and ovarian cancer cell growth through inhibition of GPCRs signaling pathways [2,11–15].

RGS10 is among the smallest of the RGS proteins and is highly expressed in a broad range of cell types [16–19]. RGS10 is an important regulator of cell survival and chemoresistance [2], and RGS10 transcript expression is significantly suppressed in multiple ovarian cancer cell lines [15]. Thus, the suppression of RGS10 proteins may contribute to chemoresistance by amplifying GPCR-mediated cell growth and survival signaling pathways. We have recently shown that suppression of RGS10 is due in part to DNA hypermethylation and to histone deacetylation, two important gene-silencing mechanisms which contribute to the progression of many cancers. DNA methylation is maintained by DNA methyl transferases (DNMTs) [20] and histone deacetylation is maintained by histone deacetylases (HDACs) [21]. Often, these two enzymes coordinately suppress transcriptional activity of genes [22,23]. Fuks *et al.* have reported that DNMT1 is associated with histone deacetylase activity and has the ability to bind HDAC1 [24]. However, the molecular mechanisms by which DNA hypermethylation and histone deacetylation suppress RGS10 and the contribution of these enzymes to acquired chemoresistance remains unknown.

We investigate here the molecular mechanisms of epigenetic regulation of RGS10 expression in ovarian cancer cells and focus on chemosensitive parental A2780 cells and their derivative cell line, chemoresistant A2780-AD. We identify two important epigenetic regulators, HDAC1 and DNMT1, which are highly associated with the RGS10 promoter in chemoresistant ovarian cancer cells. HDAC1 and DNMT1 knock down significantly increases RGS10 expression and cisplatin-stimulated cell death.

Our results suggest that HDAC1 and DNMT1 contribute to the suppression of RGS10 during acquired chemoresistance and support growing evidence that inhibition of HDAC1/DNMT1 represent novel therapeutic approaches to overcoming ovarian cancer chemoresistance.

Materials and Methods

Cell lines and reagents

The chemosensitive A2780 parental cell line and their derivative chemoresistant A2780-AD cells (derived as described [25]) were generously provided by Dr. Bob Brown, Imperial College London. These cells were maintained in RPMI 1640 medium (Mediatech Inc.) supplemented with 10% FBS and 5 mM L-glutamine. Chemoresistant cells were further maintained in 3 μM cisplatin. All cells were grown in 5 mM penicillin-streptomycin at 37°C with 5% CO_2. OV2008 and C13 cells (derived as described [26,27]) were generously provided by Dr. Patricia Kruk, University of South Florida.

5-Aza-2′-deoxycytidine (5-Aza-dC), Trichostatin A (TSA), and cisplatin were purchased from Sigma-Aldrich (St. Louis, MO). Antibodies recognizing RGS10, HDAC1, goat-anti-rat IgG-HRP (Horseradish peroxidase), and HRP conjugated rabbit antibodies were obtained from Santa Cruz (Santa Cruz, CA). Antibodies recognizing DNMT1 were obtained from Abcam (Cambridge, MA). HRP conjugated mouse antibodies were purchased from Promega (Madison, WI). Antibodies recognizing β-Actin were obtained from Cell Signaling (Beverly, MA).

siRNA constructs and transient transfection

Short interfering RNA (siRNA) pre-designed for HDAC1 (Qiagen), RGS10 and DNMT1 (Santa Cruz) were used to knock down expression of HDAC1, RGS10 or DNMT1. Scrambled All Star Control siRNA (Qiagen) was used as a control. A2780-AD cells were transfected with 10 nM of HDAC1 or DNMT1 specific siRNA or All Star scrambled control siRNA using HiPerfect transfection reagent (Qiagen) according to the manufacturer's instruction. Following indicated incubation time, cells were harvested and analyzed in western blot, RNA expression, or chromatin immunoprecipitation experiments.

RNA expression and quantitative real-time PCR

mRNA was isolated using Qiazol RNA extraction reagent (Qiagen) as described in the manufacturer's protocol. Briefly, cells were lysed in Qiazol and agitated on a 3D rotator for 5 minutes. 200 μl of chloroform was added and was incubated for three minutes at room temperature. Samples were centrifugated and the aqueous phase (400 μl) was transferred to an eppendorf tube. 500 μl of isopropanol was added and was incubated for 10 minutes at room temperature. Following centrifugation, pellets were washed with 1 mL of cold 75% ethanol, centrifuged and resuspended in 50 μl of RNAse free water. RNA was quantified and cDNA was generated from 1 μg of total extracted RNA using an Omniscript Reverse Transcription Kit (Qiagen). Following cDNA synthesis, quantitative real-time polymerase chain reaction was performed using TaqMan Universal PCR Master Mix (Roche) and specific primers and probes targeting RGS10 or GAPDH coding regions. Transcript expression was assessed using an ABI prism 7900HT Real-Time PCR System (Applied Biosystems). Reactions were normalized against GAPDH expression and calculations were performed using standard curves generated. Primers used were: RGS10 Forward: 5′-GAC CCA AGA AGG CGT GAA AAG A-3′, RGS10 Reverse: 5′-GCT GGA CAG AAA GGT CAT GTA GA-3′, RGS10 probe: 5′-AGA TAA GAC GCA GAT GCA GGA AAA GGC-3′, GAPDH Forward: 5′-GGA AGC TCA CTG GCA TGG C-3′, GAPDH Reverse: 5′-TAG ACG GCA GGT CAG GTC CA-3′ and GAPDH probe: 5′- CCC CAC TGC CAA CGT GTC AGT G-3′.

To determine the effect of 5-Aza-dC and TSA exposure on RGS10 transcript expression, 1×10^6 A2780-AD cells were plated per 10 cm^2 tissue culture plate and were incubated overnight. Cells were treated with 20 μM 5-Aza-dC or with 500 ng TSA dissolved in DMSO. TSA treated cells were incubated for 48 hours and 5-Aza-dC treated cells were incubated for three, five, or seven days, with media aspirated and replaced daily. RNA isolation and DNA synthesis were performed as described above.

Chromatin immunoprecipitation (ChIP) assay

ChIP assays were performed as previously described [15]. Briefly, cells were plated at a density of 2×10^6 in 10 cm^2 plates. Three million cells were crosslinked with 1% formaldehyde for eight minutes at room temperature. Crosslinking reactions were stopped by the addition of 0.125 M glycine. Cell nuclei were isolated and were concentrated by lysis in SDS lysis buffer (1% SDS, 10 mM EDTA, 50 mM Tris pH 8.0) plus protease inhibitors for 30 minutes on ice followed by flash freezing in liquid nitrogen. Nuclei were sonicated using a Bioruptor water bath sonicator (Diagenode) to generate an average of 500 bp of sheared DNA which was confirmed by agarose gel electrophoresis. Sonicated lysates were precleared with salmon-sperm/agarose beads (Millipore), 5% of the total lysate was stored as input for normalization. Half of the remaining lysate was immunoprecipitated with 5 μg of indicated antibody overnight at 4°C and the other half of the lysate was immunoprecipitated with a control antibody. Following an additional two hour immunoprecipitation with salmon-sperm coated agarose beads, all samples were washed with each of the following buffers: low salt buffer (0.1% SDS, 1% Triton X-100, 2 mM EDTA, 20 mM Tris pH 8.0, 150 mM NaCl), high salt buffer (0.1% SDS, 1% Triton X-100, 2 mM EDTA, 20 mM Tris pH 8.0, 500 mM NaCl), LiCl (0.25 M LiCl, 1% NP40, 1% DOC, 1 mM EDTA, 10 mM Tris pH 8.0), and 1×TE (Tris-EDTA); DNA was then eluted with SDS elution buffer (1% SDS, 0.1 M NaHCO3). Following elution, cross-links were reversed overnight with 5 M NaCl at 65°C and the immunoprecipitated DNA was isolated using phenol:chloroform:isopropanol mix (Invitrogen) as per the manufacturer's instructions. Isolated DNA was quantified by real time PCR on an ABI prism 7900 HT (Applied Biosystems, Foster City, CA) using specific primers and probes targeting RGS10 and GAPDH promoters region. Values generated from real time PCR reactions were calculated based on standard curves generated, were run in triplicate reactions, and were analyzed using the SDS 2.0 program (Applied Biosystems).

Chromatin immunoprecipitation assay in siRNA treated cells

Chemoresistant A2780-AD cells were plated at a density of 1.2×10^6 cells per 10 cm^2 tissue culture plates. Cells were treated with siRNA constructs as described above and were incubated for 72 hours. Cells were harvested and 1/10 of the cell volume was removed for analysis of knockdown efficiency by western blot analysis. ChIP assays were carried out as described above on the remaining harvested cells.

RNA expression in siRNA treated cells

Cells were plated at a density of 1×10^6 cells per 10 cm^2 tissue culture plate and were incubated overnight. The cells were then transfected with the indicated siRNA construct as described above and incubated for 72 hours, and an RNA extraction was performed as described above.

Apoptosis assay

Apoptosis of A2780-AD cells was assessed using the Annexin V: PE Apoptosis Detection Kit I (BD Pharmingen). 1×10^6 A2780-AD cells were plated on a 10 cm^2 tissue culture plate and were incubated for 24 hours at 37°C. The cells were treated with HDAC1 siRNA or with control siRNA using the HiPerfect transfection reagent. Following 48 hours incubation, 50 μM of cisplatin was added to both HDAC1 siRNA and control siRNA treated cells and the cells were incubated for an additional 48 hours. A2780-AD cells were briefly trypsinized and were harvested. A fraction of the cell volume was removed for western blot analysis and the remaining fraction of cells was washed with cold PBS twice and was resuspended in Annexin V binding buffer at a concentration of 1×10^6 cells/ml. The cells were then transferred to 5 mL culture tubes containing 5 μl of Annexin V-PE and/or 5 μl of 7-Aminoactinomycin D (7-AAD). The samples were gently mixed and were incubated for 20 minutes at room temperature. Following the addition of 400 μl of Annexin V binding buffer to each tube, samples were analyzed and quantified by flow cytometry and resulting data were analyzed using FlowJo software.

Results

Histone acetylation is suppressed at RGS10 promoters in ovarian cancer cells

We have recently shown that levels of acetylated histone H3 histone are significantly decreased at the RGS10-1 promoter in the A2780-AD cell model of ovarian cancer chemoresistance [15]. To confirm these findings in additional cell lines, chromatin immunoprecipitation (ChIP) assays were carried out in the chemosensitive ovarian cancer cell line OV2008 and in chemoresistant C13 daughter cells. While total levels of histone H3 are similar at both RGS10 and GAPDH promoters in chemosensitive and chemoresistant cells (Fig. 1A), levels of acetylated histone H3 are significantly lower at RGS10 promoters in the chemoresistant C13 ovarian cancer cells as compared to chemosensitive OV2008 cells (Fig. 1B).

Reductions in H3 lysine 18 acetylation (H3K18Ac) have been associated with aggressive cancer phenotypes and with poor patient prognosis [28,29]. We next performed ChIP assays to determine if loss of H3K18 contributes to the loss of global histone acetylation at RGS10 promoters in chemoresistant C13 cells. A significant decrease in H3K18 acetylation at RGS10 promoters was observed in chemoresistant C13 cells, while H3K18 acetylation at the GAPDH promoters in OV2008 and C13 cells remained unchanged (Fig. 1C). Together these data suggest the loss of acetylation at RGS10 promoters contributes to the loss of RGS10 expression in two independent cell models of chemoresistant ovarian cancer.

HDAC1 and DNMT1 suppress RGS10 expression in chemoresistant ovarian cancer cells

We previously demonstrated that HDAC1 proteins bind with significantly increased frequency to the RGS10 promoter in chemoresistant A2780-AD cells compared to parental chemosensitive A2780 cells [15]. To investigate molecular roles for HDAC1 in regulating RGS10 expression, a siRNA duplex was utilized to specifically knock down endogenous HDAC1 expression in A2780-AD cells. siRNA-mediated knockdown of HDAC1 resulted in a more than 3-fold increase in endogenous RGS10 transcript expression as compared to control siRNA (Fig. 2A), suggesting that HDAC1 plays a critical role in regulating RGS10 transcription. Western blot analysis confirmed HDAC1 knock down increased RGS10 protein expression (Fig.2B). In a similar experiment, A2780-AD cells were transfected with HDAC1 to determine the effects of ectopic expression of HDAC1. Overexpression of HDAC1 dramatically reduced RGS10 expression in chemoresistant A2780-AD cells (Fig. 2C–E). Together, these data indicate that HDAC1 accumulation at RGS10 promoters likely contributes to suppression of RGS10 in chemoresistant ovarian cancer cells.

The RGS10-1 promoter contains a high concentration of CpG dinucleotides making it a potential target for DNMT maintenance methylation during ovarian cancer progression. We first determined by western blot analysis that DNMT1 expression levels are similar in both A2780 and A2780-AD cell lines (Fig. 3B). To further explore the relevance of DNMT1 in the specific suppression of RGS10 expression, ChIP assays were carried out in A2780 parental and their derivative resistant A2780-AD cells. Lysates were immunoprecipitated with control or anti-DNMT1 antibody and associated DNA was analyzed via quantitative real-time PCR (qRT-PCR) using specific primers and probes spanning the RGS10 and GAPDH promoters. In contrast to total protein abundance, ChIP assays reveal that binding of DNMT1 is significantly increased at the RGS10 promoter in chemoresistant cells as compared to chemosensitive ovarian cancer cells (Fig. 3A). Together these data indicate that accumulation of DNMT1 at the RGS10 promoter likely contributes to suppression of RGS10 during ovarian cancer chemoresistance.

Accumulation of DNMT1 at the RGS10 promoter led us to determine if that accumulation affects RGS10 transcript expression level in chemoresistant cells. For this purpose, A2780-AD cells were transfected with DNMT1 siRNA or control siRNA. RNA was extracted and generated cDNA was quantified using qRT-PCR with primers and probes specific for the RGS10 coding region and normalized to housekeeping gene GAPDH expression. The data reveals that knocking down DNMT1 significantly increases endogenous RGS10 transcript expression (Fig. 3C) and protein expression (Fig. 3D) in A2780-AD cells. This increase suggests that DNMT1 functions with HDAC1 to regulate the suppression of RGS10 transcription in chemoresistant A2780-AD cells.

Inhibition of HDAC and DNMT activity enhances RGS10 expression and decreases ovarian cancer cell viability

We next sought to determine if pharmacologic inhibitors of histone deacetylation and DNA methylation can alter the expression of RGS10 in chemoresistant ovarian cancer cells. The HDAC inhibitor TSA and DNMT inhibitor 5-Aza-dC were used to inhibit HDACs and DNMTs, respectively. A2780-AD cells were treated with 500 nM TSA and were incubated for 2 days or were treated with 20 μM 5-Aza-dC and incubated for 3, 5 and 7 days. Total RNA was isolated from untreated control cells, TSA, and 5-Aza-dC treated cells. The relative expression of RGS10 transcript expression was quantified by qRT-PCR and was normalized to GAPDH transcript expression. Consistent with observations from HDAC1 and DNMT1 knock down experiments, TSA and 5-Aza-dC treatments both significantly enhanced RGS10 transcript expression in chemoresistant A2780-AD cells (Fig. 4A and 4B). To explore potential synergistic roles for

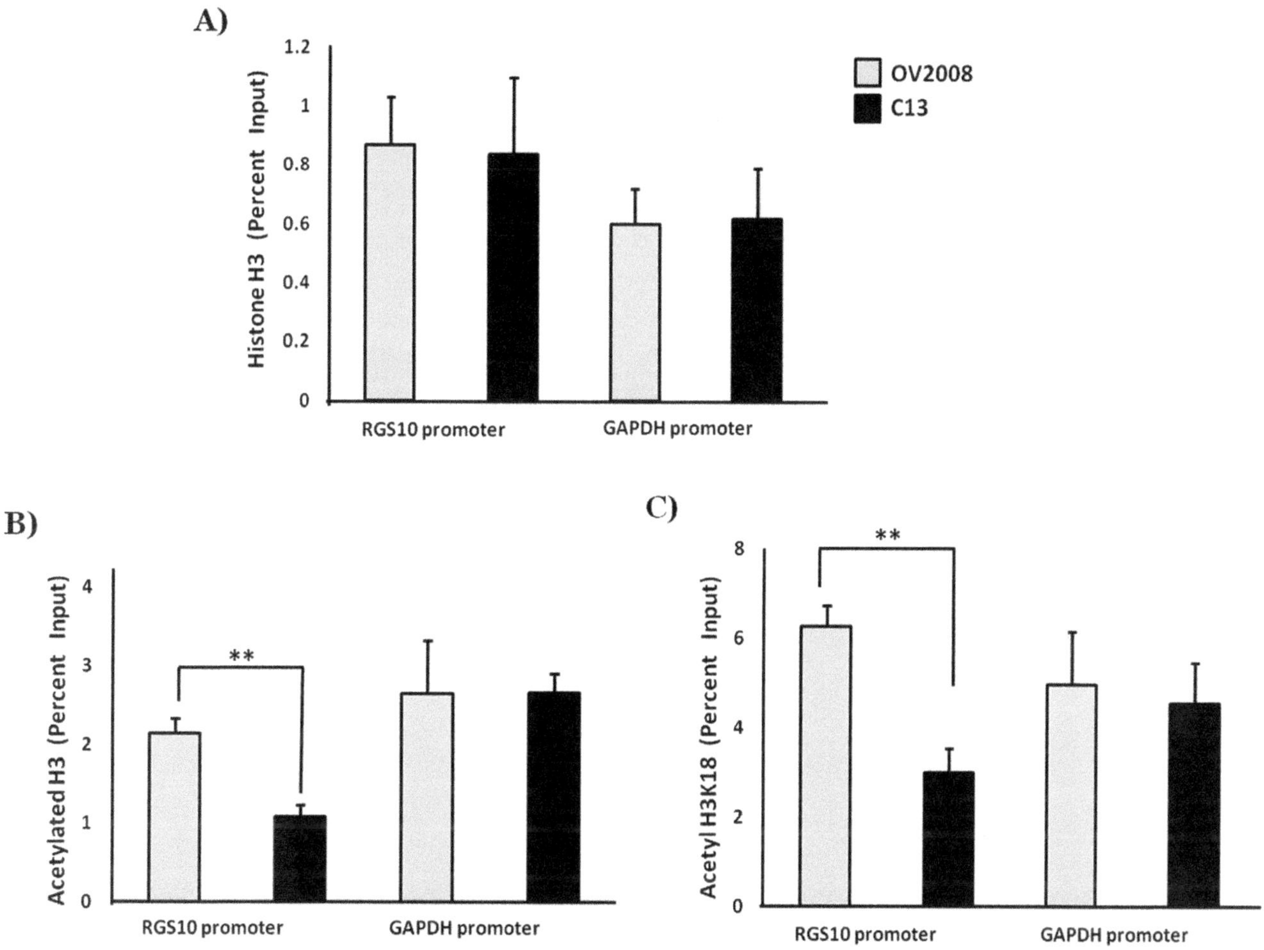

Figure 1. Histone H3 and acetylation levels at RGS10 promoters in chemoresistant C13 cells and parental OV2008 cells. ChIP assays were carried out in OV2008 parental cells and drug resistant C13 cells. Lysates were immunoprecipitated with control, anti-histone H3, anti-acetyl histone H3, or anti-acetyl H3K18 antibodies. Associated DNA was isolated and analyzed via real time PCR using primers spanning the RGS10 and GAPDH promoters. Real-time PCR values were normalized to the total amount of promoter DNA added (input). Input values represent 5% of the total cell lysate. **$p<0.005$. **A)** Global histone H3 levels associated with RGS10 and GAPDH promoters. **B)** Global levels of histone H3 acetylation associated with RGS10 and GAPDH promoters. **C)** Levels of histone H3 acetylated at lysine 18 associated with RGS10 and GAPDH promoters.

HDAC1 and DNMT1 in regulating RGS10 expression, combination studies were performed using TSA and 5-Aza-dC in chemoresistant ovarian cancer cells. Again, TSA or 5-Aza-dC alone enhanced RGS10 expression in A2780-AD cells, and the combination of these two drugs results in a fold increase in RGS10 expression greater than the sum of the individual effect, suggesting a potential cooperative effect (Fig. 4C). To investigate cooperative roles for HDAC1 and DNMT1 in cell growth and chemoresistance, A2780-AD cells were treated with TSA and/or 5-Aza-dC in the presence of cisplatin and cell viability assays were performed. 5-Aza-dC alone reduced cell growth by approximately 40%, while TSA alone had a modest but significant effect on cell viability; however, the combination of TSA and 5-Aza-dC inhibited cell viability by 90%. As expected, A2780-AD cells were resistant to cisplatin toxicity, but either TSA or 5-Aza-dC partially re-sensitized the cells to cisplatin-mediated cytotoxicity (Fig. 4D). To determine if RGS10 upregulation by TSA/5-Aza-dC combined treatment could fully account for loss of cell viability, we attempted to rescue cell viability in the presence of 5-Aza-dC and TSA with RGS10 siRNA. Not surprisingly, knock-down of RGS10 alone did not rescue cell viability, consistent with the broad range of HDAC and DNMT target genes in cancer cells (Fig. 4E). Thus, RGS10 coordinately regulates cell viability and chemosensitivity with additional HDAC and DNMT target genes.

Knocking down HDAC1 enhances cisplatin-stimulated apoptosis in chemoresistant cells

Our previous work suggests that suppression of RGS10 expression contributes to the development of chemoresistance during ovarian cancer progression through amplification of endogenous survival signaling pathways [2,15], and results presented here suggest that HDAC1 contributes to the loss of RGS10 expression in chemoresistant ovarian cancer cells. To determine HDAC1-mediated changes in cell survival of chemoresistant ovarian cancer cells, cisplatin resistant A2780-AD cells were transfected with HDAC1 siRNA. Following transfection, cells were incubated with 50 μM cisplatin and apoptosis was analyzed using an Annexin V:PE apoptosis detection kit (BD Pharmingen). Annexin V binds phosphatidylserine, which is exposed only in apoptotic cells, while the membrane impermeant DNA label 7-Aminoactinomycin D (7-AAD) selectively binds to GC regions of the DNA only in late apoptotic or dead cells with

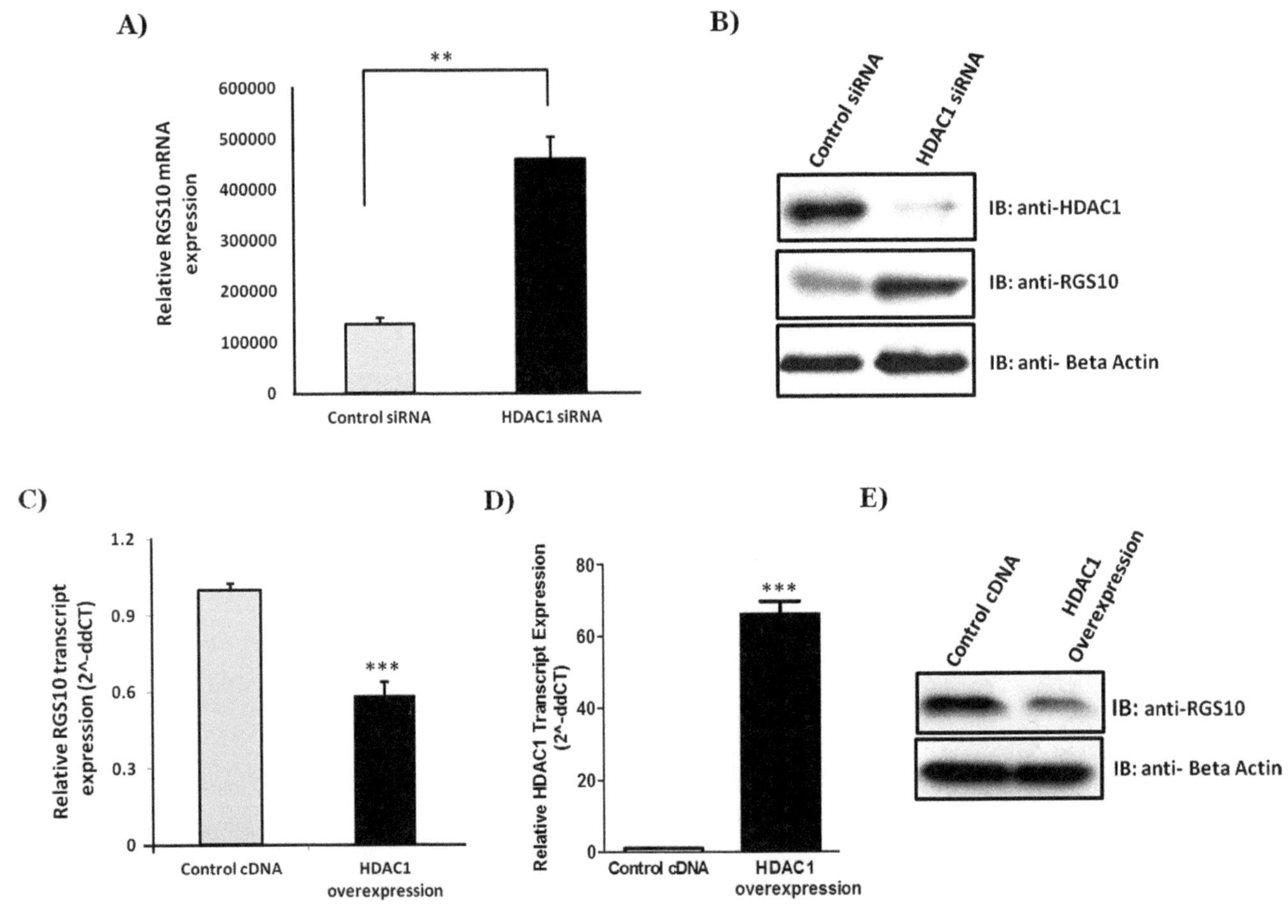

Figure 2. HDAC1 knockdown significantly increases RGS10 expression while HDAC1 overexpression decreases RGS10 expression in chemoresistant ovarian cancer cells. A) Knockdown of HDAC1 increases RGS10 mRNA transcription. A2780-AD cells were transfected with HDAC1 siRNA or control siRNA and incubated for 72 hours. RNA was extracted and cDNA was generated by using a reverse primer targeting for RGS10 or GAPDH coding region. Data was quantified using qPCR with primers and probes specific for RGS10 and GAPDH coding regions. Graphed data shows the average of three independent experiments, with error bars denoting standard error of the mean (SEM). Significance was calculated with a Student's t test $^{**}p<0.005$. **B)** Western blot analysis demonstrating efficiency of HDAC1 knockdown and RGS10 protein expression following HDAC1 knock down with Beta-Actin controls. **C–D)** HDAC1 overexpression decreases RGS10 expression in chemoresistant cells. A2780/AD cells were plated in 24-well plate and allowed to attach overnight. Cells were transfected with 500 ng HDAC1 or empty vector using FuGene 6 reagent (Promega) according to the manufacturer's protocol. Following 48 hours incubation, cells were harvested in TRIzol (Invitrogen) and the expression of RGS10 and HDAC1 genes was assessed using RT-PCR as described, and normalized to actin gene expression. Values represent mean $\pm$ SEM of four independent experiments $^{***}p<0.0005$. **E)** Western blot analysis demonstrating RGS10 protein expression following HDAC1 overexpression with Beta-Actin controls.

compromised membranes [30–32]. Thus, early apoptotic cells are stained with only annexin V-PE, while late apoptotic and dead cells are stained with both annexin V-PE and 7-AAD. Flow cytometric analysis was used to distinguish between populations of unlabeled and singly- or doubly-labeled cells. HDAC1 knock down significantly increased the population of cisplatin-stimulated cells from 12.9% to 32.1% that are positive for both annexin V-PE and 7-AAD (late apoptotic or dead cells) (Fig. 5A). The results are confirmed by three independent experiments (Fig. 5B). Knock down efficiency of HDAC1 and RGS10 protein expression following the HDAC1 knock down was confirmed in A2780-AD cells by western blot analysis (Fig. 5C). Together these data suggest that HDAC1 mediated reduction of RGS10 expression blunts the ability of cisplatin to induce cell death in A2780/AD ovarian cancer cells.

DNMT1 knock down decreases HDAC1 binding to the RGS10 promoter in chemoresistant ovarian cancer cells

HDAC1 and DNMT1 contribute to gene silencing through recruiting transcriptional repressors to promoter regions [33–35] and work together to suppress gene expression [24,36]. Our data suggest that HDAC and DNMT activities cooperatively silence RGS10 (Fig. 4C). To investigate crosstalk between these two epigenetic regulators, A2780-AD cells were transfected with DNMT1 siRNA or control siRNA and were incubated for 72 hours. HDAC1 binding to the RGS10 promoter was examined by ChIP assays in DNMT1 siRNA or control siRNA treated A2780-AD cells. DNMT1 knock down significantly decreased binding of HDAC1 to the RGS10 promoter (Fig. 6A) and western blot analysis (Fig. 6B) demonstrated successful and specific knockdown of DNMT1. The converse experiment was also performed where A2780-AD cells were transfected with HDAC1 siRNA. Western blot analysis demonstrated knockdown of HDAC1 resulted in suppression of DNMT1 protein expression

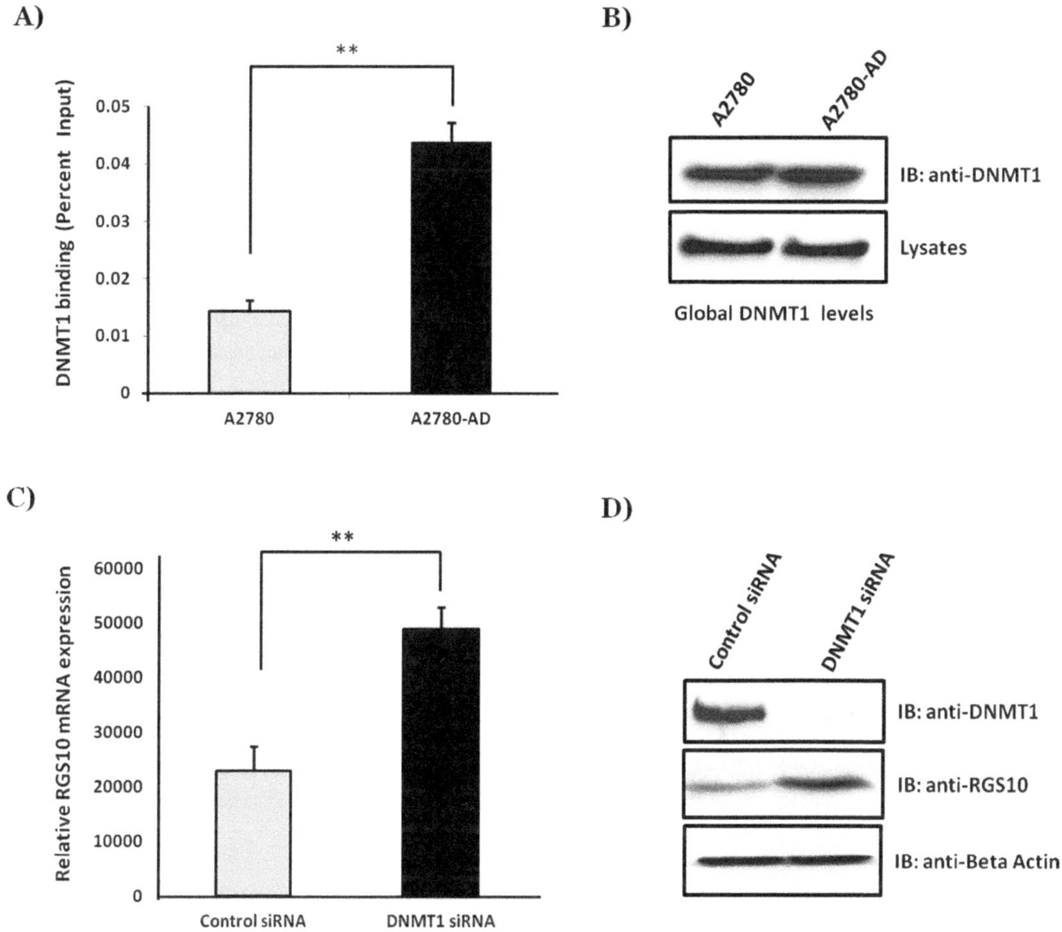

Figure 3. DNMT1 binding is increased at RGS10 promoter and DNMT1 knock down enhances the RGS10 transcript expression in chemoresistant ovarian cancer cells. A) Levels of DNMT1 associated with RGS10 promoters in A2780 and A2780-AD ovarian cancer cells. ChIP assays were carried out in A2780 parental and their derivative resistant A2780-AD cells. Lysates were immunoprecipitated with control or anti-DNMT1 antibody. Associated DNA was isolated and analyzed via real time PCR using specific primers and probes spanning the RGS10 and GAPDH promoters. Real-time PCR values were normalized to the total amount of promoter DNA added (input). Values were normalized to GAPDH and represent mean ± SEM of three independent experiments $^{**}p<0.005$. **B)** Western blot analysis of global DNMT1 levels in A2780 and A2780-AD cells. Cells were harvested and lysates were used for immunoprecipitation. Antibody-conjugated agarose beads (IP) for DNMT1 were incubated with rotation overnight. Beads were washed, eluted and subjected to western blot with respective antibodies. **C)** A2780-AD cells were transfected with DNMT1 siRNA or with control siRNA and were incubated for 72 hours. RNA was extracted and cDNA was generated by using reverse primers targeting RGS10 and GAPDH coding regions. Data generated was quantified using qRT-PCR with primers and probes specific for the RGS10 coding region. Values represent mean ± SEM of four independent experiments $^{**}p<0.005$. **D)** Western blot analysis for efficiency of knocking down DNMT1 and for RGS10 protein expression following DNMT1 knock down.

(data not shown); an observation seen by others as well [37]. These data suggest that HDAC1 is recruited to the RGS10 promoter via DNMT1 and methyl-CpG binding protein 2 (MeCP2) dependent mechanisms (Fig. 6C). MeCP2 directly interacts with DNMT1 and it is possible a MeCP2-DNMT1 complex recruits HDAC1 to RGS10 promoter via binding Sin3 [38–41] or NuRD complexes [23]. In this manner, DNMT1 and HDAC1 synergistically contribute suppression of RGS10 transcription expression as ovarian cancer progresses.

Discussion

GPCRs have been recognized as important drug targets for treatment of multiple cancers [10,42,43]. The strength of signaling pathways initiated by GPCRs is attenuated by members of the RGS protein family, including RGS10 [8,44–46]. DNA methylation and histone deacetylation are often associated with transcriptional repression of gene expression [47,48] and with decreased responsiveness to chemotherapy [49,50]. We recently linked the suppression of RGS10 expression to ovarian cancer cell survival and chemoresistance, and further showed RGS10 knock down to increase cell growth and survival [2,15]. DNA hypermethylation and histone deacetylation contribute to ovarian cancer chemoresistance through amplification of master regulators of multiple cell survival proteins [15,51–53]. Recent findings suggest epigenetic control mechanisms for cisplatin resistance in ovarian cancer, and multiple genes targets that may be subjected to epigenetic control [53]. In our current study, we demonstrate specific contribution of two important epigenetic regulators, HDAC1 and DNMT1, to the suppression of RGS10 expression in chemoresistant ovarian cancer cells.

HDACs remove acetyl groups from substrates, including the histones of chromatin. Conversely, HDAC inhibitors preserve the acetylation status of proteins and induce growth arrest and

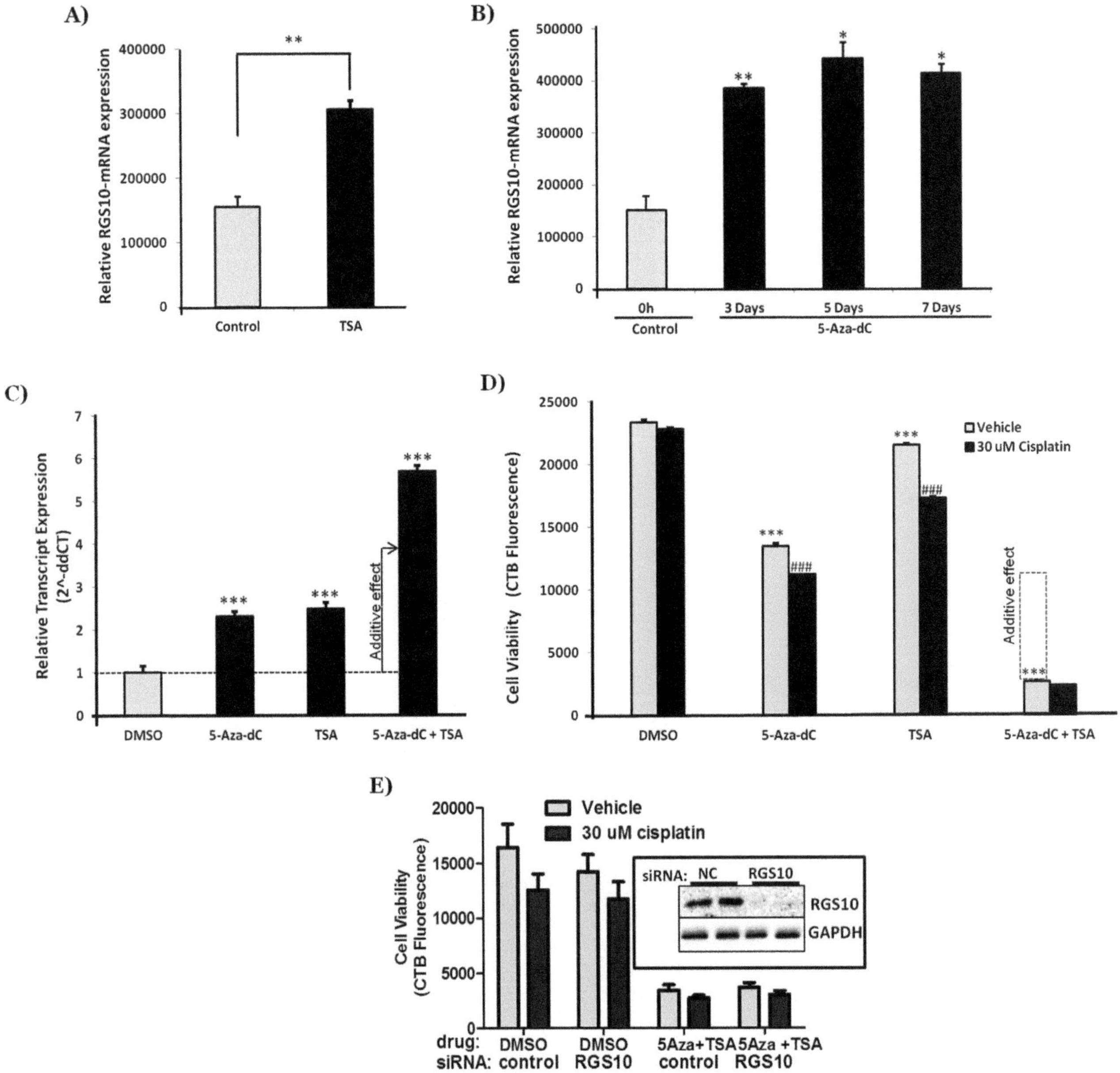

Figure 4. Effects of HDAC inhibitor trichostatin A (TSA) and DNMT inhibitor 5-Aza-2′-deoxycytidine (5-Aza-dC) on RGS10 transcript expression and cell viabilities. Total RNA was isolated from untreated control cells and TSA or 5-Aza-dC treated cells. The relative expression of RGS10 mRNA was quantified by qRT-PCR and normalized to GAPDH transcript expression * $p<0.05$; ** $p<0.005$. **A**) HDAC inhibition increases RGS10 expression in chemoresistant A2780-AD cells. The cells were plated in a 10 cm^2 plate and incubated for 24 hours. The following day, cells were treated with 500 nM TSA and were incubated for an additional 48 hours. **B**) DNMT inhibitor 5-Aza-dC enhances RGS10 expression in chemoresistant cells. Two million A2780-AD cells were seeded in 10 cm^2 plates and were incubated for 24 hours. The following day, cells were treated with 20 μM 5-Aza-dC. Media and drug were refreshed every 24 hours. After indicated incubation time (3, 5, and 7 days), cells were harvested, mRNA was isolated, and cDNA was generated and quantified using qRT-PCR with specific primers and probe. **C**) A2780-AD cells were plated in 96-well plates and treated with 5 μM 5-Aza-dC for 5 days, 500 nM TSA for 36 hours, a combination of 5 μM 5-Aza-dC for 5 days and 500 nM TSA for the final 36 hours or DMSO. Gene expression was assessed using qRT-PCR as described, and normalized to RPL13A gene expression. The arrow indicates the expression level predicted by an additive effect of TSA and 5-Aza-dC. **D**) In a parallel experiment, A2780-AD cells were treated under the same conditions as 4C with or without 30 μM cisplatin for the final 12 hours. Cell survival was assessed using CellTiter-Blue fluorimetric viability assays. ***: $p<0.001$ comparing epigenetic drug to DMSO control in the absence of cisplatin. ###: $p<0.001$ comparing vehicle versus cisplatin treatment within epigenetic drug treatment groups. The dotted box indicates the cell viability predicted by an additive effect of TSA and 5-Aza-dC. **E**) A2780/AD cells (5000 cells/well) were plated in 96-well plate and transfected with negative control or RGS10 siRNA duplexes (Ambion Grand Island, NY) as per the manufacturer's protocol using Dharmafect1 transfection reagent (Dharmacon). Cells were dosed with a combination of 5 μM 5-Aza-dC for 3 days and 500 nM TSA for the last 36 h or DMSO. 30 μM cisplatin or vehicle was added for the last 12 h. Cell survival was assessed using CellTiter-Blue fluorimetric viability assays.

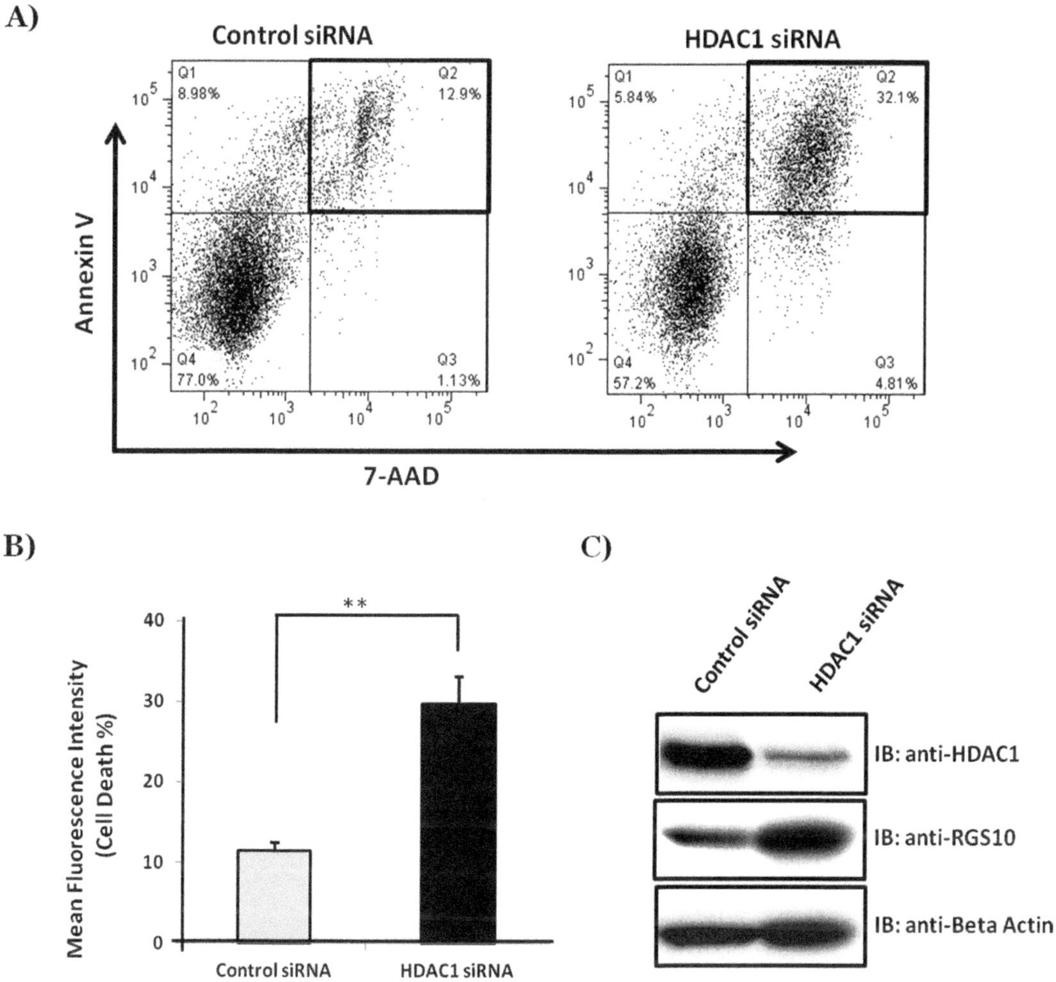

Figure 5. HDAC1 knockdown increases cisplatin stimulated apoptosis in chemoresistant cells. A2780-AD cells were treated with HDAC1 siRNA or control siRNA and were incubated for 48 hours. Following incubation, cells were treated with 50 μM cisplatin and incubated for addition 48 hours in RPMI 1640 media. An Annexin V: PE Apoptosis Detection Kit I (BD Pharmingen) was used for staining; results were quantified by Flow cytometry analysis and were analyzed using FlowJo software. Viable cells were negative for both annexin V-PE and 7-AAD; early apoptotic cells were positive for annexin V-PE and negative for 7-AAD, whereas late apoptotic dead cells were positive for both annexin V-PE and 7-AAD labeling. **A)** The relative increase of apoptotic cells in HDAC1- siRNA transfected A2780-AD cells which incorporated the Annexin V-PE and 7-AAD stains. **B)** Graph represent average of three independent experiments, with error bars denoting SEM *$p<0.05$. **C)** Western blot analysis represents efficiency of HDAC1 knockdown and RGS10 protein expression following HDAC1 knock down.

apoptosis of cancer cells [54–56]. Clinical trials show HDAC inhibitors to be effective anti-tumor drugs [57] and HDAC inhibitors have recently shown great therapeutic promise against ovarian cancer [58–60]. Our data suggest that reversal of HDAC1-mediated silencing of RGS10 likely contributes to the growth arrest initiated by HDAC inhibitors.

Multiple epigenetic modifications are commonly disrupted during carcinogenesis. Onco-genes undergo hypomethylation on DNA and acetylation and hypermethylation on histones in order to drive enhanced expression [61,62]. Conversely, DNA hypermethylation and histone deacetylation commonly occur on tumor suppressor genes [63–65]. In combination with histone deacetylase inhibition, the addition of a DNA methylation inhibitor has shown robust re-expression of silenced genes in tumor cells [66]. The data presented here further indicate DNMT1 accumulation at the RGS10 promoter suppresses RGS10 transcription in chemoresistant cells.

We previously observed that RGS10 suppressed activation of the survival factor Akt while RGS10 knock down increased activation of Akt; and thus established a causative relationship between suppression of RGS10 and reduced susceptibility to chemotherapeutic cytotoxicity [2]. Thus, RGS10 functions as a tumor suppressor by blunting endogenous survival pathways, with the level of expression of endogenous RGS10 playing a critical role in the determination of apoptosis or survival. Hence, we focused here on therapeutic approaches to decrease chemoresistance by enhancing RGS10 expression in chemoresistant ovarian cancer cells. HDAC1 knock down enhanced cisplatin-stimulated apoptosis in chemoresistant cells, suggesting that knocking down HDAC1 increases RGS10 expression and thus contributes to inhibition of GPCR-stimulated survival signaling pathways, resulting in an increase of apoptotic cells by the chemotherapeutic drug cisplatin.

DNA methylation and histone deacetylation act synergistically to silence cancer-associated genes in ovarian cancer [22–24,67]. Ovarian cancer is associated with elevated expression of DNMTs

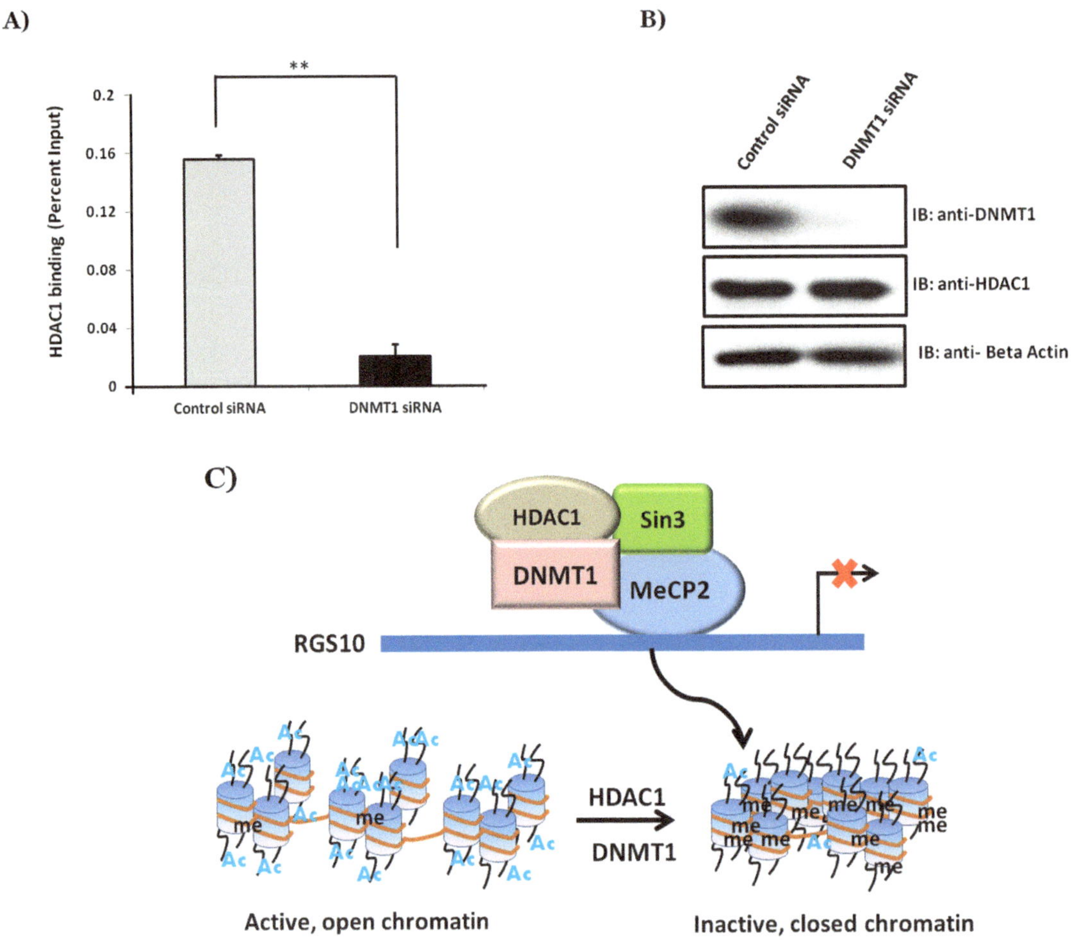

Figure 6. DNMT1 knock down decreases HDAC1 binding to RGS10 promoters in chemoresistant ovarian cancer cells. A2780-AD cells were transfected with HDAC1 siRNA or with control siRNA and were incubated for 72 hours. HDAC1 binding to RGS10 promoters was explored with ChIP assays in HDAC1 siRNA or in control siRNA treated A2780-AD cells. Lysates were immunoprecipitated with control or anti-HDAC1 antibodies. Associated DNA was isolated and analyzed via real time PCR using primers spanning the RGS10 and GAPDH promoters. Real-time PCR values were normalized to the total amount of promoter DNA added (input). Input values represent 5% of the total cell lysate ** $p<0.005$. **A)** Levels of HDAC1 associated with RGS10 promoters following DNMT1 knock-down in A2780-AD ovarian cancer cells. Data were normalized to GAPDH and values represent mean ± SEM of three independent experiments. **B)** Western blot analysis shows specificity and efficiency of DNMT1 knock down in A2780-AD cells. **C)** Model for mechanism by which RGS10 is suppressed in chemoresistant A2780-AD cells. MeCP2 binds DNA region, containing methylated CpG dinucleotides. MeCP2 directly interacts with DNMT1 to maintain DNA methylation. MeCP2-DNMT1 complex also recruits HDAC1 to RGS10 promoter via binding Sin3 complex.

and HDACs and high-level expression of DNMT1 and HDAC1 is prominent in high-grade ovarian tumors [68]. HDAC1 binds the N-terminus of DNMT1 to form a transcriptional repression complex and the MeCP2 directly interacts with DNMT1 to maintain DNA methylation [69]. To explore interactions between DNMT1 and HDAC1 at RGS10 genes, DNMT1 was knocked down and the level of HDAC1 binding to RGS10 promoters was determined by ChIP. DNMT1 knock down significantly decreased HDAC1 binding to the RGS10 promoter in chemoresistant ovarian cancer cells, indicating HDAC1 is recruited to the RGS10 promoter via DNMT1 and MeCP2 dependent mechanisms. Recent reports suggest DNMT1 and HDAC1 expression increases with ovarian cancer stage [68]. Our results further imply that the increased expression of DNMT1 and HDAC1 results in the generation of repressive complexes which target RGS10 promoters and cooperate in regulating ovarian cancer progression.

The gold standard of care for ovarian cancer is currently a combination of platinum and taxane chemotherapy which, along with second or third line chemotherapy regimens, often does not provide sufficient results [70,71]. New agents, or new agents in combination with current chemotherapeutic agents, are therefore urgently needed to overcome the drug resistance phenomenon. Gene silencing epigenetic modifications are reversible [72–74], thus inhibition of DNA hypermethylation and histone deacetylation can be considered as an adjuvant therapeutic approach for ovarian cancer treatment.

HDAC and DNMT1 inhibitors induce a potent anticancer response by inhibiting histone deacetylation and DNA hypermethylation [75–77]. We have shown that inhibition of DNMTs and HDACs by 5-Aza-dC and TSA induced significant RGS10 transcript expression in chemoresistant cells. Of note, the increase in RGS10 transcript expression was similar in HDAC1 and DNMT1 knock down experiments as in experiments with the general inhibitors TSA (HDACs) or 5-Aza-dC (DNMTs), suggesting that HDAC1 and DNMT1 are the primary enzyme subtypes responsible for suppression of RGS10 genes.

Recent reports indicate tumorigenicity and metastasis of ovarian cancer cells is significantly suppressed by the combination of HDAC inhibitor TSA and 5-Aza-dC in xenograft mouse models [78]. Thus, we determined the effects of a combination of TSA and 5-Aza-dC treatments on RGS10 expression and cell viability in chemoresistant ovarian cancer cells. The combination of these two drugs synergistically enhanced RGS10 transcript expression and chemoresistant cell viability. Further, we show that HDAC1 binding to RGS10 promoters in chemoresistant cells is dependent on DNMT activity. A likely mechanism for this suppression of RGS10 is that the DNMT1 repression complex recruits HDAC1 to RGS10 promoters.

A recent phase I clinical trial was the first to attempt to reverse platinum resistance in ovarian cancer with a combination of methylation and histone deacetylase inhibition [72,79]. These results show that changing methylation and acetylation results in changes in clinical outcomes. Further, preselecting patients based on known methylation status may optimize treatment responses [79]. Our study supports RGS10 genes as targets for demethylating and acetylating therapy and identifies RGS10 de-suppression as a likely contributing mechanism for the clinical efficacy of DNMT1 and HDAC1 inhibitors in the treatment of chemoresistant ovarian cancer.

Acknowledgments

The authors would like to thank Dr. Alex Spring for editorial assistance.

Author Contributions

Conceived and designed the experiments: EC SBH SFG. Performed the experiments: EC MWA NHB. Analyzed the data: EC MWA SBH SFG. Contributed reagents/materials/analysis tools: SBH SFG. Wrote the paper: EC SBH SFG. Read and approved the final manuscript: EC MWA NHB SBH SFG.

References

1. Siegel R, Naishadham D, Jemal A (2013) Cancer statistics, 2013. CA Cancer J Clin 63: 11–30.
2. Hooks SB, Callihan P, Altman MK, Hurst JH, Ali MW, et al. (2010) Regulators of G-Protein signaling RGS10 and RGS17 regulate chemoresistance in ovarian cancer cells. Mol Cancer 9: 289.
3. Liu B, Nash J, Runowicz C, Swede H, Stevens R, et al. (2010) Ovarian cancer immunotherapy: opportunities, progresses and challenges. J Hematol Oncol 3: 7.
4. Cai H, Xu Y (2013) The role of LPA and YAP signaling in long-term migration of human ovarian cancer cells. Cell Commun Signal 11: 31.
5. O'Hayre M, Vazquez-Prado J, Kufareva I, Stawiski EW, Handel TM, et al. (2013) The emerging mutational landscape of G proteins and G-protein-coupled receptors in cancer. Nat Rev Cancer 13: 412–424.
6. Hurst JH, Hooks SB (2009) Lysophosphatidic acid stimulates cell growth by different mechanisms in SKOV-3 and Caov-3 ovarian cancer cells: distinct roles for Gi- and Rho-dependent pathways. Pharmacology 83: 333–347.
7. Zhong H, Neubig RR (2001) Regulator of G protein signaling proteins: novel multifunctional drug targets. J Pharmacol Exp Ther 297: 837–845.
8. Shi GX, Harrison K, Han SB, Moratz C, Kehrl JH (2004) Toll-like receptor signaling alters the expression of regulator of G protein signaling proteins in dendritic cells: implications for G protein-coupled receptor signaling. J Immunol 172: 5175–5184.
9. Berman DM, Gilman AG (1998) Mammalian RGS proteins: barbarians at the gate. J Biol Chem 273: 1269–1272.
10. Hurst JH, Hooks SB (2009) Regulator of G-protein signaling (RGS) proteins in cancer biology. Biochem Pharmacol 78: 1289–1297.
11. Xie Y, Wolff DW, Wei T, Wang B, Deng C, et al. (2009) Breast cancer migration and invasion depend on proteasome degradation of regulator of G-protein signaling 4. Cancer Res 69: 5743–5751.
12. Liang G, Bansal G, Xie Z, Druey KM (2009) RGS16 inhibits breast cancer cell growth by mitigating phosphatidylinositol 3-kinase signaling. J Biol Chem 284: 21719–21727.
13. Bodle CR, Mackie DI, Roman DL (2013) RGS17: an emerging therapeutic target for lung and prostate cancers. Future Med Chem 5: 995–1007.
14. Cao X, Qin J, Xie Y, Khan O, Dowd F, et al. (2006) Regulator of G-protein signaling 2 (RGS2) inhibits androgen-independent activation of androgen receptor in prostate cancer cells. Oncogene 25: 3719–3734.
15. Ali MW, Cacan E, Liu Y, Pierce JY, Creasman WT, et al. (2013) Transcriptional suppression, DNA methylation, and histone deacetylation of the regulator of G-protein signaling 10 (RGS10) gene in ovarian cancer cells. PLoS One 8: e60185.
16. Lee JK, Chung J, Druey KM, Tansey MG (2012) RGS10 exerts a neuroprotective role through the PKA/c-AMP response-element (CREB) pathway in dopaminergic neuron-like cells. J Neurochem 122: 333–343.
17. Rivero G, Gabilondo AM, Garcia-Sevilla JA, Callado LF, La Harpe R, et al. (2013) Brain RGS4 and RGS10 protein expression in schizophrenia and depression. Effect of drug treatment. Psychopharmacology (Berl) 226: 177–188.
18. Garcia-Bernal D, Dios-Esponera A, Sotillo-Mallo E, Garcia-Verdugo R, Arellano-Sanchez N, et al. (2011) RGS10 restricts upregulation by chemokines of T cell adhesion mediated by alpha4beta1 and alphaLbeta2 integrins. J Immunol 187: 1264–1272.
19. Lu J, Gosslau A, Liu AY, Chen KY (2008) PCR differential display-based identification of regulator of G protein signaling 10 as the target gene in human colon cancer cells induced by black tea polyphenol theaflavin monogallate. Eur J Pharmacol 601: 66–72.
20. Rhee I, Jair KW, Yen RW, Lengauer C, Herman JG, et al. (2000) CpG methylation is maintained in human cancer cells lacking DNMT1. Nature 404: 1003–1007.
21. Ito K, P JB, I MA (2000) Histone acetylation and deacetylation. Methods Mol Med 44: 309-319.
22. Ghoshal K, Datta J, Majumder S, Bai S, Dong X, et al. (2002) Inhibitors of histone deacetylase and DNA methyltransferase synergistically activate the methylated metallothionein I promoter by activating the transcription factor MTF-1 and forming an open chromatin structure. Mol Cell Biol 22: 8302–8319.
23. Cai Y, Geutjes EJ, de Lint K, Roepman P, Bruurs L, et al. (2013) The NuRD complex cooperates with DNMTs to maintain silencing of key colorectal tumor suppressor genes. Oncogene.
24. Fuks F, Burgers WA, Brehm A, Hughes-Davies L, Kouzarides T (2000) DNA methyltransferase Dnmt1 associates with histone deacetylase activity. Nat Genet 24: 88–91.
25. Louie KG, Behrens BC, Kinsella TJ, Hamilton TC, Grotzinger KR, et al. (1985) Radiation survival parameters of antineoplastic drug-sensitive and -resistant human ovarian cancer cell lines and their modification by buthionine sulfoximine. Cancer Res 45: 2110–2115.
26. DiSaia PJ, Sinkovics JG, Rutledge FN, Smith JP (1972) Cell-mediated immunity to human malignant cells. A brief review and further studies with two gynecologic tumors. Am J Obstet Gynecol 114: 979–989.
27. Andrews PA, Murphy MP, Howell SB (1985) Differential potentiation of alkylating and platinating agent cytotoxicity in human ovarian carcinoma cells by glutathione depletion. Cancer Res 45: 6250–6253.
28. Manuyakorn A, Paulus R, Farrell J, Dawson NA, Tze S, et al. (2010) Cellular histone modification patterns predict prognosis and treatment response in resectable pancreatic adenocarcinoma: results from RTOG 9704. J Clin Oncol 28: 1358–1365.
29. Seligson DB, Horvath S, McBrian MA, Mah V, Yu H, et al. (2009) Global levels of histone modifications predict prognosis in different cancers. Am J Pathol 174: 1619–1628.
30. Zwaal RF, Schroit AJ (1997) Pathophysiologic implications of membrane phospholipid asymmetry in blood cells. Blood 89: 1121–1132.
31. van Engeland M, Nieland LJ, Ramaekers FC, Schutte B, Reutelingsperger CP (1998) Annexin V-affinity assay: a review on an apoptosis detection system based on phosphatidylserine exposure. Cytometry 31: 1–9.
32. Modest EJ, Sengupta SK (1974) 7-Substituted actinomycin D (NSC-3053) analogs as fluorescent DNA-binding and experimental antitumor agents. Cancer Chemother Rep 58: 35–48.
33. Ballestar E, Esteller M (2002) The impact of chromatin in human cancer: linking DNA methylation to gene silencing. Carcinogenesis 23: 1103–1109.
34. Robertson KD, Ait-Si-Ali S, Yokochi T, Wade PA, Jones PL, et al. (2000) DNMT1 forms a complex with Rb, E2F1 and HDAC1 and represses transcription from E2F-responsive promoters. Nat Genet 25: 338–342.
35. Di Croce L, Raker VA, Corsaro M, Fazi F, Fanelli M, et al. (2002) Methyltransferase recruitment and DNA hypermethylation of target promoters by an oncogenic transcription factor. Science 295: 1079–1082.
36. Fuks F, Burgers WA, Godin N, Kasai M, Kouzarides T (2001) Dnmt3a binds deacetylases and is recruited by a sequence-specific repressor to silence transcription. EMBO J 20: 2536–2544.
37. Zhou Q, Agoston AT, Atadja P, Nelson WG, Davidson NE (2008) Inhibition of histone deacetylases promotes ubiquitin-dependent proteasomal degradation of DNA methyltransferase 1 in human breast cancer cells. Mol Cancer Res 6: 873–883.
38. Vaissiere T, Sawan C, Herceg Z (2008) Epigenetic interplay between histone modifications and DNA methylation in gene silencing. Mutat Res 659: 40–48.
39. Jones PL, Veenstra GJ, Wade PA, Vermaak D, Kass SU, et al. (1998) Methylated DNA and MeCP2 recruit histone deacetylase to repress transcription. Nat Genet 19: 187–191.

40. Jones PL, Wade PA, Wolffe AP (2001) Purification of the MeCP2/histone deacetylase complex from Xenopus laevis. Methods Mol Biol 181: 297–307.
41. Nan X, Ng HH, Johnson CA, Laherty CD, Turner BM, et al. (1998) Transcriptional repression by the methyl-CpG-binding protein MeCP2 involves a histone deacetylase complex. Nature 393: 386–389.
42. Carrieri A, Perez-Nueno VI, Lentini G, Ritchie DW (2013) Recent Trends and Future Prospects in Computational GPCR Drug Discovery: From Virtual Screening to Polypharmacology. Curr Top Med Chem 13: 1069–1097.
43. Xie Y, Abel PW, Kirui JK, Deng C, Sharma P, et al. (2013) Identification of upregulated phosphoinositide 3-kinase gamma as a target to suppress breast cancer cell migration and invasion. Biochem Pharmacol 85: 1454–1462.
44. Gold SJ, Heifets BD, Pudiak CM, Potts BW, Nestler EJ (2002) Regulation of regulators of G protein signaling mRNA expression in rat brain by acute and chronic electroconvulsive seizures. J Neurochem 82: 828–838.
45. Hunt TW, Fields TA, Casey PJ, Peralta EG (1996) RGS10 is a selective activator of G alpha i GTPase activity. Nature 383: 175–177.
46. Popov S, Yu K, Kozasa T, Wilkie TM (1997) The regulators of G protein signaling (RGS) domains of RGS4, RGS10, and GAIP retain GTPase activating protein activity in vitro. Proc Natl Acad Sci U S A 94: 7216–7220.
47. Robertson KD (2005) DNA methylation and human disease. Nat Rev Genet 6: 597–610.
48. Fuks F (2005) DNA methylation and histone modifications: teaming up to silence genes. Curr Opin Genet Dev 15: 490–495.
49. Esteller M, Garcia-Foncillas J, Andion E, Goodman SN, Hidalgo OF, et al. (2000) Inactivation of the DNA-repair gene MGMT and the clinical response of gliomas to alkylating agents. N Engl J Med 343: 1350–1354.
50. Giacinti L, Vici P, Lopez M (2008) Epigenome: a new target in cancer therapy. Clin Ter 159: 347–360.
51. Zeller C, Dai W, Steele NL, Siddiq A, Walley AJ, et al. (2012) Candidate DNA methylation drivers of acquired cisplatin resistance in ovarian cancer identified by methylome and expression profiling. Oncogene 31: 4567–4576.
52. Stronach EA, Alfraidi A, Rama N, Datler C, Studd JB, et al. (2011) HDAC4-regulated STAT1 activation mediates platinum resistance in ovarian cancer. Cancer Res 71: 4412–4422.
53. Terasawa K, Sagae S, Toyota M, Tsukada K, Ogi K, et al. (2004) Epigenetic inactivation of TMS1/ASC in ovarian cancer. Clin Cancer Res 10: 2000–2006.
54. Barneda-Zahonero B, Parra M (2012) Histone deacetylases and cancer. Mol Oncol 6: 579–589.
55. Hassig CA, Schreiber SL (1997) Nuclear histone acetylases and deacetylases and transcriptional regulation: HATs off to HDACs. Curr Opin Chem Biol 1: 300–308.
56. Kruhlak MJ, Hendzel MJ, Fischle W, Bertos NR, Hameed S, et al. (2001) Regulation of global acetylation in mitosis through loss of histone acetyltransferases and deacetylases from chromatin. J Biol Chem 276: 38307–38319.
57. Marks PA, Miller T, Richon VM (2003) Histone deacetylases. Curr Opin Pharmacol 3: 344–351.
58. Arts J, Angibaud P, Marien A, Floren W, Janssens B, et al. (2007) R306465 is a novel potent inhibitor of class I histone deacetylases with broad-spectrum antitumoral activity against solid and haematological malignancies. Br J Cancer 97: 1344–1353.
59. Witt O, Deubzer HE, Milde T, Oehme I (2009) HDAC family: What are the cancer relevant targets? Cancer Lett 277: 8–21.
60. Wang C, Henkes LM, Doughty LB, He M, Wang D, et al. (2011) Thailandepsins: bacterial products with potent histone deacetylase inhibitory activities and broad-spectrum antiproliferative activities. J Nat Prod 74: 2031–2038.
61. Jin B, Yao B, Li JL, Fields CR, Delmas AL, et al. (2009) DNMT1 and DNMT3B modulate distinct polycomb-mediated histone modifications in colon cancer. Cancer Res 69: 7412–7421.
62. Muller BM, Jana L, Kasajima A, Lehmann A, Prinzler J, et al. (2013) Differential expression of histone deacetylases HDAC1, 2 and 3 in human breast cancer–overexpression of HDAC2 and HDAC3 is associated with clinicopathological indicators of disease progression. BMC Cancer 13: 215.
63. Herman JG, Baylin SB (2003) Gene silencing in cancer in association with promoter hypermethylation. N Engl J Med 349: 2042–2054.
64. Esteller M (2007) Cancer epigenomics: DNA methylomes and histone-modification maps. Nat Rev Genet 8: 286–298.
65. Nguyen CT, Gonzales FA, Jones PA (2001) Altered chromatin structure associated with methylation-induced gene silencing in cancer cells: correlation of accessibility, methylation, MeCP2 binding and acetylation. Nucleic Acids Res 29: 4598–4606.
66. Cameron EE, Bachman KE, Myohanen S, Herman JG, Baylin SB (1999) Synergy of demethylation and histone deacetylase inhibition in the re-expression of genes silenced in cancer. Nat Genet 21: 103–107.
67. Meng CF, Su B, Li W (2011) DNA demethylation is superior to histone acetylation for reactivating cancer-associated genes in ovarian cancer cells. Mol Med Rep 4: 1273–1278.
68. Gu Y, Yang P, Shao Q, Liu X, Xia S, et al. (2013) Investigation of the expression patterns and correlation of DNA methyltransferases and class I histone deacetylases in ovarian cancer tissues. Oncol Lett 5: 452–458.
69. Kimura H, Shiota K (2003) Methyl-CpG-binding protein, MeCP2, is a target molecule for maintenance DNA methyltransferase, Dnmt1. J Biol Chem 278: 4806–4812.
70. Herzog TJ, Sill MW, Walker JL, O'Malley D, Shahin M, et al. (2011) A phase II study of two topotecan regimens evaluated in recurrent platinum-sensitive ovarian, fallopian tube or primary peritoneal cancer: a Gynecologic Oncology Group Study (GOG 146Q). Gynecol Oncol 120: 454–458.
71. Dear RF, Gao B, Harnett P (2010) Recurrent ovarian cancer: treatment with pegylated liposomal doxorubicin; a Westmead Cancer Care Centre experience. Asia Pac J Clin Oncol 6: 66–73.
72. Carafa V, Nebbioso A, Altucci L (2011) Histone deacetylase inhibitors: recent insights from basic to clinical knowledge & patenting of anti-cancer actions. Recent Pat Anticancer Drug Discov 6: 131–145.
73. Espino PS, Drobic B, Dunn KL, Davie JR (2005) Histone modifications as a platform for cancer therapy. J Cell Biochem 94: 1088–1102.
74. Zhu WG, Otterson GA (2003) The interaction of histone deacetylase inhibitors and DNA methyltransferase inhibitors in the treatment of human cancer cells. Curr Med Chem Anticancer Agents 3: 187–199.
75. Johnstone RW (2002) Histone-deacetylase inhibitors: novel drugs for the treatment of cancer. Nat Rev Drug Discov 1: 287–299.
76. Takai N, Desmond JC, Kumagai T, Gui D, Said JW, et al. (2004) Histone deacetylase inhibitors have a profound antigrowth activity in endometrial cancer cells. Clin Cancer Res 10: 1141–1149.
77. Lyko F, Brown R (2005) DNA methyltransferase inhibitors and the development of epigenetic cancer therapies. J Natl Cancer Inst 97: 1498–1506.
78. Meng F, Sun G, Zhong M, Yu Y, Brewer MA (2013) Inhibition of DNA methyltransferases, histone deacetylases and lysine-specific demethylase-1 suppresses the tumorigenicity of the ovarian cancer ascites cell line SKOV3. Int J Oncol 43: 495–502.
79. Falchook GS, Fu S, Naing A, Hong DS, Hu W, et al. (2013) Methylation and histone deacetylase inhibition in combination with platinum treatment in patients with advanced malignancies. Invest New Drugs.

8

Crowdsourcing Awareness: Exploration of the Ovarian Cancer Knowledge Gap through Amazon Mechanical Turk

Rebecca R. Carter[1], Analisa DiFeo[2], Kath Bogie[3], Guo-Qiang Zhang[2], Jiayang Sun[1]*

1 Department of Epidemiology and Biostatistics, School of Medicine, Case Western Reserve University, Cleveland, Ohio, United States of America, 2 Case Comprehensive Cancer Center, Case Western Reserve University, Cleveland, Ohio, United States of America, 3 Departments of Orthopaedics and Biomedical Engineering, Case Western Reserve University, Cleveland, Ohio, United States of America

Abstract

Background: Ovarian cancer is the most lethal gynecologic disease in the United States, with more women dying from this cancer than all gynecological cancers combined. Ovarian cancer has been termed the "silent killer" because some patients do not show clear symptoms at an early stage. Currently, there is a lack of approved and effective early diagnostic tools for ovarian cancer. There is also an apparent severe knowledge gap of ovarian cancer in general and of its indicative symptoms among both public and many health professionals. These factors have significantly contributed to the late stage diagnosis of most ovarian cancer patients (63% are diagnosed at Stage III or above), where the 5-year survival rate is less than 30%. The paucity of knowledge concerning ovarian cancer in the United States is unknown.

Methods: The present investigation examined current public awareness and knowledge about ovarian cancer. The study implemented design strategies to develop an unbiased survey with quality control measures, including the modern application of multiple statistical analyses. The survey assessed a reasonable proxy of the US population by crowdsourcing participants through the online task marketplace Amazon Mechanical Turk, at a highly condensed rate of cost and time compared to traditional recruitment methods.

Conclusion: Knowledge of ovarian cancer was compared to that of breast cancer using repeated measures, bias control and other quality control measures in the survey design. Analyses included multinomial logistic regression and categorical data analysis procedures such as correspondence analysis, among other statistics. We confirmed the relatively poor public knowledge of ovarian cancer among the US population. The simple, yet novel design should set an example for designing surveys to obtain quality data via Amazon Mechanical Turk with the associated analyses.

Editor: Xiaofeng Wang, Cleveland Clinic Lerner Research Institute, United States of America

Funding: This work was supported in part by the Choose Ohio First Scholarship program in Biomedical Informatics through the EECS Department in Computer Science & Engineering at Case Western Reserve University and the Division of Medical Informatics at Case Western School of Medicine for RRC. GQZ acknowledges support from NIH/NCATS award UL1TR000439. The funders had no role in the study design, data collection and analysis, decision to publish, or preparation of the manuscript.

Competing Interests: The authors have declared that no competing interests exist.

* E-mail: jsun@case.edu

Introduction

Ovarian cancer is the most deadly gynecologic malignancy in the United States and the fifth leading cause of cancer death in women. According to the American Cancer Society's 2013 estimate, ovarian cancer is predicted to cause 22,240 new diagnoses with 14,030 deaths in the United States alone [1]. The overall 5-year survival rate for all ovarian cancer patients is 43.7% compared to 89% for all breast cancer patients. Specifically, 63% of ovarian cancer malignancies are late stage diagnoses, causing patients at this stage to experience a 5-year survival rate of only 26.9%, according to the American Congress of Obstetricians and Gynecologists (ACOG) [2]. This poor survival rate is largely due to the lack of effective, approved ovarian cancer screening tools, in contrast to the existence of mammograms and PSA tests for the screening of breast cancer and prostate cancer, respectively. Historically, ovarian cancer is known as "the silent killer," because some patients do not show disease-specific symptoms for ovarian cancer at an early stage [3]. Known symptoms include bodily changes reflected by feeling full quickly, pelvic pain, sudden weight gain or weight loss, frequent urination, bloating around the midsection, fatigue, back pain, prolonged menstrual cycles or bleeding, and fluid in the stomach [3]. In fact, more than 80% of ovarian cancer patients actually showed symptoms, even while the disease was still limited to the ovaries [4]. However, some of these symptoms can be misdiagnosed or dismissed by both patients and even some health professionals. There is a critical knowledge gap amongst both the general public and practicing physicians concerning ovarian cancer and its indicative symptoms [5].

Promotion of Survivorship with Knowledge

Cancer survival has improved during the last few decades, especially for patients diagnosed with breast cancer, the most common cancer among women. New and better combinations of treatments and screening tools for breast cancer have extended and improved the lives of survivors [6,7]. Visibility and spread of knowledge has been spearheaded by international awareness campaigns [8–10]. Social campaigns in particular, such as National Breast Cancer Awareness Month (NBCAM) have been highly successful in increasing routine screening within two years to approximately 70% of the general female population and contributed to substantial reductions in breast cancer mortality [8,11–13]. Unfortunately, ovarian cancer does not currently benefit from a widespread media-fueled awareness campaign. The lack of awareness potentially generates the majority of late stage diagnoses and consequent low survival rate. The purpose of the current study is to assess and confirm this critical knowledge gap, thereby highlighting the need for increased awareness towards the disease. Increased public awareness and a broader spread of knowledge are expected to promote early diagnoses rates and additional research in ovarian cancer, following the model successfully accomplished for breast cancer.

Assessment of the U.S. Population through Web-Based Surveys

To identify a knowledge gap, it is advisable to start by collecting data via a survey of the US population. Surveys typically can be done in two ways: a traditional paper-based survey or a web survey. Ensuring a representative sample is often a challenge in traditional survey study design. The overall goal is to achieve generalizable results, however this can entail economic obstacles due to budget, time, and manpower requirements to meet study needs [14]. Result validity, which is impacted by response rates, data-entry, and analyses, must also be considered. In the past decade, web-based surveys have been developed as a credible means of collecting data from large sample groups quickly and at minimal cost [15]. In 2004 a consortium of researchers from University of Texas at Austin, Stanford, and University of California, Berkeley addressed several concerns about data collection using the Internet, such as sample diversity, generalization, and reproducibility. In a comparison of a very large Internet sample (N = 361,703) with 510 published traditional samples, the consortium determined the Internet sample to be more diverse in demographics such as gender, socioeconomic status, geographic region, and age than traditional samples. They concluded that web-questionnaire results generalize across various survey formats, do not appear to be tainted by false data or repeat responders, and are consistent with results that use good traditional methodologies [16]. A 2012 study by Greenlaw et al. confirmed these earlier conclusions by comparing web-based and paper-based survey methods [14]. Specifically, the authors stated that there was "overwhelming support" for the cost-effectiveness and validity of web-based survey administration in comparison to traditional methods, noting the "marked reduction" of the overall cost per response as well as the effort necessary to produce and distribute surveys online.

Use of Online Crowdsourcing to Assess a Proxy of the U.S. Population

Successful surveys need to possess two important characteristics: 1) an unbiased design and 2) an excellent recruitment strategy. In our study, for 1) we designed an effective survey specifically tailored for online surveys to have both a quality control element and unbiased data, as well as good participation. For 2) we took advantage of modern crowdsourcing through the relatively new platform Amazon Mechanical Turk. The platform, released by Amazon.com in 2005, facilitates the design, dissemination, storage of data, and data analysis of web-based surveys. Amazon Mechanical Turk, hereafter referred to as **MTurk**, is a digital marketplace for work through which users can perform online "tasks" in exchange for a nominal fee. Employees (called *workers*) are recruited by employers (called *requesters*) for the execution of tasks, (known as Human Intelligence Tasks, or *HITs*). Both workers and requesters are anonymous and harness MTurk's utilities through a unique ID provided by Amazon. A requester can accept or reject results submitted by a worker, controlling whether a worker is paid or not. Data is compiled from the website into a downloadable Excel spreadsheet for analysis. The advantages of MTurk are well documented [17]. Workers tend to be from a diverse background, spanning a wide range of age, ethnicities and socioeconomic status [18]. Researchers have verified that MTurk demographic responses are accurate [19]. Furthermore, their psychometric properties are valid [20] and replicable [21–23].

In the current study, we designed a simple yet innovative survey completed at an accelerated rate of time and reduced cost compared to traditional recruitment methods. Breast cancer was chosen as the control group to compare with awareness of ovarian cancer in a representative crowdsourced sample of online respondents (See: §2 Methods). Our crowdsourcing of workers, recruited through Amazon Mechanical Turk, reflected a reasonable proxy of the US population at a minimized rate of cost and time (See: Data Collection in §3). We investigated the features of awareness of ovarian cancer among the sample (See: §3 Analyses and Results). We showed that workers consistently present a lack of awareness of ovarian cancer impact or significance. Finally, we demonstrated that in addition to presenting a lack of of ovarian cancer awareness, the worker's explicit knowledge of ovarian cancer varied widely, above and beyond simply guessing (See: §4 Discussion & Conclusions).

Methods

Design

We devised our survey with 1) an experimental control element, 2) a two-stage quality control mechanism, 3) repeated measures, and 4) additional quality control steps. The study design included basic awareness questions about ovarian cancer (using breast cancer as the control group), as listed in Table 1 (Questions 1–11), repeated measures (Questions 12–15), and additional quality control mechanisms (Questions 7a–11a) to avoid confounding factors and delineate between quality responses and possible guesses. Other quality control measurement elements consisted of pricing, timing, clear and concise user instructions, and inclusions/exclusion criterion (See: Procedure).

The justification of the design is as follows. First, simple awareness questions are quick and easy proxies to address the critical knowledge gap. Logically, if there is a severe gap in disease awareness, then there will be a severe gap in specific knowledge concerning symptoms and lifetime risk of diagnosis. Second, a control group and sound recruitment strategy specifically targeting a diverse population via the internet are the key elements in constructing a modern unbiased survey. Third, repeated questions with multiple choices arranged in a permuted order is an excellent way to assess how sure a participant is of their given answer, independent of his or her self-report of certainty in the answer. Fourth, some internet users may have a tendency to check answers

Table 1. Survey Questions and Descriptive Statistics.

Variable (Abbreviation)/Question	Response	No. (%)
1. Age (age)	18–30 Years	121 (60)
How old are you?	31–40 Years	37 (18)
(Complete distribution is shown in Figure 1)	41–50 Years	24 (12)
	51–61 Years	20 (10)
2. Gender (gender)	Male	115 (57)
	Female	87 (43)
3. Knowledge about breast cancer (kbrc)	**Very Well**	**22 (11)**
How well do you know about breast cancer?	Fairly Well	137 (68)
	Not at All	43 (21)
4. Knowledge about ovarian cancer (kovc)	**Very Well**	**5 (2)**
How well do you know about ovarian cancer?	Fairly Well	84 (42)
	Not at All	113 (56)
5. Background about breast cancer (bbrc)	**Yes**	**92 (46)**
Do you know anyone CLOSE TO YOU who has been diagnosed with breast cancer?	No	110 (54)
6. Background about ovarian cancer (bovc)	**Yes**	**24 (12)**
Do you know anyone CLOSE TO YOU who has been diagnosed with ovarian cancer?	No	178 (88)
7*. Risk of breast cancer (riskbrc)	1:8	76 (38)
What is a woman's lifetime risk of developing breast cancer?	1:70	62 (31)
The correct answer is 1:8	1:200	57 (28)
# This Q is repeated (**riskbrcr**)	1:1000	7 (3)
8* Risk of ovarian cancer (riskovc)	1:8	21 (11)
What is a woman's lifetime risk of developing ovarian cancer?	1:70	75 (37)
The correct answer is 1:70	1:200	49 (24)
# This Q is repeated (**riskovcr**)	1:1000	57 (28)
9*. Color of breast cancer ribbon (colorbrc)	Teal	2 (1)
What color is the breast cancer awareness ribbon?	Pink	197 (97.5)
The correct answer is Pink	Red	2 (1)
# This Q is repeated (**colorbrcr**)	Orange	1 (0.5)
10*. Color of ovarian cancer ribbon (colorovc)	Teal	114 (57)
What color is the ovarian cancer awareness ribbon?	Pink	25 (12)
The correct answer is Teal	Red	39 (19)
# This Q is repeated (**colorovcr**)	Orange	24 (12)
11*. Knowledge on Lethality (lethal)	Breast	34 (16)
Which cancer is more lethal than the other? Breast, Ovarian, or Same?	Ovarian	84 (42)
The correct answer is ovarian cancer	Same	84 (42)

There are 11 primary questions. Questions 7 through 11 are augmented with a follow-up self-assessment of how sure an individual is of their answer (indicated here by * and in the actual survey as Questions 7a–11a). This will provide an independent assessment of their choice certainty, confirmed via statistical analysis. Questions 7 through 10 have been augmented as repeated measures (indicated here by # and duplicated in the actual survey as Questions 12–15). These duplicated questions' answer order was permuted in order to address knowledge of disease risk and ribbon color. Results were visualized correspondence analysis in Figure 4.

to particular survey questions, therefore biasing survey results. Accordingly, clear user instructions and other quality control measures are necessary to discourage users from checking their answers and to derive a sound study.

Survey Questions

The survey began with basic demographic questions to assess age and gender. Baseline ovarian cancer knowledge was addressed by workers determining how well they knew of ovarian cancer on a 3-point Likert scale of "Very well," "Fairly Well," or "Not at All." To determine personal background and impact of ovarian cancer, workers were asked if they knew anyone close to them who had been diagnosed with ovarian cancer using a dichotomous Yes/No scale. Workers demonstrated their specific knowledge of a woman's lifetime ovarian cancer diagnosis risk by selecting from the ratio options of "1:8," "1:70," "1:200," and "1:1000." Public visibility of ovarian cancer was assessed through national cancer campaign ribbon color knowledge, where workers were asked, "What color is the ovarian cancer awareness ribbon?," with the categorical options of "Teal," "Pink," "Red," and "Orange." Last, participant estimates of comparative ovarian cancer lethality were elicited with the question of, "Which cancer is more lethal than the other?," where workers were provided the categorical options of "Breast," "Ovarian," or "Same."

An experimental control element was added to the questionnaire by replicating the ovarian cancer awareness questions for breast cancer awareness. Breast cancer was chosen as a control measure, given that the disease is the most commonly diagnosed invasive cancer in women and its advocacy efforts have greatly increased public attention to breast cancer [24]. To facilitate this control element, workers were assessed on their baseline knowledge of breast cancer first, and then subsequently assessed using the same question format on their baseline knowledge of ovarian cancer. The survey assessed workers on their knowledge of someone close to them with breast cancer, their estimations of a woman's lifetime breast cancer risk, knowledge of the breast cancer awareness ribbon color, and comparative lethality of breast cancer.

We also sought to quantify the relative certainty of workers' responses [25]. For both the control element of breast cancer and the test element of ovarian cancer, we asked workers an additional question directly: "How sure are you of the accuracy of your answer to the previous question?" (See Questions 7a to 11a). Workers were offered two response options: that they were "50% sure," implying they guessed, or "100% sure," implying absolute confidence in their previous answer. The purpose of assessing uncertainty was two-fold. One, we wanted quality control assurance; to check that workers did not cheat by using a web search engine to inform their answers. Specific details of lifetime risks of various cancers are not necessarily at the forefront of public knowledge, therefore an overwhelming number of correct responses concerning statistical knowledge of either breast or ovarian cancer would alert us to a biased survey sample. Second and more importantly, an uncertainty component in the questionnaire would provide insight into the stability of the worker's responses. Namely, it would provide a valuable opportunity to evaluate the variability of the workers questionnaire choices, and a secondary check if the correct answer was a pure guess. This was relevant to the awareness knowledge we wanted to assess.

Last, a repeated measures element was included with the cancer awareness survey [26]. The purpose of the repeated measures element was to both assess for response variance independent of the workers' self-report of certainty and to prevent bias. The repeated measure consisted of duplicating Questions 7 through 10, and permuting the order of the original response options. This avoided positioning biases, meaning that workers would not be influenced by the original question's position among the offered selections [27]. By randomizing the response order of the repeated measures, we could also be sure if workers chose the option closest to their true knowledge with a consistent answer implying a personally-held belief, and an inconsistent answer implying the opposite [25].

Procedure

The procedures to conduct a survey within MTurk are well-described [28]. For the present study, we initiated a survey using MTurk, after previously establishing an account and placing funds into the account where a 10% surcharge was assessed on all payments. The survey was uploaded on the MTurk website using the provided HTML editor, which functioned as a rudimentary webpage with the capacity to incorporate images, tables, figures, or videos. We then posted a job listing, or HIT, on the MTurk forum entitled "Cancer Awareness Survey." The short survey was advertised as taking up to 10 minutes, with a payout of $0.40 cents per fully completed survey.

The payout, or monetary incentive, was a key design component where the pay rate needed to be fair by MTurk standards to encourage a higher rate of recruitment without discouraging the more discriminating workers. The opportunity cost of MTurk has been previously described [18–23]. Another design component was the HIT filter for the workers' approval rating. We restricted participation to workers with an approval rate of at least 90%, meaning that 90% or more of the participant's previous submissions were accepted by requesters. The worker's approval rating is a system of checks and balances within MTurks, where the quality of the worker's HITs either beneficially or adversely impacts their ability to complete future HITs [15]. This predetermined approval threshold, or inclusion criteria, promoted accuracy among completed questionnaires from the MTurk population without influencing selection bias. Last, to deter respondents from using search engines to assist their accuracy during the task and to encourage HIT completion in a single sitting, a time constraint was set on the HIT to a maximum of 10 minutes. We also included text within the questionnaire to clearly explicate that true answers were appreciated and that no participant would be penalized for incorrect responses, i.e. there would be no gain from looking for the correct answer.

After agreeing to participate in the HIT, workers began the task by reading through a brief introduction to the questionnaire, which included expectations of time to complete task and clear criteria for work acceptance or rejection. Exclusion criteria were determined as follows. Respondent surveys that were incomplete or offered multiple responses for the same question were rejected. To facilitate analysis, the MTurk website compiled participant responses and formatted them into a. CSV file which was easily downloaded into an Excel spreadsheet.

Ethics Statement

The study involved the use of survey procedures obtained in such a manner that the human subjects could not be identified directly or through identifiers linked to the subjects and qualified as an exempt research activity under the Code of Federal Regulations [38 CFR 16.101(b) Section 3, Category 2].

Analysis and Results

Data Collection

Data collection was completed in 8 days (March 17th–25th, 2013), with 87% percent of subjects among the total sample pool meeting approval criteria for payment. Workers took 153.8 seconds on average to complete the survey. The working dataset is currently hosted on the website of the corresponding author, located at sr2c.case.edu/data.

Participant Characteristics

232 eligible workers were initially enrolled in the study. 202 workers were in the final sample assessment. Twelve subject surveys were rejected for multiple response entries for the same question, and 10 subject surveys were rejected for missing a question entirely. In the final sample, ages ranged from 18 years to 61 years, with a median age of 28 and mean age of 32 years (SD = 10.79, Figure 1). 115 workers were male and 87 workers were female. The age distribution is slightly right skewed, similar to the current middle segment of the US population distribution [29], though shifting slightly toward a younger demographic. The lower truncation point was at 18 years due to minimal age requirement by MTurk, while the upper truncation point reflected the average senior citizens that were less technologically savvy [22].

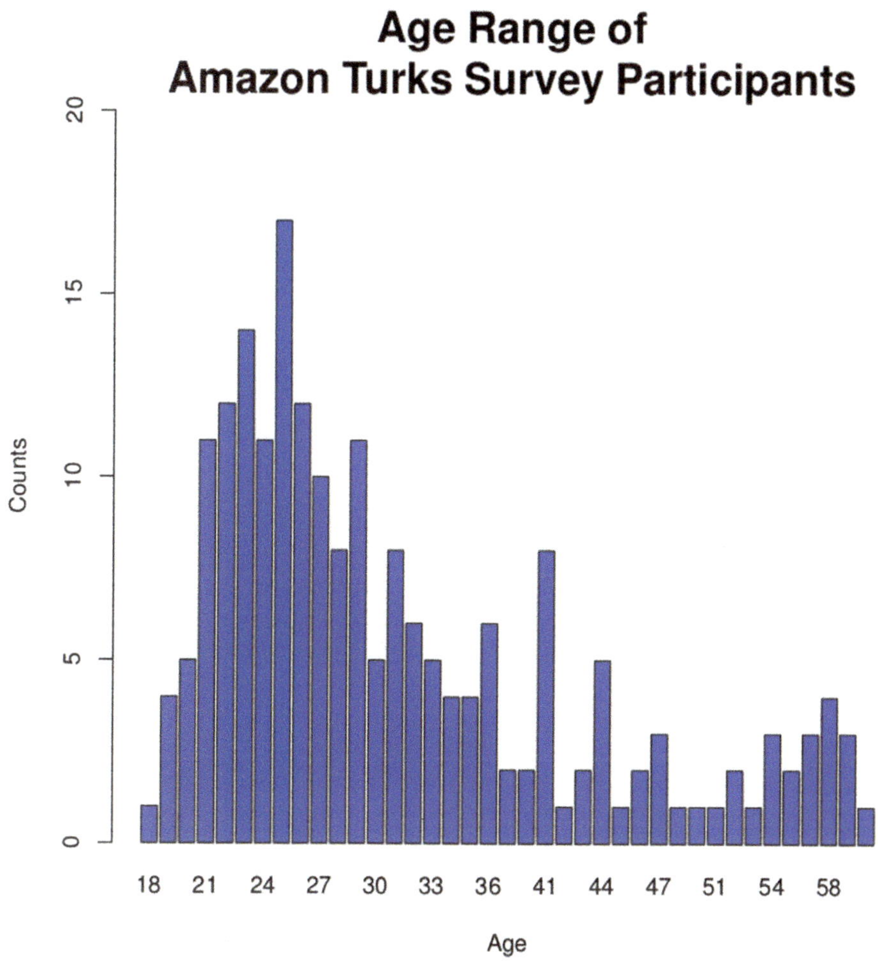

Figure 1. Age Distribution. The x-axis is age and y-axis is the frequency count. This representative population sample of 202 subjects was collected within 8 days. The median age was 28 years and the mean age was 32 years (SD = 10.79). 57% of respondents were male (N = 115), while 43% of respondents were female (N = 87).

Analysis Strategy

In addition to age and gender, the data consisted of responses from a multiple choice survey questionnaire (Table 1). Therefore the EDA summary statistics are the counts and descriptive analyses of the categorical responses. Response counts were calculated based on cross-tabulation, ratio, and frequency table descriptions. Contingency table analyses were used to evaluate relationships between worker responses for ovarian cancer (the test element), and breast cancer (the control element). Multinomial logistic regression analyses were used to determine the outcome of knowledge background while controlling for age, gender, and cancer type. Correspondence analyses were used to examine the residual differences between the repeated measures element of the survey. Group ratios were compared using a Pearson's χ^2 test and the exact multinomial test [30]. Trellis and correspondence analysis graphics were used for visualization of the results. Data were analyzed using R version 2.14.1 [31].

Baseline Knowledge Analysis

Table 2 shows a comparative projection of ovarian cancer knowledge versus breast cancer knowledge, based on cross tabulation of responses to Questions 3 and 4. Overall, the knowledge about ovarian and that of breast cancer were strongly and significantly different, with a p-value of $7.88 \cdot 10^{-13} \approx 0$, by the Pearson's Chi-squared test. Upon review of the specific differences, we found that 78.7% of all workers (N = (137+22)/202) reported they were "Fairly Well" or "Very Well" informed of breast cancer (Table 2). Conversely, over half, or 56% of workers (N = 113/202) reported *no knowledge* whatsoever of ovarian cancer. Individuals with prior knowledge of breast cancer tended to possess some knowledge of ovarian cancer: compare counts in Table 2 in the lower off-diagonal positions (70+18+1) vs those in the upper off-diagonal positions (1+2+0). Binomial comparisons of 3 individual categories between ovarian and breast cancer also showed significant differences, respectively, all with $p<0.0014$ using a 2-sample proportion test with continuity correction. The odds ratio was also strongly lopsided, with 70/1 for the odds of "Not at All" to "Fairly Well" for ovarian cancer versus breast cancer; and 2/18 for the odds of "Very Well" to "Fairly Well" for ovarian cancer versus breast cancer (Figure 2).

Familiarity/Background Analysis

Based on responses to Questions 5 and 6, 12% of workers (N = 24/202) knew someone close to them who had been diagnosed with ovarian cancer. Knowledge of someone very close with a breast cancer diagnosis accounted for 46% (N = 92/202) of

Table 2. Contingency Table of Cancer Background Knowledge.

Variable	Ovarian Cancer			
Breast Cancer	**Not at All**	**Fairly Well**	**Very Well**	**Total**
Not at All	42	**1**	0	**43**
Fairly Well	**70**	65	**2**	137
Very Well	1	**18**	3	22
Total	**113**	84	5	202

The *ij*-th entries are the number of participants who fall into the *ij*-th categories. For example, 70 people responded that they knew of breast cancer "Fairly Well," but knew nothing about ovarian cancer ("Not at All"). On the contrary, only one person claimed to know of ovarian cancer "Fairly Well," but "Not at All" for breast cancer.

workers. The difference between the familiarity proportions of two cancers is obviously significant, at a p-value of $1.734 \cdot 10^{-13} \approx 0$, using 2-sample test for equality of proportions with continuity correction.

Knowledge by Gender Analysis

We further explored knowledge of cancer on the condition of gender (Figure 2). Among the sample female population, 39% of women (N = 34/87) reported no knowledge of ovarian cancer; conversely 8% (N = 7/87) reported no knowledge of breast cancer. Almost 70% of men (N = 79/115) reported no knowledge of ovarian cancer; additionally 31% of men also reported no knowledge of breast cancer (N = 36/115). However, 92% of women reported fairly to very good knowledge of breast cancer (N = 80/87), while almost three-quarters of men reported fairly to very good knowledge of breast cancer (69%, N = 79/115). Proportions of knowledge by gender are visualized in Figure 2.

Analysis of Multi-factor Impact on Knowledge

We extended these findings by determining which predictor variables, or covariates, contributed the most to the extent of

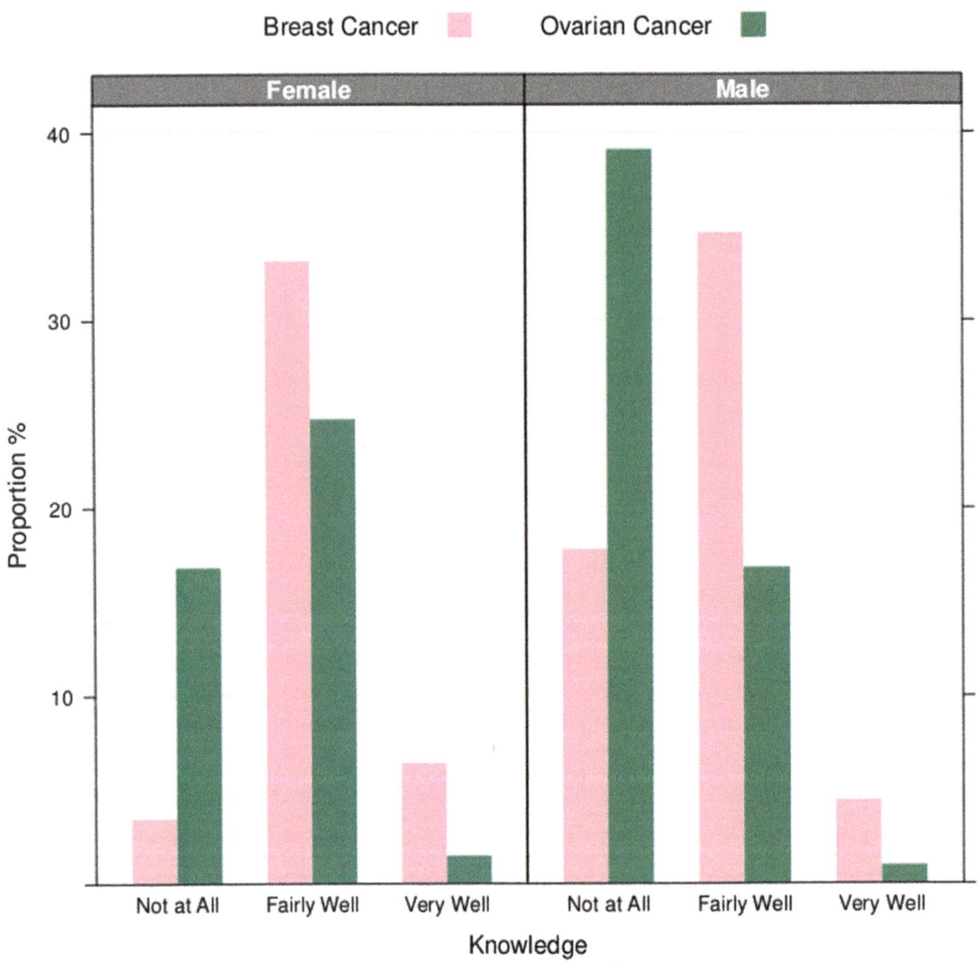

Figure 2. Gender Comparison of Diagnosis Risk Knowledge. The height of the bars are the proportion of men compared to women who knew of breast cancer or ovarian cancer "Not at All," "Fairly Well," or "Very Well," respectively. Male participants presented a strong indication of breast cancer knowledge, as evidenced by the "Fairly Well" and "Very Well" categories. Conversely, male participants had virtually no knowledge of ovarian cancer. A majority of female participants also responded that they knew of ovarian cancer "Not at All,"however most of the female participants knew of ovarian and breast cancer "Fairly Well." Both men and women did not know of breast cancer of ovarian cancer "Very Well."

cancer knowledge, and also examined the overall impact of multiple factors on the knowledge simultaneously. Therefore we conducted a multinomial logistic regression analysis. In this analysis, cancer knowledge is the polytomous response variable (call it Y), consisting of the categories: "Not at All," "Fairly Well," and "Very Well", coded as 0, 1, 2. Age, Gender, and Cancer Type are the covariates denoted as $x=(x_1,x_2,x_3)$. Here x_1 (*age*) is a continuous variable, x_2 (*gender*) is a dichotomous variable coded as 1 and 0 for male and female, and x_3 (cancer type) also coded as 1 and 0 for ovarian and breast cancer. Using the command *multinom* in the R package "nnet" [32], the resulting multinomial logistic regression relationship is

$$P(i|x)=P(Y=i|X=x)=\frac{e^{\beta_i z(x)}}{1+\sum_{j=1}^{2} e^{\beta_j z(x)}},i=1,2 \quad (1)$$

for the "Fairly Well" and "Very Well" categories, and $P(0|x)=1-P(1|x)-P(2|x)$ for the "Not at All" category. Here $z(x)=$ *(1, age, gender, cancer type, age·gender)'* was selected using the stepwise selection procedure based on AIC and represents an intercept term, linear effects in age, gender, and cancer type, as well as an interaction term between age and gender. The estimated coefficients and the associated one-sided p-values are given in Table 3. Thus, for the "Fairly Well" and "Very Well" categories, we have

$$\begin{aligned}\hat{\beta}_1 z(x)&=1.1817+0.0268^{b}\cdot\text{age}-0.0420\cdot\text{gender}-1.6189^{*}\cdot\text{type}-\\&\quad 0.0407^{\#}\cdot\text{age}\cdot\text{male}\\ \hat{\beta}_2 z(x)&=-0.6446+0.03166\cdot\text{age}-1.9903^{b}\cdot\text{gender}-\\&\quad 2.6590^{**}\cdot\text{type}+0.0096\cdot\text{age}\cdot\text{male}\end{aligned} \quad (2)$$

where * indicates a statistically *extremely significant* coefficient with a p-value $<10^{-6}$, # indicates a *significant* coefficient with a p-value <0.05, and ^{b} indicates a *slightly significant* coefficient with a p-value <0.1 (Table 3). The equations (2) and p-values in Table 3 show clearly that the cancer type is the *most* significant factor in driving the difference in knowledge, with a severe drop by the negative coefficient for ovarian cancer (from breast cancer). The interaction of age and gender (male) acts as a somewhat secondary significant factor in driving the knowledge difference for the "Fairly Well" category, indicating that Knowledge about ovarian and breast cancers is less for older male, although older people (female) seemed to be more likely to know fairly well. For the "Very Well" category, again the cancer type is the most significant factor with a much smaller probability of people who'd know ovarian cancer very well than that for breast cancer. For the "Not At All" category, everything will be reversed: there is a sharp increase for being in the "Not At All" category about the ovarian cancer, as P(0) = 1-P(1)-P(2).

Cancer Ribbon Color Awareness Analysis

We investigated public consciousness of the ovarian cancer awareness cause through identification of the national campaign's ribbon color. Table 1 summarizes the results from Questions 9 and 10, and shows that almost all responses correctly selected pink as the breast cancer awareness ribbon color (97.5%, N = 197/202). Furthermore by the secondary measure, i.e. responses to Question 9a, 94% of workers (N = 189/202) reported that their confidence in their responses were certain, or "100% sure" of their ribbon color choice for breast cancer. However, the responses for ovarian cancer ribbon color were more varied. Although over half of participants correctly selected the ovarian cancer ribbon color of teal (57%, N = 114/202), 19% of workers chose red (N = 39/202) as the correct ribbon color, 12% believed pink to also represent ovarian cancer (N = 25/202), while another 12% chose orange (N = 24/202) as a possibility. Also, by the secondary measure, the worker's confidence reveals that given just four colors, especially after a participant is sure about the color for breast cancer, only then can a significant portion of participants correctly guess the ovarian cancer ribbon color, with 93% of workers (N = 187/202) reported guessing, or being "50% sure" of their choice of ovarian cancer ribbon color.

Cancer Risk Awareness Analysis

Based on Questions 7 and 8, the worker's best estimate of a woman's lifetime ovarian cancer risk is presented in Table 1. The response patterns indicated that 37% of workers (N = 75/202) correctly determined a woman's risk of ovarian cancer to be 1 in 70, and 38% of workers (N = 38/202) correctly determined a woman's risk of breast cancer to be 1 in 8. 27% of workers correctly identified both the lifetime risk of breast and ovarian cancer (N = 55/202). However, incorrect response pairs trended towards estimates of a woman's breast cancer risk to be 1 in 200 and ovarian cancer risk to be 1 in 1000 (20%, N = 41/202), or 1 in 70 for breast cancer and 1 in 200 for ovarian cancer (13%, N = 27/202). The worker's uncertainty revealed that 87% of responses (N = 175/202) were guesses for both ovarian and breast cancer risk.

Lethality Knowledge Analysis

Figure 3 and Table 1 articulate the workers' estimation of relative cancer death among ovarian and breast cancer, in their responses Question 11. Ovarian cancer is more lethal than breast cancer, yet 58% of respondents (N = 118/202) were incorrect in their assumptions, where $p = 0.02$. Specifically, responses revealed that 41.6% of workers (N = 84/202) correctly believed ovarian

Table 3. Estimated Coefficients and Approximate 1-sided Significance.

		int	age	gender	typeov	age:male
fairlywell	β_1	**1.1817**	**0.0268**	−0.0420	**−1.6189**	**−0.0407**
	p-value	0.0234	0.0558	0.4782	1.0997e-11	0.0421
verywell	β_2	−0.6446	0.0317	**−1.9903**	**−2.6590**	0.0096
	p-value	0.2449	0.1084	0.0769	4.3918e-07	0.4028

Bolded coefficients are marginally to extremely significant from zero. Multiplying 1-sided p-values by 2 leads to 2-sided p-values. Results of this multinomial logistic regression determine that cancer type is the most significant factor related to cancer knowledge.

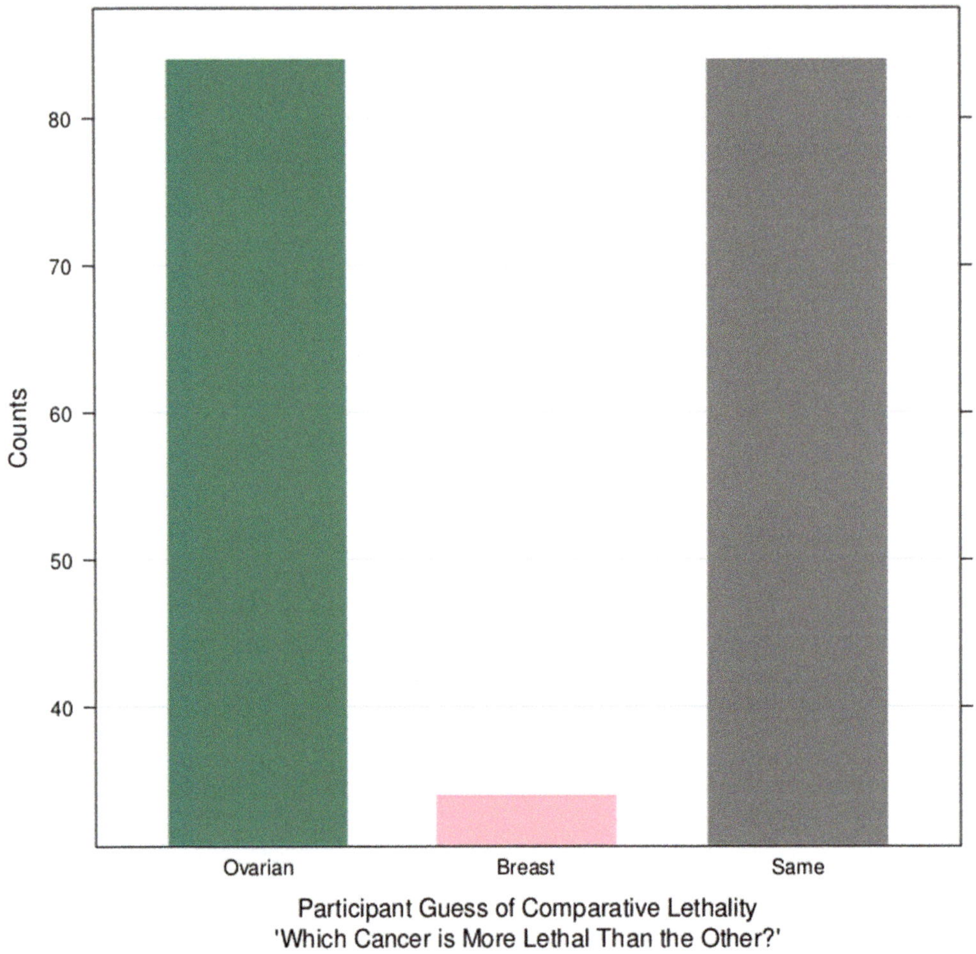

Figure 3. Knowledge of Lethality. The height of the bars are the frequency count of people who responded that ovarian cancer is more lethal, or breast cancer is more lethal, or they are of equal lethality. According to respondents, 16% believed breast cancer to be more lethal than ovarian cancer. 42% believed ovarian cancer to be more lethal than breast cancer, and 42% believed both cancers to be equally lethal. This indicates general lack of mortality knowledge, as the range of opinions varies widely.

cancer to be more lethal than breast cancer and similarly, while 41.6% of workers (N = 84/202) falsely believed both cancers to be equally lethal to women, and the remaining 16.8% of workers (N = 34/202) also falsely believed breast cancer to be more lethal than ovarian cancer (Figure 3). Over three-quarters of workers reported guessing for their response to the cancer lethality survey question across all three answer choices (83%, N = 169/202).

Knowledge Gap Analysis

Last, we examined the repeated measure residuals of the worker's responses for breast cancer and ovarian cancer risk (Figure 4). Correspondence analysis showed that workers were consistent in their responses concerning breast cancer risk, with little difference between the first time answering the question and the second time answering the question despite 88% (N = 178/202) admitting to guessing on that particular question. This was visualized by the leftmost points of Figure 4 which were very close. In contrast, the worker estimate of ovarian cancer risk varied considerably. in the first and 2nd attempts of their responses,as visualized in Figure 4 by the rightmost points in the graph. Like breast cancer, 97% (N = 195/202) of workers reported uncertainty in their estimate of ovarian cancer lifetime risk. This indicated the participant's incertitude and complete dearth of understanding of lifetime ovarian cancer risk ($p<0.001$).

Discussion and Conclusions

Our study indicates that the US population consistently presents a lack of awareness of ovarian cancer impact or significance. However, individuals with prior knowledge of breast cancer tended to possess some knowledge of ovarian cancer. We unequivocally identified the knowledge gaps in a representative sample of the US population for both specific and generalized ovarian cancer information. Given that the distribution of ovarian cancer malignancies diagnosed at an early stage are fundamentally different than that of tumors present with advanced-stage disease [33], the findings underscore the importance and need for continuing efforts to improve awareness of ovarian cancer early diagnosis endeavors and promote its research.

This is the first study we know of among the US population on the awareness of ovarian cancer. A recent survey out of the University College of London, which surveyed exclusively United Kingdom women on their levels of symptom awareness, determined that women among their sample population were unable to recall any ovarian cancer symptoms [34,35]. Their conclusions

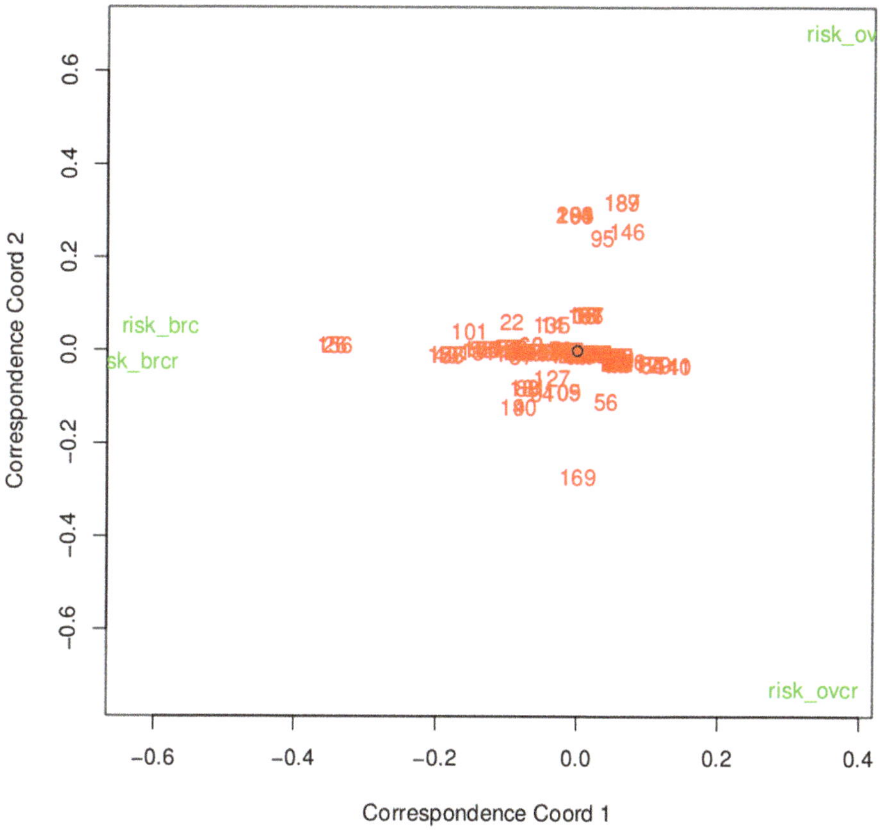

Figure 4. Correspondence Analysis of Risk. Correspondence is determined by distance away from horizontal and vertical axis. The cloud of raw data points in the middle of the graph have no relationship to one another and therefore are close to the horizontal and vertical midpoints of the graph. The points are further away from the vertical midpoint but close on the horizontal axis, which indicates a good relationship between the predictor variables. However, the points far away from the vertical midpoint and far away from the horizontal midpoint indicates a poor relationship. Therefore participants' selections for lifetime breast cancer risk were consistent in their initial and repeated survey responses. Responses for ovarian cancer lifetime risk varied widely, indicating that the participants were guessing their response selections.

coincided with ours: that there is a severe knowledge gap among the general public about ovarian cancer and more research is needed for this devastating disease. Prior studies indicate that life experience, family history and stories about family history play a key role in constructed awareness of cancer risk among individuals from hereditary cancer families [33,36–40]. The targeted population of our study, a reasonable proxy of the US population, does not necessarily possess this heuristic function of experiential ovarian cancer-related awareness to improve odds of early diagnosis. However, in future studies, it may be useful to quantify awareness of genetic risk and how it factors into public knowledge.

The current study design and implementation was performed to provide a unbiased framework with quality control and repeated measures elements. These strategies were constructed from a merger of clinical and theoretical perspectives. The cross-sectional, population-based design of the analyses were reliable, observed, and could be readily inferred.

Potential limitations in the design of the study include the MTurk worker pool. As of January 2013, MTurk no longer approves international accounts. The worker pool, once bolstered by global accounts of over 500,000 workers [41], is now restricted to individuals who must both reside in the United States and possess a valid social security number. It may be argued that MTurk workers are more technologically and Internet savvy, and have an age distribution that tends to be slightly younger than the general US population. This could unfairly bias results in general. However, given that technologically-knowledgeable internet users should be more knowledgeable, if they present a severe lack of knowledge of ovarian cancer then by extension the general US population should as well, thereby assisting our assertions [18]. Furthermore, American Amazon Turk workers have been evaluated thoroughly in the literature and are arguably closer to the US population as a whole than subjects recruited from traditional university subject pools. Last, conducting experimental research on MTurk offers benefits such as a low risk of dishonest responses, no risk of experimenter effects, and low susceptibility to coverage error in comparison to traditional studies [22].

Future studies employing our survey design will follow both specific and generalizable pathways. Greater specificity to ovarian cancer awareness will involve methodological extension as well as identification of distinct and specific early diagnostic symptom patterns. Broader application of this could involve extension of our survey design to other cancers with high mortality rates and vague symptoms, such as esophageal cancer and pancreatic cancer. Pancreatic cancer is the fourth most common cause of cancer-related death in the United States, and has an extremely poor prognosis of a 6% relative survival rate at Stage IV. Esophageal cancer, 3 to 4 times more common in men than women, also has a poor prognosis of a 3% relative survival rate at Stage IV. We advocate that the present study's survey methodology will be effective and efficient in its application beyond rare gynecological cancers, and will be particularly cost-effective for a nationwide assessment among patients diagnosed with low-prevalence diseases.

Author Contributions

Conceived and designed the experiments: JS AD GQZ KB. Performed the experiments: RRC. Analyzed the data: RRC JS. Wrote the paper: RRC JS. Revised the article critically for important intellectual content: AD KB GQZ.

References

1. Siegel R, DeSantis C, Virgo K, Stein K, Mariotto A, et al. (2012) Cancer treatment and survivorship statistics, 2012. CA Cancer J Clin 62: 220–241.
2. Slomski A (2012) Screening Women for Ovarian Cancer Still Does More Harm Than Good. JAMA 307: 2474–2475.
3. Goff Ba, Mandel LS, Drescher CW, Urban N, Gough S, et al. (2007) Development of an ovarian cancer symptom index: Possibilities for earlier detection. Cancer 109: 221–7.
4. Goff BA, Mandel LS, Melancon CH, Muntz HG (2004) Frequency of symptoms of ovarian cancer in women presenting to primary care clinics. JAMA 291: 2705–2712.
5. Baldwin LM, Trivers KF, Matthews B, Andrilla CHA, Miller JW, et al. (2012) Vignette-based study of ovarian cancer screening: Do United States physicians report adhering to evidence-based recommendations? Ann Intern Med 156: 182–194.
6. Bergh J, Jönsson PE, Glimelius B, Nygren P (2001) A systematic overview of chemotherapy effects in breast cancer. Acta Oncol 40: 253–281.
7. CTSU RI (2005) Effects of chemotherapy and hormonal therapy for early breast cancer on recurrence and 15-year survival: An overview of the randomised trials. Lancet 365: 1687–1717.
8. Catalano R, Winett L, Wallack NL, Satariano W (2003) Evaluating a campaign to detect early stage breast tumors in the United States. Eur J Epidemiol 18: 545–50.
9. Lerner BH (2002) Breast cancer activism: Past lessons, future directions. Nat Rev Cancer 2: 225–230.
10. Wu S (2003) Sickness and preventive medical behavior. J Health Econ 22: 675–689.
11. Breen N, A Cronin K, Meissner HI, Taplin SH, Tangka FK, et al. (2007) Reported drop in mammography. Cancer 109: 2405–2409.
12. Jacobsen GD, Jacobsen KH (2011) Health Awareness Campaigns and Diagnosis Rates: Evidence from National Breast Cancer Awareness Month. J Health Econ 30: 55–61.
13. Tabar L, Yen MF, Vitak B, Chen HHT, Smith RA, et al. (2003) Mammography service screening and mortality in breast cancer patients: 20-year follow-up before and after introduction of screening. Lancet 361: 1405–1410.
14. Greenlaw C, Brown-Welty S (2009) A comparison of web-based and paper-based survey methods testing assumptions of survey mode and response cost. Eval Rev 33: 464–480.
15. Schonlau M, Fricker RJ, Elliott MN (2002) Conducting research surveys via e-mail and the web. RAND: Santa Monica, MR-1480-RC.
16. Gosling SD, Vazire S, Srivastava S, John OP (2004) Should we trust web-based studies? A comparative analysis of six preconceptions about internet questionnaires. Am Psychol 59: 93–104.
17. Goodman JK, Cryder CE, Cheema A (2012) Data collection in a at world: The strengths and weaknesses of mechanical turk samples. J Behav Decis Mak.
18. Mason W, Suri S (2012) Conducting behavioral research on Amazon's Mechanical Turk. Behav Res Methods 44: 1–23.
19. Rand DG, Arbesman S, Christakis NA (2011) Dynamic social networks promote cooperation in experiments with humans. Proc Natl Acad Sci U S A 108: 19193–19198.
20. Buhrmester M, Kwang T, Gosling SD (2011) Amazon's Mechanical Turk: A New Source of Inexpensive, Yet High-Quality, Data? Perspect Psychol Sci 6: 3–5.
21. Horton JJ, Rand DG, Zeckhauser RJ (2011) The online laboratory: Conducting experiments in a real labor market. Exp Econ 14: 399–425.
22. Paolacci G, Chandler J, Ipeirotis P (2010) Running experiments on Amazon Mechanical Turk. Judgm Decis Mak 5: 411–419.
23. Suri S, Watts DJ (2011) Cooperation and contagion in web-based, networked public goods experiments. PLOS One 6: e16836.
24. Sulik GA (2007) On the receiving end: Women, caring, and breast cancer. Qual Sociol 30: 297–314.
25. Tversky A, Kahneman D (2000) Judgment under Uncertainty: Heuristics and Biases. Science 185: 1124–31.
26. Frison L, Pocock SJ (1992) Repeated measures in clinical trials: analysis using mean summary statistics and its implications for design. Stat Med 11: 1685–1704.
27. Green PE, Tull DS (1978) Research for Marketing Decisions. Englewood Cliffs, NJ: Prentice-Hall, Inc., 4th edition.
28. Berinsky AJ, Huber GA, Lenz GS (2012) Evaluating Online Labor Markets for Experimental Research: Amazon.com's Mechanical Turk. Polit Anal 20: 351–368.
29. Howden LM, Meyer JA (2011) Age and sex composition: 2010. URL www.census.gov/prod/cen2010/briefs/c2010br-03.pdf. Accessed: 2013-07-22.
30. Radlow R, Edward F (1975) An alternate multinomial assessment of the accuracy of the χ^2 test of goodness of fit. J Am Stat Assoc 70: 811–813.
31. R Development Core Team (2008) R: A Language and Environment for Statistical Computing. R Foundation for Statistical Computing, Vienna, Austria. URL http://www.R-project.org. ISBN 3-900051-07-0.
32. Venables W, Ripley B (1997) Modern Applied Statistics with S-Plus. New York: Springer, 2nd edition.
33. Köbel M, Kalloger SE, Baker PM, Ewanowich CA, Arseneau J, et al. (2010) Diagnosis of ovarian carcinoma cell type is highly reproducible: A transcanadian study. Am J Surg Pathol 34: 984–993.
34. Low E, Waller J, Menon U, Jones A, Reid F, et al. (2013) Ovarian cancer symptom awareness and anticipated time to help-seeking for symptoms among UK women. J Fam Plann Reprod Health Care 39: 163–71.
35. Simon A, Wardle J, Grimmett C, Corker E, Menon U, et al. (2012) Ovarian and cervical cancer awareness: Development of two validated measurement tools. J Fam Plann Reprod Health Care 38: 167–174.
36. Abel EK, Browner C (1998) Selective compliance with biomedical authority and the uses of experiential knowledge. Cambridge University Press, 310–26 pp.
37. D'Agincourt-Canning L (2005) The effect of experiential knowledge on construction of risk perception in hereditary breast/ovarian cancer. J Genet Couns 14: 55–69.
38. Kenen R, Ardern-Jones A, Eeles R (2003) Family stories and the use of heuristics: Women from suspected hereditary breast and ovarian cancer families. Sociol Health Illn 25: 838–865.
39. Kenen R, Arden-Jones A, Eeles R (2004) We are talking, but are they listening? communication patterns in families with a history of breast/ovarian cancer. Psychooncology 13: 335–345.
40. Mcallister M (2002) Predictive genetic testing and beyond: A theory of engagement. J Health Psychol 7: 491–508.
41. Gardner RM, Brown DL, Boice R (2012) Using Amazon's Mechanical Turk website to measure accuracy of body size estimation and body dissatisfaction. Body Image 9: 532–4.

9

In Their Own Words: Treating Very Young *BRCA1/2* Mutation-Positive Women with Care and Caution

Lindsey M. Hoskins[1], Allison Werner-Lin[2]*, Mark H. Greene[1]

1 Clinical Genetics Branch, National Cancer Institute, Bethesda, Maryland, United States of America, **2** Social Policy and Practice, University of Pennsylvania, Philadelphia, Pennsylvania, United States of America

Abstract

Purpose: Young women who have been identified as carrying a deleterious mutation in *BRCA1* or *BRCA2* face a unique set of challenges related to managing cancer risk during a demographically-dense stage of life. They may struggle with decision-making in the absence of clear age-specific guidelines for medical management and because they have not yet fully developed the capacity to make life-altering decisions confidently. This study sought a patient-centered perspective on the dilemmas faced by 18–24 year olds who completed *BRCA1/2* gene mutation testing prior to their 25th birthdays.

Patients and Method: This study integrated qualitative data from three independent investigations of *BRCA1/2*-positive women recruited through cancer risk clinics, hospital-based research centers, and online organizations. All 32 participants were women aged 21–25 who tested positive for a *BRCA1/2* gene mutation between 2 and 60 months prior to data collection. Investigators used techniques of grounded theory and interpretive description to conduct both within and cross-study analysis.

Results: Participants expressed needs for (1) greater clarity in recommendations for screening and prevention before age 25, especially with consideration of early and regular exposure to radiation associated with mammography or to hormones used in birth control, and (2) ongoing contact with providers to discuss risk management protocols as they become available.

Conclusions: Health care needs during the young adult years evolve with the cognitive capacity to address abrupt and pressing change. Specific needs of women in this population include a desire to balance autonomous decision-making with supportive guidance, a need for clear, accurate and consistent medical recommendations. Optimally, these women are best cared for by a team of genetically-oriented providers as part of a sustained program of ongoing support, rather than seen in an episodic, crisis-driven fashion. A discussion of insurance issues and provider-patient cultural differences is presented.

Editor: Redhwan Ahmed Al Naggar, Population Health and Preventive Medicine, Malaysia

Funding: This study was funded through the intramural program of the National Cancer Institute, Division of Cancer Genetics and Epidemiology, Clinical Genetics Branch. The funders had no role in study design, data collection and analysis, decision to publish, or preparation of the manuscript.

Competing Interests: The authors have declared that no competing interests exist.

* E-mail: awer@sp2.upenn.edu

Introduction

Hereditary breast and ovarian cancer risk for women aged 18–24

Deleterious mutations in the *BRCA1* or *BRCA2* genes increase a woman's lifetime risk of breast and ovarian cancer. By age 70, approximately 60–70% and 45–55% of *BRCA1* and *BRCA2* mutation carriers will develop breast cancer, respectively; 40% and 20% of *BRCA1* and *BRCA2* mutation carriers will develop ovarian cancer [1]. By age 30, however, these risks are 3.4% and 1.5% for breast cancer, and 1–2% for ovarian cancer [2–4]. While these risks are high in *relative* terms (*i.e.*, compared with age-matched women from the general population), they may be viewed quite differently if presented in *absolute* terms (*e.g.*, by age 30, 95% will *not* develop breast or ovarian cancer).

BRCA1/2 mutation testing may be offered once a woman reaches age 18 [5]. However, independent decision-making is often not well-established by this time in life [6]. Evidence-based approaches to management widely-used for older mutation carriers have not been developed (see Table 1), nor have clinical trials been undertaken for mutation-carriers <25 [7]. Women aged 18–24 who pursue *BRCA1/2* mutation testing may receive highly personal and emotionally-charged cancer risk information before they are able to confidently manage this risk. The typical primary care provider is often not equipped to bring a balanced, authoritative perspective to the extraordinary concerns faced by these women. Consequently, young carriers experience distress that is both quantitatively and qualitatively different from that of older mutation-positive women [8–9], as they adjust to their mutation status and consider limited proven risk management options.

Most extant literature regarding psychosocial aspects of *BRCA1/2*-related risk aggregates participants across the lifespan in recruitment and data analysis, obscuring development of evidence-based risk management tailored to the unique developmental needs of the youngest consumers. We sought a patient-

Table 1. A Suggested Risk Management Strategy for *BRCA1/2* Mutation-Positive Women.

BREAST CANCER RISK MANAGEMENT
By age 30, breast cancer risk is 3.4% for *BRCA1* and 1.5% for *BRCA2* mutation-positive women
Breast self-examination [BSE] starting at either 18 or 20 years of age [27].
☐ BSE not proven effective to detect early BC or to reduce mortality [28].
☐ Low sensitivity to palpable breast abnormalities in young women may result in a false sense of security [28].
Clinical breast examinations [CBE] beginning between 20 and 25 [27].
☐ Frequent biopsies may increase anxiety [16,29]
Mammography and/or MRI between ages 25 and 30, or 5–10 years earlier than youngest age at first BC diagnosis in the family [27].
☐ The relationship between ionizing radiation exposure and breast cancer risk in mutation carriers remains unclear [29–30].
☐ High density of young women's breast tissue often makes mammograms diagnostically inconclusive [31].
☐ Frequent biopsies may increase anxiety [32].
Tamoxifen
☐ 50% reduction in the risk of breast cancer in high-risk women under age 50 [33–34].
☐ Data from mutation carriers are sparse, but suggests similar benefits.
☐ Medication-related toxicities (e.g., endometrial cancer, DVT, stroke, particularly in women above the age of 50) have discouraged more widespread use [35]
Risk reducing bilateral mastectomy (RRBM)
☐ Lowers breast cancer risk by ~95% for women without a breast cancer diagnosis [36]; the breast cancer risk post-RRBM is not zero.
☐ Low acceptability for women who are single or dating [11,16]
☐ Long-term sequelae of RRBM unknown.
OVARIAN CANCER RISK MANAGEMENT
By age 30, ovarian cancer risk is 1–2% for *BRCA1/2* mutation-positive women
Ovarian Screening, starting either at age 30 or 5–10 years earlier than the earliest age of first diagnosis in the family [37].
1. Transvaginal ultrasound with color Doppler
2. CA-125 serum marker
3. Pelvic exam every six months
☐ These methods are not proven to reduce morbidity or mortality from ovarian cancer.
Risk reducing salpingo-oophorectomy (RRSO)
☐ Lowers ovarian cancer risk by 85% for women without a breast cancer diagnosis.
☐ RRSO substantially lowers lifetime risk of breast cancer for premenopausal women [38], yet it increases lifetime risk of osteoporosis and heart disease [39].
☐ Low tolerability in women who have generally not completed childbearing.
☐ Recent recognition that a significant fraction of what has been called "ovarian cancer" originated, in fact, in the fallopian tubes underscores the importance of including the fallopian tubes when RRSO is performed [23,40]
☐ Hysterectomy is not routinely performed during RRSO because endometrial cancer is not considered part of the BRCA-related spectrum of cancers [41].
Tubal Ligation
☐ 60% reduction in ovarian cancer risk in *BRCA1* carriers [42]
☐ Finding not consistently reproduced from one study to the next
☐ Preserves fertility options
Oral Contraceptives
☐ 50% reduction in sporadic ovarian cancer risk in the general population, with protective effect greater among long-term users
☐ Similar reductions observed in *BRCA1/2* mutation carriers.
☐ Concerns regarding possible increased risk of breast cancer, particularly for long-term users [22]

centered perspective on the dilemmas faced by 18- to 24-year-olds as they considered *BRCA1/2* genetic testing and risk management.

Methods

Study Participants

Data were drawn from three separate qualitative studies; each used a developmental frame to investigate the experiences of *BRCA1/2* mutation-carriers during their reproductive years. Beginning in 2003 and 2009, Werner-Lin [10–13] and Hoskins [14–17] independently recruited cancer-free, *BRCA1/2*-positive women aged 18–35 from the University of Chicago Cancer Risk Clinic and the National Cancer Institute, respectively, plus through national online organizations. All data for those studies was collected either via in-person interviews conducted in the Chicago metro area (Werner-Lin) or via telephone interview based in Bethesda, but targeting women from across the US (Hoskins)

Investigators performed these investigations after approval by appropriate local Human Investigations Committees in accord with an assurance filed with and approved by the Department of Health and Human Services, where appropriate. Investigators obtained written informed consent from each participant.

Data from participants aged 18–27 who were ≤25 when they completed genetic testing were eligible for this secondary analysis. We chose to limit analysis to only women aged 25 or younger at the time of testing in order to understand the unique needs of these very young consumers of genetic testing services; due to the absence of clear age-specific guidelines for medical management and the complex and dense demographic shifts that occur during young adulthood (e.g., unpartnered vs. partnered, nulliparous vs. parous), we hypothesized that the needs of women in this age range would be qualitatively different from those of women in their later twenties and thirties. Alphanumeric identifiers were assigned to 26 eligible individuals (see Table 2) All underwent genetic testing between1997–2010. In 2011, a focus group was convened during the national meeting of a support/advocacy organization for women with increased breast and ovarian cancer risk [18]. English-speaking (due to constraints imposed by the researchers' language ability) women aged 18–27 who considered or completed *BRCA1/2* mutation testing prior to their 25th birthday were eligible for participation. Six unaffected women aged 21–25 consented to participate.

Data Collection

In-depth interviews. Investigators independently collected in-depth, semi-structured interview data from 2004–2009. Investigators' interview guide elicited data-rich reports of: family experiences with cancer and genetic testing; impact on family, peer and romantic relationships; beliefs about how cancer risk influences individual development; family formation; and attitudes towards risk-reduction. Table 3 outlines codebook themes. Originally, these data were subsumed in each investigator's study cohort, and participants of all ages combined were analyzed as one group. Data from eligible subjects were re-analyzed to examine whether themes were similar to or different from those of the entire study cohort.

Focus group. Investigators jointly developed a focus group guide based on findings from their earlier studies to address perspectives on: learning about cancer risk before age 25; cancer risk-management; the impact of genetic testing on identity, sexuality, family and social life; and family formation. After consenting, each participant selected a pseudonym to identify herself and within eight weeks of the 90-minute focus group, all participants completed a family history phone interview.

Data Analysis

All data were audio-recorded and professionally transcribed *verbatim*. Using the *constant comparative* method, investigators independently examined a subset of transcripts from each study to generate provisional codes. Once a working list of codes was established, all transcripts were reread and coded. Grounded theory techniques were used to facilitate agreement on a set of codes that best represented each dataset. Investigators approached the separate codebooks as three waves of data collection to capture changes to standard care protocols, public policy addressing insurance and discrimination concerns, and the social perceptions of genetic susceptibility during each time frame (*i.e.*, 2004, 2009, 2011)

Table 2. Participant Demographics (N = 32).

Age at Interview	23.2 (21–27)
BRCA1 Positive	19
BRCA2 Positive	13
Relationship Status	
Single	13
In a committed relationship	15
Engaged or married	4
Childbearing Status	
Had ≥1 child	2
Desired child(ren)	24
Did not want children or undecided	6
Pregnant	0
Completed or Scheduled Risk-Reducing Bilateral Mastectomy	5
Completed or Scheduled Risk-Reducing Salpingo-Oophorectomy	0
Breast or Ovarian Cancer Diagnoses	0

Findings

Participant Demographics

Data from 32 women aged 21–27 (mean age = 23.2) were included in the current analysis. All were confirmed *BRCA1* (n = 19) or *BRCA2* (n = 13) mutation carriers. At the time of initial data collection, 13 women were single, 15 were in relationships, and 4 were engaged/married. Two had children, 24 planned to have children, and six did not want children or were undecided. None had developed breast or ovarian cancer. None were pregnant, and none reported pursuing genetic testing to inform family planning. The majority had made active lifestyle choices to support healthy living since learning their mutation status. Five had completed risk-reducing bilateral mastectomy (RRBM) or had the procedure scheduled in the coming months; none had scheduled or completed risk-reducing salpingo-oophorectomy (RRSO).

Provider recommendations

Overall, participants expressed satisfaction with the care they received from the variety of providers with whom they had contact during the process of genetic testing and initiation of risk management. Participants valued providers who acknowledged their priorities, fears, and obligations. Numbers after each participant pseudonym indicate age at the time of data collection. **Reza** (25) shared:

> *A doctor [said], "Right now there's really no reason to (have a mastectomy) In the next few years there's probably going to be advances. I'm not telling you to wait fifteen years…" Because in my head it was, why should I wait until after I get cancer? But he was, like, "Wait till you're thirty." And I was, like, "Okay, that makes sense to me."*

Pam's mother was diagnosed with breast cancer at age 32, so Pam (22) initiated screening at 21 [19]. She was satisfied with her providers' dialogue about risk-reducing surgery, reporting:

Table 3. Codebook Excerpt.

AXIAL CODES Theme = Navigation	DEFINITION & PARAMETERS OF CODES	SAMPLE PARTICIPANT QUOTES
Expectations, Anticipating Change	Captures participant conjecture, speculations, assumptions about their future lives, action and reactions in relation to cancer risk and family development.	*Automatically thought I was going to have to get rid of my breasts. I remember sitting in the shower with the shower running and sitting in there like I was taking a bath and holding my breasts and thinking, you're not worth it.*
Exploring Options	Captures the process through which participants learned about (either pro actively or passively) their option for genetic counseling or testing and cancer risk management.	*So I like to learn more and more about what I should be doing for prevention wise. Even though no one really could tell me because of my age. So that's frustrating.* *I'm still not sure what I want to do with my breasts.*
Having a Plan	Participants' expressions of behavioral intent, using prospective (future tense) language to describe alignment with specific courses of cancer risk management.	*I always wanted to be a young mom...and even more so now knowing that a lot of people with BRCA also take out their ovaries, but like I'm keeping these in until I have to take them out. I always thought that I would do that. But, now I would probably do it a lot sooner.*
Making Decisions	Participants' expressions of resolution, commitment to certain courses of action to manage cancer risk, including explanation of decision making process (or the lack there of) and rationalizations for those actions.	*And I don't want to be pushed to something that is not going to work out.* *I cried my eyes out a little bit that day when I found out the news and I decided to just take the step forward and go. They don't make me who I am and I'm just going to go ahead forth with this because at least I can do something about it now.*
Taking Action	Participant reports of steps complete towards their goals of minimizing cancer risk, engaging in protective health behaviors.	*I walked right into my ob-gyn's office and said I'm ready to get tested and they asked if – they said for insurance reasons, they asked me a couple of questions. And because I had Ashkenazi background and it got approved and that was it. I didn't have any counseling or anything before. I had that done afterwards. I did it little backwards.*
Living with it	Participant reports of the impact on identity, quality of life, relationships, and social networks of engaging with the 'cancer world' with respect to mutation status. Includes sequelae of *not* yet engaging in protective health behaviors. Includes watching loved ones cope with the impact of cancer risk, diagnosis, treatment, and mortality.	*I went through a couple of things, you know, some shock. Not shock, I don't know why. Maybe shock when you go – when you hear the statistics and the numbers, you know, it was not a good day when I found out.* *I'll be driving on the road – I drive a lot for work – and I will literally have daydreams that I had two kids. I'm gone. I have two kids and my husband is older and in therapy and I'm not there. That's pretty hard*

"They said the breasts have to go by 25. And between 30 and 35 the ovaries would need to go. I went to the surgeon and talked to her about it, and I gave her my reasons for not wanting to wait, she agreed with me. Which was nice."

Needing guidance and autonomy. Nineteen participants knew of the *BRCA1/2* mutation in their family prior to their own genetic testing. Yet, many found it difficult to have their requests for screening adequately addressed. **Monique** (25) remembered, *"...everybody was like, 'oh, you're too young to know what you want.'... the primary response was never, 'no, you shouldn't do it because medically it's not necessary."*

Incompletely developed genetic and health literacy led several participants to misunderstand their risk of inheriting a mutation, cancer risk estimates associated with being a mutation carrier, or the residual risk of cancer post surgical risk-reduction. **Linda** (23) completed genetic testing at her gynecologist's suggestion. She recalled receiving her test results:

I got a phone call from my gynecologist saying, "I was afraid of this but you tested positive." And I was like, "test positive for what? I have no idea what you're talking about." And she was like, "for the genetic mutation." Had I been smart I would have seen the genetics counselor first.

A lack of clear expectations about genetic testing and the implications of one's carrier status complicated participants' interpretation of test results. **Hannah** (19) provided an example of a common misunderstanding of statistics at they relate to genetic risk. She reported:

(T)he way the genetic counselor explained it to us ... there's only like a 25% chance of us both having it. [Since I have it], it's less likely [my sister] has it.

Hannah did not understand that one sister's mutation status was unrelated to the other's individual probability of being a mutation carrier [20,21]. Each child of a mutation-positive parent has a 50% chance of inheriting the mutation.

Participants acknowledged that incomplete health literacy increased their need for expert guidance. **Melissa** (27) stated, *"some of the research is conflicting concerning different things, and it sort of perturbed me that it wasn't presented to me that way. It was presented to me as 'never take birth control.'"* Melissa wanted her providers to directly address the uncertainty regarding birth control pills. Yet, participants also valued autonomy in making choices; they wanted to weigh differing perspectives to come to a decision that best fit their own needs, rather than having their providers make choices for them.

Inconsistent, incomplete recommendations. Participants expressed frustration at receiving inconsistent, inaccurate, ambiguous or incomplete recommendations from providers regarding their cancer risk management. During the initial phase of their mutation-positive experiences, participants reported receiving information from genetic counselors, oncologists, obstetrician/gynecologists, breast surgeons, and general practitioners, each with her/his own discipline-specific perspective and knowledge base. **Hannah** reported, *"I never took birth control because, in the beginning, they thought those hormones could actually be really negative for me. Now I hear, 'We were wrong. You should have been taking birth control all these years.'"* In the early years of managing women with *BRCA1/2* mutations, one major concern related to the possibility that exogenous hormones might further increase the risk of breast cancer – the most frequent syndrome-related malignancy. Newer data suggest that there is little evidence of increased breast cancer risk among mutation carriers using oral contraceptive formulations prescribed since 1975, while a 50% reduction in the risk of *BRCA*-related ovarian cancer is now widely accepted as an important benefit related to OC exposure [22].

Since *BRCA*-related male breast cancer penetrance is so much lower than that for females, providers and consumers often mistakenly believe hereditary risk of breast/ovarian cancer is passed only through the maternal bloodline. **Ruth** recalled a physician telling her that since cancer was present on the paternal side of her family, she *"[didn't] have anything to worry about, or maybe we'll start giving you a mammogram a little bit earlier than normal."* **Isabelle** (22), whose mother developed breast cancer at age 25, was frustrated by her inability to access screening; despite a letter signed by a doctor confirming her need for MRI, another provider refused to start screening before she turned 25. Given her family history, she perceived this to be too late.

Alysha (26), who sought out a great deal of information online, shared *"(I was) very frustrated with the conflicting information that doctors were telling me, particularly about screening – when and how often and the consequences of various tests."* Participation in the annual meeting of a consumer advocacy group validated her desire to gather information to feel well-informed. After attending the conference, she reported *"I feel much better informed about what I should be doing and what those types of screenings actually do and possible side effects and accuracy."*

Genetic testing at age 18 confirmed **Lynn** (23) carried a mutation, yet she received the message from her physician that *"you don't need a mammogram at this age."* This led her to feel out of place in the healthcare system and frustrated at her inability to access screening. Feeling "*paralyzed*" by this roadblock, she completed bilateral mastectomy at age 22, believing it to be the only way to effectively manage her cancer risk [17].

Family formation. Like older mutation-positive women in the two original study cohorts [11,13], participants were concerned about the challenges presented by HBOC risk and family formation. They discussed the need to plan for varied ways to sequence risk-management and family formation plans to attend confidently to both. Several recalled providers who suggested that they advance family formation goals quickly to support risk-management. **Tracy** (26) recalled,

> *I was talking to my genetic counselor, saying "I'm finally ready to get my breasts removed, who should I contact?" She found me the best surgeon in the state, who's wonderful. And she said "If you're still not interested in having kids, they've discovered tubal ligation can reduce your* [ovarian cancer] *risk. This might be a good option for you."*

Ashley (24) recalled that her physician told her *"...to start thinking about having kids before I'm 30 because if you breastfeed before you're 30, it reduces your risk of breast cancer"* and she reported thinking, *"oh jeez, I gotta get moving here."* **Charlotte** (25) recalled that physicians she saw in the context of a research study told her to *"start having kids at any time, get that done with..,"* contributing to her feeling of urgency to complete childbearing so that RRSO could be pursued. Although **Ashley** experienced this recommendation as informative and supportive, **Charlotte** was distressed by her perceived need to act quickly.

Reza's mother was in active chemotherapy treatment following her second ovarian cancer recurrence in three years. Reza (25) wanted to undergo RRSO, but her providers advised against it. She shared, *"Nobody would give me a reason that seemed real besides 'you're too young, you'll want to have kids someday."* **Sara** (22) also met with resistance about her decision to undergo RRSO, despite her certainty that she did not wish to have biological children. She lamented, *"I've gone to the doctor and expressed my fear of cancer. There's never been the acknowledgement of, 'okay I hear you, you don't wanna have kids; if you wanna do surgery now, that's great.'"*

Discussion

Barriers to effective utilization of the healthcare system to reduce mutation-related cancer risk lead young women to feel uncertain about risk-management, concerned about reproductive decisions, and pressured to make quick choices. Participants valued providers who addressed their priorities and obligations. They desperately wanted evidence-based guidance to inform their decisions, yet they reported receiving incomplete and inconsistent recommendations from providers with limited expertise in hereditary cancer risk assessment and management. Participants experienced being treated as too young both to know what they wanted and to make major healthcare decisions independently. Incomplete health literacy led many participants to overestimate their cancer risk, focusing on lifetime rather than shorter-term, and relative rather than absolute risk, indicating the need for providers with quantitative expertise in hereditary cancer genetics to facilitate ongoing education. The combination of inflated short-term risk perceptions, limited proven age-specific risk management strategies, and well-intentioned but inaccurate provider recommendations all created pressure to rush childbearing, so that surgical risk-reduction could be implemented. Utilization of services from genetically-oriented providers may support patients' acquisition of developmentally and medically sound knowledge of cancer risk *and* risk management. The Affordable Care Act of 2010, which requires group health plans to provide coverage for dependent children of policy-holders until their 26th birthday, may levy additional pressure to decide early about risk-reducing surgery [24].

Discrepancies in responding to cancer risk

Inaccurate cancer risk perceptions may increase distress in young women, cause them to delay genetic testing (if risk is inaccurately perceived as low), or to initiate risk-reducing surgery precipitously (if short-term risk is inaccurately perceived as very high) Rapid uptake of risk-reducing surgery following genetic testing, as seen in our sample, is driven by the perception that cancer risk is imminent. The need to accurately convey short-to-intermediate cancer risk (over 5–10 years) represents a major challenge.

Our data suggest discrepancies may exist between patient and provider responses to inherited cancer risk, further indicating the need for providers with expertise in both cancer genetics and the developmental needs of adolescents transitioning to adulthood. Providers may have difficulty believing that a 20-year-old faces similar risks to those observed in older mutation carriers. Trust in provider recommendations seemed to erode as differences between provider and consumer expectations grew. Providers may suggest women in their 20s postpone risk-reducing surgery until after childbearing to reinforce that imminent cancer risk is quite low, or because they assume young patients prioritize having children. Yet, recommendations linking risk management and family formation may signal to patients that physicians perceive short-term risk of cancer to be very high. When young adults are not ready to commit to life-long partnerships or to become parents, these well-intentioned recommendations are interpreted as a failure to be taken seriously. Striking generational and gender socialization differences may exist between patients and providers, leaving young women struggling to feel understood by those helping them make decisions about their care. Optimally, providers can convey the caring expected from an expert, while maintaining the neutrality necessary to guide patients confidently to individually-tailored and thoughtful decisions.

Implications for practice

Ideally, young women would learn all the facets of risk management early in their experience as mutation carriers, allowing them to manage risk confidently. However, our data suggest that rapid developmental changes common during the transition to adulthood may necessitate a prolonged period of care for young women, whose needs are distinct from older mutation carriers for whom standard practice guidelines and clinical trials were designed. In the context of limited evidence, young women need to work methodically with providers who are knowledgeable and non-judgmental, to avoid rushing into decisions inconsistent with their life goals. Provider recommendations may be carefully tailored to attend to developmental readiness while still providing an integrated approach to care. Such a model may enable ongoing connection with patients as shifting life circumstances precipitate interest in more aggressive risk-reduction strategies.

Limitations & Strengths

Participants received care over a thirteen-year period during which the treatment of *BRCA*-related cancer risk evolved. We maintained separate codebooks for each study to ensure temporal differences in standards of care and public policy were accounted for during analysis. All three studies recruited women who completed genetic testing before age 25. However, none recruited individuals aged 18–20 *at the time of data collection*. None enrolled racial or ethnic minority women, subpopulations which are under-represented in high-risk clinics. Uptake of genetic testing remains particularly low for women of African descent [25], and is further complicated by their higher incidence of genetic variants that are uninformative regarding risk stratification [26].

Conclusions

Young *BRCA1/2* mutation carriers comprise a unique subset of high-risk women who require particularly thoughtful individualized expert care to meet their complex needs. Insuring accurate understanding of absolute short-term cancer risk is essential to informed decision-making.

Author Contributions

Conceived and designed the experiments: LMH AWL MHG. Performed the experiments: LMH AWL. Analyzed the data: LMH AWL. Contributed reagents/materials/analysis tools: LMH AWL. Wrote the paper: LMH AWL MHG.

References

1. Clark AS, Domcheck SM (2011) Clinical management of hereditary breast cancer syndromes. J Mammary Gland Biol 16:17–25.
2. Chen S, Parmigiani G. (2007) Meta-analysis of *BRCA1* and *BRCA2* penetrance. J Clin Oncol 25(11): 1329–1333
3. Chen S, Iverson ES, Friebel T, Finkelstein D, Weber BL, et al. (2006) Characterization of *BRCA1* and *BRCA2* mutations in a large United States sample. J Clin Oncol 24(6): 863–871.
4. Evans JP, Skrzynia C, Susswein L, Harlan M. (2005–2006) Genetics and the young woman with breast cancer. Breast Disease 23: 17–19.
5. Trepanier A, Ahrens M, McKinnon W, Peters J, Stopfer J, et al. (2004) Genetic cancer risk assessment and counseling: Recommendations of the National Society of Genetic Counselors. J Genet Counseling 13(2): 83–114.
6. Arnett JJ (2004) Emerging Adulthood: The Winding Road from the Late Teens through the Twenties. Oxford, UK, Oxford University Press.
7. Samuel JC, Ollila DW (2005/2006) Prophylaxis and screening options: Recommendations for young women with *BRCA* mutations. Breast Disease 23:31–35.
8. Van Oostrom I, Meijers-Heijboer H, Lodder LN, Duivenvoorden HJ, van Gool AR, et al. (2003) Long-term psychological impact of carrying a *BRCA1/2* mutation and prophylactic surgery: A 5-year follow-up study. J Clin Oncol 21: 3867–3874.
9. Watson M, Foster C, Eeles R, Eccles D, Ashley S, et al. (2004) Psychosocial impact of breast/ovarian (*BRCA1/2*) cancer-predictive genetic testing in a UK multi-centre clinical cohort. Brit J Cancer 91(10): 1787–1794.
10. Werner Lin A (2007) Danger zones: Risk perceptions of young women from families with hereditary breast and ovarian cancer. Fam Process 46(3): 335–349.
11. Werner-Lin A (2008) Beating the biological clock: The compressed family life cycle of young women with *BRCA* mutations. Soc Work Health Care 47(4): 416–137.
12. Werner-Lin A (2008) Formal and informal support needs of young women with *BRCA* mutations. J Psychosoc Oncol 26(4): 111–133.
13. Werner-Lin A (2010) Building the cancer family: Family planning in the context of inherited breast and ovarian cancer risk. J Society for Soc Work and Res 1(1): 26–38.
14. Hoskins LM, Roy K, Peters JA, Loud J, Greene MH (2008) Disclosure of positive *BRCA1/2*-mutation status in young couples: The journal from uncertainty to bonding through partner support. Fam Syst Health 26: 296–316.
15. Hoskins LM (2010) Negotiation of health risks and risk management for young adult *BRCA1/2*-positive women: Implications for partnering and family formation. College Park, MD: UMCP.
16. Hoskins LM, Greene MH (2012) Anticipatory loss and early mastectomy for young female *BRCA1/2* mutation carriers. Qual Health Res 22(12): 1633–1646.
17. Hoskins LM, Roy KM, Greene MH (2012) Toward a new understanding of risk perception among young female *BRCA1/2* 'previvors.' Fam, Syst, Health 30(1): 32–46.
18. Facing Our Risk of Cancer Empowered, http://www.facingourrisk.org
19. Daly MB, Axilbund JE, Buys S, Crawford B, Farrell CD, et al. (2010) Genetic/familial high-risk assessment: Breast and ovarian. J Nat Comp Cancer Network, 8(5): 562–594.
20. Sivell S, Elwyn G, Gaff CL, Clarke AJ, Iredale R, et al. (2008) How risk is perceived, constructed and interpreted by clients in clinical genetics, and the effects on decision making: Systematic review. J Genet Counseling, 17:30–63.
21. Lea DH, Kaphingst KA, Bowen D, Lipkus I, Hadley DW (2011) Communicating genetic and genomic information: Health literacy and numeracy considerations. Public Health Genomics 14(4–5): 279–289.
22. Iodice S, Barile M, Rotmensz N, Feroce I, Bonanni B, et al. (2010) Oral contraceptive use and breast or ovarian cancer risk in *BRCA1/2* carriers: A meta-analysis. Eur J Cancer 46(12): 2275–2284.

23. Greene MH, Mai PL, Schwartz PE (2011) Does bilateral salpingectomy with ovarian retention warrant consideration as a temporary bridge to risk-reducing bilateral oophorectomy in *BRCA1/2* mutation carriers? Am J Obstet Gynecol 204(1): 19.e1–6.
24. Werner-Lin A, Hoskins LM, Doyle M, Greene MH (2012) 'Cancer doesn't have an age': Genetic testing and cancer risk management in *BRCA1/2* mutation-positive women aged 18–24. Health 16(6): 636–654.
25. Halbert CH, Kessler L, Wileyto EP, Weathers B, Stopfer J, et al. (2006) Breast cancer screening behaviors among African American women with a strong family history of breast cancer. Prev Med 43(5): 385–388.
26. Nanda R, Schumm LP, Cummings S, Fackenthal JD, Sveen L, et al. (2005) Genetic testing in an ethnically diverse cohort of high-risk women: A comparative analysis of *BRCA1* and *BRCA2* mutations in American families of European and African ancestry. J Amer Med Assoc 294(15): 1925–1933.
27. Pruthi S, Gostout BS, Lindor NM (2010) Identification and management of women with *BRCA* mutations or hereditary predisposition for Breast and Ovarian Cancer. Mayo Clinic Proc 85(12): 1111–1120.
28. Humphrey LL, Helfand M, Chan BK, Woolf SH (2002) Breast cancer screening: A summary of the evidence for the U.S. Preventive Services Task Force. Ann Intern Med 137 (5 Part 1): 347–360.
29. Berrington de Gonzalez A, Berg CD, Visvanathan K, Robson M (2009) Estimated risk of radiation-induced breast cancer from mammographic screening for young *BRCA* mutation carriers. J Natl Cancer Inst 101: 205–209.
30. Narod SA, Lubinski J, Ghadirian P, Lynch HT, Moller P, et al. (2006) Screening mammography and risk of breast cancer in *BRCA1* and *BRCA2* mutation carriers: a case-control study. Lancet Oncol 7: 402–406.
31. Mandelson MT, Oestreicher N, Porter PL, White D, Finder CA, et al.: Breast density as a predictor of mammographic detection: Comparison of interval- and screen-detected cancers. Journal of the National Cancer Institute 92(13): 1081–1087, 2000.
32. Newcomb PA, Weiss NS, Storer BE, Scholes D, Young BE, et al. (1991) Breast self-examination in relation to the occurrence of advanced breast cancer. J Natl Cancer Inst 83(4): 260–265.
33. Fisher B, Costantino JP, Wickerham DL, Redmond CK, Kavanah M, et al. (1998) Tamoxifen for prevention of breast cancer: report of the National Surgical Adjuvant Breast and Bowel Project P-1 Study. J Natl Cancer Inst 90: 1371–1388.
34. Gail MH, Costantino JP, Bryant J, Croyle R, Freedman L, et al. (1999) Weighing the risks and benefits of tamoxifen treatment for preventing breast cancer. J Natl Cancer Inst 91(21): 1829–1846.
35. Visvanathan K, Chlebowski RT, Hurley P, Col NF, Ropka M, et al. (2009) American Society of Clinical Oncology clinical practice guideline update on the use of pharmacologic interventions including Tamoxifen, Raloxifene, and aromatase inhibition for breast cancer risk reduction. J Clin Oncol 27(19): 3235–3258.
36. Rebbeck TR, Friebel T, Lynch HT, Neuhausen SL, van 't Veer L, et al. (2004) Bilateral prophylactic mastectomy reduces breast cancer risk in *BRCA1* and *BRCA2* mutation carriers: The PROSE study group. J Clin Oncol 22(6): 1055–1062.
37. Petrucelli N, Daly MD, Feldman GL (2010) Hereditary breast and ovarian cancer due to mutations in *BRCA1* and *BRCA2*. Genet Med 12(5): 245–259.
38. Narod SA (2002) *BRCA* mutation in the management of breast cancer: the state of the art. Nat Rev Clin Oncol 7(12): 702–707.
39. Kauff ND, Domchek SM, Friebel TM, Robson ME, Lee J, et al. (2008) Risk-reducing salpingo-oophorectomy for the prevention of *BRCA1*- and *BRCA2*-associated breast and gynecologic cancer: A multicenter, prospective study. J Clin Oncol 26: 1331–1337.
40. Crum CP (2009) Intercepting pelvic cancer in the distal fallopian tube: Theories and realities. Mol Oncol 3(2): 165–170.
41. Segev Y, Iqbal J, Libinski J, Gronwald J, Lynch HT, et al. (2013) The incidence of endometrial cancer in women with *BRCA1* and *BRCA2* mutations: An international prospective cohort study. Gynecol Oncol 130(1): 127–131.
42. Antoniou AC, Rookus M, Andrieu N, Brohert R, Chang-Claude J, et al. (2009) Reproductive and hormonal factors, and ovarian cancer risk for *BRCA1* and *BRCA2* mutation carriers: Results from the international *BRCA1/2* Carrier Cohort Study. Cancer Epidemiol Biomarkers Prev 18: 601–610.

10

Identification of Multiple Novel Protein Biomarkers Shed by Human Serous Ovarian Tumors into the Blood of Immunocompromised Mice and Verified in Patient Sera

Lynn A. Beer[1], Huan Wang[1], Hsin-Yao Tang[1], Zhijun Cao[1¤], Tony Chang-Wong[1], Janos L. Tanyi[2], Rugang Zhang[3], Qin Liu[1], David W. Speicher[1*]

1 Center for Systems and Computational Biology, and Molecular and Cellular Oncogenesis Program, The Wistar Institute, Philadelphia, Pennsylvania, United States of America, **2** Ovarian Cancer Research Center, The University of Pennsylvania, Philadelphia, Pennsylvania, United States of America, **3** Gene Expression and Regulation Program, The Wistar Institute, Philadelphia, Pennsylvania, United States of America

Abstract

The most cancer-specific biomarkers in blood are likely to be proteins shed directly by the tumor rather than less specific inflammatory or other host responses. The use of xenograft mouse models together with in-depth proteome analysis for identification of human proteins in the mouse blood is an under-utilized strategy that can clearly identify proteins shed by the tumor. In the current study, 268 human proteins shed into mouse blood from human OVCAR-3 serous tumors were identified based upon human vs. mouse species differences using a four-dimensional plasma proteome fractionation strategy. A multi-step prioritization and verification strategy was subsequently developed to efficiently select some of the most promising biomarkers from this large number of candidates. A key step was parallel analysis of human proteins detected in the tumor supernatant, because substantially greater sequence coverage for many of the human proteins initially detected in the xenograft mouse plasma confirmed assignments as tumor-derived human proteins. Verification of candidate biomarkers in patient sera was facilitated by in-depth, label-free quantitative comparisons of serum pools from patients with ovarian cancer and benign ovarian tumors. The only proteins that advanced to multiple reaction monitoring (MRM) assay development were those that exhibited increases in ovarian cancer patients compared with benign tumor controls. MRM assays were facilely developed for all 11 novel biomarker candidates selected by this process and analysis of larger pools of patient sera suggested that all 11 proteins are promising candidate biomarkers that should be further evaluated on individual patient blood samples.

Editor: Shannon M. Hawkins, Baylor College of Medicine, United States of America

Funding: This work was supported by National Institutes of Health (NIH) grant CA131582 to DWS and an institutional grant to The Wistar Institute, National Cancer Institute (NCI) Cancer Core Grant CA010813), and by the Reproductive Scientist Development Program, NIH grant 5K12HD00849 to JLT (www.nih.gov). The funders had no role in the study design, data collection and analysis, decision to publish, or preparation of the manuscript.

Competing Interests: The authors have declared that no competing interests exist.

* E-mail: speicher@wistar.org

¤ Current address: The National Center for Toxicological Research, U.S. Food and Drug Administration, Jefferson, Arizona, United States of America

Introduction

Epithelial ovarian cancer (EOC) is the fifth-leading cause of cancer-related deaths in women, with a higher fatality-to-case ratio than any other gynecologic malignancy in the United States. [1,2,3] A major problem is that greater than two-thirds of EOC cases are diagnosed at advanced stages (Stages 3 or 4), when five-year survival is about 33%. In contrast, when the disease is diagnosed at Stage 1, five-year survival is approximately 90%. [2] CA125 is the best known EOC biomarker; however, 50–60% of early-stage EOC does not express CA125. In addition, while greater than 80% of advanced EOC has elevated CA125, this is not a sufficient diagnosis, as CA125 levels are also elevated in a number of other conditions. [1,4,5,6] Due to the low incidence of ovarian cancer in the general population, the specificity and sensitivity requirements for early screening are quite high, and achieving suitable performance is likely to require a panel of biomarkers superior to most existing biomarkers. [2,7,8,9] Additional biomarkers, either instead of or in conjunction with CA125, are needed for predicting clinical outcome, stratifying therapeutic options, monitoring response to therapy, and detecting reoccurrence of the disease.

Although proteomic technologies have improved dramatically, discovering novel blood biomarkers for cancers remains formidable due to the vast complexity of the plasma proteome and the likelihood that any tumor-specific proteins will be present at very low abundance. In addition, comparison of patient and control serum or plasma to discover biomarkers is complicated by the fact that cancers and other conditions induce inflammatory responses involving changes in abundance of multiple blood proteins, and these changes are not very specific to a single disease. [10] Identifying cancer-specific changes in the context of this great complexity and inflammation-induced variability is very difficult when patient serum samples are directly analyzed to discover new biomarkers using proteomics. For this reason, many investigators have turned to alternative strategies for initial discovery of candidate biomarkers, including proteome analysis of: EOC cell lines, cell surface proteins in EOC cell lines, proteins shed by these cells into the media (the secretome), and patient ascites. [11,12,13,14,15,16] While all of these methods identify many proteins associated with EOC, a critical missing factor is that it is not apparent which of these proteins will migrate into the blood and be potential EOC serum/plasma biomarkers. Furthermore, changes in abundance levels of a protein in the tumor tissue do not necessarily correlate with their abundance levels in the blood.

The primary experimental systems where migration into the blood is assured are mouse models. Hence, one approach is to identity quantitative differences in plasma or serum of genetically engineered mice bearing murine ovarian tumors compared with appropriate controls. [17] While this model provides more consistent genetic and environmental backgrounds compared with patients, the complication of sorting protein changes caused by inflammatory host responses from proteins shed by the tumor persists. An important under-utilized alternative that circumvents the host response problem is xenograft mouse models, where in-depth proteome analysis can identify human proteins shed by the tumor into the murine blood based upon species differences in peptide sequences found in serum or plasma. Another advantage of the xenograft mouse model system, like genetically engineered mice, is a higher tumor-to-blood-volume ratio compared with patients, as well as homogeneous genetic backgrounds, environment, and diet to minimize confounding factors.

We recently identified 106 human proteins shed by a human endometrial ovarian cancer cell line (TOV-112D) into the blood of SCID mice using an in-depth 4D proteome analysis of this xenografted mouse serum. Specifically, serum was depleted of the three most abundant serum proteins followed by microscale solution isoelectrofocusing (MicroSol IEF), SDS-PAGE, and LC-MS/MS. [18] Furthermore, pilot validation of selected candidate biomarkers demonstrated that some of these proteins could be detected in human serum using multiple reaction monitoring (MRM) analysis–and three tested biomarkers were shown to be significantly elevated in cancer patients compared with normal donors. [18] Although that study identified several new biomarkers, the verification and initial validation steps were not very efficient. The success rate of establishing MRM assays for targeted candidate biomarkers using advanced EOC patient serum pools was less than 50%, and only about half of the proteins quantified using these MRM assays exhibited elevated levels in pilot analyses of advanced EOC patients using pools of patient sera ([18] and data not shown). Hence, overall, only about 20% of the TOV-112D candidate biomarkers selected for verification and initial validation in patients resulted in successful MRM assays that exhibited elevated levels in EOC in a small pilot analysis.

The current study was designed to improve ovarian cancer biomarker discovery using the xenograft mouse model system, improve the efficiency of MRM assay development and preliminary verification of biomarker candidates, and identify candidates that may include biomarkers with some degree of specificity for the serous ovarian cancer subtype. High grade serous ovarian cancers are very aggressive and account for most deaths from EOC, although they only constitute approximately half of EOC cases. Plasma from SCID mice bearing OVCAR-3 serous ovarian tumors was analyzed using an optimized 4-D plasma proteome analysis method, which resulted in identification of 268 human proteins based on two or more peptides. Parallel analysis of supernatants from the serous tumor excised from the SCID mice and incubated briefly in cell culture media increased the sequence coverage for many of the human proteins, thereby both confirming these proteins were human and providing more proteotypic peptides for MRM assay development. Selected high-priority candidate biomarkers were then compared to a dataset from a label-free quantitative comparison of serum pools from cancer patients with advanced-stage EOC and benign controls. Finally, candidate biomarkers observed to be elevated in pooled sera from advanced EOC cancer patients in the label-free analysis were selected for multiplexed assay development using targeted mass spectrometry analysis with the multiple reaction monitoring (MRM) method. MRM analysis is an alternative mass spectrometry approach utilizing the discriminating power of triple quadropole mass spectrometers, or their equivalent, to select and quantify a series of specific analytes and associated fragment ions. MRM enables rapid, quantitative measures of proteins in complex mixtures such as plasma and serum, without a dependency on the generation of antibodies or immunoassays. [19,20] Overall, the strategy used in this study proved to be highly efficient, as 100% of the proteins selected for MRM assay development resulted in successful assay development and showed elevated levels in serum pools of advanced EOC patients compared with an approximately 20% success rate in earlier studies that attempted to quantify and verify TOV-112D candidate biomarkers.

Materials and Methods

Reagents

Molecular-biology-grade ethanol (200 proof); LC-MS-grade formic acid; sodium phosphate monobasic; *N,N*-dimethylacrylamide (DMA), ammonium bicarbonate; and iodoacetamide were purchased from Sigma-Aldrich (St. Louis, MO). Sodium dodecyl sulfate (SDS), 2-mercaptoethanol, and Tris were purchased from Bio-Rad (Hercules, CA). ZOOM focusing buffers and thiourea were obtained from Invitrogen (Carlsbad, CA). PlusOne reagents dithiothreitol (DTT), 3-[(3-cholamidopropyl)dimethylammonio]-1-propanesulfonate (CHAPS), and urea were purchased from GE Healthcare (Piscataway, NJ). HPLC-grade acetonitrile was purchased from Thomas Scientific (Swedesboro, NJ). Tris(2-carboxyethyl)phosphine (TCEP) was obtained from Pierce (Rockford, IL), and sequencing-grade modified trypsin was purchased from Promega (Madison, WI).

Cell Culture

The human EOC serous cell line OVCAR-3 was obtained from the American Type Culture Collection (ATCC, Manassas, VA). The cells were maintained in a 37°C incubator with a 5% CO_2–95% air atmosphere in RPMI-1640 medium (ATCC) supplemented with 10% fetal calf serum.

Ovarian Cancer Growth *in vivo*

This study was carried out in accordance with the recommendations in the Guide for the Care and use of Laboratory Animals of the National Institutes of Health under protocol #111959 using severe combined immunodeficiency (SCID) mice. The study protocol was reviewed and approved by The Wistar Institute's Institutional Animal Care and Use Committee (IACUC). All efforts were made to minimize suffering.

Nine SCID mice were injected subcutaneously in the flank with 50 µl of OVCAR-3 cells (2×10^6) mixed 1:1 with 50 µL Matrigel (BD Biosciences, San Jose, CA). Tumors were allowed to grow until final tumor size was estimated to be at least 1 cm^3 using calipers, but less than 10% of body weight. Blood was collected, mice were euthanized, and tumors were removed at 12 weeks post-injection. Necrosis of tumor tissue was assessed by microscopic inspection of hematoxylin and eosin (H&E) stained, paraffin-embedded sections (5 µm).

SCID Mouse Plasma

Blood was collected from SCID mice containing visible OVCAR-3 tumors (see above section) by cardiac puncture under anesthesia into Microtainer 0.5 mL K_2 EDTA Blood Collection Tubes (Becton Dickinson, Franklin Lakes, NJ). The tubes were centrifuged for 3 min at room temperature, and aliquots of plasma from individual mice were snap-frozen and stored at −80°C. Plasma from the four mice that contained the largest, minimally neurotic tumors were subsequently thawed and pooled to average variations among individual mice. The pooled plasma was re-aliquoted, snap-frozen, and stored at −80°C until analysis using the 4-D fractionation method (immunoaffinity depletion/MicroSol IEF/SDS gel and trypsin digestion/LC-MS/MS). Total protein concentration of the pooled plasma was measured using a BCA Protein Assay (Pierce).

Tumor Supernatant Isolation

Immediately after removing tumors from eight of the nine SCID mice bearing the largest OVCAR-3 tumors, a section of fresh ovarian tumor tissue from each mouse was cut into small pieces (2–3 mm^3), placed in the upper chamber of a 5 μm PVDF microcentrifuge filter (Millipore, Billerica, MA), and washed three times with 400 μL of PBS for 1 min each. The tissue sections were then transferred to the upper chamber of a 0.22 μm PVDF microcentrifuge filter and incubated in 400 μL of serum-free RPMI-1640 medium for 2 h in 5% CO_2, 95% air at 37°C. After incubation, the supernatant (conditioned media) was recovered by centrifugation, then frozen and stored at −80°C until needed. For tumor supernatant analysis, 500 μL aliquots of conditioned media from tumors from four mice were thawed, pooled, and concentrated to ~30 μL by ultrafiltration using a 10 K MWCO concentration unit. Membrane rinses using 1% SDS, 50 mM Tris, pH 8.5 were combined with the concentrated sample to maximize protein recovery.

Human Serum

Human sera from normal subjects and patients with benign ovarian tumors, early-stage ovarian cancer, and late-stage ovarian cancer were collected before clinical treatment at approximately the time of diagnosis and prior to surgery as previously described. [18] Descriptions of the patients, healthy controls, and pooling strategies are summarized in **Table S2**. All research in this study involving human specimens was conducted under The Wistar Institute's Institutional Review Board (IRB) approved protocols, #2109171, #EX2110012, and #2602221 and in accordance with Health Insurance Portability and Accountability Act (HIPAA) requirements. All human samples were derived from subjects with informed written consent. Data were analyzed anonymously.

Immunoaffinity Removal of Major Blood Proteins

The pooled mouse plasma was depleted using a 4.6×100 mm MARS Mouse-3 HPLC column (Agilent Technologies, Wilmington, DE), essentially as previously described, [18] with the exception that a total of 400 μL of pooled plasma was diluted five-fold with equilibration buffer, filtered through a 0.22 μm microcentrifuge filter, and applied to the antibody column in eight serial injections of 250 μL per depletion.

Human serum samples (typically 30–60 μL) were depleted of the 20-most-abundant serum proteins using a ProteoPrep20 Immunodepletion Column (Sigma), as described previously. [21].

MicroSol IEF Fractionation

Immunodepleted and concentrated mouse plasma (2.2 mg) was fractionated by MicroSol IEF as previously described, [18,22,23] using a ZOOM-IEF fractionator (Invitrogen) where the separation chambers were defined by immobilized gel membranes having pH values of 3.0, 4.6, 5.4, 6.2, and 12.0, respectively.

SDS-PAGE/in-gel Trypsin Digestion

After evaluation of the MicroSol IEF separation on analytical SDS gels, concentrated samples were loaded onto multiple lanes of pre-cast 12% Bis-Tris NuPAGE gels (Invitrogen) and separated for discrete distances (1 or 4 cm). The concentrated tumor supernatants from both pools were loaded onto multiple lanes of pre-cast 12% Bis-Tris NuPAGE gels (Invitrogen) and separated for 6 cm. Gels were stained with Colloidal Blue (Invitrogen), each gel lane was sliced into uniform 1 mm slices, and corresponding slices from triplicate lanes were combined in a single well of a 96-well pierced digestion plate (Bio-Machines, Inc., Carrboro, NC) and digested overnight with 0.02 μg/μL of modified trypsin, as previously described. [21,24].

LC-MS/MS

Tryptic digests were analyzed using an LTQ-Orbitrap XL mass spectrometer (Thermo Scientific, Waltham, MA) interfaced with a Nano-ACQUITY UPLC system (Waters, Milford, MA), as described previously. [21] For each tryptic digest, 8 μL was injected onto a UPLC Symmetry trap column (180 μm i.d. × 2 cm packed with 5 μm C18 resin; Waters), and tryptic peptides were separated by RP-HPLC on a BEH C18 nanocapillary analytical column (75 μm i.d. × 25 cm, 1.7 μm particle size; Waters). The mass spectrometer was set to scan m/z from 400 to 2000. The full MS scan was collected at 60,000 resolution in the Orbitrap in profile mode followed by data-dependant MS/MS scans on the six most abundant ions exceeding a minimum threshold of 1000 collected in the linear trap. Monoisotopic precursor selection was enabled and charge-state screening was enabled to reject $z = 1$ ions. Ions subjected to MS/MS were excluded from repeated analysis for 60 s.

Data Processing

MS/MS spectra were extracted and searched using the SEQUEST algorithm (v. 28, rev. 13, University of Washington, Seattle, WA) in Bioworks (v. 3.3.1, Thermo Scientific) against a combined human and mouse UniRef100 protein sequence database (v. June 20,2011) to which commonly observed "contaminants" (trypsin, keratins, etc.) were added. A decoy database was produced by reversing the protein sequence of each database entry, and the entire reversed database was appended in front of the forward human and mouse databases, respectively. Spectra were searched with a partial tryptic constraint of up to two missed cleavages, 100 ppm precursor mass tolerance, 1 Da fragment ion mass tolerance, static modification of cys (+99.06840 for samples alkylated with DMA or +57.0215 Da for samples alkylated with IAM), and variable modification of methionine (+15.9949). The use of a partial tryptic constraint and 100 ppm precursor tolerance for the database search had recently been shown to enhance depth of analysis for serum and plasma proteomes. [25] Consensus protein lists were created using DTASelect (v. 2,0, licensed from Scripps Research Institute, La Jolla, CA) and the following filters were applied: full tryptic constraint, mass accuracy ≤10 ppm, and ΔCn ≥0.05. [25] FDR was estimated from the ratio of unique peptides matching reverse sequences to the number of unique peptides matching forward sequences. Non-redundant peptide totals derived from DTASelect and used for FDR calculations include variable modifications and different charge states as separate peptides. Different charge states and variable modifications of methionine oxidation were collapsed into a single unique peptide count, and peptides shared among multiple proteins were assigned to the protein having the highest sequence coverage, as previously described. [18].

Proteins identified in the database search were sorted into "human," "mouse," or "indistinguishable" based upon their species-specific sequences, as previously described. [18] To confirm species-specific assignments, putative uniquely human and mouse sequences were searched against the mouse and human UniRef100 databases (v. 6/20/11), respectively, using BLAST. Keratins and other presumed contaminants were removed from the entire dataset.

Label-free Quantitation of Patient Serum Pools

To determine whether candidate biomarkers could be detected in ovarian cancer patient sera, in-depth discovery mode analyses of patient serum pools were conducted followed by global label-free quantitative comparisons. One pool of serum from benign patients and three pools of advanced ovarian cancer patient serum samples were made as described in **Table S2**. Pools were immunodepleted and separated on a 1 D SDS gel, each serum proteome was separated into 40 fractions, and each slice was digested with trypsin and analyzed by LC-MS/MS using a 4 h gradient at 200 nL/min consisting of 5–28% B over 168 min, 28–50% B over 51.5 min, 50–80% B over 5 min, and 80% B for 4.5 min, before returning to 5% B over 0.5 min. A short blank gradient was run in between samples to minimize carryover. Full-MS and LC-MS/MS data from fractions 17–32, which encompassed the 8–50 kDa region of the gel, were analyzed using Rosetta Elucidator software (version 3.3, Rosetta Biosoftware, Seattle, WA) to compare peptide signal intensities in full MS scans. Based on peptide elution profiles and ion signal density, data for this label-free comparison was trimmed to 16–200 min. Retention time (RT) alignment, feature identification (discrete ion signals), feature extraction, and protein identifications were performed by the Elucidator system as previously described. [21,26].

Label-free Multiple Reaction Monitoring

MRM experiments were performed on a 5500 QTRAP hybrid triple quadrupole/linear ion trap mass spectrometer (AB Sciex, Foster City, CA) interfaced with a Nano-ACQUITY UPLC system with the column heater maintained at 45°C. Tryptic digests were injected using the partial loop injection mode onto a UPLC Symmetry trap column (180 μm i.d. × 2 cm packed with 5 μm C18 resin), and then separated by RP-HPLC on a BEH C18 nanocapillary analytical column (75 mm i.d. × 25 cm, 1.7 mm particle size; Waters). Chromatography was performed with solvent A, consisting of Milli-Q water with 0.1% formic acid, and solvent B, as acetonitrile with 0.1% formic acid. Peptides and transitions used for quantitation were selected from discovery results (typically the mouse tumor supernatant) and further verified by MRM-initiated detection and sequencing (MIDAS) using the 5500 QTRAP mass spectrometer. MIDAS experiments were performed at 200 nL/min with a 77-min gradient consisting of 5–28% B over 42 min, 28–50% B over 25.5 min, 50–80% B over 5 min, and 80% B for 4.5 min, before returning to 5% B over 0.5 min. To increase throughput, after optimal peptides and transitions were established, label-free MRM assays were performed with a 41-min gradient, in which peptides were eluted at 400 nL/min for 5–35% B over 38 min and 35% B for 3 min, before returning to 5% B over 0.5 min.

MRM data were acquired with a spray voltage of 3300 V, curtain gas of 20 p.s.i., nebulizer gas of 10 p.s.i., interface heater temperature of 150°C, and a pause time of 3 ms. Multiple MRM transitions were monitored per peptide at unit resolution in both Q1 and Q3 quadrupoles to maximize specificity. Scheduled MRM was used to reduce the number of concurrent transitions and maximize the dwell time for each transition. The detection window was set at 2 min, and the target scan time was set at 1.8 s. Data analysis was performed using Skyline v.1.2. [27] The transition with the strongest signal for each peptide was used for quantification unless interference from the matrix was observed. In these cases, another transition free of interference was chosen for quantification.

Results and Discussion

Overview of Discovery, Prioritization and Verification of EOC Biomarkers Using a Xenograft Serous EOC Mouse Model

The strategies used to improve ovarian cancer biomarker discovery using the xenograft mouse model system, select high priority candidate biomarkers, and improve the efficiency of MRM assay development and biomarker verification are outlined in **Figure 1**. In the discovery phase, OVCAR-3, an established human serous cell line, was grown in SCID mice. Xenograft mouse plasma pooled from four mice with the largest tumors was subjected to extensive fractionation (180 fractions) using a 4 D plasma proteome separation method developed in our laboratory which consists of immunoaffinity depletion of major serum proteins, MicroSol IEF, 1D SDS-PAGE, and LC-MS/MS. [24] Representative analytical and preparative 1D SDS gels showing MicroSol IEF fractions prior to LC-MS/MS analysis can be found in **Figure S1 B and C**, respectively. Human proteins identified in the plasma by at least two peptides, at least one of which was uniquely human, were prioritized and verified as illustrated and described in further detail below. Although this biomarker candidate discovery study used a cell line representative of a late stage tumor, our working hypothesis is that the best cancer biomarkers will be shed by the tumor into the blood and will correlate with tumor size. These biomarkers will ideally be detectable in serum or plasma at higher levels than in control subjects, even when the tumors are small, and the levels of these biomarkers will increase as the tumor grows. By utilizing the xenograft mouse model and identifying human proteins, we are assured that the candidate biomarkers are derived from the tumor and shed into the blood, at least in this model system.

Analyses of the Xenograft Mouse Plasma Proteome and Corresponding Tumor Supernatants

Plasma from four mice containing OVCAR-3 tumors that were at least 1 cm^3 was pooled and analyzed using the 4D method described above. Fractionation using MicroSol IEF and 1D SDS gels yielded 180 fractions and subsequent analysis of these fractions by LC-MS/MS produced more than 1.1 million spectra, which were searched against a combined human and mouse database. A total of 3647 non-redundant human and mouse proteins were initially identified by 22,890 peptides at a peptide FDR of 5.7% for all proteins, and a 0.5% FDR for protein identifications with two or more peptides. After species classification, 268 human proteins were identified by two or more peptides and an additional 550 by a single peptide (**Figure 2**). Because the FDR was considerably lower for proteins with ≥2 peptides in both the plasma and tumor supernatant samples, we only considered

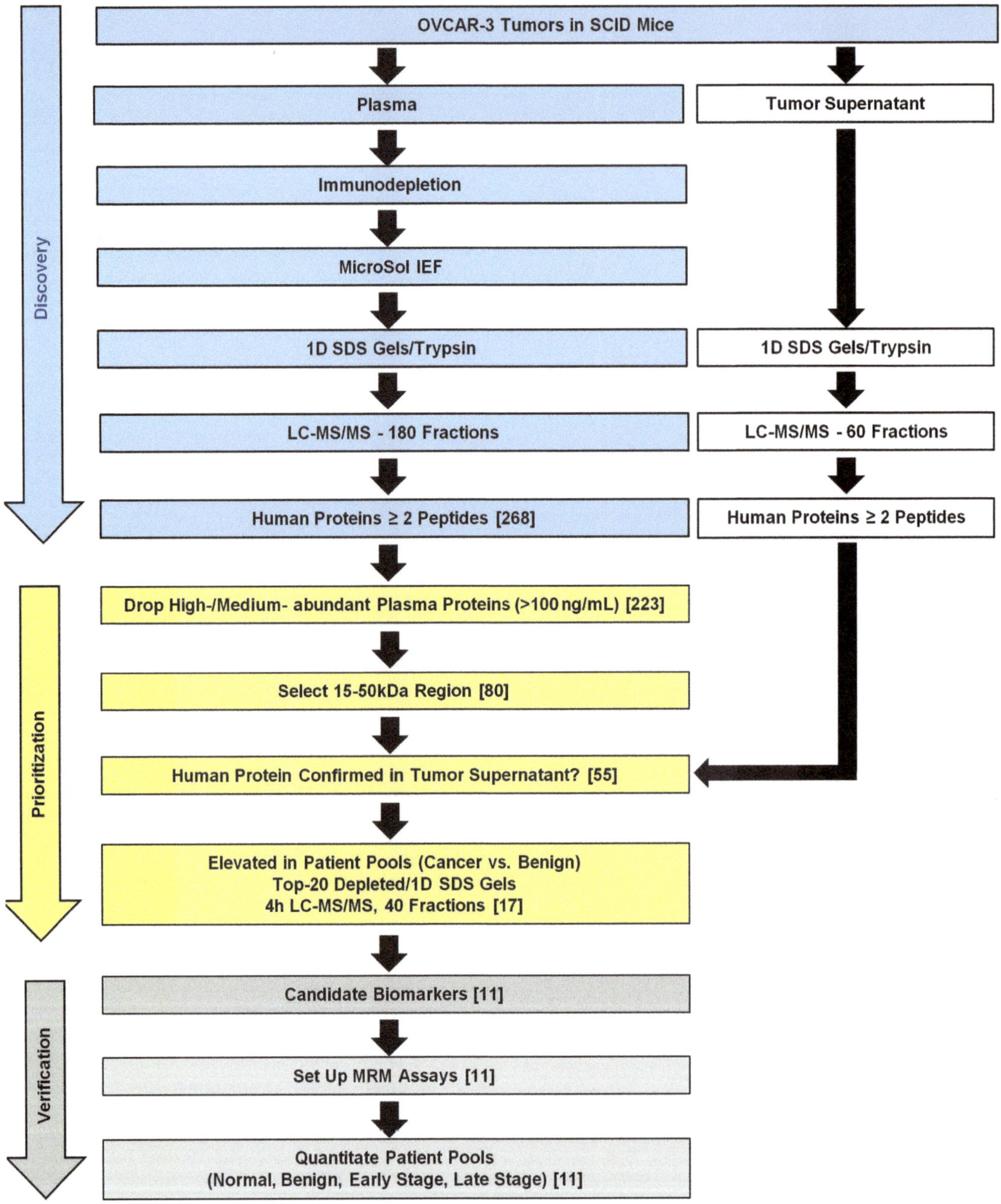

Figure 1. Scheme for ovarian cancer biomarker discovery and efficient verification using a xenograft mouse model. Candidate biomarkers were discovered in the xenograft mouse plasma using a 4D plasma proteome profiling method. Parallel analysis of the tumor supernatant was used to confirm human protein identifications and expand sequence coverage. A multi-step prioritization method ensured that only those proteins detectable in advanced EOC patient sera at elevated levels advanced to MRM assay development and verification in larger pools of patient sera.

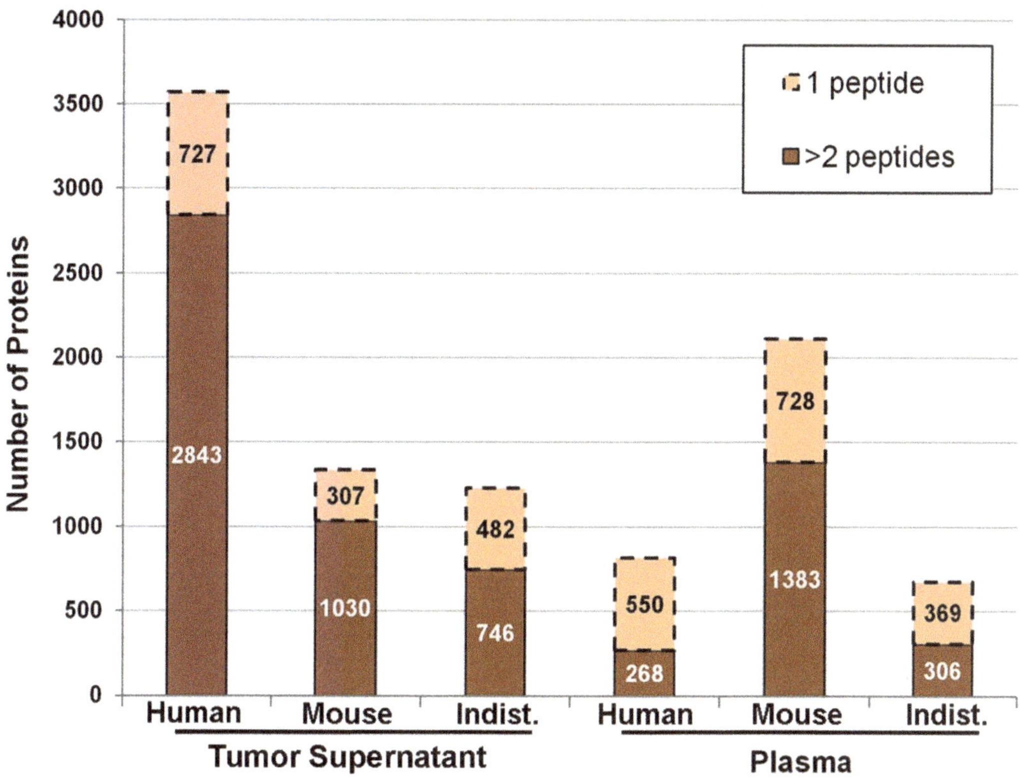

Figure 2. Proteins identified in the xenograft plasma and tumor supernatant. The numbers of unique (nonredundant) proteins identified in the OVCAR-3 xenograft tumor supernatant and mouse plasma are shown after sorting proteins based on species classification where at least one peptide was uniquely human, uniquely mouse, or indistinguishable (Indist.), that is, all detected peptides were common to human and mouse homologs.

proteins having two or more peptide identifications for downstream analyses.

Due to the difficulty of detecting low abundance human proteins in the mouse plasma, tumor supernatants from the same batch of SCID mice with OVCAR-3 tumors were analyzed to attempt to achieve more extensive sequence coverage of human proteins detected in the mouse plasma. Concentrated tumor supernatants were separated on 1D SDS gels, each lane was sliced into 60 uniform fractions (**Figure S1A**), and each sample was digested with trypsin followed by LC-MS/MS analysis resulting in 487,076 MS/MS spectra, which were searched against a combined mouse and human database. A total of 6066 unique proteins were identified from 46,111 peptides at a peptide FDR of 0.9%. Eliminating single peptide proteins resulted in 4619 unique protein entries, with a peptide FDR of 0.03%. This list of high-confidence proteins (≥2 peptides) identified from the combined human and mouse dataset is listed in **Table S1**. This complete dataset was divided into "human" and "mouse" based upon the presence of at least one peptide unique to that species, while "indistinguishable" proteins contained only peptides common to both species. A total of 2843 human proteins were identified by two or more peptides, and an additional 727 human proteins were identified by single peptides (**Figure 2**).

Interestingly, the tumor supernatant dataset provided a much greater depth of analysis both in terms of total proteins identified and sequence coverage of most proteins, despite the less extensive fractionation used. Also, the proportion of total identified proteins that could be assigned as human was far higher in the tumor supernatant. In part, this was expected because the plasma analysis was dominated by detection of high and medium abundance mouse plasma proteins. However, it also indicates that the contribution of mouse cells in the tumor, including fibroblasts and vascular cells, was relatively minor compared to shedding of proteins by the human tumor cells.

The Tumor Supernatant Increases Sequence Coverage of Human Proteins Detected in the Xenograft Mouse Plasma

Over 2800 human proteins from the tumor were identified in the supernatant and this dataset is a possible source of additional plasma biomarkers for ovarian cancer. However, unless the proteins were also detected in the mouse plasma, there is no assurance that proteins observed in the supernatant would be shed into and be detectable in the blood. Furthermore, the plasma analysis had already identified nearly 300 human proteins, which exceeds the number of proteins that could be feasibly tested in human serum. Hence, in this study, the larger tumor supernatant dataset was only used to confirm the "human" assignment of proteins identified in the mouse plasma, although this large dataset almost certainly contains additional potential plasma biomarkers that could be explored in future studies. Confirmation of apparent human proteins in the mouse plasma is important because many proteins were assigned as human based upon the detection of one human peptide and one or more peptides with sequences common to both species. A few of these apparent human proteins may be false positives while others could represent unreported mouse polymorphisms, mouse sequences not reported in the database, etc. Also, some identified proteins represent a protein family but the peptides identified in the plasma do not unambiguously define a unique isoform. Therefore, for most of the human proteins identified in the plasma, the tumor supernatant dataset improved the confidence of species assignment and in some cases more clearly defined family member(s) present in the xenograft plasma samples by confirming the original peptide and protein identifications and, in most cases, providing more extensive peptide coverage.

Examples of using the tumor supernatant data to expand the utility of data from the xenograft plasma are shown in **Figure 3**. PSMA1 (**Figure 3A**) was identified by a total of 10 peptides in the mouse plasma, but only a single one of these was a uniquely human peptide. This protein could have been de-prioritized because of its high homology to a mouse counterpart and the possibility that the single uniquely human peptide in the plasma might have been a false positive identification or unknown mouse sequence variant. However, the tumor supernatant identified an additional five peptides that were uniquely human, thus increasing the confidence of the species assignment for the original plasma identification. **Figure 3B** shows PSME2, a protein identified by two uniquely human peptides in the plasma dataset, and therefore the species assignment as human is well supported. But, the tumor supernatant analysis identified six additional human peptides, thereby providing more proteotypic peptides for setting up MRM assays.

The tumor supernatant and plasma datasets were compared to a study by Pitteri *et al.* that identified candidate biomarkers by comparing a genetically engineered mouse model and secretomes of ovarian cancer cells. [17] That study validated eight proteins found to be at higher abundance levels in ovarian cancer patients' plasma, and they also described identification of an additional nine proteins previously identified as ovarian cancer plasma biomarkers. Of the 17 candidate markers described by Pitteri *et al.*, we identified eight proteins (CTSB, FASN, IGFBP2, LCN2, MIF, THBS1, WFDC2, and NRCAM) in our tumor supernatant analysis, and three proteins (FASN, IGFBP2, and LCN1) in the high-confidence xenograft plasma dataset.

We also compared the results from the current study using OVCAR-3 cells, a serous EOC cell line to an earlier xenograft mouse study using an endometrioid EOC cell line (TOV-112D) where we identified three new biomarkers of ovarian cancer that could distinguish cancer patients from normal individuals. [18] These three biomarkers, CLIC1, CTSD, and PRDX6, were all identified in the current study.

Overall, these comparisons show that different biomarker discovery strategies result in detection of overlapping, but non-identical sets of biomarkers. These data also demonstrate that analysis of the tumor supernatant in parallel with xenograft mouse plasma is useful for confirming candidate biomarkers detected in xenograft mouse plasma.

Prioritization and Selection of Candidate Biomarkers for Verification Using Patient Sera

Efficient methods for selecting the best candidate biomarkers and economically verifying them in serum or plasma of EOC patients are needed because, some, but not all proteins shed by

A PSMA1

```
        10         20         30         40         50         60
MFRNQYDNDV TVWSPQGRIH QIEYAMEAVK QGSATVGLKS KTHAVLVALK RAQSELAAHQ

        70         80         90        100        110        120
KKILHVDNHI GISIAGLTAD ARLLCNFMRQ ECLDSRFVFD RPLPVSRLVS LIGSKTQIPT

       130        140        150        160        170        180
QRYGRRPYGV GLLIAGYDDM GPHIFQTCPS ANYFDCRAMS IGARSQSART YLERHMSEFM

       190        200        210        220        230        240
ECNLNELVKH GLRALRETLP AEQDLTTKNV SIGIVGKDLE FTIYDDDDVS PFLEGLEERP

       250        260
QRKAQPAQPA DEPAEKADEP MEH
```

B PSME2

```
        10         20         30         40         50         60
MAKPCGVRLS GEARKQVEVF RQNLFQEAEE FLYRFLPQKI IYLNQLLQED SLNVADLTSL

        70         80         90        100        110        120
RAPLDIPIPD PPPKDDEMET DKQEKKEVHK CGFLPGNEKV LSLLALVKPE VWTLKEKCIL

       130        140        150        160        170        180
VITWIQHLIP KIEDGNDFGV AIQEKVLERV NAVKTKVEAF QTTISKYFSE RGDAVAKASK

       190        200        210        220        230
ETHVMDYRAL VHERDEAAYG ELRAMVLDLR AFYAELYHII SSNLEKIVNP KGEEKPSMY
```

Highlight: Xenograft Plasma
Underline: Tumor Supernatant

Figure 3. Sequence coverage for selected human proteins from the xenograft plasma and tumor supernatants. Examples of candidate biomarkers, PSMA1 and PSME2, where increased sequence coverage is obtained from analysis of the tumor supernatant (underlined peptides) compared to the xenograft plasma (grey highlight). Tryptic sites (K or R) are indicated in red.

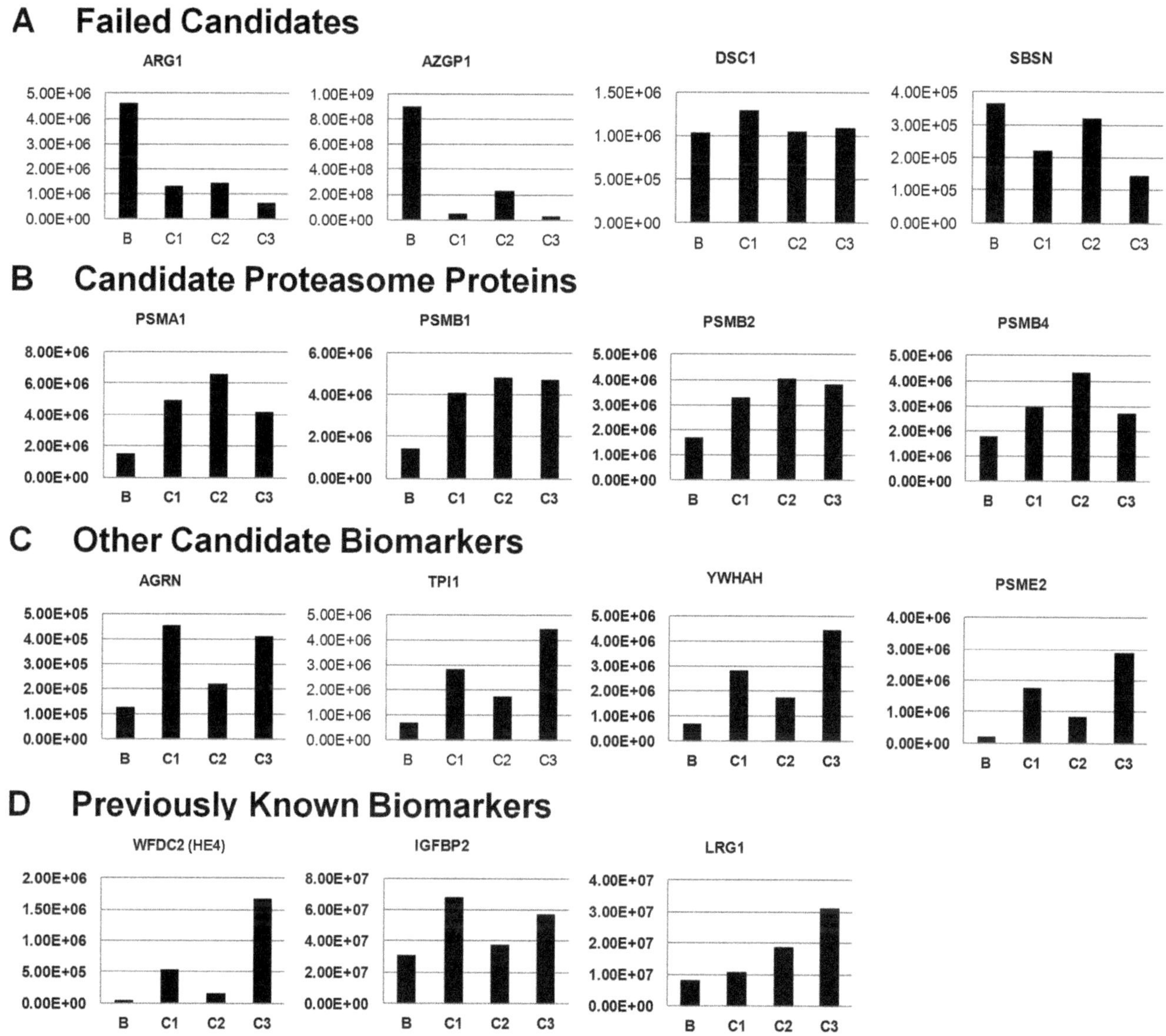

Figure 4. Quantitative comparisons of candidate biomarkers using label-free discovery mode LC-MS/MS analysis of patient serum pools. Summed protein intensities from a Rosetta Elucidator label-free analysis are shown for benign (B, n = 9) and three different late-stage ovarian cancer pools (C1, n = 9; C2, n = 9; C3, n = 5). (A) Representative proteins that failed this screen because intensities were lower or showed no difference in cancer pools compared with benign disease. (B) Four different isoforms of the proteasome complex selected for further validation because they showed elevated levels in all cancer pools compared with benign sera. (C) Additional representative proteins selected for further validation because they showed elevated levels in all cancer pools compared with benign sera. (D) Three biomarkers previously reported by others and re-discovered in the current study (see **Table 1**).

EOC tumors into blood are expected to be good biomarkers of the disease. Furthermore, some proteins detected in the xenograft mouse model may not be detectable in human blood using current methods either because the concentration in human blood is below detection limits of available assays or because in some cases the shedding may be unique to the mouse model. As noted above, when we evaluated a panel of candidate biomarkers from the TOV-112D xenograft mice tumors, the overall success in setting up MRM assays and demonstrating elevated levels of the targeted biomarker in EOC patient sera was only about 20%. Hence, an important challenge is to develop appropriate methods for more efficient triaging of candidate biomarkers and evaluating them in serum of EOC patients.

The xenograft plasma proteome was prioritized starting with the 268 human proteins identified by two or more peptides (**Figure 2**). This dataset was further refined by removing a few trypsin and keratin contaminants that were missed at the initial contaminant-removal step due to ambiguous protein descriptions or isoform differences. In addition, proteins known to be in normal human plasma at medium- to high-abundant levels (>100 ng/mL [28,29]) and hemoglobins were removed. Such proteins were not considered to be viable candidate biomarkers because the contribution of shedding from a small tumor is unlikely to be discernible above the normal variation of that protein in the general population. For example, if a protein is normally in the plasma of unaffected individuals in the 1–5 μg/mL range and the protein is also shed by a typical ovarian tumor, which contributes

Table 1. Candidate biomarkers for validation in patient serum pools.

Gene Name	Protein Description	# Peptides[a] (Supernatant)	# Peptides[a] (Plasma)
B. Previously reported biomarkers re-identified in this study			
IGFBP2	Insulin-like growth factor-binding protein 2 [38]	9/5	5/4
WFDC2 (HE4)	WAP four-disulfide core domain protein 2 [39]	2/0	0
LRG1	Leucine-rich alpha-2-glycoprotein [40]	0	1/1
A. Novel candidates identified from xenograft mouse plasma and verified in tumor supernatant			
AGRN	Agrin and agrin fragments	61/9	5/1
PSME2	Proteasome activator complex subunit 2	8/11	2/8
TPI1	Triosephosphate isomerase	7/18	4/10
DDAH2	N(G),N(G)-dimethylarginine dimethylaminohydrolase 2	7/8	1/4
GM2A	GM2 ganglioside activator protein (GM2A), mRNA	3/0	3/0
YWHAB	14-3-3 protein beta/alpha	2/8	1/12
YWHAH	14-3-3 protein eta	2/9	1/7
PSMA1	Proteasome subunit alpha type-1	6/14	1/10
PSMB1	Proteasome subunit beta type-1	3/9	1/6
PSMB2	Proteasome subunit beta type-2	1/10	1/6
PSMB4	Proteasome subunit beta type-4	3/5	2/5

[a]Number of peptides that are uniquely human/number of peptides common to mouse and human homolog.

another 50 ng/mL of that protein into the plasma, the contribution from the tumor is not detectable above normal variation.

Verification of Candidate Biomarkers in the 15–50 kDa Region Using the Tumor Supernatant and Label-free Discovery Proteomics Analysis of Patient Pools

Candidate biomarkers in the 15–50 kDa region of the gel were selected for further prioritization and verification because this was the region of the gel that contained the largest density of human proteins in the xenograft plasma analysis. By focusing on a discrete region of the gel we could increase the subsequent throughput of MRM assays by minimizing the number of fractions that need to be analyzed to quantitate the targeted group of candidate biomarkers. Candidates in this region that were identified with at least the same number of peptides in the tumor supernatant were considered further (**Figure 1** and **Table 1**). These candidate biomarkers were then compared to data from an in-depth label-free quantitative comparison of pools of patient sera using a 4 h gradient for the LC-MS/MS runs. One serum pool from patients with benign tumors (pool B, n = 9), was compared to three serum pools from patients with advanced ovarian cancer (pool C1: stage 3, n = 9; pool C2: stage 3, n = 9; pool C3: stage 4, n = 5). Descriptions of the patients and the sample pooling strategy are provided in **Table S2**. Acquisition of full MS and data-dependent MS/MS scans were identical to those described for the xenograft proteome analyses, with the exception that ions subjected to MS/MS were excluded from repeated analysis for 180 s. Xenograft plasma candidate biomarkers that could be detected in these human serum pools were quantitatively compared across pools using peptide ion signal intensities from the Rosetta Elucidator System's peptide report results. Peptides were grouped into consensus proteins by protein description and peptide intensities were summed for each protein. The criteria for selecting candidates for further validation were proteins that showed increases in all three cancer pools compared with the benign serum, and where the average intensity of the three cancer pools was at least 1.7 times that of the benign serum pool (**Figure 4**). Candidates whose protein intensities did not increase in cancer were not considered to be good biomarkers (**Figure 4A**). For example, ARG1 and AZGP1 failed because they showed decreases in cancer relative to benign disease–a trend that does not correlate with cancer burden, and DSC1 and SBSN were not further considered because the benign and cancer pools exhibited similar levels of these proteins. **Figure 4B** shows a number of proteasome subunits that exhibited increases in ovarian cancer. The proteasome complex is responsible for degradation of proteins crucial to cell cycle regulation and apoptosis and has been recognized as a potential target for cancer therapy. [30] Specific proteasome subunits, including PSMB2 and PSMB4, have been identified as upregulated in gene expression profiles of ovarian carcinomas. [31,32] Interestingly, circulating intact proteasomes have recently been reported to correlate with EOC, [33] but the assay used in that study did not distinguish specific isoforms or quantify subunits that may not have been in intact proteasomes. **Figure 4C** shows representative additional promising candidates. One candidate, AGRN, is a 215 kDa protein previously identified as being upregulated in ovarian cancer tissue samples compared with normal and non-ovarian tissue samples, [34] but it has not previously been reported to be a serum biomarker for EOC. In this study, it was identified by SDS-PAGE as both the intact 215 kDa protein and as a 43 kDa fragment from the C-terminal region of the protein in the tumor supernatant. In contrast, only the 43 kDa fragment which is presumably a proteolytic fragment produced by proteolysis either in the tumor or in the blood was detected in the xenograft plasma. The peptides quantitated in **Figure 4C** belong to the fragment and correlate with ovarian cancer in this experiment. Additionally, six proteins, including ANXA1, FABP5, PSMB3, PSMB6, PSMB8, and PSMB9 were deprioritized because they were either closely related to other selected biomarkers, or based on biology were considered unlikely to be specific to ovarian cancer. Finally, three biomarkers previously reported by others were detected in either the xenograft

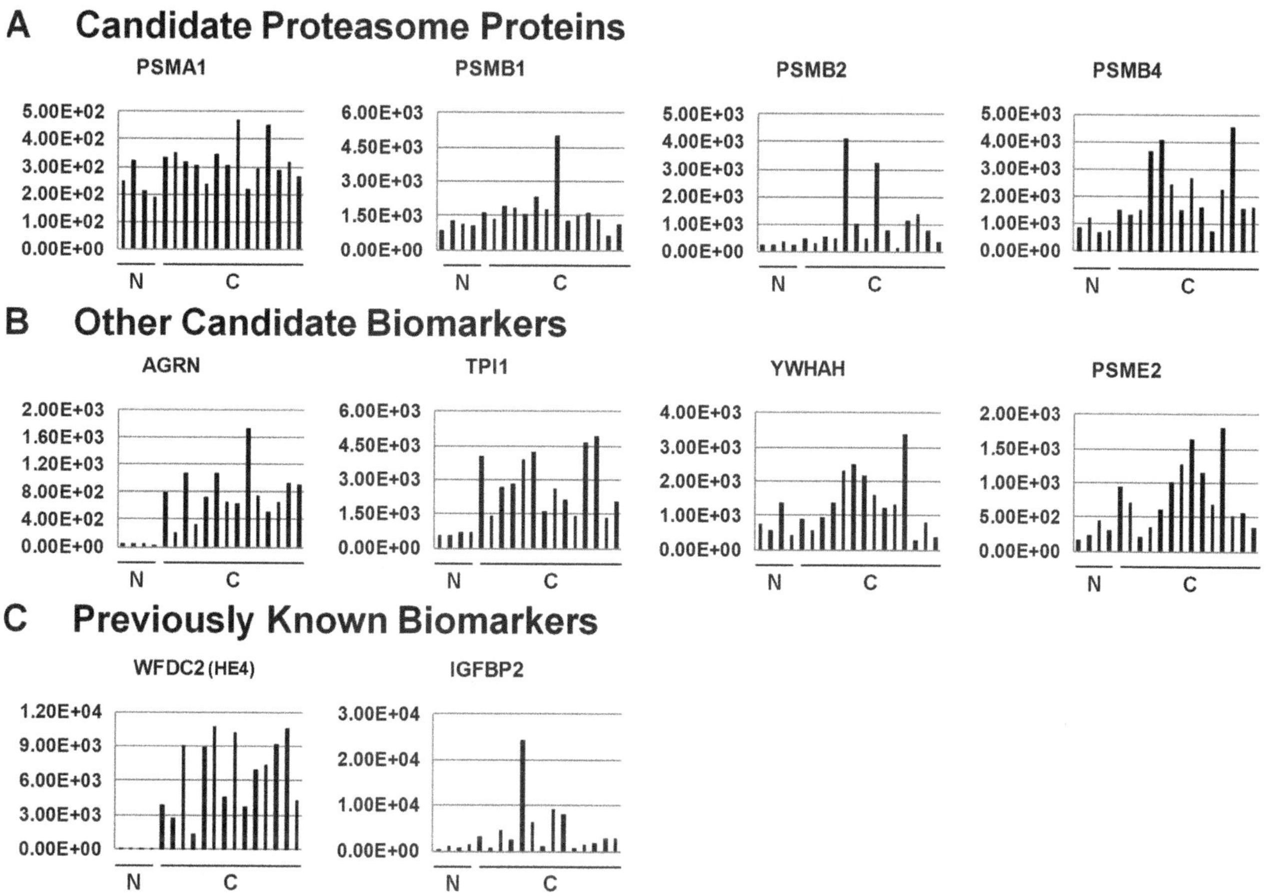

Figure 5. Gene expression of candidate biomarkers in ovarian tissues. Gene expression levels for normal ovary tissue (N; n = 4) and papillary serous ovarian carcinoma primary tumor samples (C, n = 14) are shown. (A) Representative candidate proteasome proteins. (B) Representative novel proteins identified in the xenograft mouse plasma. (C) Two previously reported ovarian cancer biomarkers that were identified in the current dataset. Microarray hybridization data were processed and scaled as previously described. [36,37] Data were extracted from www.BioGPS.org.

mouse plasma or tumor supernatant or both (**Table 1**) and were within the targeted 15–50 kDa region of the gel. These known biomarkers, which included HE4 (WFDC2) one of the two FDA approved ovarian cancer biomarkers, were included in our prioritization and verification analyses as known biomarker references. As expected, these three proteins exhibited increased levels in the cancer pools compared with the benign pool (**Figure 4D**). CA125 was not identified in the xenograft plasma, presumably due to its extensive glycosylation and low concentration as well as the high complexity of plasma; however, it was identified in the tumor supernatant by its alternative protein name 'Mucin-16′ (**Table S2**).

Potential Correlation of Biomarkers with Gene Expression

To evaluate whether gene expression in ovarian tumor tissues could be a useful indicator of whether a protein is promising serum biomarker, we queried our candidate biomarkers from **Table 1** against published microarray hybridization data using BioGPS, a centralized gene portal of combined gene annotation resources. [35] Specifically, gene expression levels for normal ovarian tissue (n = 4) and papillary serous ovarian carcinoma primary tumor samples (n = 14) [36,37] were extracted for each of the candidate markers listed in **Table 1**. **Figure 5** shows examples of gene expression patterns for some of our novel and two known ovarian cancer biomarkers. These gene expression levels can be compared with the observed levels of these same proteins in the benign and EOC patient serum pools (**Figure 4**). Some proteins show similar trends; that is, elevated levels in both the serum and tumor tissue levels for EOC, including AGRN, TPI1, and HE4. However, other proteins do not exhibit much similarity between tissue expression and serum levels. For proteins such as YWHAH and PSME2, gene expression levels overlap extensively between normal and cancer tissue, but the serum levels of these proteins show similar patterns to those for AGRN and TPI1. Also, PSMA1 exhibits similar expression levels between normal and EOC tumor samples but much higher levels in the serum of EOC patients compared with benign tumor controls. Interestingly, at the gene expression level, each of the four illustrated proteasome subunits exhibits differing expression patterns at the cancer tissue level but all four subunits show elevated serum levels in all cancer patient pools compared with the benign sera.

Overall, these comparisons suggest that gene expression levels are not reliable indicators of blood levels of a given protein, and use of gene expression levels to predict blood biomarkers is likely to be of limited value. This is not surprising because: 1) gene expression levels do not always correlate with protein abundance within cells; 2) shedding of proteins into the extracellular space and, more specifically, into the vascular system, does not necessarily depend upon the tissue levels of that protein; and 3) changes in proteolytic processing, PTM levels, or other processing

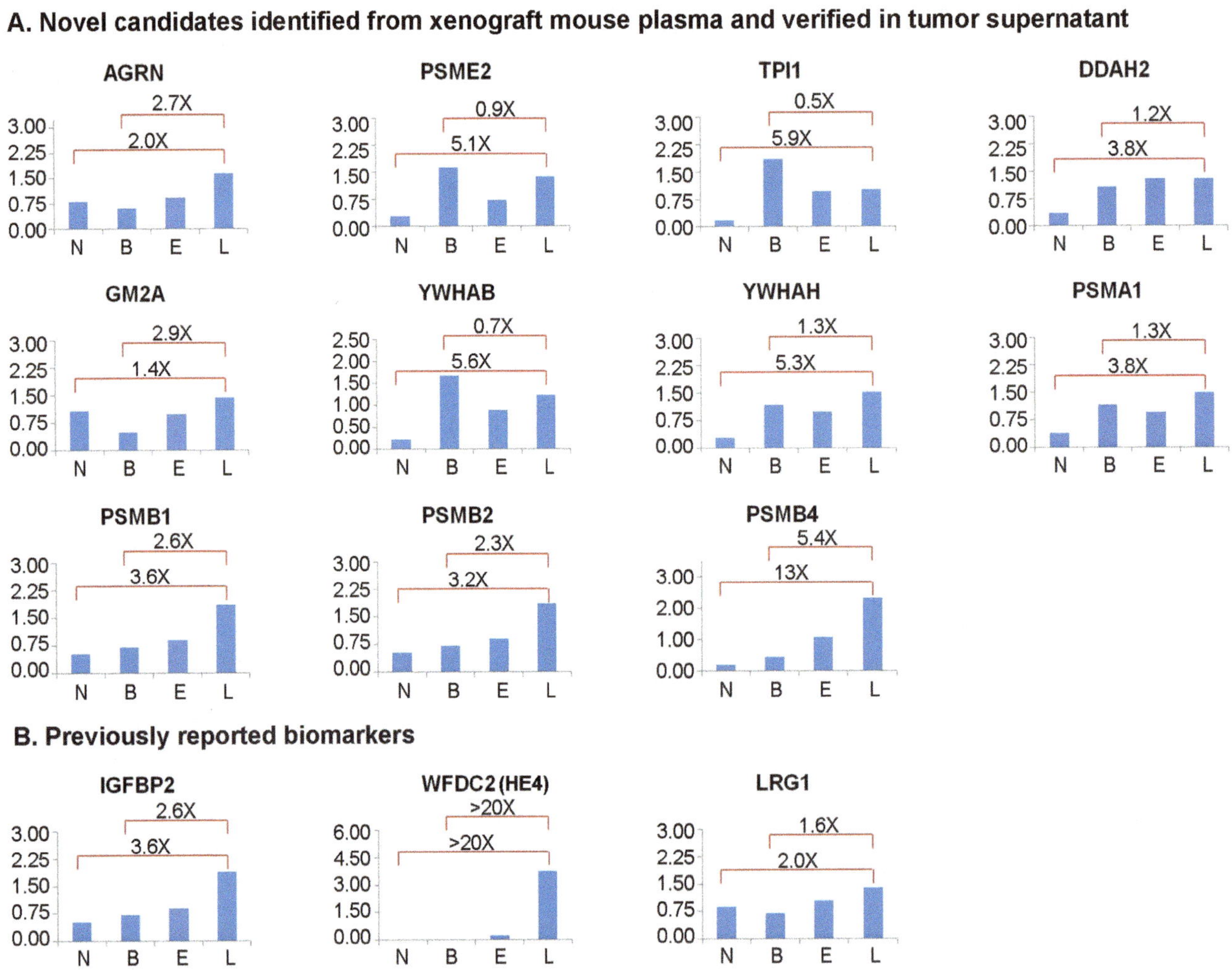

Figure 6. Verification of promising candidate biomarkers using a label-free MRM assay. Normalized relative protein amounts are shown for serum pools of normal (N; n = 9), benign (B; n = 10), early-stage ovarian cancer (E; stages 1 and 2; n = 18), and late-stage ovarian cancer (L; stage 3; n = 29). Ratios of late-stage cancer to benign disease and normal donors are shown above the histograms. (A) The 11 novel high priority biomarkers from the 15–50 kDa region of the gel. (B)Three previously reported biomarkers included as references and analyzed in parallel with the novel biomarkers.

of proteins that might affect their blood concentration may differ between normal and cancer states.

MRM Assays and Quantitation of Normal, Benign, Early Stage EOC and Late Stage EOC Serum Pools

We subsequently attempted to set up MRM assays for the 11 novel and three known biomarkers shown in **Table 1** as described in Methods. MRM assays achieve high selectivity by monitoring the combination of the specific mass/charge of a parent ion and a unique fragment ion produced after collision to quantify the targeted peptide in a complex mixture. MRM assays targeting at least two peptides per protein were successfully established for all targeted proteins. The methods were integrated into a single multiplexed MRM assay that was subsequently used to quantitate the levels of these proteins in four serum pools, including: a normal serum pool (pool N; n = 9), a benign ovarian tumor pool (pool B, n = 10), an early-stage ovarian cancer pool (pool E: stage 1 and 2, n = 18), and a late-stage cancer pool (pool L: stage 3, n = 29). The cancer pools included serum from patients with different EOC histotypes, although the majority of tumors were the serous subtype as is typically the case in groups of EOC patients. Details of the patients and samples used to prepare these pools are summarized in **Table S2**. The peptides and transitions used in the integrated multiplex MRM assay, as well as the resulting relative quantitative data for the four pools, are shown in **Table S3**. Resulting relative protein quantities for the four pools are summarized in **Figure 6A** for the 11 novel candidates. The levels in the same serum pools of the three previously reported biomarkers are shown for reference in **Figure 6B**.

These results confirm that quantitative MRM assays were established for all 11 targeted proteins and that all targeted proteins showed elevated levels in initial analysis of sera from advanced EOC. This 100% success using these two criteria is dramatically better than the 20% success rate achieved for setting up MRM assays for TOV-112D derived candidate biomarkers showing elevated levels in initial screens of sera from advanced EOC. This more efficient selection of candidate biomarkers was achieved because the current strategy utilized additional criteria prior to attempting to set up MRM assays. The key advantages of the current approach include analysis of the tumor supernatant to extend sequence coverage for putative human plasma proteins in the xenograft mouse plasma and comparison of remaining high priority candidate biomarkers to an in-depth discovery mode quantitative comparison of serum pools from benign and advanced EOC patients. This latter analysis identified those proteins detectable in patient serum as well as those proteins exhibiting elevated levels in EOC patient sera. Interestingly, approximately two-thirds of the high priority candidates from the xenograft mouse plasma both expected to be in the 15–50 kDa region and verified in the tumor supernatant, were detected in the patient pools and half of these met the criteria used above for elevated levels in EOC serum. This 20% success rate is very similar to that obtained with the TOV-112D candidate biomarkers. The major difference in the current study is that time and expenses were not invested in attempting to set up MRM assays for the 75–80% of biomarkers that would ultimately fail to be detected in patient plasma or that would not show elevated levels in advanced EOC patient serum. Although substantial mass spectrometer and analysis time was invested in conducting the in-depth discovery mode quantitative comparison of serum pools from benign and advanced EOC patients, these analyses do not need to be repeated as the same dataset can be used to screen future candidate biomarkers. Additionally, this study includes pools of mixed histotypes that approximate the mixtures of cancer subtypes typically seen clinically because the numbers of available samples and the assay throughput were too low to distinguish potential subtype specific biomarkers. One goal of future studies using higher throughput assays such as sandwich ELISA will be to carefully evaluate potential relationships between EOC subtypes and these biomarker candidates.

Conclusions

In the current study, improved strategies for both discovery and triaging novel blood biomarkers for EOC have been developed. The utility of analyzing xenograft mouse plasma and the corresponding tumor supernatant in parallel was demonstrated. The presence of human proteins in the plasma demonstrated these proteins were produced by the tumor and shed into the blood, but many of these assignments were based upon only a few peptides. Analysis of the tumor supernatant produced far more extensive sequence coverage for human proteins and confirmed many of the proteins identified in the plasma as human. In most cases an increased sequence coverage provided additional peptide candidates for potential MRM assays. A second key step in the prioritization and verification strategy was to compare candidate plasma biomarkers to an in-depth, label-free comparison of benign disease and advanced cancer patient serum pools to prescreen candidate biomarkers prior to setting up MRM assays. By extending reverse-phase gradients for the discovery mode analysis of these samples to four hours, the detection sensitivity is similar to that of MRM assays using shorter gradients. That is, if a protein cannot be detected in this dataset, it will probably not be feasible to set up an MRM assay and, therefore, effort is not wasted in assay development. Furthermore, by comparing candidate biomarker levels in the benign and advanced cancer patient pools, only those proteins showing elevated levels in the cancer sera advance to MRM assay development. This new approach reduces the effort invested in setting up MRM assays by about four-fold relative to the biomarkers detected in advanced EOC patient sera at elevated levels. Based upon initial screening of large pools of normal, benign, early, and advanced ovarian cancer sera, all of the biomarkers selected for MRM assay development in the current study should move forward and be further evaluated using serum or plasma from individual patients and controls. Although the fold changes observed in the pooled samples for most of these candidate biomarkers are not as large as HE4, the ranges of values for these biomarkers in individual EOC and control sera need to be determined in order to compare their diagnostic capacities to HE4 and CA125. While it is unlikely that most individual biomarkers will prove to be superior to HE4 or CA125, it is more likely that combinations with each other or with CA125 and HE4 could outperform the use CA125 or HE4 alone. Finally, the strategies developed in this study demonstrate that in-depth analysis of xenograft mouse plasma with efficient pilot verification using multiplexed assays can efficiently identify multiple promising candidate EOC biomarkers. This approach can be readily applied to further in-depth analysis of the OVCAR-3 cell line, as well as other EOC cell lines to identify additional EOC plasma biomarkers.

Supporting Information

Figure S1 Analysis of OVCAR-3 xenograft plasma and tumor supernatant. (A) SDS-PAGE of concentrated media from the OVCAR-3 tumor supernatant. The sample was separated for 6 cm, the gel lane was sliced into 60 uniform fractions, digested with trypsin and analyzed by LC-MS/MS. (B) Analytical SDS-PAGE of unfractionated, depleted mouse plasma (DP), and MicroSol IEF fractions (F1–F4) and membrane extractions (M1–M5). (C) Representative preparative SDS-PAGE of the samples shown in panel B. Distances samples were separated are indicated and gel lanes were cut into 1 mm slices for trypsin digestion and subsequent LC-MS/MS analysis.

Table S1 Proteins identified in the OVCAR-3 tumor supernatant by two or more unique peptides.

Table S2 Sample classification for ovarian cancer patient sera.

Table S3 Peptide transitions monitored by MRM.

Acknowledgments

We gratefully acknowledge Dr. Dionyssios Katsaros, University of Turin, Turin, Italy, for providing benign and ovarian cancer sera. We gratefully acknowledge the Proteomics Core, the Histotechnology Core, and the Animal Facility of the Wistar Institute for their assistance in this project. The administrative assistance of Mea Fuller is gratefully acknowledged.

Author Contributions

Advice and critical evaluation of manuscript: RZ. Conceived and designed the experiments: LAB HYT DWS. Performed the experiments: LAB HW HYT ZC TCW. Analyzed the data: LAB HYT ZC QL DWS. Contributed reagents/materials/analysis tools: JLT. Wrote the paper: LAB HYT DWS.

References

1. Jemal A, Siegel R, Ward E, Hao Y, Xu J, et al. (2008) Cancer statistics, 2008. CA Cancer J Clin 58: 71–96.
2. Clarke-Pearson DL (2009) Clinical practice. Screening for ovarian cancer. N Engl J Med 361: 170–177.
3. Cannistra SA (2004) Cancer of the ovary. N Engl J Med 351: 2519–2529.
4. Jacobs I, Bast RC (1989) The CA125 tumour-associated antigen: a review of the literature. Hum Reprod 4: 1–12.

5. Woolas RP, Xu FJ, Jacobs IJ, Yu YH, Daly L, et al. (1993) Elevation of multiple serum markers in patients with stage I ovarian cancer. J Natl Cancer Inst 85: 1748–1751.
6. Bast RC Jr, Klug TL, St John E, Jenison E, Niloff JM, et al. (1983) A radioimmunoassay using a monoclonal antibody to monitor the course of epithelial ovarian cancer. N Engl J Med 309: 883–887.
7. Sasaroli D, Coukos G, Scholler N (2009) Beyond CA125: the coming of age of ovarian cancer biomarkers. Are we there yet? Biomark Med 3: 275–288.
8. Cramer DW, Bast RC Jr, Berg CD, Diamandis EP, Godwin AK, et al. (2011) Ovarian cancer biomarker performance in prostate, lung, colorectal, and ovarian cancer screening trial specimens. Cancer Prev Res (Phila) 4: 365–374.
9. Zhu CS, Pinsky PF, Cramer DW, Ransohoff DF, Hartge P, et al. (2011) A framework for evaluating biomarkers for early detection: validation of biomarker panels for ovarian cancer. Cancer Prev Res (Phila) 4: 375–383.
10. Hoffman SA, Joo WA, Echan LA, Speicher DW (2007) Higher dimensional (Hi-D) separation strategies dramatically improve the potential for cancer biomarker detection in serum and plasma. J Chromatogr B Analyt Technol Biomed Life Sci 849: 43–52.
11. Gortzak-Uzan L, Ignatchenko A, Evangelou AI, Agochiya M, Brown KA, et al. (2008) A proteome resource of ovarian cancer ascites: integrated proteomic and bioinformatic analyses to identify putative biomarkers. J Proteome Res 7: 339–351.
12. Faca VM, Ventura AP, Fitzgibbon MP, Pereira-Faca SR, Pitteri SJ, et al. (2008) Proteomic analysis of ovarian cancer cells reveals dynamic processes of protein secretion and shedding of extra-cellular domains. PLoS One 3: e2425.
13. Kuk C, Kulasingam V, Gunawardana CG, Smith CR, Batruch I, et al. (2009) Mining the ovarian cancer ascites proteome for potential ovarian cancer biomarkers. Mol Cell Proteomics 8: 661–669.
14. Amon LM, Law W, Fitzgibbon MP, Gross JA, O'Briant K, et al. (2010) Integrative proteomic analysis of serum and peritoneal fluids helps identify proteins that are up-regulated in serum of women with ovarian cancer. PLoS One 5: e11137.
15. Zhang Y, Xu B, Liu Y, Yao H, Lu N, et al. (2012) The ovarian cancer-derived secretory/releasing proteome: A repertoire of tumor markers. Proteomics 12: 1883–1891.
16. Faca VM, Hanash SM (2009) In-depth proteomics to define the cell surface and secretome of ovarian cancer cells and processes of protein shedding. Cancer Res 69: 728–730.
17. Pitteri SJ, JeBailey L, Faca VM, Thorpe JD, Silva MA, et al. (2009) Integrated proteomic analysis of human cancer cells and plasma from tumor bearing mice for ovarian cancer biomarker discovery. PLoS One 4: e7916.
18. Tang HY, Beer LA, Chang-Wong T, Hammond R, Gimotty P, et al. (2012) A xenograft mouse model coupled with in-depth plasma proteome analysis facilitates identification of novel serum biomarkers for human ovarian cancer. J Proteome Res 11: 678–691.
19. Kuhn E, Wu J, Karl J, Liao H, Zolg W, et al. (2004) Quantification of C-reactive protein in the serum of patients with rheumatoid arthritis using multiple reaction monitoring mass spectrometry and 13C-labeled peptide standards. Proteomics 4: 1175–1186.
20. Anderson L, Hunter CL (2006) Quantitative mass spectrometric multiple reaction monitoring assays for major plasma proteins. Mol Cell Proteomics 5: 573–588.
21. Beer LA, Tang HY, Sriswasdi S, Barnhart KT, Speicher DW (2011) Systematic discovery of ectopic pregnancy serum biomarkers using 3-D protein profiling coupled with label-free quantitation. J Proteome Res 10: 1126–1138.
22. Zuo X, Echan L, Hembach P, Tang HY, Speicher KD, et al. (2001) Towards global analysis of mammalian proteomes using sample prefractionation prior to narrow pH range two-dimensional gels and using one-dimensional gels for insoluble and large proteins. Electrophoresis 22: 1603–1615.
23. Tang HY, Speicher DW (2005) Complex proteome prefractionation using microscale solution isoelectrofocusing. Expert Rev Proteomics 2: 295–306.
24. Tang HY, Ali-Khan N, Echan LA, Levenkova N, Rux JJ, et al. (2005) A novel four-dimensional strategy combining protein and peptide separation methods enables detection of low-abundance proteins in human plasma and serum proteomes. Proteomics 5: 3329–3342.
25. Wang H, Tang HY, Tan GC, Speicher DW (2011) Data analysis strategy for maximizing high-confidence protein identifications in complex proteomes such as human tumor secretomes and human serum. J Proteome Res 10: 4993–5005.
26. Liu Q, Tan G, Levenkova N, Li T, Pugh EN Jr, et al. (2007) The proteome of the mouse photoreceptor sensory cilium complex. Mol Cell Proteomics 6: 1299–1317.
27. MacLean B, Tomazela DM, Shulman N, Chambers M, Finney GL, et al. (2010) Skyline: an open source document editor for creating and analyzing targeted proteomics experiments. Bioinformatics 26: 966–968.
28. Anderson L (2005) Candidate-based proteomics in the search for biomarkers of cardiovascular disease. J Physiol 563: 23–60.
29. Polanski M, Anderson NL (2007) A list of candidate cancer biomarkers for targeted proteomics. Biomark Insights 1: 1–48.
30. Voorhees PM, Dees EC, O'Neil B, Orlowski RZ (2003) The proteasome as a target for cancer therapy. Clin Cancer Res 9: 6316–6325.
31. Yue W, Sun LY, Li CH, Zhang LX, Pei XT (2004) [Screening and identification of ovarian carcinomas related genes]. Ai Zheng 23: 141–145.
32. Nowee ME, Snijders AM, Rockx DA, de Wit RM, Kosma VM, et al. (2007) DNA profiling of primary serous ovarian and fallopian tube carcinomas with array comparative genomic hybridization and multiplex ligation-dependent probe amplification. J Pathol 213: 46–55.
33. Heubner M, Wimberger P, Dahlmann B, Kasimir-Bauer S, Kimmig R, et al. (2011) The prognostic impact of circulating proteasome concentrations in patients with epithelial ovarian cancer. Gynecol Oncol 120: 233–238.
34. Tchagang AB, Tewfik AH, DeRycke MS, Skubitz KM, Skubitz AP (2008) Early detection of ovarian cancer using group biomarkers. Mol Cancer Ther 7: 27–37.
35. Wu C, Orozco C, Boyer J, Leglise M, Goodale J, et al. (2009) BioGPS: an extensible and customizable portal for querying and organizing gene annotation resources. Genome Biol 10: R130.
36. Welsh JB, Zarrinkar PP, Sapinoso LM, Kern SG, Behling CA, et al. (2001) Analysis of gene expression profiles in normal and neoplastic ovarian tissue samples identifies candidate molecular markers of epithelial ovarian cancer. Proc Natl Acad Sci U S A 98: 1176–1181.
37. Su AI, Welsh JB, Sapinoso LM, Kern SG, Dimitrov P, et al. (2001) Molecular classification of human carcinomas by use of gene expression signatures. Cancer Res 61: 7388–7393.
38. Baron-Hay S, Boyle F, Ferrier A, Scott C (2004) Elevated serum insulin-like growth factor binding protein-2 as a prognostic marker in patients with ovarian cancer. Clin Cancer Res 10: 1796–1806.
39. Hellstrom I, Raycraft J, Hayden-Ledbetter M, Ledbetter JA, Schummer M, et al. (2003) The HE4 (WFDC2) protein is a biomarker for ovarian carcinoma. Cancer Res 63: 3695–3700.
40. Andersen JD, Boylan KL, Jemmerson R, Geller MA, Misemer B, et al. (2010) Leucine-rich alpha-2-glycoprotein-1 is upregulated in sera and tumors of ovarian cancer patients. J Ovarian Res 3: 21.

11

Stem Cell-Like Gene Expression in Ovarian Cancer Predicts Type II Subtype and Prognosis

Matthew Schwede[1], Dimitrios Spentzos[3], Stefan Bentink[1,4], Oliver Hofmann[2], Benjamin Haibe-Kains[1,6], David Harrington[1,2], John Quackenbush[1,2,5], Aedín C. Culhane[1,2]*

1 Biostatistics and Computational Biology, Dana-Farber Cancer Institute, Boston, Massachusetts, United States of America, 2 Biostatistics, Harvard School of Public Health, Boston, Massachusetts, United States of America, 3 Division of Hematology/Oncology, Department of Medicine, Beth Israel Deaconess Medical Center, Boston, Massachusetts, United States of America, 4 Exosome Diagnostics GmbH, Martinsried, Germany, 5 Cancer Biology, Dana-Farber Cancer Institute, Boston, Massachusetts, United States of America, 6 Integrative Systems Biology, Institut de recherches cliniques de Montréal, Montreal, Quebec, Canada

Abstract

Although ovarian cancer is often initially chemotherapy-sensitive, the vast majority of tumors eventually relapse and patients die of increasingly aggressive disease. Cancer stem cells are believed to have properties that allow them to survive therapy and may drive recurrent tumor growth. Cancer stem cells or cancer-initiating cells are a rare cell population and difficult to isolate experimentally. Genes that are expressed by stem cells may characterize a subset of less differentiated tumors and aid in prognostic classification of ovarian cancer. The purpose of this study was the genomic identification and characterization of a subtype of ovarian cancer that has stem cell-like gene expression. Using human and mouse gene signatures of embryonic, adult, or cancer stem cells, we performed an unsupervised bipartition class discovery on expression profiles from 145 serous ovarian tumors to identify a stem-like and more differentiated subgroup. Subtypes were reproducible and were further characterized in four independent, heterogeneous ovarian cancer datasets. We identified a stem-like subtype characterized by a 51-gene signature, which is significantly enriched in tumors with properties of Type II ovarian cancer; high grade, serous tumors, and poor survival. Conversely, the differentiated tumors share properties with Type I, including lower grade and mixed histological subtypes. The stem cell-like signature was prognostic within high-stage serous ovarian cancer, classifying a small subset of high-stage tumors with better prognosis, in the differentiated subtype. In multivariate models that adjusted for common clinical factors (including grade, stage, age), the subtype classification was still a significant predictor of relapse. The prognostic stem-like gene signature yields new insights into prognostic differences in ovarian cancer, provides a genomic context for defining Type I/II subtypes, and potential gene targets which following further validation may be valuable in the clinical management or treatment of ovarian cancer.

Editor: Vincenzo Coppola, Ohio State University Comprehensive Cancer Center, United States of America

Funding: Funding for this work was provided by the National Institutes of Health 1U19CA148065 (J.Q., B.H.K.), Dana-Farber Cancer Institute Women's Cancers Program (awarded to A.C.C; M.S, A.C.C.) and the Claudia Adams Barr foundation (J.Q. and A.C.C.). The funders had no role in study design, data collection and analysis, decision to publish, or preparation of the manuscript.

Competing Interests: SB is an employee of Exosome Diagnostics GmbH; JQ is Exosome Diagnostics Scientific Advisory Board Member and has minimal stock options in the company.

* E-mail: aedin@jimmy.harvard.edu

Introduction

Ovarian cancer is the fifth most common cause of cancer deaths among women and is the leading cause of death from gynecological neoplastic disease [1]. The vast majority of initially responsive ovarian cancers eventually relapse [2], and this may be explained by a sub-population of stem cell-like chemotherapy-resistant tumors cells [3–5].

In breast cancer, there are widely-accepted molecular subtypes. Approximately 15% of breast cancers are estrogen receptor (ER)-negative, high-grade and often basal-like breast cancer that are enriched in cells expressing putative stem cell markers $CD44^{+}/CD24^{-}$ [6] and over-expresses genes associated with embryonic stem cell gene signatures [7]. This "stemness" may be explained, in part, by the observation that BRCA1, which is reported to regulate mammary stem cell fate [8], is often mutated in basal-like tumors [9].

In contrast, ovarian cancer has no consensus molecular subtype classification. Tothill et al. used k-means clustering of microarray data and described six molecular subtypes of serous and endometrioid ovarian cancer [10]. The Cancer Genome Atlas (TCGA) consortium identified four molecular subtypes of high grade serous ovarian cancers [11]. However, others have proposed pathology-site of origin based subtyping of ovarian cancer into Type I tumors, which are low-grade and histologically heterogeneous, and Type II tumors, which are high-grade and mostly serous [12,13]. Type II is believed to arise largely in the fallopian tube epithelium while Type I's site of origin is thought to be the ovary, although the cell of origin remains unclear [12,13]. No Type I/II molecular signature exists, and classifying tumors as Type I or Type II based on clincopathologic analysis is generally but not always straightforward [14].

Here we report the identification of ovarian cancer subtypes based on the expression of genes associated with stem cell signatures. Using a computational approach, we demonstrate the presence of a poor prognosis, stem cell-like subtype in ovarian cancer that aligned closely with the cell of origin classification and provides the first genomic definition of Type I/II ovarian cancer. This gene expression profile does not demonstrate the existence of a subpopulation of cancer stem cells in these tumors. Instead it discovers common molecular pathways expressed by these cancers and stem cells. Tumors displaying expression of stem-like genes may have a less differentiated phenotype. Discovery of this stem cell subtype provides us a more complete understanding of ovarian cancer's molecular diversity and opens up the potential for new and more directed approaches to treating and managing the disease.

Methods

Data

Stem-like cluster discovery was applied to ovarian cancer gene expression data published by Tothill et al. [10], as part of the Australian Ovarian Cancer Study (AOCS) data, and which were downloaded from Gene Expression Omnibus (GEO) [15] (GSE9891). AOCS samples (n = 206), were obtained from the Royal Brisbane Hospital (n = 22), Westmead Hospital (**n** = 54), and Netherlands Cancer Institute (NKI-AVL; n = 3) [10], and gene expression was assayed on Affymetrix GeneChip U133 plus 2.0 arrays [10]. Raw data were normalized using RMA [16] with custom cell description files (CDFs) based on Ensembl gene mapping (version 12) as provided by the Microarray Lab at the University of Michigan [17]. Custom CDFs were used because updated probe set definitions provide better precision and accuracy compared to Affymetrix probe set definitions [18].

The four validation ovarian cancer gene expression datasets used in this analysis were from Dressman et al. [19]; Wu et al. (GSE6008) [20]; Tone et al. (GSE10961) [21]; and Crijns et al. [22]. The three validation breast cancer datasets were from Miller et al. (GSE3494) [23]; Desmedt et al. (GSE7390) [24]; and a merged dataset combining GSE2034 [25] and GSE5327 [26], which we called "Veridex." All datasets were downloaded from GEO, except the Crijns dataset, which was received from the authors in normalized form as described in their paper [22], and the Dressman dataset was downloaded from the authors' website [19]. TCGA ovarian cancer microarray dataset (n = 518) was downloaded from the TCGA data portal [11]. All datasets other than the Crijns, Wu, and Tone datasets were RMA-normalized with custom Ensembl CDF's [17].

RMA-normalization was used in most datasets because of its highly reproducible results and correlation with RT-PCR data [27]. However, due to the inclusions of normal fallopian tube in the Tone dataset and normal ovarian surface epithelium samples in the Wu dataset, these datasets were normalized using the Invariant Set normalization method [28] to avoid the assumption within RMA of equivalent gene expression distribution. All validation data had been collected on Affymetrix GeneChip U133a arrays, except for the Tone and Crijns datasets, which had been collected on Affy U133 Plus 2.0 chips and Operon human v3 ~35 K 70-mer two-color oligonucleotide microarrays, respectively.

In the Desmedt and Veridex breast cancer datasets, we predicted molecular subtypes as described by Desmedt et al. (2008) [29]. Specifically, subtypes based on gene markers ESR1, ERBB2, and AURKA were generated using the *subtype.cluster* function with model *scmgene* in Bioconductor package genefu. This entailed using mixture modeling to group patients into HER2+, ER−/HER2- (basal-like), or ER+/HER2- (luminal) [29]. While triple-negative breast cancer is not equivalent to basal-like breast cancer [30–32], most triple-negative breast cancer classify to the basal-like molecular subtype [32] leading us to regard prediction of ER−/HER2- an approximation of "basal-like".

Statistical Analysis

Statistical analyses, unless otherwise described, were performed using all available data and standard functions in R version 2.10.1. The ISIS algorithm [33] was applied to the AOCS dataset to generate unsupervised candidate bipartitions of the patients. For each candidate bipartition, ISIS calculates a diagonal linear discriminant (DLD) score with the most significant genes supporting the bipartition. Default parameters of the R implementation of ISIS were used, except that the number of genes used for scoring ("p") was 100, a level which has been previously used [34]. We also took advantage of another paramater ("p.offs") by ignoring the top 5 most related genes in order to reduce the effects of high leverage genes on scoring, resulting in a 95-gene signature used for scoring each bipartition.

To diminish confounding effects from differential stroma and non-tumor cells in different arrayed sites (e.g. peritoneal or ovary) (unpublished data), only AOCS arrays of ovarian mRNA from malignant, serous, and primary site ovarian tumors from patients that did not receive neoadjuvant therapy were included, reducing the dataset from 285 to 145 patients. Analyses of the AOCS dataset were performed on this subset unless we specify the "entire" AOCS dataset (n = 285) or "remaining" AOCS data (n = 140), which were tumors not used for ISIS class discovery.

Genes used for subtype cluster discovery were limited to 83 mouse and human gene signatures of adult, cancer, or embryonic stem cells obtained from GeneSigDB [35] that had at least 5 and at most 1,000 genes. For each gene signature, we retrieved the article describing the gene signature to confirm its description and association with adult, cancer, or embryonic stem cells. Stem-like gene signatures frequently contain proliferation genes [7]. To avoid dividing patients based on proliferation, we also removed genes (n = 580, Table S1 in Methods S1) associated with proliferation (see Methods S1), similar to analyses by Ben-Porath we al. [7].

The resulting matrix of 2,632 stem-like genes was subject to ISIS bipartition discovery. The highest scoring bipartition that was significantly ($p<0.05$) associated with grade and disease-free survival was selected for further investigation. These criteria were based on the finding that the stem cell-like sub-population of breast cancer tumors discovered by Ben-Porath et al. was characterized by high grade and poor prognosis [7]. The association with prognosis was secondary since the Ben-Porath et al. analysis primarily described association between stem cell-like gene expression and higher grade [7]. We selected the bipartition that most closely satisfied the criteria and called this bipartition the "stemness bipartition". Leave-one-out cross-validation was used to refine the gene list defining the stemness bipartition, and the genes which were in each 95-gene list in all 145 folds formed an ovarian cancer "51-gene stemness signature" (Table S2 in Methods S1).

Gene-Set-Enrichment Analysis (GSEA) with nonparametric inference for linear models as implemented in *gsealmPerm* in the package gsealm in Bioconductor [36] was performed with curated gene sets (C2) and Gene Ontology (GO) gene sets (C5) from the gene set database MSigDB version 3.0 [37]. GSEA was also performed using the 13 stem cell gene sets of Ben-Porath et al.: two describing embryonic stem cells; four activated by Nanog, Oct4, and/or Sox2; four bound by the Polycomb repressive complex 2 PRC2; and two activated by c-Myc [7].

Class Prediction

To confirm the presence of the stem-like subtype in ovarian cancer, the stem-like subtype classification was applied to multiple independent microarray datasets. In order to predict the class of new tumors, we first needed generate a "stemness molecular classifier," a model of gene weight which discriminated the stem-like and differentiated tumors. Diagonal linear discriminant (DLD) analysis [38] was used to train this gene classifier using expression profiles of the 51 genes in the AOCS dataset (Table S2 in Methods S1). To predict the subtype of new tumors, expression profiles were projected as supplementary points onto the DLD axis, and the DLD score was the weighted sum of the expression of the genes. As the DLD scores of new ovarian tumors projected on this axis were bimodally distributed (Figure S1 in Methods S1), Gaussian mixture modeling [39] was used to define the two populations and assign new tumors to either the stem-like or differentiated subtype. The DLD score is the linear combination of weighted expression of many genes, and although we did not investigate the effect of batch-specific technical variation [40] in depth, we found it robust to mild noise from missing data and outliers in the datasets tested. This stemness molecular classifier was applied to each validation dataset.

The ovarian cancer datasets used for validation are phenotypically and clinically heterogeneous, and contain different histological subtypes, grades, prognoses, treatments and follow-up protocols. Unless stated we did not control for phenotype variation; instead we exploited the heterogeneity in datasets, in particular histology and grade, to explore how the bipartition associated with phenotypes beyond those represented in the AOCS dataset and to determine the extent to which the stemness molecular classifier could be generalized.

Results

Discovery of a Stem Cell-like Subtype in Ovarian Cancer

To explore whether ovarian cancer has a stem-like component, we tested whether genes reported to be expressed by stem cells are also expressed in a subset of ovarian tumors. To do this, we extracted the union of all adult, cancer, or embryonic stem (ES) cell gene expression signatures in GeneSigDB [35] as described in Methods S1 to generate a list of 2,632 stem-like genes (Table S3 in Methods S1).

We then took the AOCS ovarian cancer gene expression data (n = 145 patients) and considered only the 2,632 genes reported to be expressed in stem cells. To this, we applied ISIS [33], an unsupervised bipartition clustering algorithm that randomly partitions samples into two subsets and selects the genes that most significantly associate with the partition. ISIS identified twenty-eight separate distinct, statistically significant patient bipartitions of the data, and each of which was further tested for association with grade and disease-free survival.

The top scoring bipartition, hereafter referred to as the ovarian cancer stemness bipartition differentiated two distinct subgroups of ovarian cancer patients: a set of 121 patients with worse disease free ($p = 0.0541$), overall survival ($p = 0.102$), and higher grade ($p = 0.00326$) that was interpreted as more "stem cell-like" as these tumors over-expressed a number of genes known to be associated with stemness, and a smaller group of 24 patients with better survival and lower grade that we refer to as the "differentiated" subgroup (Figure 1).

Leave-one-patient-out cross-validation was performed to extract the most robust gene signature of this bipartition, resulting in a 51-gene stemness signature (Table S2 in Methods S1). Although the bipartition's association with overall survival showed a trend and did not reach conventional statistical significance, the signature was significantly prognostic in subsequent analyses when the sample size was larger (see below).

To provide further support for the phenotypes revealed by the bipartition, we tested if gene targets known to be expressed in stem cells were differentially regulated between the stem-like and differentiated subtypes using gene set enrichment analysis (GSEA). Thirteen lists of genes (Table S4 in Methods S1) which have been previously used to characterize stem cells [7] but were not among the initial 83 signatures used to discover the stem-like ovarian subtype were examined. Activation targets of Nanog, Oct4, Sox2 and c-Myc, which are up-regulated in stem cells, were also up-regulated in the stem-like subtype, and eight of nine of these gene lists were significantly ($p<0.05$) different across the subtypes (Table 1). Four sets of Polycomb-regulated genes, which characterize more differentiated cells, were up-regulated in the differentiated subtype when compared to the stem-like subtype and were close to significance ($p<0.10$). Since some of these gene sets are reported to be dependent on proliferation genes [7], we also performed a modified gene set analysis with proliferation genes excluded as previously described [7]. Even with this modification, the stem-like subtype was enriched in gene expression of ES [41] ($p<0.0001$), Nanog [42] ($p<0.05$), and c-Myc [43] ($p<0.05$) targets. High expression of the same ES gene set is reported in high-grade, estrogen receptor (ER)-negative breast tumors [7].

Identification of Functional Links to Basal-like Breast Cancer

To further characterize tumors in the stem-like subtype, we performed GSEA using all of the gene sets in MSigDB [37] to identify which gene sets were enriched in genes differentially expressed between tumors in the stem-like and differentiated subtypes (again, these sets did not include the gene sets initially utilized to discover the bipartition). Genes over-expressed by stem-like tumors were especially enriched ($p<0.0001$) for gene sets describing poor prognosis and undifferentiated cancers; high-grade, invasive ovarian cancer; Myc targets; and embryonic stem cells, BRCA1 mutation, estrogen receptor (ER)-negative status, and the basal-like subtype in breast cancer (Table S5). In contrast, gene sets strongly enriched in the differentiated subtype included those related to cellular projections (Table S6), ER-positive breast cancer, and low malignant potential (LMP) and low-grade ovarian cancer (Table S5 in Methods S1).

Both high-grade, serous ovarian and basal-like breast cancer are seen in women with mutant BRCA1 [9,44]. To investigate the GSEA prediction that the stem-like serous ovarian cancer molecular subtype is enriched for genes also expressed in high grade basal-like breast cancer, we applied diagonal linear discriminant analysis [38] to the AOCS ovarian cancer data to train a stemness molecular classifier and predicted the "stem-like" or "differentiated" classification of tumors in two published breast gene expression datasets (Desmedt [24] and Veridex [25,26] datasets). The gene list we applied to the breast cancer datasets was not optimized for breast cancer, and the DLD scores did not exhibit bimodal distributions. However to maintain consistency with the methodology applied to ovarian cancer data, we used the same Gaussian mixture modeling approach to dichotomize the DLD scores of breast cancers defining them as stem-like or differentiated. The resulting stemness classification of breast tumors confirmed the gene set analysis predictions; breast tumors assigned to the stem-like subtype were significantly enriched in basal-like molecular subtype and high-grade (logistic regression likelihood ratio test $p = 1.42 \times 10^{-9}$ and $p = 0.00964$, Desmedt and Veridex datasets respectively – Table 2) breast cancer.

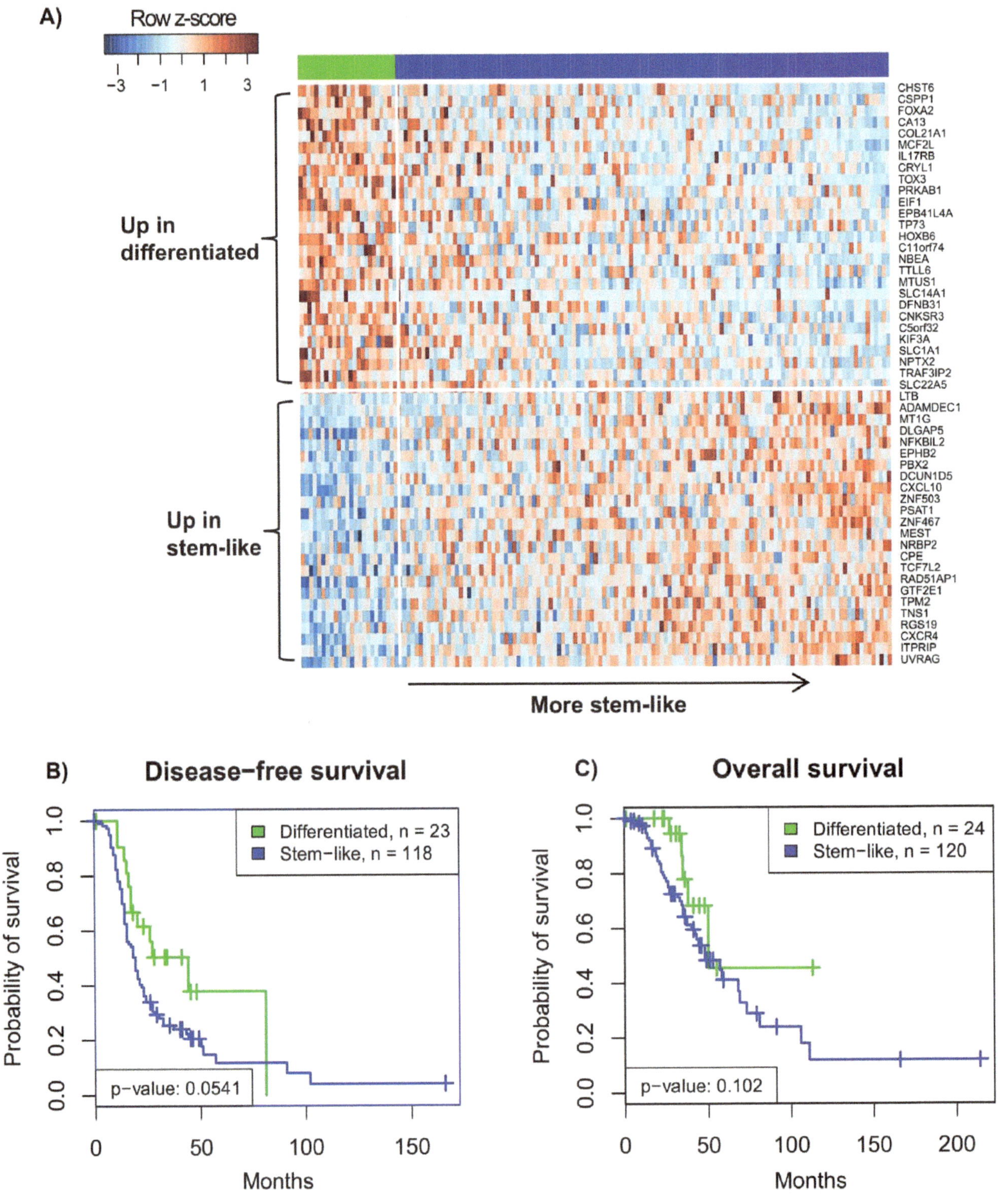

Figure 1. Heatmap of gene expression and Kaplan-Meier survival curves for the stemness bipartition. (A) A heatmap of gene expression profiles of the 24 differentiated (green) and 121 stem-like (blue) tumors from the AOCS dataset [10]. The tumors are ordered by increasing stemness molecular subtype score, and the 51 classifier genes are ordered from top to bottom by increasing over-expression in the stem-like subtype according to a pooled *t*-test. The Kaplan-Meier curves are with respect to (B) disease-free survival and (C) overall survival and are not significant at $p<0.05$, but this is possibly due to the small size of the differentiated subtype.

Table 1. The stem-like and differentiated subtypes are enriched in stem cell and differentiated gene sets respectively.

	Gene Set	Enrichment	P-value	Adjusted P-value*
Embryonic stem cell genes	ES exp1	Stem-like	0.00002	0.00004
	ES exp2	Stem-like	0.00031	0.01671
NOS targets	Nanog targets	Stem-like	0.00115	0.01573
	Oct4 targets	Stem-like	0.01509	0.07951
	Sox2 targets	Stem-like	0.02296	0.12607
	NOS targets	Stem-like	0.00969	0.10489
	NOS TFs	Stem-like	0.09596	0.13822
Myc targets	Myc targets1	Stem-like	0.01144	0.03774
	Myc targets2	Stem-like	0.01349	0.10387
Polycomb targets	Suz12 targets	Differentiated	0.05251	0.05508
	Eed targets	Differentiated	0.06293	0.05605
	H3K27 bound	Differentiated	0.05046	0.06329
	PRC2 targets	Differentiated	0.08553	0.09058

*Analysis was repeated after removing proliferation-related genes from the gene sets, as described by Ben-Porath et al. [7]. No multiple testing correction was performed.

Reproducibility of the "Stemness" Phenotypes in Independent Datasets

To validate our ovarian stem-like and differentiated molecular subtypes, we applied the stemness DLD molecular classifier to three independent ovarian cancer microarray datasets and the "remaining AOCS data" ($n = 140$) not used in the initial bipartition discovery. Two datasets, Crijns et al. [22] and Dressman et al. [19], consisted of high-stage, serous tumors, while the other two, the Wu et al. dataset [20] and the remaining AOCS data [10] were histologically heterogeneous.

First, we confirmed the association between grade and the stem-like molecular subtype. In these independent data, stem-like tumors had higher grade in the Wu ($n = 103$, logistic regression $p = 1.63 \times 10^{-5}$), remaining AOCS ($n = 140$, $p = 1.16 \times 10^{-7}$), and Dressman ($n = 118$, $p = 0.073$) datasets.

Next we explored which histological subtypes of ovarian cancer were classified as stem-like. Serous is the most common histological form of epithelial ovarian tumor, but epithelial ovarian cancer is a heterogeneous disease with mixed malignancy potentials and histological subtypes, including endometrioid, clear cell, and mucinous [12,13]. Despite initial classification being performed only on malignant, serous tumors, the stemness molecular classifier discriminated between different histological subtypes. In the Wu dataset [20], most serous tumors (29/41) were "stem-like", but most endometrioid (22/37), almost all clear cell (7/8), and all mucinous (13/13) tumors, as well as all four (4/4) "normal" ovarian surface epithelium samples were "differentiated."

Table 2. The stem-like subtype is significantly overrepresented in basal-like breast cancer.

	Desmedt***		Veridex***	
	Basal	**Non-basal**	**Basal**	**Non-basal**
Stem-like	35	14	90	63
Differentiated	11	138	12	179

***Fisher's exact test $p = 3.50 \times 10^{-18}$ and $p = 1.11 \times 10^{-27}$, Desmedt and Veridex datasets respectively.

To further evaluate association with histological subtype, we examined the entire AOCS dataset ($n = 285$). This larger dataset was comprised of the serous AOCS discovery dataset ($n = 145$) and the remaining AOCS data ($n = 140$), which included LMP serous tumors and malignant endometrioid and serous tumors arrayed from sites other than the ovary. We observed that the differentiated subtype was significantly enriched in endometrioid tumors (9/20, Fisher's test $p < 0.05$ after FWER correction [45]). Of note, the stemness DLD scores were significantly lower in the LMP serous tumors (Wilcoxon rank-sum test p-value $= 1.09 \times 10^{-4}$) than in the malignant, differentiated tumors, and almost all (17/18) LMP tumors were classified as differentiated. Additionally, within the stem-like subtype the DLD score was significantly associated with higher grade ($p = 0.00159$), though it was not correlated ($p > 0.05$ after FWER correction) with stage, overall survival, or disease-free survival, suggesting that further investigation into the clinical value of the continuous DLD score within subtypes is warranted.

The stem-like subtype classification was not equivalent to the classification recently proposed by Tothill et al. in which serous and endometrioid tumors are identified as one of six molecular subtypes, C1–C6 [10]. The stem-like tumors ($n = 233$) were not classified into a single molecular subtype but instead were mostly distributed among poor prognosis subtypes C1 ($n = 80$), C2 ($n = 48$), C4 ($n = 39$), C5 ($n = 29$) and Not Classified ($n = 30$). A considerable number of differentiated tumors were in good prognosis molecular subtypes C3 ($n = 25$) and C6 ($n = 4$), and the remaining 23 differentiated tumors were distributed among the other subtypes (Table 3). So, while the bipartition roughly separated better prognosis low-grade subtypes C3 and C6 from the others and overlap with the molecular subtype classification was significant, no combination of AOCS subtypes fully explained the bipartition. However, it should be noted that the C1–C6 subtype classification was arrived at using *k*-means clustering [10], a method that is not deterministic in the sense that re-running the algorithm can produce different clusters, so the assignments by the

Table 3. Clinical characteristics of patients in stem-like and differentiated subtypes.

Dataset			Differentiated	Stem-like	P-value
Wu et al	Stage	I	31	4	***
(n = 103)		II	6	5	
		III	13	31	
		IV	4	5	
	Grade	1	18	1	***
		2	9	8	
		3	14	24	
	Histology	Clear Cell	7	1	***
		Endometrioid	22	15	
		Mucinous	13	0	
		OSE	4	0	
		Serous	12	29	
Entire AOCS	Type	LMP	17	1	***
(n = 285)		Malignant	35	232	***
	Stage	I	15	9	
		II	8	10	
		III	28	189	
		IV	1	21	
	Grade	1	14	5	***
		2	19	78	
		3	17	147	
	Histology	Adenocarcinoma	0	1	*
		Endometrioid	9	11	
		Serous	43	221	
	Primary site	Fallopian tube	0	8	**
		Ovary	52	191	
		Peritoneum	0	34	
	Arrayed Site	Other	0	14	***
		Ovary	50	150	
		Peritoneum	2	69	
	Age	Median age	56.3	59.3	*
	Residual disease	<1 cm	43	118	**
		>1 cm	5	76	
	Molecular subtype	C1	3	80	***
		C2	2	48	
		C3	25	3	
		C4	7	39	
		C5	7	29	
		C6	4	4	
		NC	4	30	

**p-value <0.01,
***p-value <0.001. OSE Ovarian surface epithelium, NC not classified. In each dataset, p-values were corrected for family-wise error rate using Hommel's method [46], except for the test for association with the Tothill et al. molecular subtypes.

AOCS should be considered only approximate.Prognostic value of the stem-like phenotype.

In the three independent validation datasets and the remaining AOCS data, tumors with the stem-like subtype had worse prognosis (Figure 2). The stem-like subtype had both significantly worse overall survival (log-rank test $p = 4.41 \times 10^{-7}$) and disease-free survival ($p = 0.00127$) in the remaining AOCS dataset ($n = 140$) and worse overall survival in the Crijns ($n = 157$, $p = 0.021$) and Dressman datasets ($n = 118$, $p = 0.0354$). Although the Wu dataset [20] did not include survival information, the stem-like subtype's tumors had significantly higher stage ($n = 103$, $p = 1.03 \times 10^{-6}$), which suggests worse prognosis.

A finding of potential clinical importance is that the stemness molecular classifier may also be prognostic within high-grade,

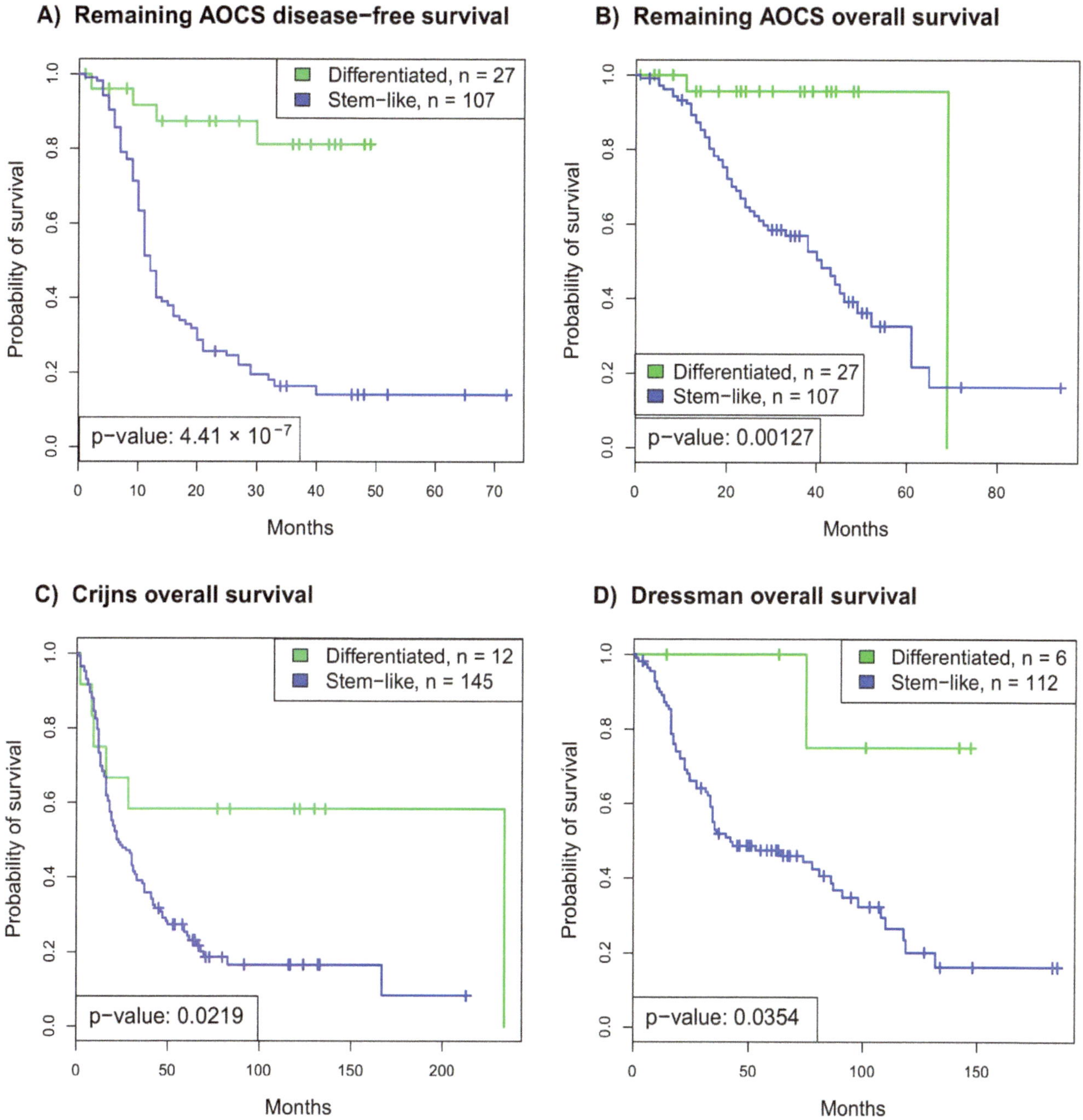

Figure 2. Validation of the stemness bipartition in independent ovarian cancer microarray datasets, as well as in the remaining AOCS dataset. In the remaining AOCS dataset, the stem-like subtype has strongly worse (A) disease-free survival ($p<0.001$) and (B) overall survival ($p=0.00127$). In the (C) Crijns and (D) Dressman datasets, the stem-like subtype has significantly worse overall survival ($p=0.022$ and $p=0.035$, respectively).

high-stage serous ovarian cancer. The stem-like subtype had worse disease-free ($p=0.0053$) and overall survival ($p=0.0299$) in high-grade, malignant tumors of the entire AOCS dataset. In independent analysis of each histology, the stem-like subtype was associated with poorer disease-free survival in high-grade serous ($p=0.0447$), but was not a significant predictor in high-grade endometrioid tumors ($p=0.278$). In the Crijns and Dressman datasets, which were exclusively high-stage serous tumors, the stemness molecular classifier identified a small subset of differentiated subtype tumors with better overall survival (Figure 2). Equally, across datasets the differentiated subtype included a small number of high-grade tumors (grades 2 or 3) [14] with better prognosis. Further analysis is needed to determine if this classification is useful in identifying high-grade tumors more likely to have a favorable outcome.

The stem-like subtype was associated with phenotypes often predictive of poor outcome (Table 3), but the stem-like subtype's prognostic ability is not fully explained by these common clinical variables. In the entire AOCS dataset the stem-like subtype was a strong predictor of outcome (univariate analysis DFS

$p=3.23\times10^{-6}$, OS $p=0.00122$), was associated with greater patient age ($p<0.05$), and was strongly ($p<0.001$ after FWER correction [46]) associated with high stage; peritoneal arrayed site, a site to which high-grade ovarian cancer frequently spreads; and greater residual disease after surgery.

Despite these associations, in multivariate analysis, the stemness bipartition remained a strong predictor of worse disease-free survival. The bipartition remained a significant predictor of disease-free survival when adjusting for one ($p<0.005$) or two variables among stage, grade, and residual disease (Table 4) or any combination of two variables ($p<0.05$) in Table 3, with the exception of adjusting for both stage and low malignancy potential ($p=0.0785$). Notably, the stem-like subtype had significantly worse disease-free survival ($p=0.0143$) in multivariate analysis adjusting for grade, histological subtype, and low malignancy potential. Even when adjusting for stage, low malignancy potential, histological subtype, and grade, the stem-like subtype still had a 54% increased odds of relapse, although this was not significant ($p=0.126$).

Stem-like Tumors have Characteristics of Type II Ovarian Cancer

A recent pathogenesis model of ovarian cancer divides tumors into Type I, which is low-grade and histologically diverse, and Type II, which is high-grade and mostly serous [12,13]. A gene signature-based molecular classification for Type I/II ovarian cancer has not yet been described, and Type I/II are distinguished largely based on their morphological properties (Table 5). In comparing our molecular subtypes to these morphological classifications, we found stem-like tumors to possess characteristics of Type II ovarian tumors and the differentiated tumors to be similar to Type I (Table 5).

Both Type II and the stem-like subtype are associated with poor prognosis, high-grade serous tumors (Table 5). Although formal evaluation of the stem-like and differentiated subtypes' prevalence and lethality would require prospective random sampling of ovarian carcinomas and subsequent classification, the stem-like subtype properties would appear to be consistent with the reports Type II's relative prevalence and lethality (Table 5).

Mutations characteristic of Type II ovarian cancer are found in the stem-like subtype. Type II tumors are thought to arise from precursor lesions in fallopian tube epithelium and have "p53 signatures" that have strong p53 immunoreactivity and usually p53 mutations [13]. It is reported that most Type II ovarian tumors (>80%) have p53 mutation [12]. TCGA ovarian cancer data consists of 489 high-grade serous ovarian adenocarcinomas and almost all have TP53 mutation (96%) [11]. In our analysis stemness molecular subtype scores of TCGA ovarian cancers lacked bimodality and most tumors were classified into one subtype which was more stem-like (data not shown). The mutation status of almost all samples in other ovarian microarray datasets are unknown but Wu et al. [20] reported p53 mutation status of endometrioid tumors ($n=37$), and these endometrioid tumors with p53 mutations were overrepresented in the stem-like subtype ($p=0.016$). In addition, we observed that genes expressed by the stem-like ovarian cancer subtype are enriched for two gene sets that are over-expressed by p53-mutant breast cancers relative to breast cancer without p53 mutation [47,48] (GSEA p-values 0.00008 and 0.00004, respectively in AOCS dataset–Table S7 in Methods S1). To confirm this association, we applied the stemness bipartition classification to a breast cancer dataset in which the p53 status of tumors is known [23], and the stem-like subtype had strong overlap with p53-mutant tumors (Fisher's exact test $p=1.36\times10^{-12}$).

Differentiated Tumors have Characteristics of Type I Ovarian Cancer

In contrast, "differentiated" tumors and Type I tumors describe histologically diverse and mostly (although not exclusively) low-grade and LMP tumors (Table 5). Type I tumors are characterized by other mutations (including KRAS, BRAF, PTEN, and PIK3CA and others shown in Table 5) [12], and we observed

Table 4. Multivariate Cox proportional hazards models of the stemness bipartition to predict relapse-free survival when adjusting for two prognostic variables (A) residual disease and stage, (B) grade and stage or (C) grade and residual disease.

Variable	Hazard ratio	Lower limit (95% CI)	Upper limit (95% CI)	P-value
(A) Adjusting for residual disease and stage				
Stem-like subtype	1.75	1.00	3.05	0.0498*
Residual disease	1.43	1.02	2.00	0.0374*
Stage[1]	7.30	2.57	20.8	0.000195***
(B) Adjusting for grade and stage				
Stem-like subtype	2.17	1.22	3.85	0.00818**
Grade[1]	1.16	0.586	2.29	0.674
Stage[1]	7.72	2.80	21.2	7.64×10^{-5} ***
(C) Adjusting for grade and residual disease				
Stem-like subtype	2.36	1.32	4.22	0.00370**
Grade[1]	1.42	0.672	3.01	0.358
Residual disease	1.76	1.26	2.46	0.000872***

*$p<0.05$,
**$p<0.01$,
***$p<0.001$.
[1]In regression analyses, the ordinal variables stage and grade were broken into multiple components using default functions in R. However, only the linear components (levels treated as a continuous variable) are displayed in the table because the other components were not significant. Grade was also coded as a quadratic component (grade 2 vs. grades 1 and 3) and stage as both quadratic (stages 2 and 3 vs. stages 1 and 4) and cubic (stage 2> stage 4> stage 1> stage 3) components.

Table 5. Shared characteristics of Types I and II ovarian cancer and the stem-like and differentiated subtypes [12].

	Type I	Type II	Stemness bipartition
Presence of ciliated cells	Possibly	No	Differentiated subtype is enriched in genes related to cilia and more similar to normal fallopian tube.
Histological subtypes	Serous, endometrioid, mucinous, clear cell	Mostly serous	Stem-like subtype overrepresented serous ovarian cancer while the differentiated subtype had mixed histology (Table 3).
Mutations	KRAS, BRAF PTEN, CTNNB1, ERBB2, PIK3CA	Mostly p53	Stem-like subtype is enriched in p53-mutant tumors and p53 mutation-associated genes. Differentiated subtype is enriched in other mutations.
Benign tumors	Sometimes	No	Almost all 18 of the LMP tumors were classified as differentiated in entire AOCS dataset.
Grade	Low grade	High grade	Stem-like subtype has higher grade across datasets.
% epithelial ovarian carcinomas	25%	75%	Original stem-like subtype comprises 83% of the tumors and in entire AOCS dataset, 77% of tumors.
% ovarian cancer deaths	10%	90%	Stem-like consists of 91% of deaths in original bipartition and 94% in entire AOCS dataset.

that all 15 endometrioid tumors in the Wu dataset with CTNNB1, PTEN, or PIK3CA mutations were characterized as differentiated. Moreover, all 13 tumors in this dataset with β-catenin accumulation were differentiated, which is consistent with aberrations in Wnt signaling seen in low-grade endometrioid tumors [12]. Thus, the subtype classification was consistent with reported mutation status of Type I/II tumors.

Type I tumors purportedly arise from either ovarian surface epithelium that undergoes metaplasia or epithelium of fallopian tube, endometrium, or peritoneum that proliferates after being trapped in ovarian cortical inclusion cysts [13] with the cell of origin possibly being normal fallopian tube epithelium (FTE) that sheds by endosalpingiosis [12,13]. We tested whether the differentiated subtype's gene expression patterns are similar to that of normal FTE by applying our stemness classification to the Tone et al. dataset [21] in which the authors compared expression profiles of serous ovarian cancer and normal FTE from women with and without BRCA1/2 mutation. Our stemness classification assigned 13/13 ovarian cancer samples to the stem-like group and 24/24 FTE samples to the differentiated. Although all four normal OSE samples in the Wu dataset [20] were also classified as "differentiated," these results suggest substantial similarity in gene expression profiles between FTE and the differentiated subtype.

Consistent with the hypothesis that Type I (but not Type II) tumors are enriched for expression of genes associated with cilia [12], the differentiated subtype of the AOCS dataset (n = 145) was enriched in gene sets associated with cilia, such as apical projections gene sets (Table S6 in Methods S1) and FOXJ1, which is required for ciliogenesis [49] and has been proposed as a marker for ciliated fallopian tube cells [50]. FOXJ1 is not in the 51-gene stemness signature but was strongly up-regulated in the differentiated subtype compared to the stem-like subtype (*t*-test $p = 4.87 \times 10^{-7}$). These observations provide evidence for the hypothesis that Type II/high-grade serous ovarian cancer arises from non-ciliated epithelial cells [13].

Therefore, the Type I/II and stemness classifications are similar in terms of grade, histological subtype, prevalence, and lethality, in addition to cell of origin, presence of ciliated cells, and mutation status (Table 5). From a gene expression point of view, Type II ovarian tumors may be more stem-like in their gene expression. If this molecular definition holds in further prospective studies, our stem-like classification would represent a molecular classification system that could establish the Type I/II system and provide insight into possible mechanism and therapies for these subtypes.

Biological Basis of the Stem-like Gene Classifier

Of the 51 genes used for classification, 37 were present in all four ovarian cancer datasets used for clinical validation (remaining AOCS, Wu, Dressman, and Crijns), because the gene expression profiling was performed on different technological platforms. Of these, a subset of 12 were consistently over-expressed ($p<0.05$ after FDR correction) in either the stem-like or differentiated subtypes across the four datasets and are thus most robustly expressed. The six stem-like subtype genes were UVRAG, CXCR4, RGS19, RAD51AP1, PSAT1, and CXCL10, and the six differentiated subtype genes were FOXA2, EIF1, MTUS1, DFNB31, TRAF3IP2, and SLC22A5. Despite enrichment in gene expression of the targets of Nanog, Oct4, and Sox2 in the stem-like subtype (Table 1), we did not find that that these genes were differentially expressed between the stem-like and differentiated subtypes.

Discussion

The cancer stem cell theory proposes that a subpopulation of cells inherit or acquire stem-like properties that enable them to survive therapy and drive recurrent tumor growth, but the function and identification of such stem cells is controversial both in normal and malignant ovarian and fallopian tube tissue [51–53]. We have not demonstrated the existence of cancer stem cells in ovarian cancer; instead our analysis identified a subtype of ovarian cancer with stem-like gene expression which provides a new molecular subtype classification of ovarian cancer, a genomic context for further investigation of type I/II ovarian cancers and insights into why ovarian cancer is so likely to be fatal despite aggressive therapy.

Tumors identified as being of the stem-like subtype have higher tumor grade and significantly worse prognosis, properties that were reproducible in independent and heterogeneous ovarian cancer microarray datasets; the associations between stem cell-like gene expression and grade or survival have been observed before but has not been explored in ovarian cancer [7,54]. In our analysis, stemness was also a significant predictor of disease-free survival in multivariate analyses that adjusted for prognostic variables, such as grade and stage. Thus, this classification's prognostic value may be independent of confounding clinical variables.

The classification is also valuable because of similarity to and support for a subtype classification associated with distinct pathogenesis pathways. Type I ovarian cancer, which includes low-grade and histologically heterogeneous tumors that may arise in the ovary, is similar to the differentiated subtype while Type II, which includes high-grade and mostly serous tumors that arise in the fallopian tube, is similar to the stem-like subtype [12,13]. This is the first potential gene expression-based description of Type I and II ovarian tumors (a distinction that up to now was mainly morphologic), and thus it provides rationale for new biologic and treatment hypotheses.

Our signature classified a low number of high-grade, serous tumors, which would normally be classified as Type II, as Type I. The identification of good prognosis, high-grade serous carcinomas may reflect novel biological insight or gene expression patterns of tumors that were originally low-grade and became high-grade [55]. Alternatively, these tumors may reflect initial misclassification in tumor grade because such clinical pathological classification of Type I and II tumors is mostly not always straightforward [14].

The 51 classification genes we identified may provide insight into pathogenesis of Type I and II ovarian cancer. FOXA2, which is consistently up in the differentiated subtype, is an inhibitor of the epithelial-mesenchymal transition associated with invasion and metastasis [56,57]. On the other hand, CXCR4, which is consistently highly expressed in the stem-like subtype, is implicated in ovarian cancer metastasis [58], and is a potential therapeutic target of drugs such as CXCR4 antagonists AMD3100 [58] and CTCE-9908 [59]. Other genes including UVRAG and RAD51AP1 are implicated in DNA damage response, which has been recently linked to cell differentiation status [60].

The stem-like subtype was enriched in stem cell-related gene sets, including gene targets of stem cell markers Oct4 and Nanog, which are reported to be associated with grade and stage in serous ovarian cancer [61,62]. Although many common markers of stem cells or EMT were not up-regulated in stem-like ovarian cancer, expression of stem cell markers were also not observed in the stem cell-like high-grade, ER-negative breast cancer [7]. This may be because stem cell markers are up-regulated in a minority of cancer stem cells which would not be reflected in gene expression profiling of whole tumor. Kim et al. proposed that Myc activity explains the apparent contradiction between the predictive power of stem cell-related transcriptional programs and the absence of canonical stem cell gene expression [61,62]. In our analysis, we observed an enrichment of the Kim et al. Myc module in the stem-like subtype, but without an over-expression of Myc (AOCS dataset t-test $p = 0.445$).

The stem-like subtype was predominant in high grade serous ovarian and basal-like breast cancer supporting common biological connections between these cancers that also share BRCA1 dysfunction [9,44] and p53 mutation [63].Molecular similarities between basal-like breast cancer and high-grade serous ovarian cancer have been described in other studies, including the recent study by the Cancer Genome Atlas Network [64]. Inactivation of p53 in breast cancers has been shown to correlate with stem cell transcriptional signatures [65] and the basal-like subtype [9] in breast cancer. The guardian of the genome, p53 maintains DNA integrity and DNA repair processes but also plays an important role in stem cell and cell state reprogramming. While the majority of ovarian cancer patients (~ 80%) have tumors of the stem-like subtype, the stem-like is observed in only 15% of breast cancers which may partially explain the relatively poor prognosis in ovarian cancer [1]. Our analysis provides additional support that therapies effective in basal-like breast may also be may also be effective in high grade serous ovarian cancer. Poly(ADP-ribose) polymerase (PARP) inhibitors, which are especially effective in cancer associated with BRCA1 or BRCA2 mutation [66], have shown considerable promise in triple-negative breast cancer [67] and may be valuable in treating high-grade serous Type II ovarian cancer [68].

We present a prognostic stem-like subtype classification of ovarian cancer which provides a genomic context for the Type I/II classification. Though it does not explain all variation in survival, in combination with other clinical indicators, it may have the potential to explain prognosis with greater accuracy than currently used clinical variables can alone. This classification requires further experimental validation in a large cohort of patients to characterize the properties of each molecular subtype, their association with Types I and II ovarian cancer and demonstrate possible clinical application. Our study provides support for the recently described Type I/II model of ovarian cancer and provides a molecular signature for stratification of these subtypes.

Supporting Information

Methods S1 This file contains: Figure S1 Distributions of stemness bipartition diagonal linear discriminant (DLD) scores in each dataset. In the ovarian cancer datasets, the DLD scores were all bimodal, and Gaussian mixture modeling [39] of the score was used to classify the lower scoring group as differentiated and the higher scoring group as stem-like. In the breast cancer datasets, mixture modeling was still used to discover approximate stem-like and differentiated classes, despite lack of clear bimodality. The range of scores is inconsistent in different datasets, because genes were often lost when crossing microarray platforms and potentially because of batch effects across datasets. Table S1 Proliferation genes (see Supplementary Methods) that were removed from the set of 83 GeneSigDB [35] gene signatures that were used for class discovery with ISIS [33]. After removing these genes, 2,632 genes were still used for class discovery.Table S2 Genes used to generate the stemness bipartition and their corresponding weights when predicting the bipartition in other datasets, as well as pooled t-statistics for differential expression between the stem-like and differentiated subtypes. Negative weights correspond to the differentiated subtype and positive weights correspond to the stem-like subtype. Table S3. A list of the 83 gene signatures from GeneSigDB [35] that are reported to be associated with stem cells. Table S4 The 13 gene sets used by Ben-Porath et al. to characterize classes of cancer as stem cell-like or differentiated. Genes in these gene sets were limited to those that were in the DNA microarray platform (Affy U133 Plus 2.0 platform) of the AOCS data [10]. Table S5 Gene-Set-Enrichment p-values for enrichment in stem-like and differentiated subtypes for all of the curated gene sets on MSigDB v 3.0. No multiple testing correction was used. Table S6 Gene-Set-Enrichment p-values for enrichment in stem-like and differentiated subtypes for all of the Gene Ontology gene sets on MSigDB v 3.0. No multiple testing correction was used. Table S7 Genes over-expressed in breast cancer cells containing wild type and mutant p53 from Figure 5 of Troester et al. [47] and Table 1 of Takahashi et al. [48] and whether they are over-expressed in the stem-like or differentiated subtype. P-value is for over-expression in either the stem-like or differentiated class and was calculated with the likelihood ratio test for logistic regression. Only genes in the AOCS dataset were considered. No multiple testing correction was performed. In the

Troester et al., the Gene-Set-Enrichment p-value for enrichment of mutant p53 genes in stem-like subtype was 0.00004 and p-value for enrichment of WT p53 genes in differentiated subtype was 0.00005. These p-values were 0.00008 and 0.05144, respectively, in the Takahashi et al. signature.

Acknowledgments

We thank Professor Ronny Drapkin and Dr. Panos Konstantinopoulos for useful discussions. We are grateful to Professor Win Hide and his group for assistance in curation of stem cell gene signatures and for interpretation of results and Ms. Renee Rubio and Ms. Hui-Ying Piao for technical support.

Author Contributions

Conceived and designed the experiments: ACC MS DH. Performed the experiments: MS ACC. Analyzed the data: MS ACC SB. Contributed reagents/materials/analysis tools: OH SB BHK JQ. Wrote the paper: MS ACC DS JQ.

References

1. Jemal A, Siegel R, Xu J, Ward E (2010) Cancer statistics, 2010. CA Cancer J Clin 60: 277–300.
2. Jazaeri AA, Awtrey CS, Chandramouli GV, Chuang YE, Khan J, et al. (2005) Gene expression profiles associated with response to chemotherapy in epithelial ovarian cancers. Clin Cancer Res 11: 6300–6310.
3. Rizzo S, Hersey JM, Mellor P, Dai W, Santos-Silva A, et al. (2011) Ovarian cancer stem cell-like side populations are enriched following chemotherapy and overexpress EZH2. Mol Cancer Ther 10: 325–335.
4. Hu L, McArthur C, Jaffe RB (2010) Ovarian cancer stem-like side-population cells are tumourigenic and chemoresistant. Br J Cancer 102: 1276–1283.
5. Curley MD, Garrett LA, Schorge JO, Foster R, Rueda BR (2011) Evidence for cancer stem cells contributing to the pathogenesis of ovarian cancer. Front Biosci 16: 368–392.
6. Honeth G, Bendahl PO, Ringner M, Saal LH, Gruvberger-Saal SK, et al. (2008) The CD44+/CD24− phenotype is enriched in basal-like breast tumors. Breast Cancer Res 10: R53.
7. Ben-Porath I, Thomson MW, Carey VJ, Ge R, Bell GW, et al. (2008) An embryonic stem cell-like gene expression signature in poorly differentiated aggressive human tumors. Nat Genet 40: 499–507.
8. Liu S, Ginestier C, Charafe-Jauffret E, Foco H, Kleer CG, et al. (2008) BRCA1 regulates human mammary stem/progenitor cell fate. Proc Natl Acad Sci U S A 105: 1680–1685.
9. Manie E, Vincent-Salomon A, Lehmann-Che J, Pierron G, Turpin E, et al. (2009) High frequency of TP53 mutation in BRCA1 and sporadic basal-like carcinomas but not in BRCA1 luminal breast tumors. Cancer Res 69: 663–671.
10. Tothill RW, Tinker AV, George J, Brown R, Fox SB, et al. (2008) Novel molecular subtypes of serous and endometrioid ovarian cancer linked to clinical outcome. Clin Cancer Res 14: 5198–5208.
11. Cancer Genome Atlas Research Network (2011) Integrated genomic analyses of ovarian carcinoma. Nature 474: 609–615.
12. Kurman RJ, Shih Ie M (2010) The origin and pathogenesis of epithelial ovarian cancer: a proposed unifying theory. Am J Surg Pathol 34: 433–443.
13. Karst AM, Drapkin R (2010) Ovarian cancer pathogenesis: a model in evolution. J Oncol 2010: 932371.
14. Ayhan A, Kurman RJ, Yemelyanova A, Vang R, Logani S, et al. (2009) Defining the cut point between low-grade and high-grade ovarian serous carcinomas: a clinicopathologic and molecular genetic analysis. Am J Surg Pathol 33: 1220–1224.
15. Edgar R, Domrachev M, Lash AE (2002) Gene Expression Omnibus: NCBI gene expression and hybridization array data repository. Nucleic Acids Res 30: 207–210.
16. Irizarry RA, Hobbs B, Collin F, Beazer-Barclay YD, Antonellis KJ, et al. (2003) Exploration, normalization, and summaries of high density oligonucleotide array probe level data. Biostatistics 4: 249–264.
17. Dai M, Wang P, Boyd AD, Kostov G, Athey B, et al. (2005) Evolving gene/transcript definitions significantly alter the interpretation of GeneChip data. Nucleic Acids Res 33: e175–e175.
18. Sandberg R, Larsson O (2007) Improved precision and accuracy for microarrays using updated probe set definitions. BMC Bioinformatics 8: 48.
19. Dressman HK, Berchuck A, Chan G, Zhai J, Bild A, et al. (2007) An integrated genomic-based approach to individualized treatment of patients with advanced-stage ovarian cancer. J Clin Oncol 25: 517–525.
20. Wu R, Hendrix-Lucas N, Kuick R, Zhai Y, Schwartz DR, et al. (2007) Mouse model of human ovarian endometrioid adenocarcinoma based on somatic defects in the Wnt/beta-catenin and PI3K/Pten signaling pathways. Cancer Cell 11: 321–333.
21. Tone AA, Begley H, Sharma M, Murphy J, Rosen B, et al. (2008) Gene expression profiles of luteal phase fallopian tube epithelium from BRCA mutation carriers resemble high-grade serous carcinoma. Clin Cancer Res 14: 4067–4078.
22. Crijns AP, Fehrmann RS, de Jong S, Gerbens F, Meersma GJ, et al. (2009) Survival-related profile, pathways, and transcription factors in ovarian cancer. PLoS Med 6: e24.
23. Miller LD, Smeds J, George J, Vega VB, Vergara L, et al. (2005) An expression signature for p53 status in human breast cancer predicts mutation status, transcriptional effects, and patient survival. Proc Natl Acad Sci U S A 102: 13550–13555.
24. Desmedt C, Piette F, Loi S, Wang Y, Lallemand F, et al. (2007) Strong time dependence of the 76-gene prognostic signature for node-negative breast cancer patients in the TRANSBIG multicenter independent validation series. Clin Cancer Res 13: 3207–3214.
25. Wang Y, Klijn JG, Zhang Y, Sieuwerts AM, Look MP, et al. (2005) Gene-expression profiles to predict distant metastasis of lymph-node-negative primary breast cancer. Lancet 365: 671–679.
26. Minn AJ, Gupta GP, Padua D, Bos P, Nguyen DX, et al. (2007) Lung metastasis genes couple breast tumor size and metastatic spread. Proc Natl Acad Sci U S A 104: 6740–6745.
27. Millenaar FF, Okyere J, May ST, van Zanten M, Voesenek LA, et al. (2006) How to decide? Different methods of calculating gene expression from short oligonucleotide array data will give different results. BMC Bioinformatics 7: 137.
28. Li C, Wong WH (2001) Model-based analysis of oligonucleotide arrays: expression index computation and outlier detection. Proc Natl Acad Sci U S A 98: 31–36.
29. Desmedt C, Haibe-Kains B, Wirapati P, Buyse M, Larsimont D, et al. (2008) Biological processes associated with breast cancer clinical outcome depend on the molecular subtypes. Clin Cancer Res 14: 5158–5165.
30. Foulkes WD, Smith IE, Reis-Filho JS (2010) Triple-negative breast cancer. N Engl J Med 363: 1938–1948.
31. Carey L, Winer E, Viale G, Cameron D, Gianni L (2010) Triple-negative breast cancer: disease entity or title of convenience? Nat Rev Clin Oncol 7: 683–692.
32. Lehmann BD, Bauer JA, Chen X, Sanders ME, Chakravarthy AB, et al. (2011) Identification of human triple-negative breast cancer subtypes and preclinical models for selection of targeted therapies. J Clin Invest 121: 2750–2767.
33. von Heydebreck A, Huber W, Poustka A, Vingron M (2001) Identifying splits with clear separation: a new class discovery method for gene expression data. Bioinformatics 17 Suppl 1: S107–114.
34. Bentink S, Haibe-Kains B, Risch T, Fan JB, Hirsch MS, et al. (2012) Angiogenic mRNA and microRNA gene expression signature predicts a novel subtype of serous ovarian cancer. PLoS One 7: e30269.
35. Culhane AC, Schwarzl T, Sultana R, Picard KC, Picard SC, et al. (2009) GeneSigDB–a curated database of gene expression signatures. Nucleic Acids Res.
36. Jiang Z, Gentleman R (2007) Extensions to gene set enrichment. Bioinformatics 23: 306–313.
37. Subramanian A, Tamayo P, Mootha VK, Mukherjee S, Ebert BL, et al. (2005) Gene set enrichment analysis: a knowledge-based approach for interpreting genome-wide expression profiles. Proc Natl Acad Sci U S A 102: 15545–15550.
38. Dudoit S, Fridlyand J, Speed TP (2002) Comparison of Discrimination Methods for the Classification of Tumors Using Gene Expression Data. Journal of the American Statistical Association 97: 77–87.
39. Fraley CaR, Adrian E (2002) Model-Based Clustering, Discriminant Analysis, and Density Estimation. Journal of the American Statistical Association 97: 611–631.
40. Leek JT, Scharpf RB, Bravo HC, Simcha D, Langmead B, et al. (2010) Tackling the widespread and critical impact of batch effects in high-throughput data. Nat Rev Genet 11: 733–739.
41. Assou S, Le Carrour T, Tondeur S, Strom S, Gabelle A, et al. (2007) A meta-analysis of human embryonic stem cells transcriptome integrated into a web-based expression atlas. Stem Cells 25: 961–973.
42. Boyer LA, Lee TI, Cole MF, Johnstone SE, Levine SS, et al. (2005) Core transcriptional regulatory circuitry in human embryonic stem cells. Cell 122: 947–956.
43. Fernandez PC, Frank SR, Wang L, Schroeder M, Liu S, et al. (2003) Genomic targets of the human c-Myc protein. Genes Dev 17: 1115–1129.
44. Turner NC, Reis-Filho JS, Russell AM, Springall RJ, Ryder K, et al. (2007) BRCA1 dysfunction in sporadic basal-like breast cancer. Oncogene 26: 2126–2132.
45. Benjamini Y, Hochberg Y (1995) Controlling the False Discovery Rate: A Practical and Powerful Approach to Multiple Testing. Journal of the Royal Statistical Society Series B (Methodological) 57: 289–300.
46. Hommel G (1988) A Stagewise Rejective Multiple Test Procedure Based on a Modified Bonferroni Test. Biometrika 75: 383–386.

47. Troester MA, Herschkowitz JI, Oh DS, He X, Hoadley KA, et al. (2006) Gene expression patterns associated with p53 status in breast cancer. BMC Cancer 6: 276.
48. Takahashi S, Moriya T, Ishida T, Shibata H, Sasano H, et al. (2008) Prediction of breast cancer prognosis by gene expression profile of TP53 status. Cancer Sci 99: 324–332.
49. Okada A, Ohta Y, Brody SL, Watanabe H, Krust A, et al. (2004) Role of foxj1 and estrogen receptor alpha in ciliated epithelial cell differentiation of the neonatal oviduct. J Mol Endocrinol 32: 615–625.
50. Levanon K, Crum C, Drapkin R (2008) New insights into the pathogenesis of serous ovarian cancer and its clinical impact. J Clin Oncol 26: 5284–5293.
51. Burgos-Ojeda D, Rueda BR, Buckanovich RJ (2012) Ovarian cancer stem cell markers: prognostic and therapeutic implications. Cancer Lett 322: 1–7.
52. Wang Y, Sacchetti A, van Dijk MR, van der Zee M, van der Horst PH, et al. (2012) Identification of quiescent, stem-like cells in the distal female reproductive tract. PLoS One 7: e40691.
53. Zhang H, Zheng W, Shen Y, Adhikari D, Ueno H, et al. (2012) Experimental evidence showing that no mitotically active female germline progenitors exist in postnatal mouse ovaries. Proc Natl Acad Sci U S A 109: 12580–12585.
54. Shats I, Gatza ML, Chang JT, Mori S, Wang J, et al. (2011) Using a stem cell-based signature to guide therapeutic selection in cancer. Cancer Res 71: 1772–1780.
55. Dehari R, Kurman RJ, Logani S, Shih Ie M (2007) The development of high-grade serous carcinoma from atypical proliferative (borderline) serous tumors and low-grade micropapillary serous carcinoma: a morphologic and molecular genetic analysis. Am J Surg Pathol 31: 1007–1012.
56. Tang Y, Shu G, Yuan X, Jing N, Song J (2011) FOXA2 functions as a suppressor of tumor metastasis by inhibition of epithelial-to-mesenchymal transition in human lung cancers. Cell Res 21: 316–326.
57. Song Y, Washington MK, Crawford HC (2010) Loss of FOXA1/2 is essential for the epithelial-to-mesenchymal transition in pancreatic cancer. Cancer Res 70: 2115–2125.
58. Kajiyama H, Shibata K, Terauchi M, Ino K, Nawa A, et al. (2008) Involvement of SDF-1alpha/CXCR4 axis in the enhanced peritoneal metastasis of epithelial ovarian carcinoma. Int J Cancer 122: 91–99.
59. Kwong J, Kulbe H, Wong D, Chakravarty P, Balkwill F (2009) An antagonist of the chemokine receptor CXCR4 induces mitotic catastrophe in ovarian cancer cells. Mol Cancer Ther 8: 1893–1905.
60. Sherman MH, Bassing CH, Teitell MA (2011) Regulation of cell differentiation by the DNA damage response. Trends Cell Biol.
61. Zhang J, Li YL, Zhou CY, Hu YT, Chen HZ (2010) Expression of octamer-4 in serous and mucinous ovarian carcinoma. J Clin Pathol 63: 879–883.
62. Pan Y, Jiao J, Zhou C, Cheng Q, Hu Y, et al. (2010) Nanog is highly expressed in ovarian serous cystadenocarcinoma and correlated with clinical stage and pathological grade. Pathobiology 77: 283–288.
63. Bowtell DD (2010) The genesis and evolution of high-grade serous ovarian cancer. Nat Rev Cancer 10: 803–808.
64. Koboldt DC, Fulton RS, McLellan MD, Schmidt H, Kalicki-Veizer J, et al. (2012) Comprehensive molecular portraits of human breast tumours. Nature 490: 61–70.
65. Mizuno H, Spike BT, Wahl GM, Levine AJ (2010) Inactivation of p53 in breast cancers correlates with stem cell transcriptional signatures. Proc Natl Acad Sci U S A 107: 22745–22750.
66. Fong PC, Boss DS, Yap TA, Tutt A, Wu P, et al. (2009) Inhibition of poly(ADP-ribose) polymerase in tumors from BRCA mutation carriers. N Engl J Med 361: 123–134.
67. Anders CK, Winer EP, Ford JM, Dent R, Silver DP, et al. (2010) Poly(ADP-Ribose) polymerase inhibition: "targeted" therapy for triple-negative breast cancer. Clin Cancer Res 16: 4702–4710.
68. Banerjee S, Kaye SB, Ashworth A (2010) Making the best of PARP inhibitors in ovarian cancer. Nat Rev Clin Oncol 7: 508–519.

12

On the Reproducibility of TCGA Ovarian Cancer MicroRNA Profiles

Ying-Wooi Wan[1,2,4], Claire M. Mach[2,3], Genevera I. Allen[1,7,8], Matthew L. Anderson[2,4,5]*, Zhandong Liu[1,5,6,7]*

1 Department of Pediatrics, Baylor College of Medicine, Houston, Texas, United States of America, **2** Department of Obstetrics and Gynecology, Baylor College of Medicine, Houston, Texas, United States of America, **3** College of Pharmacy, University of Houston, Houston, Texas, United States of America, **4** Department of Pathology and Immunology, Baylor College of Medicine, Houston, Texas, United States of America, **5** Dan L. Duncan Cancer Center, Baylor College of Medicine, Houston, Texas, United States of America, **6** Computational and Integrative Biomedical Research (CIBR) Center, Baylor College of Medicine, Houston, Texas, United States of America, **7** Neurological Research Institute, Texas Children's Hospital, Houston, Texas, United States of America, **8** Department of Statistics and Electrical & Computer Engineering, Rice University, Houston, Texas, United States of America

Abstract

Dysregulated microRNA (miRNA) expression is a well-established feature of human cancer. However, the role of specific miRNAs in determining cancer outcomes remains unclear. Using Level 3 expression data from the Cancer Genome Atlas (TCGA), we identified 61 miRNAs that are associated with overall survival in 469 ovarian cancers profiled by microarray ($p<0.01$). We also identified 12 miRNAs that are associated with survival when miRNAs were profiled in the same specimens using Next Generation Sequencing (miRNA-Seq) ($p<0.01$). Surprisingly, only 1 miRNA transcript is associated with ovarian cancer survival in both datasets. Our analyses indicate that this discrepancy is due to the fact that miRNA levels reported by the two platforms correlate poorly, even after correcting for potential issues inherent to signal detection algorithms. Corrections for false discovery and microRNA abundance had minimal impact on this discrepancy. Further investigation is warranted.

Editor: Amanda Ewart Toland, Ohio State University Medical Center, United States of America

Funding: This work is supported in part through the Collaborative Advances in Biomedical Computing Seed Funding Program at the Ken Kennedy Institute for Information Technology at Rice University supported by the John and Ann Doerr Fund for Computational Biomedicine and through the Center for Computational and Integrative Biomedical Research Seed Funding Program at Baylor College of Medicine. GA is also partially supported by NSF DMS-1209017. ZD is supported by the Houston Bioinformatics Endowment and NSF DMS-1263932. The funders had no role in study design, data collection and analysis, decision to publish, or preparation of the manuscript.

Competing Interests: The authors have declared that no competing interests exist.

* E-mail: Zhandonl@bcm.edu (ZL); matthew@bcm.edu (MLA)

Introduction

MicroRNAs (miRNAs) are endogenous RNA transcripts that regulate diverse patterns of gene expression [1]. Most human miRNAs are transcribed as long precursors known as pri-miRNAs. Starting in the nucleus, pri-miRNAs undergo a series of processing events that ultimately result in the cytoplasmic release of mature transcripts ~22 nucleotides in length. Mature miRNAs catalyze translational inhibition by directly binding to messenger RNAs (mRNAs) and promoting their degradation [2]. Recent data indicate that miRNAs can inhibit translation independent of their ability to induce mRNA degradation.

Patterns of miRNA expression have been extensively profiled in human tissues. It is now clear that dysregulated miRNA expression is a feature of many different cancers, including carcinomas of the breast, ovary and lung [3–5]. However, determining the mechanisms by which individual miRNAs contribute to cancer outcomes remains a key challenge for biologists hoping to exploit their power. Recently, the Cancer Genome Atlas Consortium (TCGA) reported that ovarian cancers cluster into distinct molecular subtypes based on their patterns of gene and microRNA expression [6]. However, we have discovered an alarming lack of consistency between the microRNA (miRNA) expression profiles initially used by the TCGA and a subsequent profile of miRNA expression generated by this group for the same ovarian cancer specimens using miRNA-Seq. As these observations challenge the validity of the underlying data, they also suggest that scientific discoveries based solely on this data should be interpreted with caution.

Results

To delineate miRNAs associated with ovarian cancer patient survival, we performed a univariate Cox regression analysis using Level 3 TCGA miRNA data for 469 ovarian cancers profiled using Agilent microarray technology. Initial regression analysis was further refined by use of the Benjamini–Hochberg (BH) procedure to adjust for multiple hypothesis testing [7]. We found that 16 mature miRNAs are significantly associated with ovarian cancer survival ($FDR<0.01$) (Figure 1A). Of these, miR-505, miR-652 and miR-551b* demonstrate the most robust associations. Hazard ratios (HR) calculated for these miRNAs were -1.73, -1.8, and 9.3, respectively. This result indicates that each of these miRNAs potentially plays an important role in determining ovarian cancer survival.

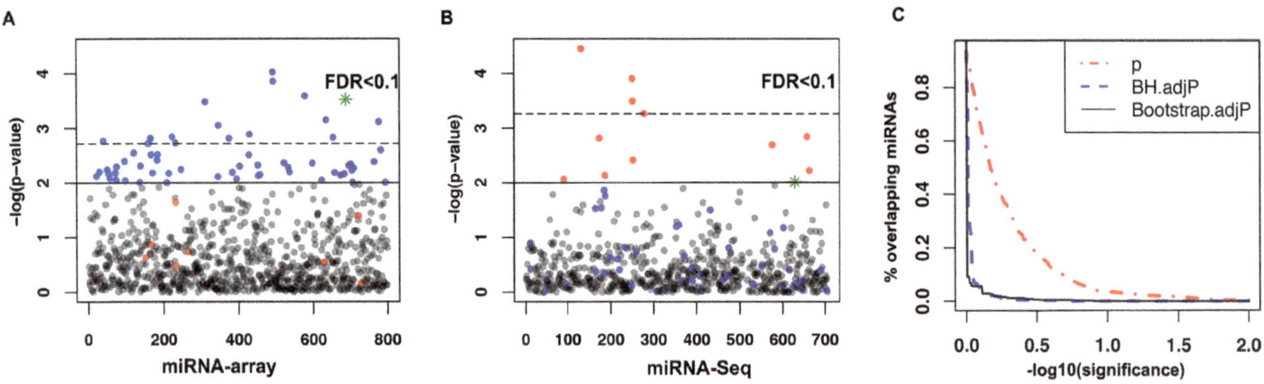

Figure 1. MicroRNAs associated with ovarian cancer survival. P-value plots of univariate Cox regression for microRNAs associated with ovarian cancer survival identified by microarray (A) or miRNA-Seq (B) data. P-value<0.01 (Solid line). False discovery rate (FDR)<0.1 (Dotted line). In both A&B, blue dots indicate miRNAs associated with survival by miRNA array, while red dots indicate miRNAs associated with survival by miR-Seq. Green stars are miRNAs associated with survival in both datasets. (C) percentage of overlapping miRNAs between the array and NGS seq platform at different cut-off threshold for Cox p-values, BH adjusted FDR, and Storey q-values.

To validate these observations, we next interrogated a second dataset of miRNA expression generated for the same ovarian cancer specimens using Next Generation Sequencing (miRNA-Seq). The TCGA ovarian cancer project is unique in that miRNA expression has been profiled using both miRNA array and miRNA-Seq. These technically distinct platforms create a unique opportunity to validate discoveries made using one dataset against the other. Ideally, the results obtained should correlate well. Using Cox Proportional Hazards analysis, we found that 4 miRNA transcripts are associated with survival when miRNAs were profiled in ovarian cancers using miRNA-Seq at an identical FDR level (Figure 1B). There is no overlap between the results obtained from these two platforms, despite the fact that both datasets were generated from the same samples.

To determine whether the microarray and Next Gen platforms will give more consistent results when analyzed using a relaxed threshold, we reduced the p-value threshold used for our analyses to 0.01. This resulted in more miRNAs significantly associated with patient survival in both datasets. For example, we identified 61 miRNAs from data generated using the array platform. However, the hazard ratios estimated for the 12 miRNAs identified from miRNA-Seq data are all very close to 1.0. Only miR-652 is associated with survival in both the miRNA-Seq and microarray datasets. To correct for multiple hypothesis testing, we adjusted our Cox model p-values using Benjamini–Hochberg procedure [7]. After completing these analyses, no miRNAs are correlated with survival in both datasets when the false discovery rate was set at 10%.

To determine whether choice of a multiple hypothesis adjustment procedure contributes to these results, we re-analyzed the TCGA data using an alternative q-value estimation procedure [8]. In addition, we computed the percentage of overlapping miRNAs at different FDR or p-value cut-off. Our results indicate that the limited number of overlapping miRNAs between the two platforms is independent of the choice of multiple hypothesis adjustment procedure or cut-off thresholds (Figure 1C).

To elucidate potential causes for this unexpected discrepancy, we examined the reproducibility of miRNA expression between the two TCGA files that describe this data. Pearson correlation coefficients (r) were calculated for each of the 359 mature human miRNAs for which Level 3 expression data was available in both the miRNA-Seq and microarray databases. We found that correlation coefficients for levels of individual miRNAs reported by each technique varied widely. For example, miR-505 is the miRNA most robustly associated with patient outcome in our analyses of the miRNA array data (HR = −1.7, p<9e-5). However, when assessed using sequencing data, the hazard ratio for mir-505 was 0.998 (p = 0.03). Levels of miR-505 measured by miRNA-array and miRNA-Seq data correlated only modestly (r = 0.59) (Figure 2B). Discrepancies were also observed in a number of other miRNAs that have been previously implicated in ovarian cancer, such as miR-143 [9]. The correlation coefficient for miR-143 in our analyses was 0.39 (Figure 2C). Another miRNA well-studied in ovarian cancer is miR-141, which has been previously reported to target p38α and modulate the oxidative stress response [10,11]. However, the correlation between levels of miR-141 in TCGA microarray and miRNA-Seq expression data is only 0.32 (Figure 2D). Overall, we found that correlation coefficients for ~72% of miRNAs profiled in both datasets were ≤0.5 (Figure 3A, 3C), indicating poor reproducibility. Only 22% of the mRNAs measured by Agilent microarray and Illumina HiSeq using the same ovarian cancer specimens correlate poorly (r≤0.5; Figure 3B, 3C). Thus, the discrepancy we report here appears to be limited to the TCGA miRNA dataset.

One potential cause for poor reproducibility may be the signal detection algorithm used to report levels of miRNA expression. Level 3 TCGA miRNA data are reported in two formats. The first, labeled as a "Quantification Data," reports levels for individual human miRNAs. However, one of the advantages of miRNA-Seq is that transcripts retrieved by this technique can be precisely mapped. A second file, labeled as "Isoform Data," has also been released by the TCGA. This file reports read counts for transcripts according to their genomic location. As part of this file, transcripts are identified as either mature miRNA, miRNA* (3p arms of human miRNAs), stem-loop transcript or precursor. While working through this data, we learned that miRNA levels reported in the TCGA quantification file include read counts for miRNA precursors as well as mature miRNAs. Because miRNA precursors are currently thought to lack biologic activity, inclusion of precursors with counts for mature miRNAs could confound survival analyses. To address this issue, we retrieved read counts for mature miRNAs only from the isoform data file and repeated our analyses. However, the proportion of miRNA correlation coefficients ≤0.5 remained as high as 71% despite the use of this more precisely defined data.

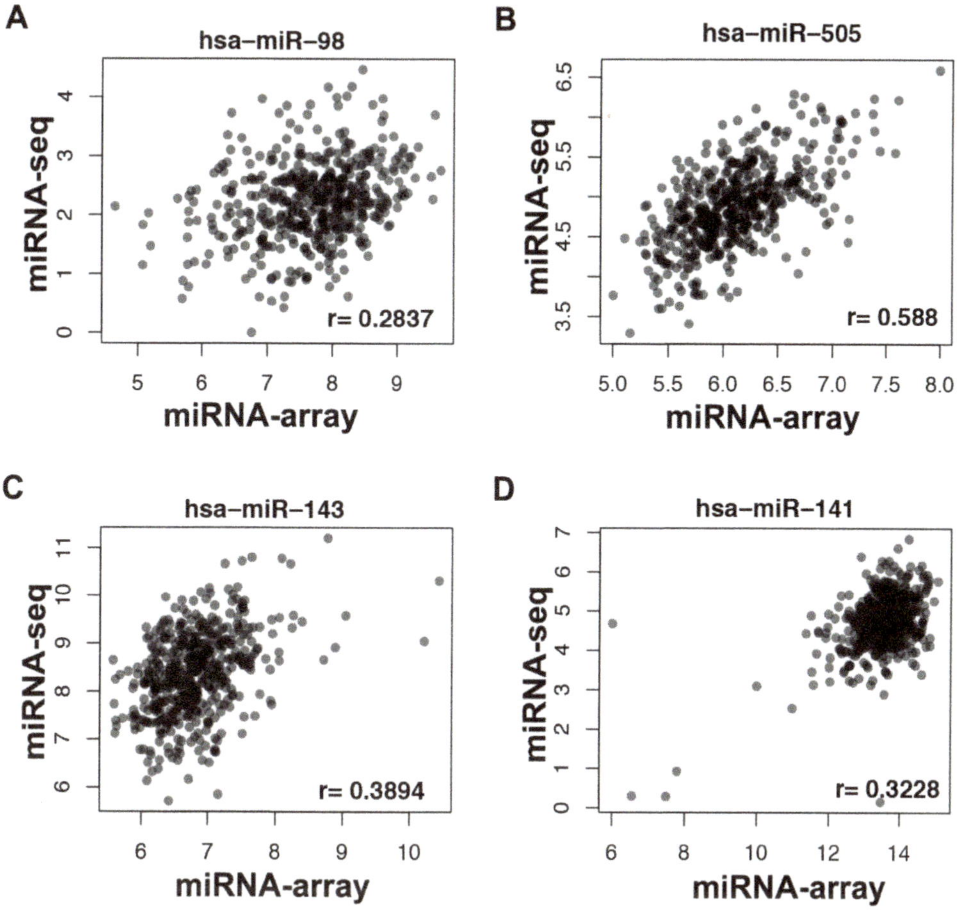

Figure 2. Scatter-plots of microRNA expression measured by microarray and miRNA-Seq. (A) miR-98, (B) miR-505 (C) miR-143 and (D) miR-141.

A second possible explanation for the observed discrepancy might be that correlations between measures of miRNA expression depend on the frequency with which individual miRNA transcripts are expressed. If so, infrequently expressed miRNAs might be reported by one or both of the platforms used to profile miRNA expression randomly or inaccurately. To explore this hypothesis,

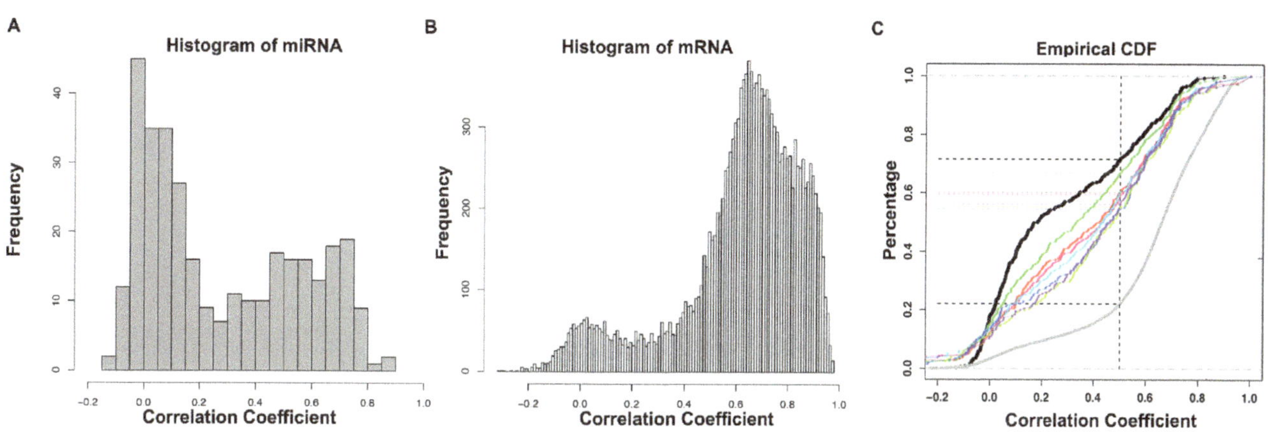

Figure 3. Distribution of correlations between microarray and sequencing profiles for miRNA and gene expression. (A) Histogram of correlation coefficients for individual miRNAs measured by miRNA-Seq and miRNA array. (B) Histogram of correlation coefficients for mRNAs profiled by Illumina HiSeq and mRNA array. (C) The empirical cumulative distribution function (ECDF) of the correlation between array and sequencing for miRNA (black), filtered miRNA (color) and mRNA (gray) measurements. Nearly, 72% of miRNAs demonstrate a correlation coefficient ≤0.5 whereas 22% of RNAs have a correlation coefficient ≤0.5. When filtered based on expression level, the percentage of miRNAs with correlation ≤0.5 saturated to 56%.

we re-calculated correlation coefficients for each miRNA identified by both platforms after excluding any transcript in the miRNA-Seq dataset with a read count less than 5. This reduced the number of distinct miRNAs available for analysis in the miRNA-Seq data file from 705 to 380. However, the proportion of miRNAs with correlation coefficients ≤0.5 also decreased from 72% to 56%. Similarly removing poorly expressed transcripts from the pool of mRNAs profiled by Illumina HiSeq reduces the proportion of mRNAs whose correlation coefficients ≤0.5 from 22% to 20%. These observations indicate that problems detecting infrequently expressed miRNA may impact the ability or one or both platforms to reliably report miRNA expression. However, the fact that more than half of miRNA transcripts still had correlation coefficients ≤0.5 even after correcting for this issue indicates that poorly expressed transcripts are not solely responsible for the discordant patterns of miRNA expression reported by the two platforms.

To explore this issue more in depth, we calculated the range of log2 transformed expression levels for all microRNAs in the two datasets. We also developed an algorithm that allowed us to vary the threshold of expression acceptable for inclusion for analysis from a minimum value (0) to the mean log2 transformed expression level of all transcripts. For each threshold, we only considered microRNAs expressed above the threshold and recomputed the correlation between the two platforms. This analysis reveals that the exclusion of miRNA transcripts expressed less frequently than the mean only slightly improves the overall correlation between the two platforms used to profile miRNA expression (Figure 3C). As shown graphically, we found that 71% of the miRNA demonstrate correlation less than 0.5 without the use of any filtering. By utilizing an expression level filter as described, we found that the proportion of transcripts with correlation coefficients across the two platforms saturated at 56%. This is still far higher than the 22% observed with mRNA expression profiling systems.

Discussion

Much to our surprise, our analyses indicate that the microRNAs associated with survival in ovarian cancer depend highly on whether specimens were profiled by the TCGA using microarray or miRNA-Seq. Our analyses indicate that this discrepancy exists because miRNA-Seq and microarray have generated very different profiles of miRNA expression, even though the data is based on the same ovarian cancer specimens. We do not currently have a clear explanation for why miRNA expression profiles reported by the TCGA are discordant. However, understanding this discrepancy will ultimately be important for identifying which miRNAs if any are important for determining ovarian cancer outcomes.

A variety of DNA microarray technologies have been previously validated by investigators examining within platform and cross-platform reproducibility [12–14]. Spearman correlation coefficients reported in these studies range from 0.59 to 0.94 with a mean of 0.82. These results are similar to what we have observed for correlations between patterns of gene expression profiled using microarray and Illumina HiSeq platforms by the TCGA. Both miRNA-Seq and microarray technologies are associated with multiple technical limitations that might account for the differences we have observed. For example, cross-hybridization is a well-recognized issue that can reduce signal specificity when profiling RNA transcripts by microarray [15]. However, it seems unlikely that cross-hybridization is a primary cause of the discrepancy we observed, as the number of transcripts correlated with survival by array is greater than the number associated with survival by miRNA-Seq. One alternate explanation might be that the signal extraction algorithm used to analyze miRNA-Seq data does not accurately report miRNA levels. In general, miRNA-Seq allows for precise transcript mapping with much greater confidence. The signal extraction algorithm currently used by the TCGA to report miRNA levels includes read counts for both a mature miRNA and its corresponding precursor. Our analyses indicate that precursors account for fewer than 1% of the total miRNA counts in the TCGA isoform file. This likely reflects the use of size-fractionated RNA to prepare libraries for miRNA-Seq [5]. Thus, their inclusion or exclusion in analyses of the TCGA dataset likely has little bearing on which miRNAs are associated with ovarian cancer survival.

Collectively, these observations underscore the urgent need for well-defined algorithms for processing signals generated by miRNA-Seq and transcriptional profiling platforms. Our understanding is that the same analyses have been performed by TCGA for other cancers, including colon, breast and lung [16–18]. Because miRNA expression in these other cancers has not been profiled by microarray, it is not possible to repeat our analyses to determine whether the discrepancy we report is observed in other cancers. Ultimately, consistent and reliable genomic data is critical for constructing testable hypotheses and achieving the full potential of the TCGA. Our observations identify an important hazard of which investigators should be aware as they utilize the TCGA miRNA data to study ovarian cancer. For the short term, knowledge of this hazard underscores the need to validate observations made with one or both of TCGA miRNA datasets. However, for the long term, resolution of this discrepancy will be important for determining the most effective platform and signal extraction algorithms for profiling miRNA expression as part of large scale genomic profiling efforts.

Materials and Methods

Gene and microRNA Expression Data

Level 3 data documenting patterns of gene expression for 296 ovarian cancer specimens profiled using Agilent G4502A arrays and Illumina HiSeq were downloaded from the TCGA data portal. Level 3 microRNA expression data were also retrieved for 469 ovarian cancer specimens profiled using the Agilent 4X15k array and miRNA-Seq. Level 3 miRNA data profiled by miRNA-Seq were retrieved from both the miRNA quantification and isoform files available at the TCGA data portal along with metafiles annotating each dataset. Permission to access all data was obtained from the Data Access Committee for the National Center for Biotechnology Information Genotypes and Phenotypes Database (dbGAP) at the National Institutes of Health.

Survival Analyses

Coded patient survival data was extracted from the TCGA clinical information file. A Cox Proportional Hazards model was used to estimate association between levels of individual miRNAs. Patient survival was calculated as time in months elapsed from date of diagnosis until date of last contact.

Statistical Analyses

Spearman's rank correlation coefficients, histograms, and the empirical cumulative distribution were computed and plotted for each miRNA and gene using r. Sequencing data were log transformed for plotting. Both direct read counts and counts normalized according to millions of miRNAs were examined as part of our analyses. All analyses were performed using both raw and normalized read counts reported as part of the TCGA miRNA-Seq datasets.

Acknowledgments

The authors gratefully acknowledge communication from David Wheeler, Rehan Akban, Gordon Robertson and Andy Chu regarding TCGA miRNA data analysis algorithms.

Author Contributions

Conceived and designed the experiments: ZL MA GA. Performed the experiments: YWW. Analyzed the data: YWW. Contributed reagents/materials/analysis tools: YWW CM. Wrote the paper: ZL MA GA YWW CM.

References

1. Wu L, Belasco JG (2008) Let me count the ways: mechanisms of gene regulation by miRNAs and siRNAs. Mol Cell 29: 1–7.
2. Bartel DP (2009) MicroRNAs: target recognition and regulatory functions. Cell 136: 215–233.
3. Eder M, Scherr M (2005) MicroRNA and lung cancer. The New England journal of medicine 352: 2446–2448.
4. Zhang L, Huang J, Yang N, Greshock J, Megraw MS, et al. (2006) microRNAs exhibit high frequency genomic alterations in human cancer. Proc Natl Acad Sci U S A 103: 9136–9141.
5. Creighton CJ, Fountain MD, Yu Z, Nagaraja AK, Zhu H, et al. (2010) Molecular profiling uncovers a p53-associated role for microRNA-31 in inhibiting the proliferation of serous ovarian carcinomas and other cancers. Cancer Res 70: 1906–1915.
6. (2011) Integrated genomic analyses of ovarian carcinoma. Nature 474: 609–615.
7. Benjamini Y, Hochberg Y (1995) Controlling the False Discovery Rate: A Practical and Powerful Approach to Multiple Testing. Journal of the Royal Statistical Society Series B (Methodological) 57: 289–300.
8. Storey JD, Taylor JE, Siegmund D (2004) Strong control, conservative point estimation and simultaneous conservative consistency of false discovery rates: a unified approach. Journal of the Royal Statistical Society: Series B (Statistical Methodology) 66: 187–205.
9. Marchini S, Cavalieri D, Fruscio R, Calura E, Garavaglia D, et al. (2011) Association between miR-200c and the survival of patients with stage I epithelial ovarian cancer: a retrospective study of two independent tumour tissue collections. The lancet oncology 12: 273–285.
10. Mateescu B, Batista L, Cardon M, Gruosso T, de Feraudy Y, et al. (2011) miR-141 and miR-200a act on ovarian tumorigenesis by controlling oxidative stress response. Nature Medicine 17: 1627–1635.
11. Yang D, Sun Y, Hu L, Zheng H, Ji P, et al. (2013) Integrated Analyses Identify a Master MicroRNA Regulatory Network for the Mesenchymal Subtype in Serous Ovarian Cancer. Cancer Cell 23: 186–199.
12. Sato F, Tsuchiya S, Terasawa K, Tsujimoto G (2009) Intra-platform repeatability and inter-platform comparability of microRNA microarray technology. PLoS One 4: e5540.
13. Yauk CL, Rowan-Carroll A, Stead JD, Williams A (2010) Cross-platform analysis of global microRNA expression technologies. BMC Genomics 11: 330.
14. Shi L, Reid LH, Jones WD, Shippy R, Warrington JA, et al. (2006) The MicroArray Quality Control (MAQC) project shows inter- and intraplatform reproducibility of gene expression measurements. Nature Biotechnology 24: 1151–1161.
15. Wu C, Carta R, Zhang L (2005) Sequence dependence of cross-hybridization on short oligo microarrays. Nucleic Acids Research 33: e84.
16. (2012) Comprehensive molecular characterization of human colon and rectal cancer. Nature 487: 330–337.
17. (2012) Comprehensive genomic characterization of squamous cell lung cancers. Nature 489: 519–525.
18. (2012) Comprehensive molecular portraits of human breast tumours. Nature 490: 61–70.

13

Exploiting the Synergy between Carboplatin and ABT-737 in the Treatment of Ovarian Carcinomas

Harsh Vardhan Jain[1]*, Alan Richardson[2], Michael Meyer-Hermann[3,4], Helen M. Byrne[5,6]

1 Department of Mathematics, Florida State University, Tallahassee, Florida,United States of America, **2** Institute for Science and Technology in Medicine, Keele University, Stoke-on-Trent, United Kingdom, **3** Department of Systems Immunology, Helmholtz Centre for Infection Research, Braunschweig, Germany, **4** Bio Centre for Life Science, Braunschweig University of Technology, Braunschweig, Germany, **5** Oxford Centre for Collaborative and Applied Mathematics, Mathematical Institute, University of Oxford, Oxford, United Kingdom, **6** Department of Computer Science, University of Oxford, Oxford, United Kingdom

Abstract

Platinum drug-resistance in ovarian cancers mediated by anti-apoptotic proteins such as Bcl-xL is a major factor contributing to the chemotherapeutic resistance of recurrent disease. Consequently, concurrent inhibition of Bcl-xL in combination with chemotherapy may improve treatment outcomes for patients. Here, we develop a mathematical model to investigate the potential of combination therapy with ABT-737, a small molecule inhibitor of Bcl-xL, and carboplatin, a platinum-based drug, on a simulated tumor xenograft. The model is calibrated against *in vivo* experimental data, wherein xenografts established in mice were treated with ABT-737 and/or carboplatin on a fixed periodic schedule. The validated model is used to predict the minimum drug load that will achieve a predetermined level of tumor growth inhibition, thereby maximizing the synergy between the two drugs. Our simulations suggest that the infusion-duration of each carboplatin dose is a critical parameter, with an 8-hour infusion of carboplatin given weekly combined with a daily bolus dose of ABT-737 predicted to minimize residual disease. The potential of combination therapy to prevent or delay the onset of carboplatin-resistance is also investigated. When resistance is acquired as a result of aberrant DNA-damage repair in cells treated with carboplatin, drug delivery schedules that induce tumor remission with even low doses of combination therapy can be identified. Intrinsic resistance due to pre-existing cohorts of resistant cells precludes tumor regression, but dosing strategies that extend disease-free survival periods can still be identified. These results highlight the potential of our model to accelerate the development of novel therapeutics such as BH3 mimetics.

Editor: Natalia L. Komarova, University of California-Irvine, United States of America

Funding: Funding came from a National Science Foundation grant DMS 0931642 and Award No. KUK-C1-013-04 made by the King Abdullah University of Science and Technology (KAUST). The funders had no role in study design, data collection and analysis, decision to publish, or preparation of the manuscript.

Competing Interests: The authors have declared that no competing interests exist.

* E-mail: hjain@fsu.edu

Introduction

Although ovarian cancer accounts for only 3% of cancers in women, it is the fifth most common cause of cancer death in women in the developed world [1]. Primary treatment for advanced ovarian cancer consists of cytoreductive surgery followed by adjuvant chemotherapy. The chemotherapeutic regimen typically combines a taxane such as paclitaxel with a platinum-based drug such as carboplatin, which causes cell death by inducing DNA damage. While patients initially respond well to therapy, most ultimately relapse, with recurrent disease being associated with progressive resistance to platinum-based therapy [2,3]. Consequently, 5-year survival rates for women with advanced ovarian cancer are only 30–40% [4].

Several factors may contribute to platinum drug-resistance (for a comprehensive review, see [5,6]). Here, we are concerned with the contribution of the anti-apoptotic protein Bcl-xL to drug-resistance. Bcl-xL belongs to the Bcl-2 family of intracellular proteins that regulates programmed cell death, or apoptosis [7]. Previous studies have revealed a significant correlation between Bcl-xL expression and carboplatin-resistance [8–10], and increased sensitivity to standard chemotherapeutic agents of ovarian cancer cell lines when Bcl-xL expression is inhibited [11–13]. Therefore, concomitant inhibition of Bcl-xL in combination with adjuvant chemotherapy may improve treatment outcomes for ovarian cancer patients.

In [13], Witham et al. assess the therapeutic potential of treating ovarian cancer that express Bcl-xL with carboplatin and ABT-737, a small-molecule inhibitor of Bcl-xL. Results from *in vitro* cell proliferation assays revealed synergistic inhibition of cell-growth and more rapid apoptosis when carboplatin was combined with ABT-737, than when it was administered as a single agent. Further, the times at which the two drugs are administered were also shown to be an important determinant of therapy efficacy, with an ABT-737 dose immediately following carboplatin found to yield the greatest extent of cell death. To understand better these experimental findings, we have previously developed a biochemically-motivated model for the growth of *in vitro* ovarian cancer [14], that was validated against available experimental data. A key prediction of our model is that the experimentally observed synergy between ABT-737 and carboplatin is due to the increased dependence of DNA-damaged cells intracellular Bcl-xL.

Here, we develop a mathematical model of ovarian cancer xenograft growth to test the efficacy of combining ABT-737 and carboplatin for the treatment of ovarian cancers growing *in vivo*. While models of cancer therapy involving platinum-based compounds [15,16] or drugs targeting the Bcl-2 family [17,18] have been proposed, to the best of our knowledge this is the first attempt to model the effect of a combination of these drugs on tumor growth. We carefully account for the pharmacodynamics of both drugs. Further, since the active processing of administered drugs by the body may have a significant effect on their efficacy and how they interact, we also need to incorporate the pharmacokinetics of carboplatin and ABT-737 in our model. The model is parametrized using experimental data reported in [13], wherein monoclonal ovarian tumor xenografts established in mice were treated with fixed doses of carboplatin and ABT-737 administered periodically and time-courses of tumor growth inhibition recorded. The validated model is then used to identify dosing strategies for the treatment of monoclonal tumors, which either lead to fastest times to minimal residual disease or minimize total drug load to achieve a predetermined level of tumor growth inhibition. The infusion time of carboplatin doses is predicted to be an important determinant of the long-term response of tumors to therapy, this testable prediction underscoring the practical significance of our results.

As mentioned earlier, a major cause of long-term treatment failure in ovarian cancer patients is the emergence of carboplatin-resistance. Given its synergistic action with carboplatin, ABT-737 co-therapy has the potential to prevent or delay treatment failure. We investigate this potential in the case when resistance to carboplatin is driven by genetic or epigenetic aberrations. Such aberrations arise in two different ways. In *acquired resistance*, genetic mutations emerge after the administration of chemotherapy, as a result of a failure in DNA repair in cells treated with carboplatin. Alternatively, in *intrinsic resistance*, a small population of resistant cells may already be present before the administration of chemotherapy. By distinguishing between these alternative scenarios of drug resistance, our model represents a useful tool with which to design individualized treatment protocols targeted against carboplatin-resistance.

Results

Our model of ovarian cancer xenograft growth and its response to carboplatin and ABT-737 therapy can be described in mathematical terms by a coupled system of ordinary and partial differential equations (further details are included in the Section S1 in File S1), which govern the temporal dynamics of the following key variables: the numbers of proliferating and arrested cancer cells; the concentrations of carboplatin and ABT-737 in circulatory and cancer tissue/intracellular compartments; and the intracellular concentrations of two members of the Bcl-family (Bcl-xL and Bax). A schematic detailing the response of the cancer cells to therapy is shown in Figure 1A, while Figure 1B depicts intracellular reactions between ABT-737 and Bcl-family proteins.

We calibrate our model by fitting time-course tumor xenograft growth inhibition data taken from [13], wherein ovarian cancer (IGROV-1 cell) xengrafts were established in mice and treatment in the form of 30 mg/kg carboplatin administered weekly, or 100 mg/kg ABT-737 administered daily, or a combination of both, started 19 days post-transplantation. The results of these fits are plotted in Figure 1. Following model calibration, a series of numerical experiments are carried out to identify dosing strategies that exploit the synergy between carboplatin and ABT-737. Since our model formulation is based on experiments that studied the response of monoclonal xenografts to therapy, we start by considering a tumor that comprises a homogenous population of carboplatin-sensitive cells. A major aim of our model is to investigate the potential of co-treatment with ABT-737 to prevent or delay the onset of carboplatin-resistance that is a leading cause of treatment failure. We therefore also simulate the treatment of a tumor that consists of carboplatin-sensitive and -resistant cells. The emergence of resistance under two distinct scenarios is considered: (i) acquired resistance resulting from faulty DNA damage repair; and (ii) intrinsic resistance resulting from a pre-existing population of resistant cells.

Following [13], in all simulations carboplatin is assumed to be administered on a weekly schedule and ABT-737 on a daily schedule. When simulating monoclonal xenograft treatment, the initial number of tumor cells is calculated from the size of tumors at the initiation of therapy. As can be seen from the cell number time-courses in Figure 1D, the weekly administration of carboplatin induces oscillations in tumor size. Therefore, cell numbers averaged over the period of carboplatin administration (7 days) are used to make quantitative comparisons between tumor responses to various treatment strategies (see Figures 2–5). Tumors are assumed to have achieved a steady-state average size if the relative change in average tumor cell numbers between successive weeks is less than 0.001% and time to minimal residual disease (T_m) is defined as the period for which therapy must be administered so that the average number of cells is less than 1.

Optimal Relative Doses for Monoclonal Tumors

We consider the following optimization problem in the treatment of cancers with a combination of two or more drugs – "What drug doses achieve a predetermined level of cell kill while minimizing patient drug load?"

For illustrative purposes, we use our model to predict the optimal doses of carboplatin and ABT-737 required to achieve a 67% growth inhibition in monoclonal tumors at the end of 4 weeks of therapy (that is, the treatment time reported in [13]). Note that minimizing the drug load is equivalent to minimizing the Combination Index (CI) of the two drugs, defined as $CI_{67}=(C/C_{67})+(A/A_{67})$ [19], subject to the constraint that 4 weeks post-therapy, tumor size is 33% of its untreated value. Here, C_{67} and A_{67} are the amounts of drugs required to achieve a 67% growth inhibition when administered as single-agents, C is the weekly bolus dose of carboplatin and A is the daily bolus dose of ABT-737 when these drugs are used in combination. C is varied between 0 and C_{67}, and the constraint used to generate values of A. This represents an optimization problem for the function CI_{67} in a single variable C that assumes values on a closed and bounded interval and, hence, CI_{67} attains its minimum therein.

A phase diagram of the drug doses required to inhibit tumor growth by 67% after 4 weeks is shown in Figure 2A, with ABT-737 doses plotted along the abscissa and carboplatin doses plotted along the ordinate. CI_{67} values for various dose combinations are enumerated along the curve. A weekly bolus of 17.8 mg/kg carboplatin combined with a daily bolus dose of 86.5 mg/kg ABT-737 is predicted to minimize the CI_{67} (dashed lines). We remark that similar curves can be computed for other levels of tumor growth inhibition at the end of a fixed time period, and for other treatment strategies. The tumor cell time-course data corresponding to these optimal doses presented in Figure 2B reveal that the levels of tumor growth inhibition after 4 weeks of treatment with either 86.5 mg/kg ABT-737 administered as a single agent or 17.8 mg/kg carboplatin administered weekly as a single agent are 31.4% and 28.9% respectively. The predicted level of growth inhibition when these doses are combined is 67%.

Simulating treatment for periods longer than 4 weeks with drug doses fixed at the above values further underscores the synergy between the two drugs. Figure 2C shows that if the tumor is allowed to reach its (average) steady state size, the levels of tumor

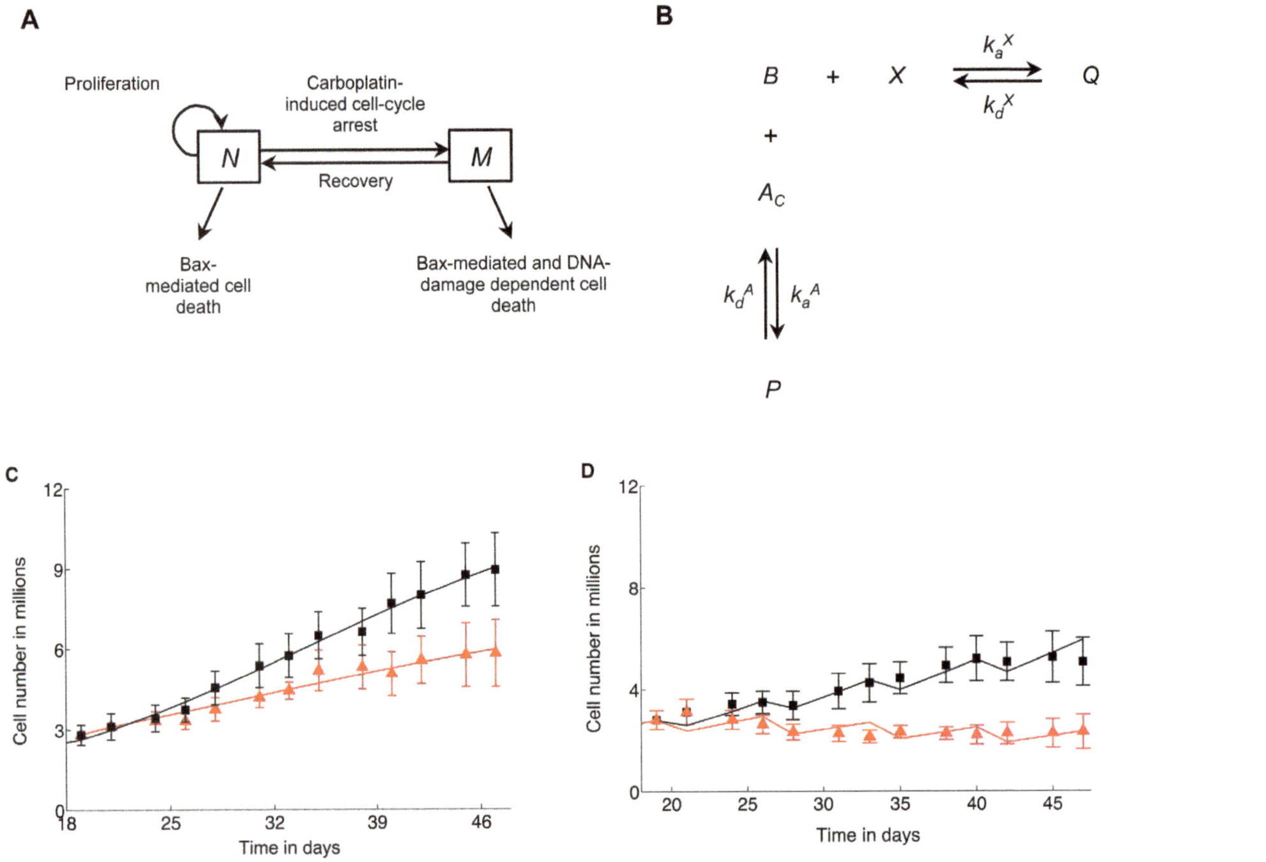

Figure 1. Model schematic and fits to experimental data. A, Model schematic. Ovarian cancer cells, $N(t)$ proliferate and undergo apoptosis at a rate dependent on intracellular Bax concentration. Administration of carboplatin induces DNA damage, leading to cell cycle arrest. Arrested cells, $M(t,a)$ subsequently undergo apoptosis at a rate proportional to the amount of DNA damage sustained at the time of arrest and on their intracellular Bax concentration, and may also recover to the proliferating population. The rates at which N and M undergo cell death are elevated on application of ABT-737, which leads to increased levels of intracellular Bax. **B**, Intracellular reaction diagram of the heterodimerization reaction between Bcl-xL (B) and Bax (X) molecules, and the inhibition of Bcl-xL by intracellular ABT-737 (A_C). **C, D**, Fit to time-course tumor xenograft growth inhibition data taken from [13]. Briefly, ovarian cancer (IGROV-1 cell) xengrafts were established in mice and treatment started 19 days post-transplantation. Levels of tumor growth inhibition were recorded periodically. Experimental data is represented by black squares and red triangles, while solid curves show best fits. Values represent mean and standard deviation (from experimental data). **C**, Weekly treatment with vehicle (black squares and curve) or daily treatment with 100 mg/kg of ABT-737 (red triangles and curve). **D**, Weekly treatment with 30 mg/kg carboplatin (black squares and curve) or a combination of carboplatin and ABT-737 (red triangles and curve).

growth inhibition decrease to 31.7% and 23.1% when ABT-737 or carboplatin are applied as monotherapy, respectively, whereas combination treatment results in a 79.2% tumor growth inhibition in the long term.

Optimal Dose Scheduling for Monoclonal Tumors

We next use our model to identify an optimal dose-delivery strategy when monoclonal tumors are treated with a combination of ABT-737 and carboplatin for long times. Following the experimental protocol in [13], the doses of carboplatin and ABT-737 are fixed at 30 mg/kg and 100 mg/kg, respectively. In particular, the dependence of tumor response on two key parameters, the carboplatin infusion time T_i, and the sensitivity ρ_s of arrested cells to changes in intracellular Bax, is investigated.

With ρ_s fixed at its baseline value ($\rho_s = 135$), steady-state values of average cell number are calculated as T_i varies between 0 hours (bolus dose) and 120 hours. Figure 3A reveals that minimal survival of tumor cells is predicted for $1 \le T_i \le 25$. If $T_i < 1$ hour, even though significant levels of long-term tumor growth inhibition can be achieved (see inset), complete remission is not possible. Additionally, for $T_i > 25$ hours, the level of growth inhibition decreases rapidly as T_i increases. In Figure 3B, we show how Tm, the length of time for which treatment must be administered in order to achieve minimal survival of tumor cells varies when $1 \le T_i \le 25$. As Ti increases from $T_i = 1, T_m$ decreases, attaining a minimum of 215 days when carboplatin is administered via weekly infusions lasting 8 hours, and then increases for larger values of T_i.

T_m depends not only on the carboplatin infusion time T_i, but also on ρ_s, the sensitivity of arrested cells to changes in intracellular Bax. For each value of ρ_s between 0 and 600, the minimum of T_m is calculated as T_i is varied between 0 and 120 hours. Figure 3C shows that this minimum decreases rapidly as ρ_s increases from $\rho_s = 0$, plateauing at a value of 215 days for large values of ρ_s. In all considered cases, T_m attains its minimum for $T_i = 8$ hours (data not shown).

Emergence of Acquired Resistance

We now investigate the potential of ABT-737 co-therapy to prevent or delay the emergence of carboplatin-resistance. Since

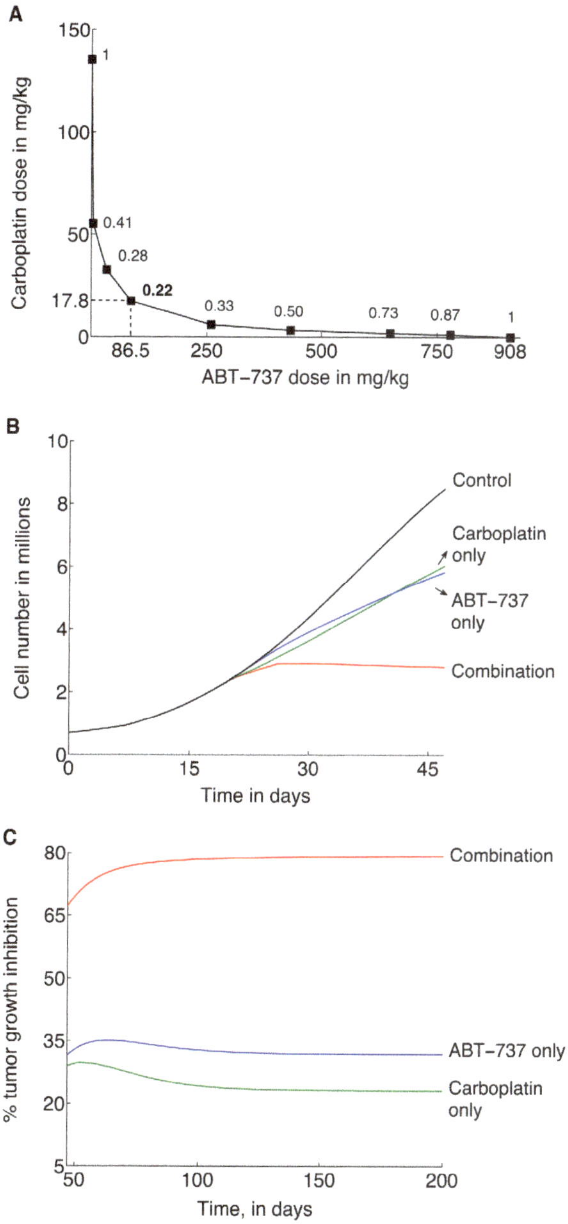

Figure 2. Optimizing carboplatin and ABT-737 doses when given in combination. A, Predicted Combination Index (CI) values computed for a desired tumor growth inhibition level of 67%, for various combinations of carboplatin and ABT-737. Following the experimental protocol in [13], treatment is initiated at 19 days post-transplantation and continued for 4 weeks. Simulations indicate that a combination of 17.8 mg/kg carboplatin given weekly combined with a daily dose of 86.5 mg/kg ABT-737 minimizes the CI and hence maximizes the synergy between the two drugs (dashed lines). **B**, Predicted tumor growth dynamics corresponding to the optimal dose combination found above. Plots show tumor cell numbers averaged over 7 days (the period of carboplatin administration) versus time. **C**, Predicted time-courses of tumor growth inhibition levels as compared to the control (no treatment) case, corresponding to the optimal dose combination found above.

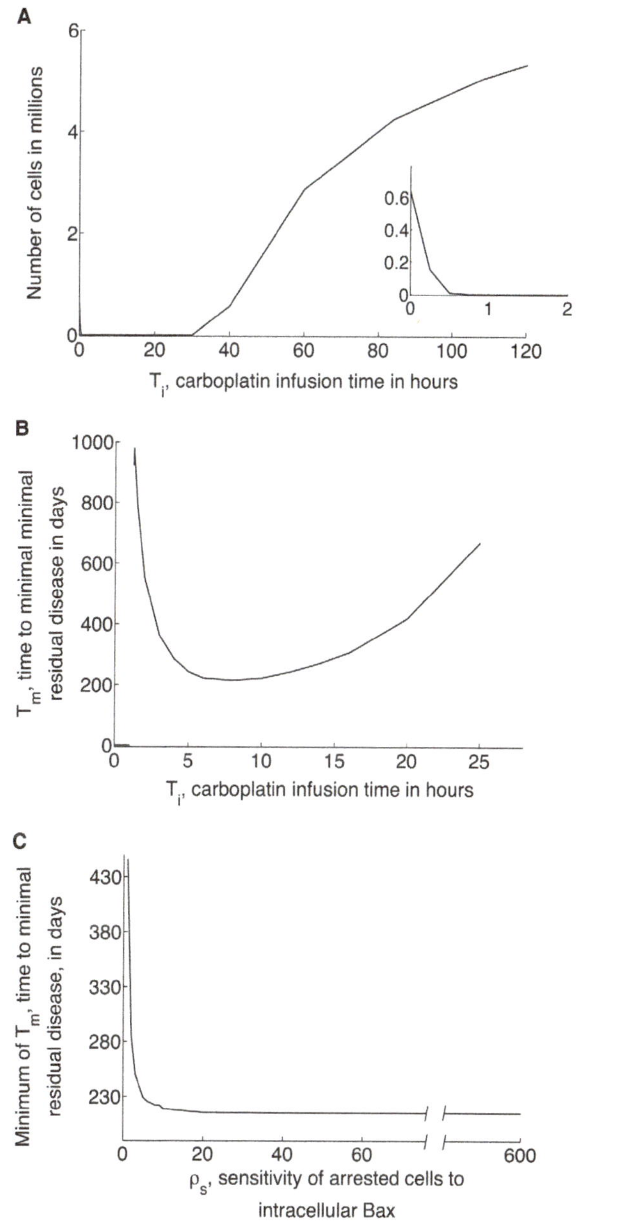

Figure 3. imulations showing long-term tumor xenograft response to combination therapy. Following the experimental protocol in [13], the administration of a weekly dose of 30 mg/kg carboplatin together with a daily dose of 100 mg/kg ABT-737 is simulated, and simulations allowed to run until tumor cell numbers averaged over 7 days (the period of carboplatin administration) achieve a steady-state. **A**, Predicted steady states of average tumor cell numbers as a function of carboplatin infusion time T_i. As T_i is increased from 0 hours (corresponding to a bolus dose) to 120 hours, the average tumor cell number steady-state decreases rapidly to <1 (see inset), and then increases, with minimal survival of tumor cells predicted for $1 \leq T_i \leq 25$. **B**, Predicted values of T_m, the length of time therapy must be administered to achieve minimal residual disease (defined as <1 cell remaining) as T_i is varied between 1 and 25 hours. A minimum value of $T_m = 215$ days is predicted for weekly carboplatin infusions lasting 8 hours. **C**, Minimum values of T_m are predicted to decrease to 215 days as ρ_s, the arrested cell sensitivity to intracellular Bax is increased. In all cases, a carboplatin infusion time of 8 hours minimized the cure time.

ovarian cancers are frequently diagnosed at a late stage [20], we simulate the application of therapy to tumors that have already attained their maximal untreated size (carrying capacity). As several carboplatin-sensitive and resistant ovarian cancer cell lines

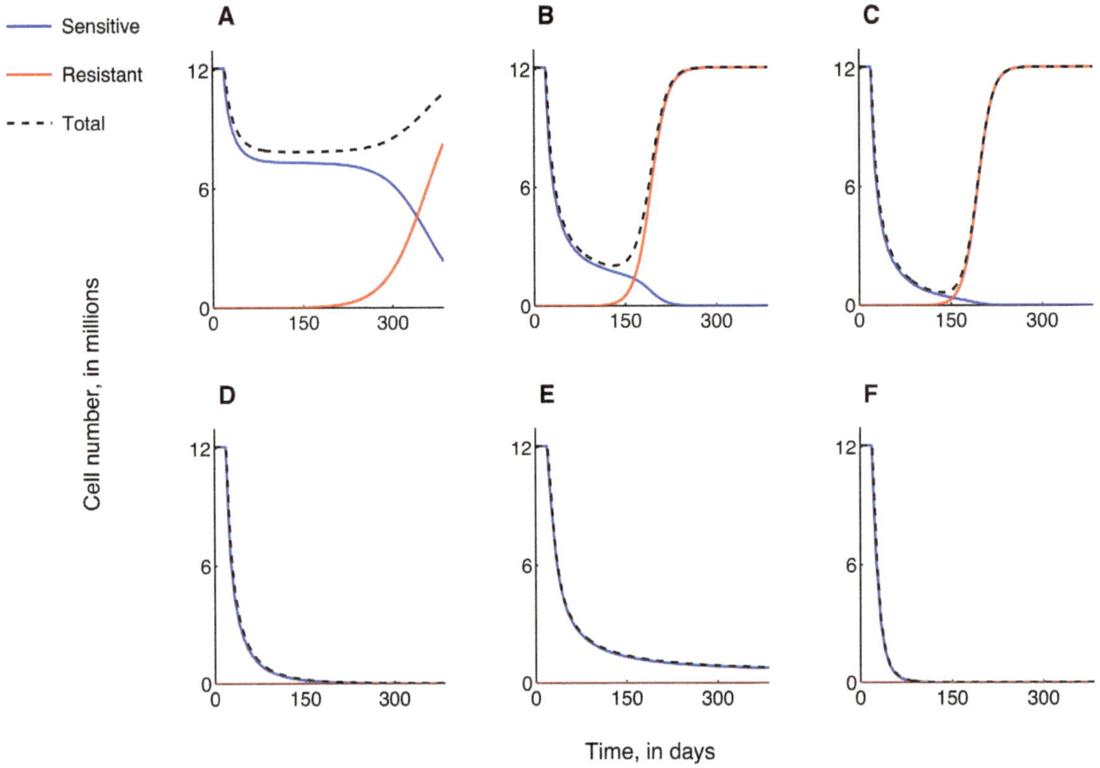

Figure 4. The emergence of acquired resistance to carboplatin therapy. DNA-mismatch repair in arrested cells recovering to the proliferating population is assumed to be the cause of resistance. The treatment of a late-stage tumor is simulated. Plots show 7 day-averages of carboplatin-sensitive (blue curve), carboplatin-resistant (red curve) and total (dashed black curve) tumor cell numbers versus time, as treatment strategy is varied. In all cases, therapy is administered for a period of 1 year. Increasing the weekly bolus dose of carboplatin administered as a single agent from **A**, 30 mg/kg, **B**, 300 mg/kg, to **C**, 800 mg/kg, cannot prevent the emergence of carboplatin-resistance. **D**, In fact, a weekly dose of 1300 mg/kg carboplatin is required to induce tumor regression. **E**, A combination of 30 mg/kg carboplatin delivered weekly as a bolus together with 100 mg/kg ABT-737 delivered daily is predicted to prevent the emergence of resistance and lead to tumor growth control at 6.5% of pre-treatment levels. **F**, The same combination dose, with carboplatin delivered via a 8-hour infusion is predicted to induce tumor regression within 150 days.

have been shown to have similar sensitivity to ABT-737 [13], carboplatin-sensitive and -resistant tumor cells are assumed to be equally sensitive to ABT-737 in our model.

We first assume that there is a small probability that cells recovering from a carboplatin-induced state of arrest experience DNA damage, resulting in a resistant phenotype. We assume further that no resistant cells exist at the start of treatment. Figure 4A–D shows predicted average cell number time-courses for a tumor treated with increasing weekly bolus doses of carboplatin only. A weekly dose of 1300 mg/kg is required to affect a cure and prevent the emergence of resistance (Figure 4D). Smaller doses result in transient decreases in tumor size, with the tumor eventually recovering to its untreated size (Figure 4A–C) due to the dominance of resistant cells. In contrast, Figure 4E reveals that a weekly bolus dose of 30 mg/kg carboplatin combined with a daily dose of 100 mg/kg ABT-737 may prevent the onset of carboplatin-resistance and result in tumor-growth control at 6.5% of its untreated level at steady-states. Significantly, the same combination, with carboplatin administered as an 8-hour infusion instead of as a bolus, is predicted to result in tumor remission within 150 days of treatment (Figure 4F).

Optimal Dose Scheduling for Monoclonal Tumors

Finally, we consider the response of a tumor which contains a small population of carboplatin-resistant cells at the start of treatment. Figure 5A–C shows predicted average cell number time-courses when the tumor is treated with increasing weekly bolus doses of carboplatin alone. Now, even doses in excess of 1300 mg/kg (Figure 5C) are unable to induce sustained tumor regression. Further, in contrast to the case of acquired resistance, a weekly bolus dose of 30 mg/kg carboplatin combined with a daily dose of 100 mg/kg ABT-737 is unable to prevent the onset of carboplatin-resistance (Figure 5D), with the tumor recovering to 65.2% of its untreated size after a transient decline in cell numbers. Figure 5E shows that administering carboplatin as an 8-hour infusion results in the tumor reaching a much lower minimum at around day 150 of treatment, indicating a possible period of disease-free survival, defined as clinically undetectable disease. However, resistant cells eventually dominate and the tumor escapes from therapy-induced growth control. Increasing the daily ABT-737 dosage to 500 mg/kg in combination with 30 mg/kg carboplatin given as a 8-hour infusion is predicted to increase the disease-free survival time, and lead to a greater level of long-term growth control (Figure 5F).

Discussion

The development of carboplatin-resistance is a major factor hampering the successful treatment of ovarian cancer with standard chemotherapy (carboplatin+paclitaxel). This resistance may be mediated in part by members of the Bcl-2 family that regulate cellular apoptosis. Consequently, it has recently been

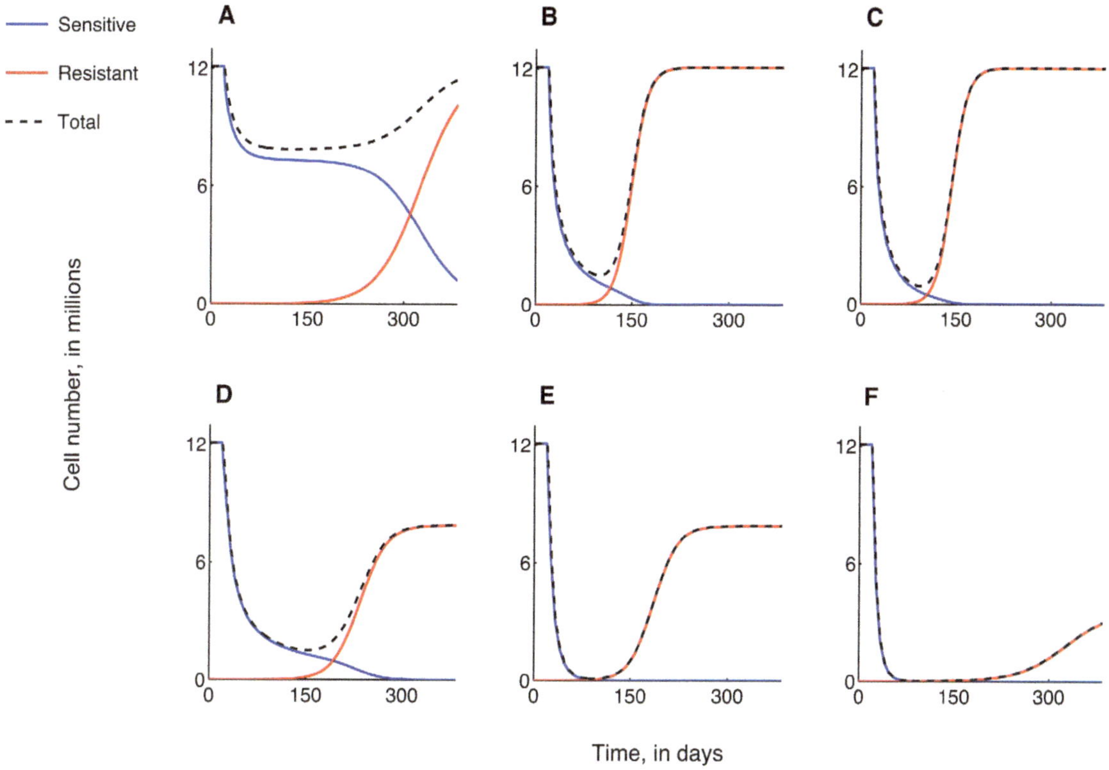

Figure 5. Intrinsic resistance to carboplatin therapy. A small fraction (1 in 60,000) of carboplatin-resistant cells is assumed to be present prior to treatment initiation. The treatment of a late-stage tumor is simulated. Plots show 7 day-averages of carboplatin-sensitive (blue curve), carboplatin-resistant (red curve) and total (dashed black curve) tumor cell numbers versus time, as treatment strategy is varied. In all cases, therapy is administered for a period of 1 year. Increasing the weekly bolus dose of carboplatin administered as a single agent from **A**, 30 mg/kg, **B**, 600 mg/kg, to **C**, 1300 mg/kg, cannot prevent the onset of carboplatin-resistance, with overall tumor size returning to pre-treatment levels eventually. **D, E, F**, In fact, a combination therapy of 30 mg/kg carboplatin delivered weekly as a bolus (**D**) or via 8-hour infusion (**E, F**) together ABT-737 delivered daily at a dose of 100 mg/kg (**D, E**) or 500 mg/kg (**F**) is also unable to prevent the emergence of resistance. However, combination therapy is predicted to result in partial tumor growth control, with a steady-state tumor size reaching 65.2% of pre-treatment levels for a combination of 30 mg/kg carboplatin and 100 mg/kg ABT-737 (**D, E**). Increasing ABT-737 dosage to 500 mg/kg is predicted to induce extended periods of disease-free survival, as evidenced by a dip in the total tumor size graph (**F**).

proposed [13] that inhibiting anti-apoptotic proteins such as Bcl-xL may improve the efficacy of carboplatin. A critical challenge in the development of such novel therapeutics is to arrive at treatment strategies that maximally exploit any synergy between the drugs, and to identify patients who might benefit from such a combination.

In this article, we have presented a mathematical model of the growth of an ovarian cancer xenograft and its treatment with carboplatin, and ABT-737, a small molecule inhibitor of Bcl-xL. The main goal of this research was to identify protocols for the treatment of ovarian cancer *in vivo* that exploit the molecular basis of synergy between the two drugs. To this end, we explicitly incorporated the intracellular regulation of apoptosis by the Bcl-2 family of proteins, and introduced a cell-age structured model to simulate the effect of carboplatin on cell fate. Further, to reflect the *in vivo* setting, detailed pharmacokinetics of carboplatin and ABT-737 were also included. The model was validated by fitting time-courses of ovarian cancer xenograft growth inhibition reported in [13]. The good agreement between model simulations and experimental data give confidence that the model is able accurately to describe the underlying biology.

We first simulated the treatment of tumors that consist of a monoclonal population of cells. Doses of carboplatin and ABT-737 required for a certain level of tumor growth inhibition were calculated, which minimize patient drug load and hence maximize the synergy between the two drugs. The method we describe here can in principle be applied to any drug combination and can easily be tailored to account for side effects of the drugs under evaluation, once appropriate data is available to support the model. Using our approach, physicians can estimate the impact of different doses of drugs in combination on the therapeutic response of patients. As combination therapies are increasingly being applied in oncology, models such as the one we present here can lead to significant time and cost savings by minimizing the choices that need to be examined experimentally. Further, such modeling can also be used to arrive at optimal individualized treatment strategies for evaluating combinations of chemotherapeutic drugs in clinical trials.

An equally important application of the model is predicting the long-term response to therapy. An exhaustive search of parameter space revealed a control parameter that is predicted to be a critical determinant of tumor growth dynamics when prolonged administration of carboplatin and ABT-737 co-therapy is simulated. This is the infusion time of the weekly dose of carboplatin. Carboplatin is typically administered as an infusion lasting 15 minutes or more when given in combination with paclitaxel. In fact, it has been proposed that the efficacy of carboplatin is directly linked to its AUC (Area Under the Curve) value, and the Calvert formula currently used to determine its clinical doses makes use of this fact [21]. However, our model simulations suggest that when combined with ABT-737, the efficacy of combination therapy is determined not only by the AUC of carboplatin, but also by the duration of drug infusion. Our simulations predict that weekly carboplatin infusions lasting between 1 and 25 hours combined with daily doses of ABT-737 result in the minimal survival of tumor cells. This is because, when administered as a rapid infusion, the peak tissue concentration of carboplatin is high, and a high level of DNA damage is induced in cancer cells from which they are unlikely to recover, irrespective of changes in intracellular Bcl-xL levels. Consequently, the synergy between the carboplatin and ABT-737 is muted. Equally, slower infusions of carboplatin result in extremely low tissue concentrations of the drug, so that the level of DNA damage induced in cells is minimal, and even with inhibited Bcl-xL levels, arrested cells are likely to recover to the proliferating pool. Note that since ABT-737 was simulated to be administered daily and has a slow clearance rate, its intracellular concentration rapidly achieves a non-zero mean (see Figure S2D). Therefore, changing the infusion time of ABT-737 administration is not predicted to alter our predictions.

Further, numerical simulations were carried out to identify the carboplatin infusion time that results in the fastest time to minimal residual disease. These times were observed to decrease rapidly to a minimum value as the sensitivity of arrested cells to intracellular Bax concentration (ρ_s) was increased. The parameter ρ_s is a quantitative measure of the synergy between the carboplatin and ABT-737 and can be important in identifying a subclass of patients who would most benefit from such a combination of drugs. However, ?s cannot be directly measured from experiments. As demonstrated here, we can infer its value by fitting model simulations to tumor xenograft growth inhibition data when both drugs are given in combination.

ABT-737 co-therapy is now being developed to improve the efficacy of carboplatin, and may aid in delaying the onset of chemoresistance in ovarian cancers. We therefore investigated the therapeutic potential of combinations of ABT-737 and carboplatin to treat ovarian cancers in which carboplatin-resistance arises in two distinct scenarios. Genetic mutations leading to resistance may be acquired as a result of faulty DNA damage repair when cells try to recover from carboplatin administration. Carboplatin-resistance may also be an intrinsic property of the cancer, stemming from resistant cells present when treatment starts. A key strength of our approach is the ability to distinguish between these scenarios. For instance, in the case of acquired resistance, model simulations predicted that preventing cells that have undergone carboplatin-induced DNA-damage from recovering and returning to the proliferating population precludes the emergence of resistance. However, the amount of carboplatin required to achieve this as a single-agent may be toxic for the host and thus not feasible. In contrast, combination therapy at low doses, with carboplatin administered optimally as described earlier, is sufficient to prevent the onset of resistance. When resistance to carboplatin is intrinsic, tumor remission is no longer feasible, but our model can be applied to identify dosing strategies that extend periods of disease-free survival. It has been proposed that the development of chemoresistance may result from insufficient exposure of tumor cells to drugs [22], and our simulations further accentuate the dangers of under-treatment.

The model presented in this article has the potential to accelerate the translation from bench-to-bedside of novel therapeutics such as ABT-737, and to reduce the costs associated with drug development. However, the eventual clinical application of our model will require the validation of its predictions with further experiments. For instance, tumor xenograft growth inhibition experiments with varying doses of carboplatin and ABT-737 alone, and in combination would be extremely helpful in fine-tuning the functional responses of cancer cells to therapy. Measuring the relative constitutive expression levels of the Bcl-2 family would improve the accuracy of the quantitative description of the ABT-737-targeted intracellular apoptosis pathway. Detailed pharmacokinetic studies of ABT-737, which include the temporal dynamics of its intracellular concentration, would help in a better parameterization of our model. Finally, experimentally validating our model predictions relating to the optimal time of infusion of carboplatin when co-administered with ABT-737 could constitute a significant breakthrough in the treatment of ovarian cancers, and solid tumors in general.

A limitation of our approach is that while we have incorporated carboplatin-resistance by simulating a completely resistant cell line, in practice a human tumor may contains many different populations of cells with varying levels of resistance to carboplatin, and sensitivities to ABT-737. Further, resistance to therapy can arise from multiple mechanisms. Consequently, in future versions of our model we will incorporate a greater diversity of cellular phenotypes. We also plan to include the administration of paclitaxel as a third drug in the combination chemotherapy of ovarian cancers, and replace ABT-737 with ABT-263, its orally available analogue currently under phase I clinical trials for the treatment of a number of solid tumors [23,24].

Finally, the work presented here illustrates how mathematical modeling has the potential to support the preclinical and clinical development of novel cancer therapeutics. There are numerous parameters that affect the outcome of drug evaluation, and it may not be feasible to address all of these experimentally. Quantitative modeling represents a powerful resource to optimize the likelihood of the successful development of targeted therapies.

Materials and Methods

Model Foundation

our model of ovarian cancer xenograft growth and treatment consists of a coupled system of ordinary and partial differential equations (full model equations are listed in section S1 in File S1), which govern the temporal dynamics of the following key variables: N(t) and M(t,a), the numbers of proliferating and arrested cancer cells (in millions) respectively; $C_{perit}(t)$, $C_P(t)$ and $C_T(t)$, the concentrations in μM of intraperitoneal, plasma and tissue carboplatin respectively; $A_{perit}(t)$, $A_P(t)$ and $A_C(t)$, the concentrations in nM of intraperitoneal, plasma and intracellular ABT-737 respectively; and $B(t)$, $X(t)$, $Q(t)$ and $P(t)$, the intracellular concentrations in nM of Bcl-xL, Bax, Bcl-xLBax complex and Bcl-xLABT-737 complex respectively. Here, time t is measured in days, and a is a time-like variable, representing the period of time a cell has spent in a growth-arrested state. A schematic detailing the response of the cancer cells to therapy is shown in Figure 1A. In the sections that follow, the principles underlying our model formulation are introduced.

Dynamics of Proliferating Cells

Equation A models the growth of proliferating ovarian cancer cells, $N(t)$.

Equation A :

$$\frac{dN}{dt} = \lambda_N N\left(1 - \frac{T}{K}\right) - \delta_N(X)N - \alpha_C(C_T)N + M(t,a=a_r).$$

The growth rate of untreated tumor xenografts is typically exponential at early times, and plateaus as they become larger [25]. Consequently, we assume that ovarian cancer cells grow logistically in the absence of treatment, with growth rate λ_N and carrying capacity K. We remark that models of periodic chemotherapy based on the logistic equation have been proposed previously [26–29]. Arrested cells ($M(t,a)$) are assumed to compete for space with proliferating cells so that $T(t)$ is the total (proliferating+arrested) number of cancer cells at time t. The parameters λ_N and K are chosen by fitting time-courses of cell numbers to data from untreated tumor xenografts in [13], as shown in Figure 1C (black curve).

We account for the regulation of cell death by the Bcl-2 family of proteins in the following way. For simplicity, and in the absence of appropriate experimental data, we represent each of the pro- and anti-apoptotic sub-families of the Bcl-2 family by single variables. Given the specificity of ABT-737 for Bcl-2 and Bcl-xL, and its similar binding affinity for both these molecules [30], we represent the anti-apoptotic members of the Bcl-2 family by Bcl-xL. Further, Bax is taken to represent the pro-apoptotic proteins since it is the members of the Bax-like subfamily which controls the release of cytochrome c from the mitochondria that leads to caspase activation, that is followed by cell death [7]. The rate of cell death $\delta_N(X)$ is consequently assumed to be an increasing function of free intracellular Bax ($X(t)$).

Pharmacologic therapy is applied periodically in the form of ABT-737 or carboplatin, alone or in combination. ABT-737 increases the rate of cell death δ_N, while carboplatin induces DNA damage and subsequent cell arrest at a rate $\alpha_C(C_T)$, which depends on tissue carboplatin concentration $C_T(t)$. The final term in Equation A represents the rate at which arrested cells recover and return to the proliferating pool.

We now describe the effect on the growing tumor of the application of carboplatin and ABT-737.

Effect of ABT-737 on Proliferating Cells. Upon application, ABT-737 enters the proliferating tumor cells where it binds to, and occupies Bcl-xL (see Figure 1B). This results in a build-up of free Bax that was previously sequestered in the form of Bcl-xLBax heterodimers, thereby increasing the rate of cell death. Parameters relating to the death rate δ_N of proliferating cells are chosen by fitting time-courses of estimated cell numbers to tumor xenograft growth inhibition data taken from [13], wherein IGROV-1 xenografts established in mice were treated daily with a fixed dose of ABT-737 administered intraperitoneally for 4 weeks. The best fit is shown in Figure 1C (red curve). The reaction diagram in Figure 1B representing ABT-737 pharmacodynamics is translated into a system of ordinary differential equations using the principle of mass balance.

Effect of Carboplatin on Proliferating Cells. The cytotoxicity of carboplatin is primarily due to damage induced by the formation of intra- and interstrand adducts at the nucleophilic N7 sites in the DNA. This damage stimulates the activation of downstream pathways that lead to cell cycle arrest, followed by either survival if the DNA damage is repairable, or apoptosis [6]. Consequently, upon drug application, proliferating cells are assumed to undergo cell cycle arrest at a rate α_C that is assumed to be an increasing and saturating function of the tissue carboplatin concentration, $C_T(t)$, so that as the drug dose (and correspondingly the level of DNA damage) increases, the rate of cell cycle arrest also increases up to a maximum level.

An Age-structured Model of Arrested Cell Dynamics

The arrested cells are removed to a separate compartment, where they either undergo apoptosis or recover and return to the proliferating population (a schematic is shown in Figure 1A). In [13], the initiation of apoptosis was routinely observed in cells 12–16 hours post carboplatin administration. Consequently, arrested cell dynamics are described by the following partial differential equation derived by applying the general McKendrick equation that is widely used to model age-structured populations [31].

$$\text{Equation A}: \quad \frac{\partial M}{\partial t}+\frac{\partial M}{\partial a}=-\delta_M(C_T(t-a,X(t),a)M.$$

Here the rate of arrested cell death δ_M is taken to be a function of the time a for which the cells have been arrested. Cell cytotoxicity has been found to correlate linearly with the amount of platinum bound to the DNA, and hence the extent of DNA damage [6]. Accordingly, the rate of arrested cell death is taken to be linearly proportional to $C_T(t-a)$, the amount of tissue carboplatin at the time of cell-cycle arrest. Next, as in the case of proliferating cells, when ABT-737 is co-administered with carboplatin, it is taken up by the arrested cells where it binds to, and occupies Bcl-xL (see Figure 1B), causing a build-up of free Bax, $X(t)$. Further, in [14] the observed synergy between carboplatin and ABT-737 was shown to be due to an increased dependence of DNA-damaged cells on Bcl-xL for survival. Accordingly, the rate of arrested cell death δ_M is taken also to be proportional (with constant of proportionality ρ_s) to $X(t)$. ρ_s is an important parameter in our model: it represents the sensitivity of the arrested cells to changes in Bax, and hence provides a quantitative measure of the degree of synergy between carboplatin and ABT-737. Equation B is solved subject to the boundary condition:

$$M(t,0)=\alpha_C(C_T)N,$$

which represents the rate of cell arrest (see Equation A). Finally, the length of time for which a cell can remain in an arrested state is limited. We therefore assume that cells that have not undergone apoptosis after a characteristic time $a_r=48$ hours recover and return to the proliferating population, this return being instantaneous so that $M(t,a)=0$ for $a>a_r$. Additionally, the number of arrested cells at time t is given by $\int_{t-a_r}^{t} M(t,a)da$.

Parameters relating to the rate at which proliferating cells become growth arrested α_C and the rate at which arrested cells die δ_M are chosen by fitting time-courses of estimated numbers of cells to tumor xenograft growth inhibition data taken from [13], wherein IGROV-1 xenografts established in mice were treated weekly with a fixed dose of carboplatin administered intravenously for 4 weeks as a single agent, or in combination with a fixed daily dose of ABT-737. The best fits are shown in Figure 1D.

The functional forms used in our model for the response of proliferating and arrested cells to carboplatin and ABT-737 also account for their pharmacokinetics, which are described below.

Carboplatin Pharmacokinetics

Carboplatin was administered intraperitoneally on a weekly schedule in [13] and its pharmacokinetics are assumed to be governed by the following 3-comparment model. Experimental evidence suggests that small molecular weight drugs (molecular weight of carboplatin = 371.2 Da [32]) delivered intraperitoneally are readily absorbed through the peritoneal vasculature to enter systemic circulation [33,34]. Consequently, the peritoneal cavity is taken to be the first compartment. Since the time-activity curve of carboplatin in the blood plasma of mice has been shown to be biphasic [32], the circulatory system together with highly vascularized and well-perfused organs are taken to be the second or central compartment, and the peripheral organs and tissues with relatively poor vascular perfusion account for the third compartment. As tumor vasculature is characterized by its poor functional quality, and is highly disorganized [35], we assume that the tumor resides in the peripheral pharmacokinetic compartment of carboplatin. Details regarding carboplatin pharmacokinetics and pharmacodynamics are provided in section S3 in File S1 and Figure S2. Related parameter values are provided in Table S3.

We investigate the effect on tumor response of administering the same dose of carboplatin as either a rapid infusion or bolus, or a continuous infusion lasting several hours, when given in combination with ABT-737. In fact, the time of infusion (T_i) of each dose of carboplatin is predicted to be a critical parameter in determining the therapeutic efficacy of combination therapy.

ABT-737 Pharmacokinetics

ABT-737 was administered intraperitoneally on a daily schedule in [13] and its pharmacokinetics are assumed to be governed by the following 3-comparment model. Since ABT-737 is a low molecular weight drug (molecular weight = 813.4 Da [24]), as in the case of carboplatin, the peritoneal cavity is taken as the first compartment, and the systemic circulation as the central (and second) compartment. In our model, we explicitly account for the regulation of cell death by the Bcl-2 family of proteins. Therefore, a third intracellular compartment, into which the drug permeates from the systemic circulation, is included. Details regarding ABT-737 pharmacokinetics and the intracellular regulation of cell death are provided in section S2 in File S1 and Figure S1. Related parameter values are provided in Tables S1 and S2.

We remark that given that the circulation half-life of ABT-737 is several hours (see File S1), administering it daily ensures that carboplatin-arrested cells are exposed to it, irrespective of the time of cell arrest.

The emergence of carboplatin-resistance. When considering the emergence of resistance to carboplatin, the proliferating cell population is subdivided into two classes - carboplatin-sensitive and carboplatin-resistant. Following [13] where ovarian cancer cell lines with different sensitivities to carboplatin were observed to be comparably responsive to ABT-737, both carboplatin-sensitive and resistant cells are assumed to be equally sensitive to ABT-737.

Model Parametrization and Simulation

Details of parameter estimation described in this section, and a list of parameter values can be found in section S5 in File S1 and Table S4. All model simulations are carried out in Matlab, a technical computing language, the numerical methods being described in Section S4 of the supplemental File S1. Figure S3 shows typical model simulations. A sensitivity analysis on the estimated parameter values can be found in Figure S4 and section S5 of the supplemental File S1.

Supporting Information

Figure S1 ABT-737 pharmacokinetics in a mouse. A, ABT-737 is periodically administered intraperitoneally (i.p.), into the peritoneal cavity from where it enters the systemic circulation. From here, ABT-737 enters the intracellular compartment, and is also cleared from the body. Figures showing **B**, intraperitoneal, **C**, plasma and **D**, intracellular ABT-737 concentration time-courses when 100 mg/kg of the drug is administered daily starting on day 5. **E**, Resultant intracellular Bcl-xL (black curve) and Bax (red curve) concentration time-courses.

Figure S2 Carboplatin pharmacokinetics in a mouse. A, Carboplatin is periodically administered intraperitoneally (i.p.), into the peritoneal cavity from where it enters the systemic circulation. From here, carboplatin is distributed to peripheral organs and tissues with poor vascular perfusion, and is also cleared from the body. Figures showing plasma (black curve) and peripheral tissue (red curve) carboplatin concentration time-courses corresponding to a dose of 30 mg/kg, given **B**, as a bolus, or **C**, as a continuous infusion lasting 12 hours.

Figure S3 Tumor xenograft response to 30 mg/kg of carboplatin-only therapy. Carboplatin administration as a bolus dose every 7 days, starting on day 19 (black arrow) is simulated. Figure shows total cell number (red curve) and total cell number averaged over the period of therapy administration (black curve) versus time.

Figure S4 Parameter sensitivity analysis. A–E, Model sensitivity to key parameters. Variation of the parameters from their baseline values is plotted on the x-axis. The % change in the Euclidean norm of the error over its value from performing fits of the model to experimental data (see Figures 1B,C in main manuscript) is plotted on the y-axis. **F**, Predicted average total (black curve), proliferating (red curve) and growth arrested (blue curve) tumor cell numbers at the end of 4 weeks of treatment of a tumor xenograft with 30 mg/kg carboplatin administered weekly, as the time of infusion of each dose is varied.

File S1 Supplementary Information. Section S1: Model Equations. Section S2: ABT-737 Pharmacokinetics and the Intracellular Regulation of Cell Death. Section S3: Carboplatin Pharmacokinetics. Section S4: Simulation Methodology. Section S5: Parameter Estimation for Monoclonal Tumor Xenograft Growth Treatment.

Table S1 List of parameter values relating to ABT-737 pharmacokinetics and pharmacodynamics.

Table S2 List of non-dimensional parameter values relating to ABT-737 pharmacokinetics and pharmacodynamics.

Table S3 List of parameter values relating to carboplatin pharmacokinetics.

Table S4 List of parameter values relating to xenograft growth and treatment.

Acknowledgments

The authors thank Dr. Marisa Eisenberg and Dr. Paul Hurtado for many helpful discussions.

Author Contributions

Conceived and designed the experiments: HVJ AR MM HMB. Performed the experiments: AR. Analyzed the data: HVJ MM HMB. Wrote the paper: HVJ AR MM HMB.

References

1. Evans MA, Evans P (2009) Ovarian cancer: an overview. Am Fam Physician 80: 609–616.
2. Bookmans MA (2010) The addition of new drugs to standard therapy in the first-line treatment of ovarian cancer. Ann Oncol 21: vii211–vii217.
3. Vasey PA (2003) Resistance to chemotherapy in advanced ovarian cancer: mechanisms and current strategies. Br J Cancer 89(Suppl 3): S23–S28.
4. Bukowski RM, Ozols RF, Markman M (2007) The management of recurrent ovarian cancer. Semin Oncol 34: S1–S15.
5. Galluzzi L, Senovilla L, Vitale I, Michels J, Martins I, et al. (2012) Molecular mechanisms of cisplatin resistance. Oncogene 31: 1869–1883.
6. Siddik ZH (2003) Cisplatin: mode of cytotoxic action and molecular basis of resistance. Oncogene 22: 7265–7279.
7. Adams JM, Cory S (2007) The Bcl-2 apoptotic switch in cancer development and therapy. Oncogene 26: 1324–1337.
8. Liu JR, Fletcher B, Page C, Hu C, Nunez G, et al. (1998) Bcl-xL is expressed in ovarian carcinoma and modulates chemotherapy-induced apoptosis. Gynecol Oncol 70: 398–403.
9. Minn AJ, Rudin CM, Boise LH, Thompson CB (1995) Expression of Bcl-xL can confer a multidrug resistance phenotype. Blood 86: 1903–1910.
10. Williams J, Lucas PC, Griffith KA, Choia M, Fogorosa S, et al. (2005) Expression of Bcl-xL in ovarian carcinoma is associated with chemoresistance and recurrent disease. Gynecol Oncol 96: 287–295.
11. Brotin E, Meryet-Figuière M, Simonin K, Duval RE, Villedieu M, et al. (2010) Bcl-xl and MCL-1 constitute pertinent targets in ovarian carcinoma and their concomitant inhibition is sufficient to induce apoptosis. Int J Cancer 126: 885–895.
12. Villedieu M, Louis MH, Dutoit S, aand H Lincet EB, Duigou F, et al. (2007) Absence of Bcl-xL down-regulation in response to cisplatin is associated with chemoresistance in ovarian carcinoma cells. Gynecol Oncol 126: 31–44.
13. Witham J, Valenti MR, De-Haven-Brandon AK, Vidot S, Eccles SA, et al. (2007) The Bcl-2/Bcl- xL family inhibitor ABT-737 sensitizes ovarian cancer cells to carboplatin. Clin Cancer Res 13: 7191–7198.
14. Jain HV, Meyer-Hermann M (2011) The molecular basis of synergism between carboplatin and ABT-737 therapy targeting ovarian carcinomas. Cancer Res 71: 705–715.
15. El-Kareh AW, Labes RE, Secomb TW (2008) Cell cycle checkpoint models for cellular pharmacology of paclitaxel and platinum drugs. AAPS J 10: 15–34.
16. El-Kareh AW, Secomb TW (2003) A mathematical model for cisplatin cellular pharmacodynamics. Neoplasia 5: 161–169.
17. Jain HV, Nor JE, Jackson TL (2009) Quantification of endothelial cell-targeted anti-Bcl-2 therapy and its suppression of tumor growth and vascularization. Mol Cancer Ther 8: 2926–2936.
18. Jain HV, Nor JE, Jackson TL (2008) Modeling the VEGF-Bcl-2-CXCL8 pathway in intratumoral angiogenesis. Bull Math Biol 70: 89–117.
19. Chou TC, Talalay P (1984) Quantitative analysis of dose-effect relationships: the combined effects of multiple drugs or enzyme inhibitors. Adv Enzyme Regul 22: 27–55.
20. Despierre E, Lambrechts D, Neven P, Amant F, Lambrechts S, et al. (2010) The molecular genetic basis of ovarian cancer and its roadmap towards a better treatment. Gynecol Oncol 117: 358–365.
21. Calvert AH, Newell DR, Gumbrell LA, O'Reilly S, Burnell M, et al. (1989) Carboplatin dosage: prospective evaluation of a simple formula based on renal function. J Clin Oncol 7: 1748–1756.
22. Tan DSP, Ang JE, Kaye SB (2008) Ovarian cancer: can we reverse drug resistance? Adv Exp Med Biol 622: 153–167.
23. Gandhi L, Camidge DR, de Oliveira MR, Bonomi P, Gandara D, et al. (2011) Phase I study of Navitoclax (ABT-263), a novel Bcl-2 family inhibitor, in patients with small-cell lung cancer and other solid tumors. J Clin Oncol 29: 909–916.
24. Stamelos VA, Robinsona E, Redmanc CW, Richardson A (2013) Navitoclax augments the activity of carboplatin and paclitaxel combinations in ovarian cancer cells. Gynecol Oncol 128: 377–382.
25. Bonate PL (2011) Modeling tumor growth in oncology. In: Bonate PL, Howard DR, editors, Pharmacokinetics in drug development, New York: Springer Verlag, volume 3. pp. 1–11.
26. Panetta JC (1995) A logistic model of periodic chemotherapy. Appl Math Lett 8: 83–86.
27. Panetta JC, Adam J (1995) A mathematical model of cycle-specific chemotherapy. Math Comput Model 22: 67–82.
28. Panetta JC (1997) A logistic model of periodic chemotherapy with drug resistance. Appl Math Lett 10: 123–127.
29. Jain HV, Byrne HM (2012) Qualitative analysis of an integro-differential equation model of periodic chemotherapy. Appl Math Lett 25: 2132–2136.
30. Whitecross KF, Alsop AE, Cluse LA, Wiegmans A, Banks KM, et al. (2009) Defining the target specificity of ABT-737 and synergistic antitumor activities in combination with histone deacetylase inhibitors. Blood 113: 1982–1991.
31. Keyfitz BL, Keyfitz N (1997) The mckendrick partial differential equation and its uses in epidemiological studies. Math Comput Modell 26: 1–9.
32. Siddik ZH, Newell DR, Boxall FE, Harrap KR (1987) The comparative pharmacokinetics of carboplatin and cisplatin in mice and rats. Biochem Pharmacol 36: 1925–1932.
33. Bajaj G, Yeo Y (2010) Drug delivery systems for intraperitoneal therapy. Pharm Res 27: 735–738.
34. Lukas G, Brindle SD, Greengard P (1971) The route of absorption of intraperitoneally administered compounds. J Pharmacol Exp Ther 178: 562–566.
35. Siemann DW (2011) The unique characteristics of tumor vasculature and preclinical evidence for its selective disruption by Tumor-Vascular Disrupting Agents. Cancer Treat Rev 37: 63–74.

14

Tim-3 Expression Defines Regulatory T Cells in Human Tumors

Jing Yan[1], Yi Zhang[2], Jing-Ping Zhang[1], Jing Liang[2], Lian Li[2], Limin Zheng[1,2]*

1 State Key Laboratory of Oncology in South China, Sun Yat-sen University Cancer Center, Guangzhou, P. R. China, **2** State Key Laboratory of Biocontrol, School of Life Sciences, Sun Yat-sen University, Guangzhou, P. R. China

Abstract

Tim-3, a member of the novel Tim (T cell immunoglobulin and mucin domain) family, has been reported to negatively regulate the immune responses against viral infection and had implications for autoimmune disease. However, the nature and role of Tim-3$^+$ CD4 T cells in human tumors remain largely unknown. In the present study, we characterized Tim-3$^+$ CD4 T cells in 100 specimens from human hepatocellular, cervical, colorectal and ovarian carcinoma patients. Compared with peripheral blood and nontumor-infiltrating lymphocytes, the lymphocytes isolated from the corresponding tumor tissues of hepatocellular, cervical, colorectal and ovarian carcinoma patients contained significantly greater proportion of Tim-3$^+$ CD4 T cells. The majority of tumor-derived Tim-3$^+$ CD4 T cells exhibited an impaired capacity to produce IFN-γ and IL-2, but expressed higher levels of CD25, Foxp3, CTLA-4 and GITR than their Tim-3$^-$ CD4 T cell counterparts. In contrast, most Tim-3$^+$ CD4 T cells isolated from the paired nontumor tissues and peripheral blood did not express these molecules. Moreover, tumor-derived Tim-3$^+$ CD4 T cells, but not tumor-derived Tim-3$^-$ CD4 T cells, significantly suppressed the proliferation of autologous CD8$^+$ T cells *in vitro*. Notably, multi-color immunofluorescence and confocal microscopy demonstrated that Tim-3$^+$Foxp3$^+$CD4$^+$ cells were preferentially distributed in the tumor nest rather than the peritumoral stroma of hepatocellular carcinoma. Together, our data indicate that Tim-3-expressing CD4 T cells in human tumors could represent the functional regulatory T cells which contribute to the formation of the immune-suppressive tumor micromilieu.

Editor: Jacques Zimmer, Centre de Recherche Public de la Santé (CRP-Santé), Luxembourg

Funding: This work was supported by project grants from the National Basic Research Program of China (2010CB529904 and 2011CB811305; http://www.973.gov.cn/Default_3.aspx), the National Natural Science Foundation of China (81230073 and 91029737; http://www.nsfc.gov.cn/Portal0/default152.htm), and the Ministry of Health of China (2012ZX10002-011; http://www.moh.gov.cn/publicfiles//business/htmlfiles/wsb/index.htm). The funders had no role in study design, data collection and analysis, decision to publish, or preparation of the manuscript.

Competing Interests: The authors have declared that no competing interests exist.

* E-mail: zhenglm@mail.sysu.edu.cn

Introduction

Tim-3, a member of the novel T cell immunoglobulin and mucin domain (Tim) family, was originally identified as a negative immune regulator which is expressed on T helper 1 (Th1) cells, but not Th2 cells [1]. The interaction between Tim-3 and its ligand galectin-9 inhibits Th1 responses and induces peripheral tolerance [2–4]. However, growing evidence indicates that Tim-3 is also expressed on multiple cell types [5,6] and is involved in the pathogenesis of autoimmune disease and virus infection [7]. For example, T cell clones isolated from multiple sclerosis patients expressed lower levels of Tim-3 but secreted higher amounts of IFN-γ [8]. Upregulation of Tim-3 expression has been observed on exhausted CD8 T cells isolated from patients infected with human immunodeficiency virus (HIV), Hepatitis B virus (HBV), Hepatitis C virus (HCV) and Herpes simplex virus (HSV), and correlated with inefficient antiviral activity [9–13]. Recently, Tim-3 expression on Foxp3$^+$ Tregs was found in mouse skin transplantation model and chronic HCV-infected patients [14,15]. Such dysregulation of Tim-3 expression in disease settings indicates that Tim-3 may play an important role in adaptive immune responses.

Increased expression of Tim-3 has been recently detected in tumor-infiltrating lymphocytes (TILs) [16–20]. In murine tumor models, coexpression of Tim-3 and Programmed death 1 (PD-1) in CD8 T cells marks the most exhausted population of tumor-infiltrating T cells [17]. Simultaneous blockade of Tim-3 and PD-1 could effectively restore the antitumor activity of these exhausted T cells, resulted in complete tumor regression, and remained tumor free even after rechallenge [17]. In addition, expression of Tim-3 on T cells has been shown to promote the expansion of immunosuppressive myeloid-derived suppressor cells in mice bearing T-cell lymphomas [21], suggesting that Tim-3 is an inhibitory regulatory molecule important for the induction of immune tolerance in tumors microenvironment. Nonetheless, other studies have indicated that Tim-3 also plays a positive role in the antitumor immune response [22–24]. The Tim-3 ligand galectin-9 was found to prolong the survival of tumor-bearing mice by inducing cytotoxicity in CD8$^+$Tim-3$^+$ T cells, as well as facilitating the maturation of Tim-3$^+$ dendritic cells [24]. Although these findings suggest that Tim-3$^+$ cells have a potential impact in murine tumors, the nature and role of Tim-3$^+$ CD4 T cells in human tumors are still largely unknown [7].

In the current study, we report that Tim-3$^+$ CD4 T cells accumulate in human tumor tissues, and that Tim-3 expression defines a subset of regulatory T cells (Tregs) in several types of human tumors. Tim-3$^+$ Tregs from human hepatocellular carcinoma (HCC) suppressed autologous CD8 T cell proliferation and cytokine production *in vitro*. Additionally, Tim-3$^+$ Tregs specifically accumulated in the tumor nest, where Tim-3$^+$ CD4 cells had close contact with the Tim-3 ligand galectin-9. Together, our results suggest that the Tim-3-galectin-9 pathway may contribute to the suppressive tumor microenvironment in human cancer by promoting regulatory T cells.

Materials and Methods

Patients and Specimens

A total of 90 patients with pathologically confirmed hepatocellular carcinoma and 10 patients with cervical, colorectal or ovarian carcinoma from Sun Yat-sen University Cancer Center were enrolled in this study. None of the patients had received antitumor therapy before sampling. Paired tumor and nontumor tissue samples from 46 HCC patients and 10 patients with cervical, colorectal or ovarian carcinoma were processed to isolate fresh tissue infiltrating leukocytes. Fresh blood samples from 31 HCC patients were processed to isolate peripheral blood mononuclear cells (PBMCs). Paraffin-embedded samples from 13 HCC patients were used for immunofluorescence staining. Control blood samples were obtained from 36 healthy donors attending Guangzhou Blood Center, all of whom were negative for HBV, HCV, HIV and syphilis. The clinical and pathological characteristics of the patients are summarized in Table 1 and Tables S1, S2, S3.

Ethics Statement

Written informed consent was obtained from all patients and all samples were coded anonymously, in strict accordance with local ethical guidelines and as stipulated by the Declaration of Helsinki. Before the study, the protocol was approved by the Review Board of Sun Yat-sen University Cancer Center.

Cell Isolation

Peripheral blood leukocytes were isolated by Ficoll density gradient centrifugation. Fresh tumor and nontumor tissues were washed, cut into small pieces and digested in RPMI 1640 supplemented with 0.05% collagenase IV (Sigma-Aldrich, St. Louis, MO), 0.002% DNase I (Roche, Basel, Switzerland), and 20% FBS (HyClone Laboratories, Logan, UT) at 37°C for 30 minutes. Dissociated cells were filtered through a 150-μm mesh. Tumor-infiltrating lymphocytes (TILs) and nontumor-infiltrating lymphocytes (NILs) were obtained after Ficoll density gradient centrifugation [25–28].

Flow Cytometric Analysis

The fluorochrome-conjugated antibodies (Abs) and isotype-matched controls used in this study are described in Table S4. The non-specific staining for Tim-3 expression was shown in Figure S1. For intracellular cytokine staining, the cells were stimulated for 4 h with Leukocyte Activation Cocktail (BD Biosciences, San Diego, CA) and then stained with extracellular Abs, fixed and permeabilized with IntraPre Reagent (Beckman Coulter, Fullerton, CA), and finally stained with intracellular Abs [25]. To be noticed, stimulation with Leukocyte Activation Cocktail for 4 h did not affect Tim-3 expression on T cell surface. Intracellular staining for Foxp3 was performed by using a Foxp3 staining kit (eBioscience, San Diego, CA) according to the manufacturer's instructions. Data were acquired using a Gallios multicolor flow cytometer (Beckman Coulter, Brea, CA) and analyzed with FlowJo software (TreeStar, San Carlos, CA).

Immunofluorescence

Paraffin-embedded samples were cut into 5-μm sections and processed for immunofluorescence staining, as previously described [27]. Sections were dewaxed in xylene and rehydrated in a series of graded alcohols according to histopathological standards. Antigen retrieval was achieved by pressure cooking in EDTA antigen retrieval buffer (pH 9.5, Zhongshan golden bridge, China) for 10 min and cooling them to room temperature. Slides were then incubated in PBS containing 5% BSA and 0.1% Triton X-100 for 30 minutes to block unspecific binding. HCC tissue sections were stained with rabbit-anti-human CD4 (Spring Bioscience, Fremont, CA) or mouse-anti-human CD4 (NeoMarker, Freemont, CA), goat-anti-human Tim-3 (R&D Systems, Minneapolis, MN), mouse anti-human Foxp3 (Abcam, Cambridge, UK), mouse anti-human CD68 (Dako, Glostrup, Denmark) and rabbit anti-human galectin-9 (Abcam), followed by Alexa Fluor 488-, 555-, or 647-conjugated donkey anti-mouse IgG, Alexa Fluor 555- or 647-conjugated donkey anti-rabbit IgG, or Alexa Fluor 488-

Table 1. Clinical and pathological characteristics of the HCC patients.

Variable	Fresh tissue	Peripheral blood	Paraffin section
Cases (*n*)	46	31	13
Age, years (median, range)	51, 22–79	59, 22–76	59, 36–80
Gender (male/female)	43/3	25/6	13/0
HBsAg (negative/positive)	3/43	7/24	3/10
Cirrhosis (absent/present)	10/36	5/26	3/10
ALT, units/L (median, range)	38, 14–303	37, 16–69	60, 29–82
AFP, ng/ml (≤25/>25)	13/33	10/21	4/9
Tumor multiplicity (solitary/multiple)	32/14	22/9	9/4
Tumor size, cm (≤5/>5)	11/35	17/14	2/11
Vascular invasion (absent/present)	38/8	25/6	12/1
TNM stage (I–II/III–IV)	25/21	19/12	8/5
Tumor differentiation (I–II/III–IV)	19/27	14/17	6/7

Note: HBsAg, hepatitis B surface antigen; ALT, alanine aminotransferase; AFP, a-fetoprotein; TNM, tumor-node-metastasis.

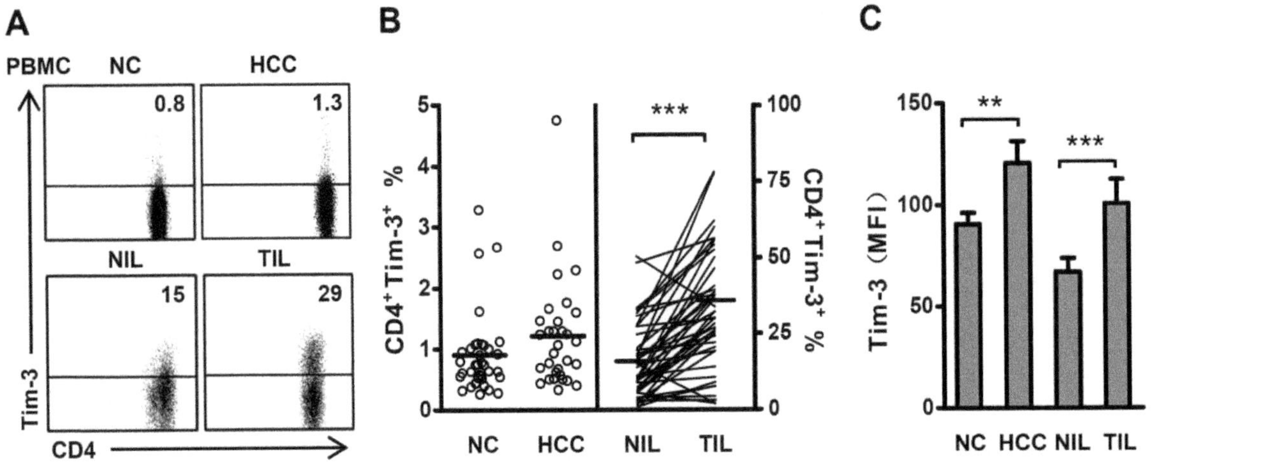

Figure 1. Tim-3 is upregulated on CD4 T cells in HCC tumor tissues. A. Representative FACS analysis of Tim-3 expression in CD4 T cells isolated from the PBMCs of normal healthy controls (NC) and HCC patients (HCC), and nontumor-infiltrating lymphocytes (NILs) and tumor-infiltrating lymphocytes (TILs) from HCC patients. Flow cytometry data are representative of at least 31 samples in each group. **B**. Statistical analysis of the proportion of Tim-3^+ CD4 T cells in NC (n = 36), HCC (n = 31), NILs and TILs (n = 46). Each circle or thin line represents a single case. Horizontal lines indicate the mean of an individual group. **C**. Mean fluorescence intensity (MFI) for Tim-3 on $CD4^+$Tim-3^+ T cells in each group. NC (n = 36), HCC (n = 31), NILs and TILs (n = 46). Bars indicate the SEM; **, $P<0.01$; ***, $P<0.001$.

conjugated donkey anti-goat IgG, as appropriate (Molecular Probes, Carlsbad, CA). Negative control staining was performed by replacing the primary antibodies with isotype-matched control antibodies. Nuclei were stained with 40-6-diamidino-2-phenylindole (DAPI). Images were viewed and assessed using an Olympus confocal laser microscope (Fluoview; Tokyo, Japan). For the quantification of $CD4^+$Tim-$3^{+/-}$Foxp$3^{+/-}$ subset cells, $CD4^{+/-}$galectin-$9^{+/-}$ subset cells, or $CD68^{+/-}$galectin-$9^{+/-}$ subset cells, slides were first screened for CD4 or CD68 hot-spots. Then 8 images per slide were taken with 40× oil-immersed objective lens. Numbers of each subset cell per field were counted manually by two independent, blinded observers.

Suppression Assay

The suppression assay was performed as previously described with minor modifications [29]. TILs were first gated on $CD45^+$ cells to exclude non-hematopoietic $CD45^-$ cells. $CD4^+$Tim-3^+, $CD4^+$Tim-3^- and $CD4^-$ T cells were sorted using a FACS Aria II (BD Biosciences, San Diego, CA); cell purity was over 90%. For suppression assay using carboxyfluorescein diacetate succinimidyl ester (CFSE; Molecular Probes), 5×10^4 $CD4^-$ T cells (responder) were labeled with 1 μM CFSE and cultured with autologous $CD4^+$Tim-3^+ cells, $CD4^+$Tim-3^- T cells or medium alone. Cells were first stimulated with anti-CD3 (0.2 μg/ml) and anti-CD28 (0.4 μg/ml) mAbs for 2 days, cultured in the presence of IL-2 (20 U/ml) for another 3 days, and then cell proliferation was analyzed by flow cytometry. For the BrdU incorporation assay, the cells were cultured as stated above and then pulsed with BrdU during the last 6 h using the BrdU kit (Roche, Mannheim, Germany). Cell proliferation was quantified by measuring the optical density (OD) of each group. Culture supernatants were collected for quantification of the IFN-γ concentration by ELISA (eBioscience, San Diego, CA).

Statistical Analysis

Data are presented as the mean ± SEM. Comparisons between groups were performed using the Student's t-test. The association between indexes of Tim-3^+ Tregs and the TNM stages were evaluated using Fisher's exact test. Statistical analyses were performed using SPSS software (version 13.0; SPSS Inc., Chicago, IL).

Results

Tim-3 Expression is Upregulated on CD4 T cells in the Tumor Tissues of Cancer Patients

To explore the potential role of Tim-3 in tumor immunopathology, we first examined the distribution of Tim-3 in lymphocytes freshly isolated from the paired tumor and nontumor tissues of 46 HCC patients, as well as lymphocytes isolated from the peripheral blood of 31 HCC patients and 36 healthy donors. Approximately 5% of the circulating Tim-3^+ lymphocytes in both healthy donors and HCC patients were CD4 T cells. This proportion was significantly elevated in tumor-infiltrating lymphocytes (TIL) compared with nontumor-infiltrating lymphocytes (NIL) (19.9±2.7% vs. 5.3±0.9%, $P<0.001$, Figure S2). With respect to CD4 T cells, Tim-3 was only expressed on a small fraction of the circulating CD4 T cells in healthy individuals, with slightly higher levels of circulating Tim-3^+ CD4 T cells observed in HCC patients (Figure 1A and 1B). In contrast, we detected substantial numbers of Tim-3-expressing CD4 T cells in both nontumor and tumor tissues. The frequency of Tim-3^+ CD4 T cells and mean fluorescence intensity (MFI) for Tim-3 were significantly higher in TILs than the NILs of the same HCC patients (32.9±2.8% vs. 16.5±1.9% for frequency; 100.7±11.7 vs. 67.1±6.7 for MFI, respectively; both $P<0.001$, Figure 1B and 1C).

To investigate whether these findings are confined to HCC, we also examined Tim-3-expressing T cells in other human tumors. Compared with the corresponding nontumor tissues, the levels of Tim-3-expressing CD4 T cells were also significantly higher in tumors from patients with colorectal, cervical or ovarian carcinoma (Figure S3A). These data indicated that Tim-3-expressing cells comprise a significant subset of CD4 T helper cells, which are selectively enriched in human tumors.

Tumor-derived Tim-3$^+$ CD4 T cells Exhibit Impaired Production of IFN-γ and IL-2

CD4 T helper (Th) cells play a central role in orchestrating host immune responses through cytokine production and expression of membrane-bound molecules [30–32]. To evaluate the functional status of Tim-3$^+$ CD4 T cells, we examined their capacity to produce IFN-γ, IL-2, IL-4 and IL-17. In TILs isolated from HCC tissues, Tim-3$^+$ CD4 T cells produced significantly less IFN-γ and IL-2 than the Tim-3$^-$ CD4 T cells (22.1±6.4% vs. 43.9±6.9%, $P<0.01$ for IFN-γ; 7.8±2.8% vs. 41.7±3.7%, $P<0.001$ for IL-2, respectively; Figure 2A and 2B). The frequency of Tim-3$^+$ CD4 T cells from TILs was also significantly lower in IFN-γ$^+$ or IL-2$^+$ cells than their IFN-γ$^-$ or IL-2$^-$ counterparts (13.0±3.5% vs. 33.1±6.8% for IFN-γ; 3.1±1.5% vs. 19.7±4.9% for IL-2, both $P<0.01$, Figure 2A and 2B). In contrast, we found little or no difference in IL-2 or IFN-γ production between Tim-3$^+$ and Tim-3$^-$ CD4 T cells derived from NILs, whereas circulating Tim-3$^+$ CD4 T cells produced even more IFN-γ than Tim-3$^-$ cells (Figure 2A), suggesting that the tumor environment can profoundly affect the phenotype of Tim-3$^+$ CD4 T cells. Sorted Tim-3$^+$ CD4 T cells also secreted less amounts of IFN-γ and IL-2 compared with Tim-3$^-$ CD4 T cells (data not shown). In addition, most Tim-3$^+$ CD4 T cells did not produce IL-4 or IL-17 (Figure S4). Similar results were observed in samples isolated from human patients with colorectal, cervical and ovarian carcinoma, including the selective impairment of IFN-γ and IL-2 production in Tim-3$^+$ CD4 T cells isolated from TILs (data not shown). These data provide the first indication that Tim-3-expressing CD4 T cells might represent a population of dysfunctional Th1 cells (or another cell type) in human tumor tissues.

To determine whether tumor-derived Tim-3$^+$ CD4 T cells are dysfunctional Th1 cells, we quantified expression of the Th1-specific transcription factor T-bet [33] and the well-recognized exhausted/anergic marker PD-1 [34,35] on Tim-3$^+$ CD4 T cells. The majority of Tim-3$^+$ CD4 T cells isolated from TILs did not express T-bet (Figure 2C), suggesting that the majority of these cells were different to Th1 cells. In contrast, approximately 80% of the Tim-3$^+$ CD4 T cells isolated from TILs co-expressed PD-1 (Figure 2D), a marker for exhausted or anergic T cells.

Tim-3 is Preferentially Expressed by CD25$^+$CD127^{low}Foxp3$^+$ T cells in Human Tumors

To further characterize the phenotype of Tim-3$^+$ CD4 T cells, we examined the expression of CD25 and CD127. As shown in Figure 3A, Tim-3$^+$ CD4 T cells isolated from TILs expressed significantly higher levels of CD25 than the Tim-3$^-$ cells isolated from TILs (63.2±5.0% vs. 13.1±2.1%, $P<0.001$, Figure S5A). Interestingly, the majority (82.9±4.7%) of Tim-3$^+$ CD4 T cells in TILs were CD127^{low} (Figure S5B). The frequency of Tim-3$^+$ CD4 T cells was also significantly higher among CD25$^+$ or CD127^{low} cells than their CD25$^-$ or CD127^{high} counterparts (Figure 3A and S5); these characteristics are also shared by human Treg cells [30,36–38]. Thus, we next determined the correlation between expression of Tim-3 and Foxp3, a transcription factor generally used as a marker for Treg cells [39]. As shown in Figure 3B, Foxp3 expression was significantly higher in Tim-3$^+$ CD4 T cells from TILs than the Tim-3$^-$ cells (61.7±4.5% vs. 13.1±3.2%, $P<0.001$), at a level similar to CD4$^+$CD25$^+$ T cells (65.5±4.7%). Back gating of Foxp3 in TILs showed that ~70% of the CD4$^+$Foxp3$^+$ T cells were Tim-3$^+$, compared with ~20% of the CD4$^+$Foxp3$^-$ T cells. Similar results were obtained in the samples from colorectal, cervical and ovarian carcinoma patients, including the expression of high levels of Foxp3 and CD25, and

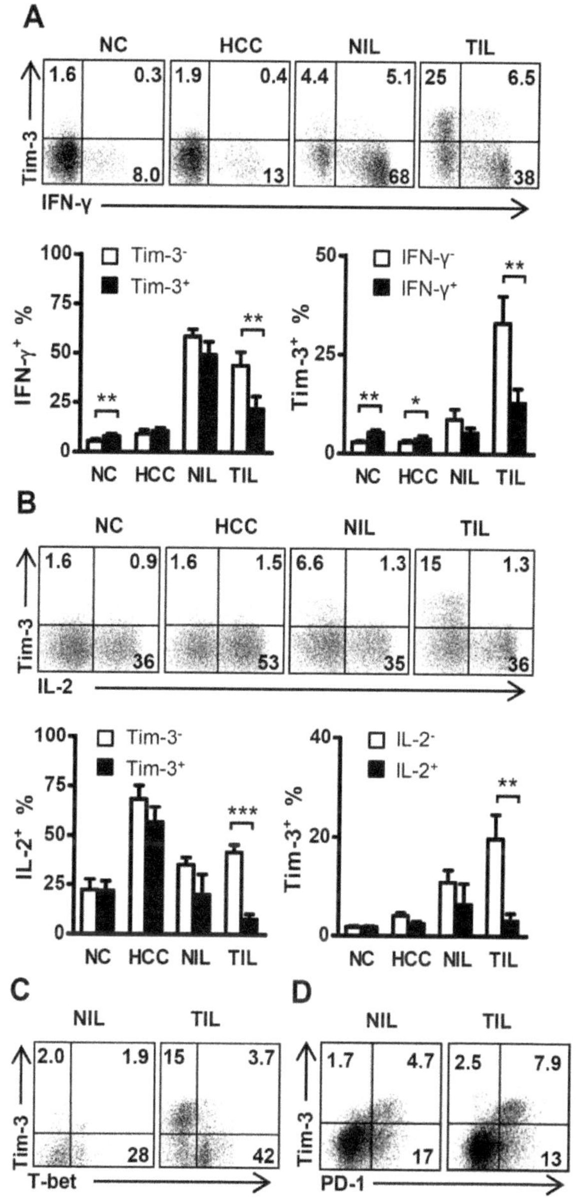

Figure 2. Tumor-infiltrating Tim-3$^+$ CD4 T cells exhibit impaired ability to produce Th1-type cytokines. A. Representative FACS analysis illustrating the association between IFN-γ and Tim-3 expression in CD4 T cells isolated from the PBMCs of normal healthy controls (NC, $n=15$) and HCC patients (HCC, $n=10$), and nontumor-infiltrating lymphocytes (NILs, $n=6$) and tumor-infiltrating lymphocytes (TILs, $n=6$) from HCC patients. Statistical analysis showed the mean percentage of IFN-γ$^+$ cells in the Tim-3 positive or negative CD4 T cell subsets (left), and the proportion of Tim-3$^+$ cells in the IFN-γ positive or negative CD4 T cell subsets (right). **B.** Relationship between the expression of Tim-3 and IL-2 in CD4 T cells, At least 4 samples were tested in each group. Bars indicate the SEM; *, $P<0.05$; **, $P<0.01$; ***, $P<0.001$. **C.** The majority of Tim-3$^+$ CD4 T cells isolated from TILs did not express the Th1-specific transcription factor T-bet, $n=4$. **D.** Correlation of Tim-3 and PD-1 expression in tumor tissues, $n=4$.

lower levels of CD127 on Tim-3$^+$ CD4 T cells from TILs (Figure S3B and data not shown). These data strongly indicate that Tim-3 could represent a novel surface marker to define the regulatory T cell subset of CD4 T cells in human tumors.

In contrast, the majority of Tim-3$^+$ CD4 T cells isolated from the peripheral blood of healthy donors and cancer patients did not express the Treg-related molecules CD25 and Foxp3. Although a trend toward increased levels of these Treg-related molecules was observed on Tim-3$^+$ CD4 T cells in NILs, their frequency and intensity were markedly lower than the levels observed on the corresponding TILs (Figure 3 and S5). The differential phenotypic features of Tim-3-expressing cells in blood, NILs and TILs suggest that upregulation of Tim-3 on CD4 T cells may occur in the tumor environment, and in turn, the regulatory properties of these cells may contribute to the immunosuppressive environment in tumors.

A recent study using mouse skin transplantation model showed that the presence of Tim-3$^+$PD-1$^+$ Tregs *in situ* were crucial for induction of tolerance and restraining allograft rejection [14]. To determine whether Tim-3$^+$PD-1$^+$ Tregs exist in human tumor tissues, we compared the expression of Foxp3 in Tim-3 single positive (Tim-3 SP), PD-1 single positive (PD-1 SP), Tim-3 and PD-1 double positive cells (DP) and Tim-3 and PD-1 double negative (DN) cells. Interestingly, Tim-3 and PD-1 DP cells isolated from both NILs and TILs expressed Tim-3 at comparable levels to Tim-3 SP cells, while the PD-1 SP as well as Tim-3 and PD-1 DN cells expressed negligible levels of Foxp3 (Figure S6). Therefore, Tim-3, but not PD-1, marks the population of Foxp3$^+$ T cells in the tumor microenvironment. On the other hand, PD-1$^+$Tim-3$^-$ cells may represent the *bona fide* population of exhausted CD4 T cells in tumor tissue.

Another recent study showed that Tim-3$^+$ TILs expressed negligible levels of Foxp3 [16]; the discrepancy between this previous report and the results of this study may be due to differences in the clinical stages of the patients and the anatomic regions of the specimens analyzed. Therefore, we examined the distribution of Tim-3$^+$ CD4 cells throughout the tumor tissues using multi-color immunofluorescence, paying particular attention to their micro-anatomic location. The majority of Tim-3$^+$ CD4 T cells in the peritumoral stroma did not express Foxp3, whereas most Tim-3$^+$ CD4 T cells in the cancer nest co-stained brightly with Foxp3 (Figure 3C). The accumulation of Tim-3$^+$Foxp3$^+$ CD4 T cells in the cancer nest other than in peritumoral stroma implied that Tim-3$^+$ Tregs could be induced during tumor progression. In support of this hypothesis, we found that the percentage of Foxp3$^+$/Tim-3$^+$ CD4 T cells (Foxp3$^+$/Tim-3$^+$%) in TILs correlated positively with the TNM stage of the HCC patients. The 18 patients for whom Tim-3 and Foxp3 data were available were divided into two groups, according to the median Foxp3$^+$/Tim-3$^+$% value in TILs. In the group with a low Foxp3$^+$/Tim-3$^+$%, 8 out of 9 patients had an early TNM stage. In contrast, 7 out of the 9 patients from the high Foxp3$^+$/Tim-3$^+$% group belonged to the advanced TNM stages group ($P = 0.015$, Table S5). Similar trends were also observed using other parameters of Tim-3$^+$ Tregs as the comparison index, albeit the P values for these analyses did not reach statistical significance (Table S5).

CD4$^+$Tim-3$^+$ Cells Isolated from TILs Exhibit Suppressive Activity

To determine whether tumor-derived Tim-3$^+$ CD4 T cells are functional Tregs, we first examined the expression of functional inhibitory markers of Tregs on these cells [30,38]. Tim-3$^+$ CD4 T cells from TILs expressed high levels of Cytotoxic T lymphocyte antigen-4 (CTLA-4) and glucocorticoid-induced TNF-related receptor (GITR) whereas Tim-3$^+$ CD4 T cells from NILs did not express high levels of these inhibitory markers (Figure 4A), implying that tumor-derived Tim-3$^+$ CD4 T cells are functional Tregs. To confirm the inhibitory activity of Tim-3$^+$ Tregs, we examined their ability to suppress the proliferation and IFN-γ production of autologous tumor-infiltrating CD8$^+$ T cells. Tumor-derived CD4 T cells were sorted into Tim-3$^+$ and Tim-3$^-$ subsets, and then cocultured with responder cells on anti-CD3/CD28 stimulation for 5 days. The CFSE assay showed that tumor-derived Tim-3$^+$CD4$^+$ cells inhibited the proliferation of CD8$^+$ T cells, whereas Tim-3$^-$CD4 T cells had no effect on the proliferation of CD8$^+$ T cells (Figure 4B). In contrast to the robust proliferation of Tim-3$^-$ counterparts, tumor-derived Tim-3$^+$CD4 T cells were anergic to anti-CD3/CD28 stimulation, characteristics shared by "classical" human Treg cells [40]. Similar results were obtained in complementary experiments using the BrdU incorporation assay (Figure 4C). Furthermore, we observed that tumor-derived Tim-3$^+$CD4$^+$ cells, but not their Tim-3$^-$ counterparts, suppressed production of IFN-γ by T cells (Figure 4C). Thus, Tim-3 can be used as a biomarker to identify functional Treg cells in human tumor tissues.

Notably, we observed that Tim-3$^+$ CD4 T cells isolated from peripheral blood did not suppress the proliferation and IFN-γ production of T cells (data not shown), which is in line with our data indicating that circulating Tim-3$^+$ CD4 T cells exhibit different functional and phenotypic features to tumor-derived Tim-3$^+$ cells (Figure 2, 3 and 4A).

To further compared between Tim-3$^+$ and Tim-3$^-$ Foxp3$^+$ CD4 T cells, we examined the expression of CTLA-4, GITR and PD-1 in these two populations. The results showed that Tim-3$^+$Foxp3$^+$ CD4 T cells expressed higher levels of CTLA-4, GITR and PD-1 in comparison with Tim-3$^-$Foxp3$^+$ CD4 T cells (Figure S7). These data suggest that Tim-3$^+$Foxp3$^+$ CD4 T cells in tumor tissue might represent a group of Tregs different from the Tim-3$^-$Foxp3$^+$ CD4 T cells.

Close Interaction between Tim-3$^+$CD4$^+$ Cells and Galectin-9$^+$ Cells in HCC

The Tim-3 ligand, galectin-9, has been linked with tumor progression [41]. To explore the potential effect of galectin-9 on Tim-3$^+$ cells in tumors *in situ*, we examined the distribution of galectin-9 and Tim-3 in HCC tumor tissues using multi-color immunofluorescence and confocal microscopy. Interestingly, we found that many immune cells infiltrating the tumors coexpressed Tim-3 and galectin-9 (Figure 5A), implying that Tim-3 and galectin-9 may interact with each other in an autocrine manner. Both the tumor-infiltrating CD4$^+$ cells and macrophages expressed abundant levels of galectin-9 (Figure 5B–5E). Typically, a direct interaction between the Tim-3$^+$CD4$^+$ cells and galcetin-9$^+$ cells was observed (Figure 5A), indicating that Tim-3 interacts with its ligand galectin-9 *in vivo*.

Discussion

Tim-3 has recently been identified as an important player in the CD8 T cell exhaustion that occurs in chronic disease states such as chronic viral infection and cancer [13,17,19]. The present study showed that the expression of Tim-3 is upregulated on tumor-infiltrating CD4 T cells. These Tim-3$^+$ CD4 T cells produced lower levels of Th1-type cytokines whereas expressed higher levels of CD25, Foxp3, CTLA-4 and GITR, compared with Tim-3$^-$ CD4 T cells. Moreover, Tim-3$^+$ CD4 T cells significantly suppressed autologous CD8 T cells. Interestingly, Tim-3$^+$Foxp3$^+$ CD4 T cells were preferentially distributed in the tumor nest, rather than the peritumoral stroma. These findings indicate that Tim-3 expression on tumor-derived CD4 T cells defines regulatory T cells which can contribute to the immunosuppressive tumor micromilieu.

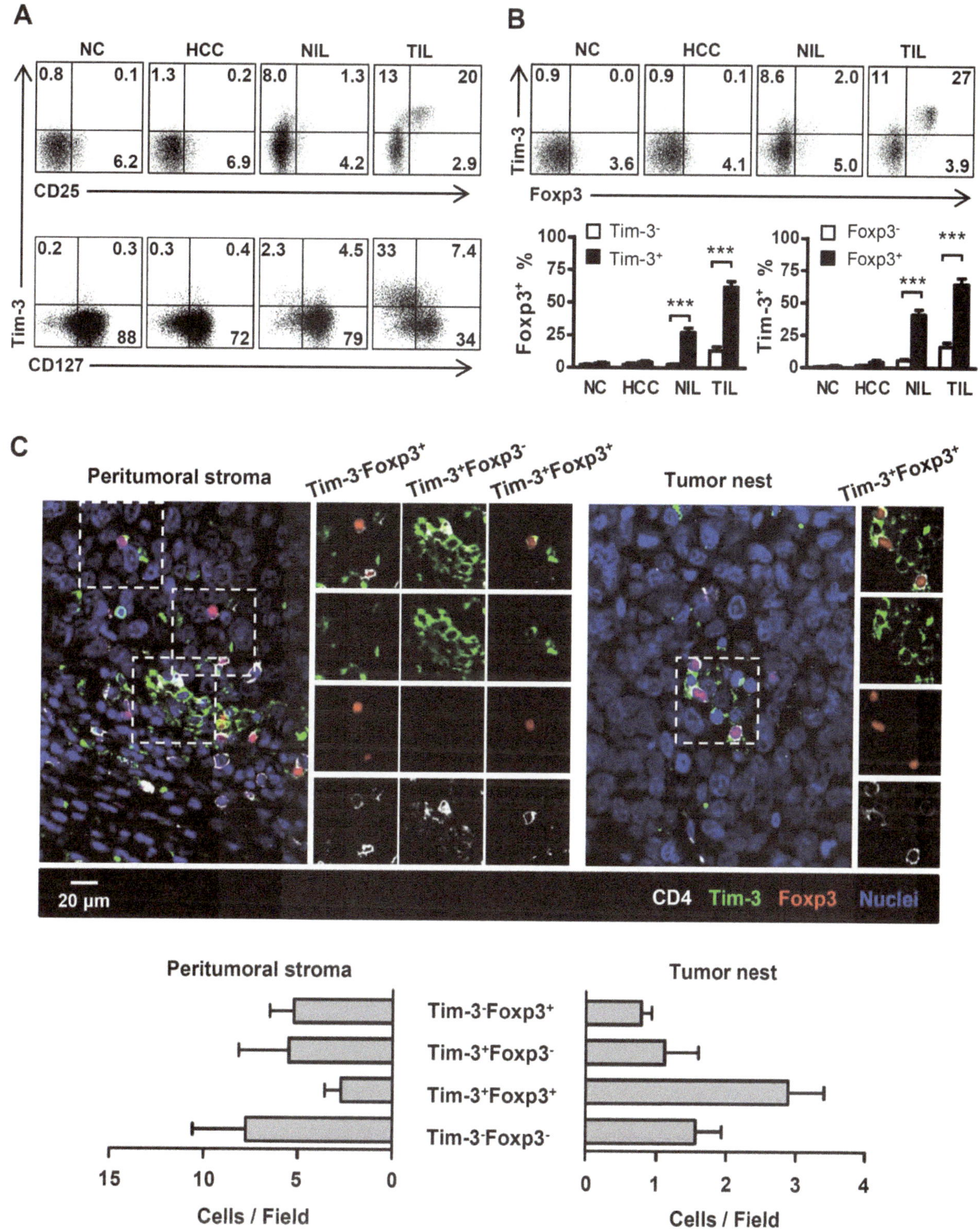

Figure 3. Tim-3 expression defines a population of CD4 T cells with Treg characteristics in TILs. A. Representative FACS analysis showing the association of CD25, CD127 and Tim-3 expression in CD4 T cells isolated from the PBMCs of normal healthy controls (NC, $n=7$) and HCC patients (HCC, $n=6$), and nontumor-infiltrating lymphocytes (NILs, $n=18$) and tumor-infiltrating lymphocytes (TILs, $n=18$) from HCC patients. **B.** FACS and statistical data showing that most tumor-infiltrating Tim-3$^+$ CD4 T cells expressed the Treg-specific transcription factor Foxp3. Bars indicate the SEM; ***, $P<0.001$. **C.** Paraffin-embedded HCC sections were subjected to multi-color immunofluorescence staining for CD4 (white), Tim-3 (green), Foxp3 (red) and nuclei (DAPI, blue). Confocal microscopic analysis revealing the different distribution of Tim-3$^+$Foxp3$^+$CD4$^+$ cells in the peritumoral stroma and tumor nest of HCC. Images are representative of 13 samples. For the quantification of CD4$^+$Tim-3$^{+/-}$Foxp3$^{+/-}$ cells, eight CD4 hot-spot fields per slide were taken with 40× oil-immersed objective lens. Numbers of each subset cells were counted manually by two independent, blinded observers.

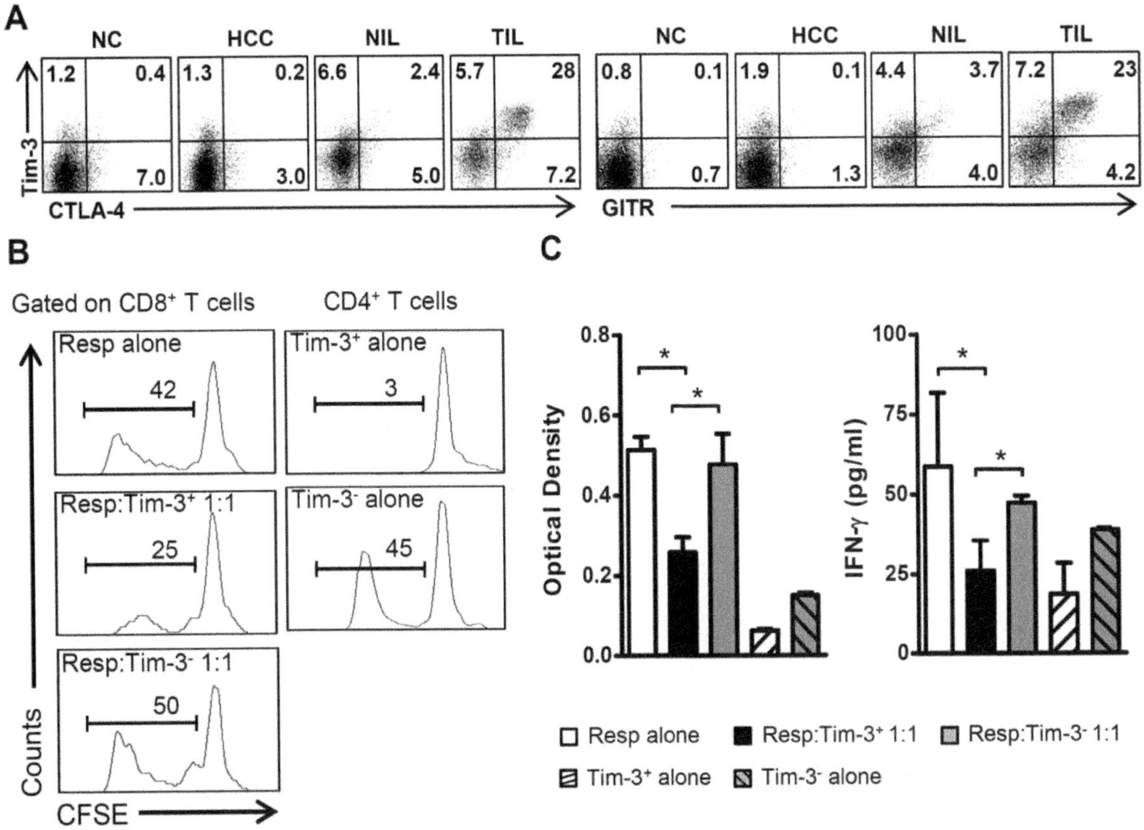

Figure 4. CD4⁺Tim-3⁺ T cells isolated from TILs exhibit suppressive activity. A. Representative FACS analysis showing that most tumor-infiltrating Tim-3⁺ CD4 T cells expressed the Treg functional markers CTLA-4 (left) and GITR (right), $n = 6$. **B.** CD4⁺Tim-3⁺ T cells suppressed autologus tumor-infiltrating CD8⁺ T cells. CD4⁺Tim-3⁺, CD4⁺Tim-3⁻ and CD8⁺ T cells were sorted from TILs, and the suppression assay was performed as described in Materials and Methods. The ratios of responder to suppressor cells were indicated. Cell proliferation was tracked by monitoring the decrease in CFSE fluorescence, $n = 4$. The numbers in the histograms indicate the percentage of proliferating cells. **C.** The BrdU incorporation assay supported the suppressive function of CD4⁺Tim-3⁺ T cells isolated from TILs. IFN-γ production in the indicated culture supernatants was quantified by ELISA, $n = 4$. Bars indicate the SEM; *, $P<0.05$.

Immunosuppression mediated by Tregs is a key facilitator of tumor immune evasion [30,42,43]; however, knowledge of the phenotypic characteristics of tumor-associated Tregs in human tumors remains limited [44,45]. In the current study, we demonstrated that Tim-3 can serve as a novel surface marker to define tumor-infiltrating Tregs. Tim-3⁺ CD4 TILs produced lower levels of IFN-γ and IL-2, relative to their Tim-3⁻ counterparts. In contrast, over 60% of tumor-infiltrating Tim-3⁺ CD4 T cells expressed CD25, and ~80% of Tim-3⁺ CD4 TILs were $CD127^{low}$, two characteristics shared by human Treg cells [30,36–38]. Most of the Tim-3⁺ CD4 TILs expressed the Treg-specific transcription factor Foxp3, and exhibited suppressive activity. Unlike CD25 and CD127, which characterize Treg in both peripheral blood and tumor tissues, Tim-3 is not expressed by circulating Foxp3⁺ CD4 T cells, indicating that Tim-3 is specifically expressed on tumor associated Tregs. In addition, tumor-infiltrating Tim-3⁺Foxp3⁺ CD4 T cells expressed higher levels of CTLA-4, GITR and PD-1 compared with Tim-3⁻Foxp3⁺ CD4 T cells. It has been reported that Tim-3 expression on Tregs was upregulated upon TCR activation [18]. Activated tumor-infiltrating Tregs were found to express higher levels of CTLA-4, GITR and PD-1 [46–48], which were observed in the Tim-3⁺Foxp3⁺ CD4 T cells. Therefore, it's possible that Tim-3⁺ Foxp3⁺ CD4 T cells in tumor tissue might represent the highly activated Tregs that possess potent inhibitory activity. In support of our results, a recent study illustrated the accumulation of Tim-3⁺PD-1⁺ Tregs in the tumor tissues of lung cancer patients [18]. Similar to these findings, Tim-3⁺Foxp3⁺ Tregs have also been observed under other circumstances characterized by persistent antigen stimulation, such as during chronic viral infection and allograft rejection [14,15]. Together, these studies imply that Tim-3-expressing Tregs may be involved in a diverse range of human diseases. The Tim-3 ligand galectin-9 has been found to promote the expansion of regulatory T cells; however, the exact mechanism by which galectin-9 regulates Tregs is not clear [13,15,49,50]. In this study, we found that Tim-3 is specifically expressed on tumor-associated Tregs, which may render these cells susceptible to regulation by galectin-9. In support of this hypothesis, we observed that Tim-3⁺ cells were in close contact with galectin-9⁺ immune cells in tumors *in vivo*. The galectin-9 expression level correlated positively with the Foxp3 expression level in tumors *in situ* (data not shown). Treatment of T cells with galectin-9 augmented Foxp3 expression *in vitro*, as previously reported (data not shown). Hence, galectin-9 may promote Treg expansion through the Tim-3-galectin-9 interaction. In contrast, galectin-9 eliminates Tim-3⁺ effector T cells (Teffs) by triggering their apoptosis [7,51,52]. In this case, the Treg-to-Teff ratio would increase, coinciding with our finding that a higher Foxp3/Tim-3 ratio was associated with less favorable clinical parameters in HCC patients. Thus, the Tim-3-galectin-9 pathway could regulate

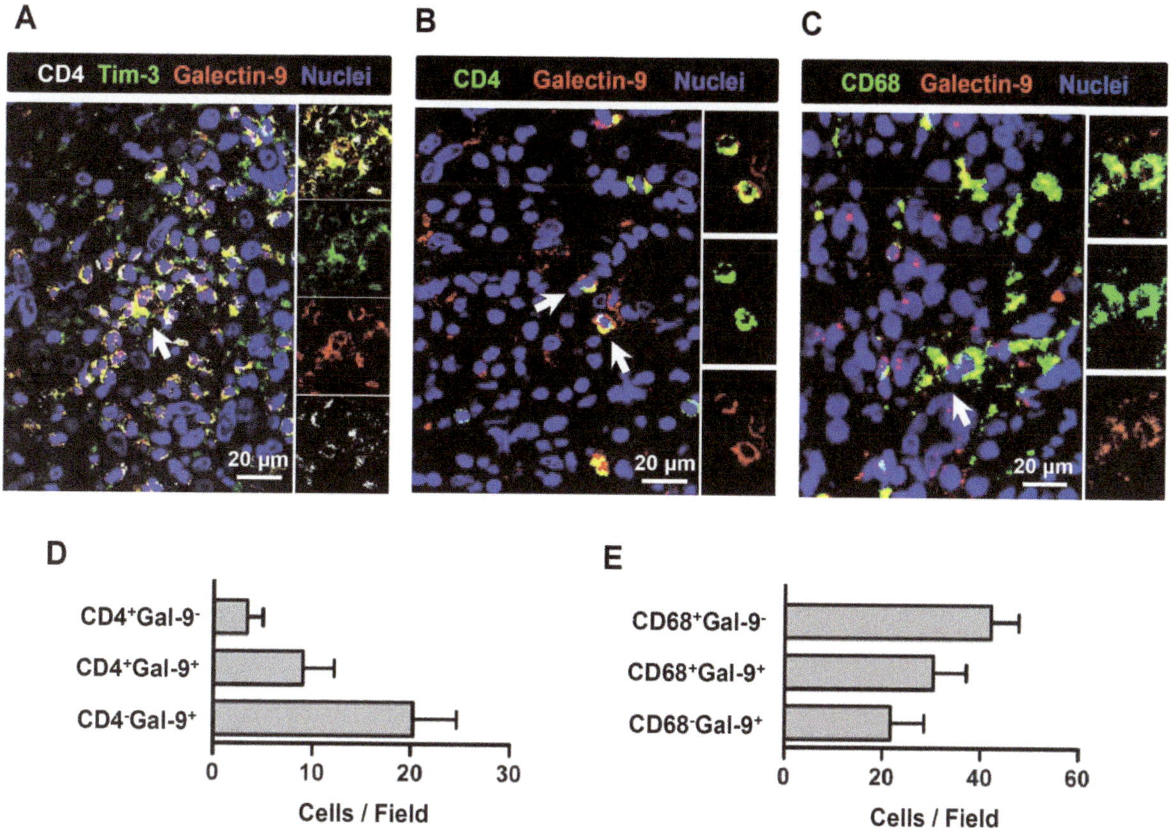

Figure 5. Close interaction between Tim-3^{+}CD4^{+} cells and galectin-9^{+} cells in HCC tumor tissue. **A**. Paraffin-embedded HCC tumor sections were subjected to multi-color immunofluorescence staining for CD4 (white), Tim-3 (green), galectin-9 (red) and nuclei (DAPI, blue). Confocal analysis showed that Tim-3^{+}CD4^{+} cells were in close contact with galectin-9^{+} cells in the tumor nest. **B.** Paraffin-embedded HCC tumor sections were subjected to multi-color immunofluorescence staining for CD4 (green), galectin-9 (red) and nuclei (DAPI, blue). Confocal analysis indicated that galectin-9 was expressed by the tumor-infiltrating CD4^{+} cells. **C.** Paraffin-embedded HCC tumor sections were subjected to multi-color immunofluorescence staining for CD68 (green), galectin-9 (red) and nuclei (DAPI, blue). Confocal analysis indicated that galectin-9 was expressed by tumor-infiltrating CD68^{+} macrophages. White arrows in A–C indicate the magnified cells. Images are representative of 13 samples. For the quantification of CD4$^{+/-}$galectin-9$^{+/-}$ cells **(D)** or CD68$^{+/-}$galectin-9$^{+/-}$ **(E)** cells, eight CD4 or CD68 hot-spot fields per slide were taken with 40× oil-immersed objective lens. Numbers of each subset cells were counted manually by two independent, blinded observers. Gal-9 in D and E is short for galectin-9.

homeostasis of the immune response by balancing the Treg and Teff responses in the tumor microenvironment.

The specific nature of the tumor micromilieu can profoundly determine the phenotype and function of immune cells in tumor pathology [26,27,53,54]. Our previous studies showed that activated monocytes in the peritumoral stroma can promote the expansion of proinflammatory Th17 cells [27]; whereas macrophages in the tumor nest induce immunosuppressive Tregs [28]. Paying particular attention to the micro-anatomic location in tumor tissues, here we observed that the majority of Tim-3^{+}CD4^{+} cells in the peritumoral stroma were Foxp3^{-}, whereas the majority of Tim-3^{+}CD4^{+} cells in the cancer nest co-expressed Foxp3. Furthermore, fewer Tim-3^{+}Foxp3^{+} CD4 T cells were observed in the tumors of early TNM stage HCC patients, consistent with another report of negligible Tim-3 expression by Foxp3^{+} TILs isolated from relatively early-stage HCC patients [16]. We propose that Tim-3^{+} CD4 T cells exhibit different phenotypes and functions during the process of tumor progression. Early activated Tim-3^{+} Teffs in the peritumoral stroma can secrete effector cytokines such as IFN-γ, which may exert an antitumor effect in this area [53,55]. However, IFN-γ-induced expression of galectin-9 in tumor-associated macrophages [16] promotes Tim-3^{+} Treg expansion, which in turn eliminates and dampens the effects of Teffs in the tumor nest. Therefore, different tissue contexts may determine whether Tim-3^{+} CD4 T cells exert a beneficial or detrimental effect on tumor immunopathogenesis.

Emerging Tim-3 function in tumor immunity is being discovered [7,51,52]. Treatment with anti-Tim-3 Ab alone or in combination with anti-CTLA-4 and/or PD-1 Abs significantly suppressed tumor growth in mice [17,19,21,56]. In addition to the inhibitory role of Tim-3 in the immune response, Tim-3 has also been found to exert an antitumor immune response [22–24]. The results of the present study reveal that different tissue contexts may determine the phenotype and function of Tim-3^{+} CD4 T cells in the tumor microenvironment. Fine-tuning the Tim-3 pathway could potentially help to develop a novel antitumor therapy, to simultaneously restore the functions of Teffs and restrain the immunosuppressive effects of Tregs.

Supporting Information

Figure S1 Isotype control for Tim-3 expression. Isotype controls for Tim-3 were shown for CD4 T cells isolated from PBMCs from normal controls (NC), PBMCs from HCC patients (HCC), nontumor-infiltrating lymphocytes (NIL) and tumor-infiltrating lymphocytes (TILs). Images are representative of at least 31 samples in each group.

Figure S2 Proportion of Tim-3$^+$ lymphocyte subsets in Tim-3$^+$ cells. Frequency of T cells (CD3$^+$), CD4 T cells (CD3$^+$CD4$^+$), CD8 T cells (CD3$^+$CD8$^+$), NKT cells (CD3$^+$CD56$^+$) and NK cells (CD3$^-$CD56$^+$) in Tim-3$^+$ lymphocytes isolated from PBMCs from normal controls (NC), PBMCs from HCC patients (HCC), nontumor-infiltrating lymphocytes (NIL) and tumor-infiltrating lymphocytes (TILs). At least 12 samples were tested in each group. Bars indicate the SEM. *, $P<0.05$, ***, $P<0.001$.

Figure S3 Tim-3 is upregulated on tumor-infiltrating Foxp3$^+$ CD4 T cells isolated from colon carcinoma, cervical cancer and ovarian cancer patients. A. Proportion of Tim-3$^+$ CD4 T cells isolated from paired non-tumor-infiltrating lymphocytes (NILs) and tumor-infiltrating lymphocytes (TILs). Each line represents a single case; *, $P<0.05$. **B.** Representative FACS analysis of Tim-3 and Foxp3 expression in NILs and TILs isolated from patients with colon carcinoma ($n=4$), cervical cancer ($n=3$) and ovarian cancer ($n=3$).

Figure S4 Proportion of Th2, Th17, Th1 and Treg cells in Tim-3$^-$ and Tim-3$^+$ CD4 T cells. Statistical analysis showed the percentage of IL-4$^+$, IL-17$^+$, IFN-γ^+, IL-2$^+$ and Foxp3$^+$ cells in Tim-3$^-$ and Tim-3$^+$ CD4 T cells from non-tumor-infiltrating lymphocytes (NIL) and tumor-infiltrating lymphocytes (TIL) isolated from HCC patients. At least 6 samples were tested in each group. Bars indicate the SEM; **, $P<0.01$; ***, $P<0.001$.

Figure S5 Statistical analysis showed the mean percentage of CD25$^+$ cells (A) and CD127^{low} cells (B) in the Tim-3 positive or Tim-3 negative CD4 T cell subsets (left), and the proportion of Tim-3$^+$ cells in the CD25 (A) and CD127 (B) high or negative/low CD4 T cell subsets (right) isolated from HCC patients. At least 12 samples were tested in each group. Bars indicate the SEM. *, $P<0.05$; **, $P<0.01$; ***, $P<0.001$.

Figure S6 Frequency of Foxp3 expression in Tim-3 single positive (Tim-3 SP), Tim-3 and PD-1 double positive (DP), PD-1 single positive (PD-1 SP), and Tim-3 and PD-1 double negative (DN) CD4 T cell subsets from non-tumor-infiltrating lymphocytes (NIL, $n=4$) and tumor-infiltrating lymphocytes (TIL, $n=4$) isolated from HCC patients. Bars indicate the SEM; *, $P<0.05$; **, $P<0.01$; ***, $P<0.001$.

Figure S7 Expression of CTLA-4, GITR and PD-1 in Tim-3$^+$Foxp3$^+$ and Tim-3$^-$Foxp3$^+$ CD4 T cells. Tumor-infiltrating lymphocytes were first gated on CD4$^+$Foxp3$^+$ T cells. Expression of CTLA-4, GITR and PD-1 were compared between Tim-3$^+$Foxp3$^+$ and Tim-3$^-$Foxp3$^+$ CD4 T cells. FACS images are representative of 4 samples. Bars indicate the SEM; *, $P<0.05$; **, $P<0.01$.

Table S1 Clinical characteristics of the four colon cancer patients.

Table S2 Clinical characteristics of the three cervical cancer patients.

Table S3 Clinical characteristics of the three ovarian cancer patients.

Table S4 Fluorochrome-conjugated antibodies used in flow cytometry.

Table S5 Correlation between Tim-3$^+$ Tregs and TNM stages in HCC.

Author Contributions

Conceived and designed the experiments: JY YZ JPZ LZ. Performed the experiments: JY YZ JPZ. Analyzed the data: JY YZ JPZ JL LL LZ. Contributed reagents/materials/analysis tools: JL LL. Wrote the paper: JY LZ.

References

1. Monney L, Sabatos CA, Gaglia JL, Ryu A, Waldner H, et al. (2002) Th1-specific cell surface protein Tim-3 regulates macrophage activation and severity of an autoimmune disease. Nature 415: 536–541.
2. Sanchez-Fueyo A, Tian J, Picarella D, Domenig C, Zheng XX, et al. (2003) Tim-3 inhibits T helper type 1-mediated auto- and alloimmune responses and promotes immunological tolerance. Nat Immunol 4: 1093–1101.
3. Sabatos CA, Chakravarti S, Cha E, Schubart A, Sanchez-Fueyo A, et al. (2003) Interaction of Tim-3 and Tim-3 ligand regulates T helper type 1 responses and induction of peripheral tolerance. Nat Immunol 4: 1102–1110.
4. Zhu C, Anderson AC, Schubart A, Xiong H, Imitola J, et al. (2005) The Tim-3 ligand galectin-9 negatively regulates T helper type 1 immunity. Nat Immunol 6: 1245–1252.
5. Wiener Z, Kohalmi B, Pocza P, Jeager J, Tolgyesi G, et al. (2007) TIM-3 is expressed in melanoma cells and is upregulated in TGF-beta stimulated mast cells. J Invest Dermatol 127: 906–914.
6. Gleason MK, Lenvik TR, McCullar V, Felices M, O'Brien MS, et al. (2012) Tim-3 is an inducible human natural killer cell receptor that enhances interferon gamma production in response to galectin-9. Blood 119: 3064–3072.
7. Sakuishi K, Jayaraman P, Behar SM, Anderson AC, Kuchroo VK (2011) Emerging Tim-3 functions in antimicrobial and tumor immunity. Trends Immunol 32: 345–349.
8. Koguchi K, Anderson DE, Yang L, O'Connor KC, Kuchroo VK, et al. (2006) Dysregulated T cell expression of TIM3 in multiple sclerosis. J Exp Med 203: 1413–1418.
9. Jones RB, Ndhlovu LC, Barbour JD, Sheth PM, Jha AR, et al. (2008) Tim-3 expression defines a novel population of dysfunctional T cells with highly elevated frequencies in progressive HIV-1 infection. J Exp Med 205: 2763–2779.
10. Ju Y, Hou N, Zhang XN, Zhao D, Liu Y, et al. (2009) Blockade of Tim-3 pathway ameliorates interferon-gamma production from hepatic CD8$^+$ T cells in a mouse model of hepatitis B virus infection. Cell Mol Immunol 6: 35–43.
11. Wu W, Shi Y, Li S, Zhang Y, Liu Y, et al. (2012) Blockade of Tim-3 signaling restores the virus-specific CD8(+) T-cell response in patients with chronic hepatitis B. Eur J Immunol 42: 1180–1191.
12. Golden-Mason L, Palmer BE, Kassam N, Townshend-Bulson L, Livingston S, et al. (2009) Negative immune regulator Tim-3 is overexpressed on T cells in hepatitis C virus infection and its blockade rescues dysfunctional CD4$^+$ and CD8$^+$ T cells. J Virol 83: 9122–9130.
13. Sehrawat S, Reddy PB, Rajasagi N, Suryawanshi A, Hirashima M, et al. (2010) Galectin-9/TIM-3 interaction regulates virus-specific primary and memory CD8 T cell response. PLoS Pathog 6: e1000882.
14. Gupta S, Thornley TB, Gao W, Larocca R, Turka LA, et al. (2012) Allograft rejection is restrained by short-lived TIM-3$^+$PD-1$^+$Foxp3$^+$ Tregs. J Clin Invest 122: 2395–2404.
15. Moorman JP, Wang JM, Zhang Y, Ji XJ, Ma CJ, et al. (2012) Tim-3 pathway controls regulatory and effector T cell balance during hepatitis C virus infection. J Immunol 189: 755–766.
16. Li H, Wu K, Tao K, Chen L, Zheng Q, et al. (2012) Tim-3/galectin-9 signaling pathway mediates T-cell dysfunction and predicts poor prognosis in patients with hepatitis B virus-associated hepatocellular carcinoma. Hepatology 56: 1342–1351.

17. Sakuishi K, Apetoh L, Sullivan JM, Blazar BR, Kuchroo VK, et al. (2010) Targeting Tim-3 and PD-1 pathways to reverse T cell exhaustion and restore anti-tumor immunity. J Exp Med 207: 2187–2194.
18. Gao X, Zhu Y, Li G, Huang H, Zhang G, et al. (2012) TIM-3 expression characterizes regulatory T cells in tumor tissues and is associated with lung cancer progression. PLoS One 7: e30676.
19. Fourcade J, Sun Z, Benallaoua M, Guillaume P, Luescher IF, et al. (2010) Upregulation of Tim-3 and PD-1 expression is associated with tumor antigen-specific $CD8^+$ T cell dysfunction in melanoma patients. J Exp Med 207: 2175–2186.
20. Yang ZZ, Grote DM, Ziesmer SC, Niki T, Hirashima M, et al. (2012) IL-12 upregulates TIM-3 expression and induces T cell exhaustion in patients with follicular B cell non-Hodgkin lymphoma. J Clin Invest 122: 1271–1282.
21. Dardalhon V, Anderson AC, Karman J, Apetoh L, Chandwaskar R, et al. (2010) Tim-3/galectin-9 pathway: regulation of Th1 immunity through promotion of $CD11b^+Ly\text{-}6G^+$ myeloid cells. J Immunol 185: 1383–1392.
22. Simmons WJ, Koneru M, Mohindru M, Thomas R, Cutro S, et al. (2005) Tim-3^+ T-bet^+ tumor-specific Th1 cells colocalize with and inhibit development and growth of murine neoplasms. J Immunol 174: 1405–1415.
23. Geng H, Zhang GM, Li D, Zhang H, Yuan Y, et al. (2006) Soluble form of T cell Ig mucin 3 is an inhibitory molecule in T cell-mediated immune response. J Immunol 176: 1411–1420.
24. Nagahara K, Arikawa T, Oomizu S, Kontani K, Nobumoto A, et al. (2008) Galectin-9 increases Tim-3^+ dendritic cells and $CD8^+$ T cells and enhances antitumor immunity via galectin-9-Tim-3 interactions. J Immunol 181: 7660–7669.
25. Zhang JP, Yan J, Xu J, Pang XH, Chen MS, et al. (2009) Increased intratumoral IL-17-producing cells correlate with poor survival in hepatocellular carcinoma patients. J Hepatol 50: 980–989.
26. Kuang DM, Zhao Q, Peng C, Xu J, Zhang JP, et al. (2009) Activated monocytes in peritumoral stroma of hepatocellular carcinoma foster immune privilege and disease progression through PD-L1. J Exp Med 206: 1327–1337.
27. Kuang DM, Peng C, Zhao Q, Wu Y, Chen MS, et al. (2010) Activated monocytes in peritumoral stroma of hepatocellular carcinoma promote expansion of memory T helper 17 cells. Hepatology 51: 154–164.
28. Zhou J, Ding T, Pan W, Zhu LY, Li L, et al. (2009) Increased intratumoral regulatory T cells are related to intratumoral macrophages and poor prognosis in hepatocellular carcinoma patients. Int J Cancer 125: 1640–1648.
29. Fu J, Xu D, Liu Z, Shi M, Zhao P, et al. (2007) Increased regulatory T cells correlate with CD8 T-cell impairment and poor survival in hepatocellular carcinoma patients. Gastroenterology 132: 2328–2339.
30. Zou W (2006) Regulatory T cells, tumour immunity and immunotherapy. Nat Rev Immunol 6: 295–307.
31. Chen M, Guo Z, Ju W, Ryffel B, He X, et al. (2012) The development and function of follicular helper T cells in immune responses. Cell Mol Immunol 9: 375–379.
32. Biswas SK, Mantovani A (2010) Macrophage plasticity and interaction with lymphocyte subsets: cancer as a paradigm. Nat Immunol 11: 889–896.
33. Szabo SJ, Kim ST, Costa GL, Zhang X, Fathman CG, et al. (2000) A novel transcription factor, T-bet, directs Th1 lineage commitment. Cell 100: 655–669.
34. Blank C, Mackensen A (2007) Contribution of the PD-L1/PD-1 pathway to T-cell exhaustion: an update on implications for chronic infections and tumor evasion. Cancer Immunol Immunother 56: 739–745.
35. Keir ME, Butte MJ, Freeman GJ, Sharpe AH (2008) PD-1 and its ligands in tolerance and immunity. Annu Rev Immunol 26: 677–704.
36. Seddiki N, Santner-Nanan B, Martinson J, Zaunders J, Sasson S, et al. (2006) Expression of interleukin (IL)-2 and IL-7 receptors discriminates between human regulatory and activated T cells. J Exp Med 203: 1693–1700.
37. Liu W, Putnam AL, Xu-Yu Z, Szot GL, Lee MR, et al. (2006) CD127 expression inversely correlates with FoxP3 and suppressive function of human $CD4^+$ T reg cells. J Exp Med 203: 1701–1711.
38. Sakaguchi S, Miyara M, Costantino CM, Hafler DA (2010) $FOXP3^+$ regulatory T cells in the human immune system. Nat Rev Immunol 10: 490–500.
39. Zheng Y, Rudensky AY (2007) Foxp3 in control of the regulatory T cell lineage. Nat Immunol 8: 457–462.
40. Li L, Godfrey WR, Porter SB, Ge Y, June CH, et al. (2005) $CD4^+CD25^+$ regulatory T-cell lines from human cord blood have functional and molecular properties of T-cell anergy. Blood 106: 3068–3073.
41. Wiersma VR, de Bruyn M, Helfrich W, Bremer E (2011) Therapeutic potential of Galectin-9 in human disease. Med Res Rev.
42. Hu G, Liu Z, Zheng C, Zheng SG (2010) Antigen-non-specific regulation centered on $CD25^+Foxp3^+$ Treg cells. Cell Mol Immunol 7: 414–418.
43. Abastado JP (2012) The next challenge in cancer immunotherapy: controlling T-cell traffic to the tumor. Cancer Res 72: 2159–2161.
44. Piersma SJ, Welters MJ, van der Burg SH (2008) Tumor-specific regulatory T cells in cancer patients. Hum Immunol 69: 241–249.
45. He J, Tang XF, Chen QY, Mai HQ, Huang ZF, et al. (2012) Ex vivo expansion of tumor-infiltrating lymphocytes from nasopharyngeal carcinoma patients for adoptive immunotherapy. Chin J Cancer 31: 287–294.
46. Woo EY, Yeh H, Chu CS, Schlienger K, Carroll RG, et al. (2002) Cutting edge: Regulatory T cells from lung cancer patients directly inhibit autologous T cell proliferation. J Immunol 168: 4272–4276.
47. Gobert M, Treilleux I, Bendriss-Vermare N, Bachelot T, Goddard-Leon S, et al. (2009) Regulatory T cells recruited through CCL22/CCR4 are selectively activated in lymphoid infiltrates surrounding primary breast tumors and lead to an adverse clinical outcome. Cancer Res 69: 2000–2009.
48. Raimondi G, Shufesky WJ, Tokita D, Morelli AE, Thomson AW (2006) Regulated compartmentalization of programmed cell death-1 discriminates $CD4^+CD25^+$ resting regulatory T cells from activated T cells. J Immunol 176: 2808–2816.
49. Mengshol JA, Golden-Mason L, Arikawa T, Smith M, Niki T, et al. (2010) A crucial role for Kupffer cell-derived galectin-9 in regulation of T cell immunity in hepatitis C infection. PLoS One 5: e9504.
50. Seki M, Oomizu S, Sakata KM, Sakata A, Arikawa T, et al. (2008) Galectin-9 suppresses the generation of Th17, promotes the induction of regulatory T cells, and regulates experimental autoimmune arthritis. Clin Immunol 127: 78–88.
51. Ngiow SF, Teng MW, Smyth MJ (2011) Prospects for TIM3-Targeted Antitumor Immunotherapy. Cancer Res 71: 6567–6571.
52. Anderson AC (2012) Tim-3, a negative regulator of anti-tumor immunity. Curr Opin Immunol 24: 213–216.
53. Fridman WH, Pages F, Sautes-Fridman C, Galon J (2012) The immune contexture in human tumours: impact on clinical outcome. Nat Rev Cancer 12: 298–306.
54. Bjorkstrom NK, Ljunggren HG, Sandberg JK (2010) CD56 negative NK cells: origin, function, and role in chronic viral disease. Trends Immunol 31: 401–406.
55. Gao Q, Wang XY, Qiu SJ, Zhou J, Shi YH, et al. (2011) Tumor stroma reaction-related gene signature predicts clinical outcome in human hepatocellular carcinoma. Cancer Sci 102: 1522–1531.
56. Fourcade J, Sun Z, Pagliano O, Guillaume P, Luescher IF, et al. (2012) CD8(+) T cells specific for tumor antigens can be rendered dysfunctional by the tumor microenvironment through upregulation of the inhibitory receptors BTLA and PD-1. Cancer Res 72: 887–896.

15

Characterization of an Italian Founder Mutation in the RING-Finger Domain of *BRCA1*

Laura Caleca[1*⁹], Anna Laura Putignano[2,3⁹], Mara Colombo[1], Caterina Congregati[2], Mohosin Sarkar[4], Thomas J. Magliery[4], Carla B. Ripamonti[1], Claudia Foglia[1], Bernard Peissel[5], Daniela Zaffaroni[5], Siranoush Manoukian[5], Carlo Tondini[6], Monica Barile[7], Valeria Pensotti[8,9], Loris Bernard[8,10], Laura Papi[2¶], Paolo Radice[1¶]

1 Unit of Molecular Bases of Genetic Risk and Genetic Testing, Department of Preventive and Predictive Medicine, Fondazione IRCCS Istituto Nazionale dei Tumori (INT), c/o Amadeolab, Milano, Italy, **2** Department of Biomedical, Experimental and Clinical Sciences, University of Florence, Florence, Italy, **3** FiorGen Foundation for Pharmacogenomics, Sesto Fiorentino, Italy, **4** Department of Chemistry and Department of Biochemistry, The Ohio State University, Columbus, Ohio, United States of America, **5** Unit of Medical Genetics, Department of Preventive and Predictive Medicine, Fondazione IRCCS Istituto Nazionale dei Tumori, Milan, Italy, **6** Unit of Medical Oncology, Azienda Ospedaliera Papa Giovanni XXIII, Bergamo, Italy, **7** Division of Cancer Prevention and Genetics, Istituto Europeo di Oncologia, Milan, Italy, **8** COGENTECH-Cancer Genetic Testing Laboratory, Milan, Italy, **9** Fondazione Istituto FIRC di Oncologia Molecolare, Milan, Italy, **10** Department of Experimental Oncology, Istituto Europeo di Oncologia, Milan, Italy

Abstract

The identification of founder mutations in cancer predisposing genes is important to improve risk assessment in geographically defined populations, since it may provide specific targets resulting in cost-effective genetic testing. Here, we report the characterization of the *BRCA1* c.190T>C (p.Cys64Arg) mutation, mapped to the RING-finger domain coding region, that we detected in 43 hereditary breast/ovarian cancer (HBOC) families, for the large part originating from the province of Bergamo (Northern Italy). Haplotype analysis was performed in 21 families, and led to the identification of a shared haplotype extending over three *BRCA1*-associated marker loci (0.4 cM). Using the DMLE+2.2 software program and regional population demographic data, we were able to estimate the age of the mutation to vary between 3,100 and 3,350 years old. Functional characterization of the mutation was carried out at both transcript and protein level. Reverse transcriptase-PCR analysis on lymphoblastoid cells revealed expression of full length mRNA from the mutant allele. A green fluorescent protein (GFP)-fragment reassembly assay showed that the p.Cys64Arg substitution prevents the binding of the BRCA1 protein to the interacting protein BARD1, in a similar way as proven deleterious mutations in the RING-domain. Overall, 55 of 83 (66%) female mutation carriers had a diagnosis of breast and/or ovarian cancer. Our observations indicate that the *BRCA1* c.190T>C is a pathogenic founder mutation present in the Italian population. Further analyses will evaluate whether screening for this mutation can be suggested as an effective strategy for the rapid identification of at-risk individuals in the Bergamo area.

Editor: Klaus Brusgaard, Odense University Hospital, Denmark

Funding: This study was partially supported by funds from the Italian Association for Cancer Research (AIRC, http://www.airc.it/), grant no. 11897. The funder had no role in study design, data collection and analysis, decision to publish, or preparation of the manuscript. No additional external funding was received for this study.

Competing Interests: The authors have declared that no competing interests exist.

* E-mail: laura.caleca@istitutotumori.mi.it

⁹ These authors contributed equally to this work.

¶ These authors also contributed equally to this work.

Introduction

Inactivating germline mutations of *BRCA1* and *BRCA2* genes account for approximately 15% to 20% of hereditary breast and/or ovarian cancer (HBOC) cases [1,2]. The majority of alterations identified throughout the whole sequence of both genes are private or detected in few families only [3], but a number of specific mutations that appear repeatedly in ethnically defined groups or in populations enriched with genetic isolates, because of a shared common ancestry (founder mutations), have been reported [4].

The identification of founder mutations in various ethnic groups and their geographical distribution has important implications for designing mutational screening. For example, three founder mutations in the Ashkenazi Jewish (*BRCA1* c.68_69delAG, *BRCA1* c.5266dupC, *BRCA2* c.5946delT) and one in the Icelanders (*BRCA2* c.771_775del5), account for virtually all HBOC families linked to BRCA genes in these populations [5–8], where, therefore, it is worthwhile to test high-risk patients specifically for these mutations, before considering the more expensive complete sequence analysis of both genes. Furthermore, the identification of recurrent genomic rearrangements of the *BRCA1* and *BRCA2* genes, due to founder effects, has provided a strong rational for including the screening for these alterations in the diagnostic setting. For instance, in the Dutch population two distinct deletions involving exons 13 and 22 account for approximately 25% of all *BRCA1*-positive families [9], while approximately 9% of *BRCA1*-positive families in the United Kingdom carry a common exon 13 duplication [10]. As a result, in these populations screening for specific *BRCA1* rearrangements is now part of routine genetic testing of HBOC families. Notably, the knowledge of founder *BRCA1* or *BRCA2* mutations may provide more precise estimates of the prior probability of carrying a mutation in either genes and of the likelihood of a mutation carrier developing cancer [11].

To date, a few BRCA founder mutations have been reported also in the Italian population, where they appear to be limited to geographically restricted areas (reviewed in ref. 4).

Here, we report the characterization of the *BRCA1* c.190T>C missense mutation (p.Cys64Arg), located in the gene region coding for the RING-finger motif of the protein, which segregates with the disease in Italian HBOC families, mostly originating from the province of Bergamo (Northern Italy).

Materials and Methods

Ethics Statement

All subjects included in the study received genetic counseling and provided a written informed consent for BRCA gene mutation testing and for the use of their biological samples for research purposes: This study was approved by the ethical committee of the Fondazione IRCCS Istituto Nazionale dei Tumori (INT) of Milan.

Case Material

The study includes 43 apparently unrelated families carrying the c.190T>C (p.Cys64Arg) mutation in *BRCA1* exon 5, identified among those referred for BRCA gene testing from December 1995 to December 2012 by the following institutions: Fondazione IRCCS Istituto Nazionale dei Tumori (INT) and Istituto Oncologico Europeo (IEO) of Milan, Azienda Ospedaliera Papa Giovanni XXIII of Bergamo (AO-BG) and University of Florence (Department of Biomedical, Experimental and Clinical Sciences). The presence of the mutation was ascertained in family probands by either denaturing high performance liquid chromatography (DHPLC) and/or direct sequencing of all coding exons and adjacent intronic regions of the *BRCA1* and *BRCA2* genes. Sequencing of *BRCA1* exon 5 was performed to identify additional mutation carriers among the probands' relatives.

Microsatellite analysis

A total of 76 individuals, including 43 mutation carriers and 33 non carriers, from 21 of the above families were genotyped at the *BRCA1* locus as previously described [12].

Haplotyping and estimate of mutation age

Haplotypes were constructed manually from microsatellite analyses, assuming the least number of possible recombinations. Age estimate of the *BRCA1* c.190T>C mutation was carried out with the DMLE+2.2 software program (URL: http://www.dmle.org) [13]. The DMLE input file included the full haplotypes of mutations carriers and of non-carriers, used as controls from the general population, for the 6 examined markers, chromosome map distances derived from the Marshfield and/or Genéthon sex-average genetic maps (URL: http://www.ncbi.nlm.nih.gov/mapview/), an estimate of population growth rate per generation and an estimate of the proportion of sampled mutation-carrying chromosomes. The population growth rates per generation (r) were estimated as described [12], based on available demographic data (Italian National Statistics Institute, ISTAT; URL: http://www.istat.it) and assuming a time interval of 25 years per generation. The r value for the province of Bergamo from the year 1300 to present was estimated to be 0,0526. This index was subsequently used for mutation age estimates. Three separate analyses were then performed, each using a different estimate for the proportion of sampled mutation-carrying chromosomes: 0.015, 0.01, and 0.005.

Transcript analysis

Epstein-Barr virus (EBV)-immortalized human lymphoblastoid cell lines (LCLs) were established and cultured as described [14]. Four *BRCA1* mutant and six wild-type LCLs were grown in the absence and in the presence of cycloheximide (CHX) (100 µg/ml) for 4 hours to account for potential degradation of unstable transcripts via nonsense mediated mRNA decay. Total RNA was purified and reverse transcribed into cDNA as described [14]. The PCR reaction was performed with a forward primer in *BRCA1* exon 5 (5′-GCATGCTGAAACTTCTCAAC-3′), and a reverse primer in exon 6 (5′-TCCAAACCTGTGTCAAGCTG-3′). The reverse primer was labeled with 6-carboxyfluorescein (6-FAM). The fluorescent amplification products were run on a 3130 Genetic Analyzer (Applied Biosystems) using the GeneScan 500 ROX Size Standard (Applied Biosystems) as internal marker. Size calling and quantification of peak areas were performed with GeneMapper Software v4.0 (Applied Biosystems). The molecular nature of the peaks was confirmed by sequencing.

Statistical Analysis

The ratios of the peak areas of the *BRCA1* Δexon5q and full-length mRNA isoforms in different samples were compared by two-tailed Student t test using GraphPad Prism version 5.0 software and 95% confidence interval (CI).

Plasmid construction

The pET11a-NfrGFP-Z and pMRBAD-Z-CfrGFP expression vectors, encoding anti-parallel leucine zipper motifs (Z) fused to the N-terminal or C-terminal fragment of Green Fluorescent Protein (NfrGFP, CfrGFP, respectively) and the plasmids encoding N-terminal RING domains of BARD1 (amino acids 26–140) and BRCA1 (amino acids 1–109) attached via a linker sequences to the NfrGFP (pET11a-NfrGFP-BARD1) or CfrGFP (pMRBAD-BRCA1-CfrGFP), were created as described [15]. The pET11a-NfrGFP-Z and pET11a-NfrGFP-BARD1 vectors also encode a hexahistidine (H_6)-tag at the N-terminus of the NfrGFP useful for rapid purification of the H_6-tagged protein. The pMRBAD-Z-CfrGFP and pMRBAD-BRCA1-CfrGFP (both as wild-type and mutant forms) bear an HA epitope at the C-terminus of the CfrGFP as a detection tag. The *BRCA1* c.190T>C (p.Cys64Arg), c.199G>T (p.Asp67Tyr) and c.181T>G (p.Cys61Gly) mutants were obtained by direct mutagenesis of pMRBAD-BRCA1-CfrGFP using the QuikChange XL Site-directed Mutagenesis Kit (Stratagene) according to the manufacturer's instruction. Recombinant clones were checked by DNA sequencing.

GFP-fragment reassembly screening

Compatible pairs of plasmids [pET11a-NfrGFP-Z and pMRBAD-Z-CfrGFP; pET11a-NfrGFP-BARD1 and pMRBAD-BRCA1-CfrGFP (both as wild-type or mutant forms)] were co-transformed into BL21-(DE3) *E. coli* competent cells by electroporation. Single colonies were screened for the occurrence of GFP-fragment reassembly as previously described [15].Fluorescence was observed after excitation with long-wave (365 nm) UV light in combination with the short pass (SP) emission filter using a Syngene image capture system (SYNGENE) as specified by the manufacturer.

Purification of the reassembled GFP complexes

The H_6-NfrGFP-Z/Z-CfrGFP-HA and H_6-NfrGFP-BARD1/BRCA1-CfrGFP-HA (both as wild-type or mutant forms) complexes were purified from the soluble fraction of co-transformed *E. coli* strain BL21-(DE3) by Immobilized Metal Affinity Chromatography (IMAC) using nickel nitrilotriacetic (Ni-NTA) agarose resin (QIAGEN), following the protocol described [15]. The protein complexes were subjected to 13% SDS-PAGE and visualized by Western blotting using a polyclonal anti-GFP antibody (# 600-101-215; Rockland). Unpurified cell lysates from induced *E. coli* BL21-(DE3) bacteria were similarly resolved and visualized to detect expression levels of both NfrGFP-BARD1 and CfrGFP-BRCA1 recombinant proteins.

Clinical and pathological characteristics

Clinical and pathological data of affected mutation carriers were collected at genetic counseling and from medical records. Loss of heterozygosity (LOH) at *BRCA1* locus in tumor DNA was performed as previously described [16].

Results

Geographical distribution and frequency of the *BRCA1* c.190T>C families

The birth places of the probands of the 43 *BRCA1* c.190T>C positive families are shown in Figure 1. The majority were from the city of Bergamo and its province (n = 23) or from neighboring provinces of the Lombardy region (n = 16). The frequencies of c.190T>C positive families on the total number of families tested for *BRCA1* and *BRCA2* mutations and on the total number of BRCA-positive families were 8.7% and 30.2%, respectively, in cases recruited in Bergamo and 0.8% and 3.2%, respectively, in cases recruited in Milan (Table 1).

Haplotype analysis

Fragment analysis of 6 microsatellite marker loci intragenic and flanking *BRCA1* identified a shared haplotype extending over 3 marker loci (0.4 cM) in carriers of the *BRCA1* c.190T>C from 20 families for which DNA of more than one member was available (Figure 2). In one additional mutated family with only one individual available for the analysis, the observed genotypes were compatible with the shared haplotype.

Age estimate of the *BRCA1* c.190T>C mutation

The DMLE+2.2 program was used to estimate the age of the *BRCA1* c.190T>C mutation based on haplotype data from mutation carriers and non carriers.

Three separate analyses were performed, using a population growth rate per generation of 0.052 and different estimates of the proportion of sampled mutation-carrying chromosomes (0.015, 0.01 and 0.005). The resulting age estimates were 124 generations (95% credible set: 79–170), 130 generations (95% credible set: 91–170) and 134 generations (95% credible set: 97–171), respectively (data not shown). Assuming an interval of 25 years per generation, this corresponds to the mutation being 3,100, 3,250 and 3,350 years old, respectively. Thus, age estimates were only slightly affected by the actual proportion of sampled mutation-carrying chromosomes.

Evaluation of the effect of the *BRCA1* c.190T>C variant on mRNA transcripts

The *BRCA1* c.190T>C variant is mapped to an alternatively used donor splice site. The usage of this site leads to the synthesis of a naturally occurring isoform missing 22 bp at the 3′-end of exon 5 (Δexon5q) [17,18]. To evaluate the putative effect of the mutation on Δexon5q and full-length transcription levels, the cDNA region encompassing the mutation site was amplified and analyzed by capillary electrophoresis. The ratio between the peak areas of the Δexon5q and the full-length isoforms in LCLs carrying the c.190T>C, cultured in the presence and in the absence of

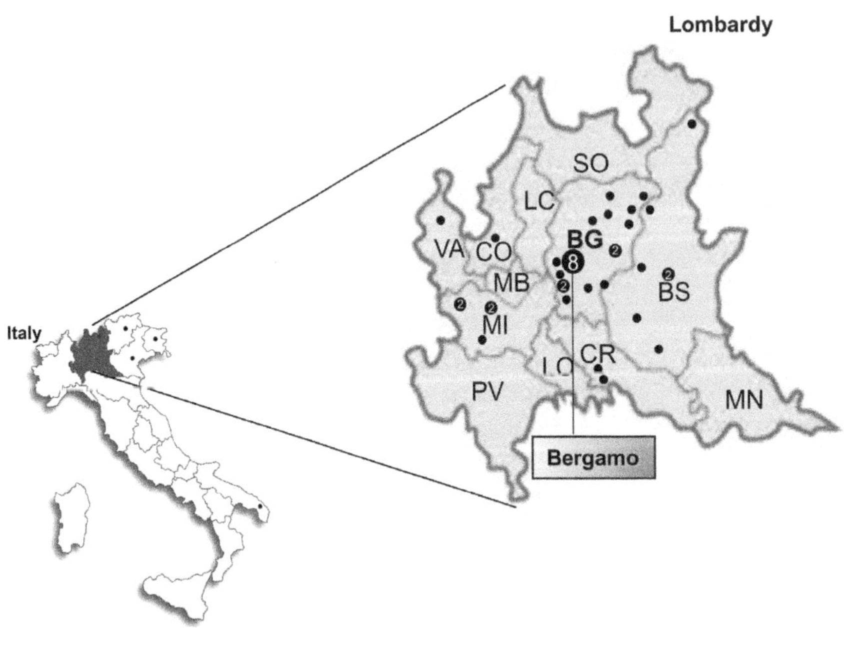

Figure 1. Geographical distribution of *BRCA1* c.190T>C (p.Cys64Arg) mutation carriers. Symbol ("•") indicates the birth places of index case from families segregating the mutation.

Table 1. Number and frequencies of *BRCA1* c.190T>C positive families among those recruited at three Italian institutions and tested for BRCA mutations.

Institution	No. identified	% on total tested families*	% on BRCA1/2 families
INT	22	1,03 (22/2140)	3,98 (22/553)
IEO	4	0,39 (4/1013)	1,54 (4/260)
INT+IEO	26	0,82 (26/3153)	3,20 (26/813)
AO-BG	16	8,74 (16/183)	30,19 (16/53)

*Intake criteria for BRCA testing are described in Manoukian et al [38].

cycloheximide, was calculated and compared with those of wild-type LCLs (Figure 3). The LCL carrying the *BRCA1* c.212G>A mutation previously reported to up-regulate the Δexon5q isoform [14] was used as internal control. A significant decrease in the ratio of the Δexon5q vs. full length expression levels was observed in the c.190T>C LCLs compared to normal controls (0,45, 95% CI = 0.44–0.46 and 0.52, 95%, CI = 0.50–0.54, for the CHX-untreated and treated samples, respectively). Sequence analyses detected the presence of the mutation in the full length cDNA (data not shown). These results indicate that the c.190T>C mutation does not impair the synthesis of full-length mRNA and are consistent with a sustained expression of the mutated protein.

Evaluation of the effect of the c.190T>C mutation on the interaction of BRCA1 with BARD1

The BRCA1 protein displays an E3 ubiquitin ligase activity mediated by the interaction with BARD1 through its N-terminal RING-finger domain [19,20], where the c.190T>C (p.Cys64Arg) is located.

To assess whether the mutation affects the BRCA1/BARD1 complex formation, we carried out a GFP-fragment reassembly screening, a Bimolecular Fluorescence Complementation-based assay (BiFC) [21]. In this assay, the GFP is dissected into two fragments (NfrGFP and CfrGFP) that, when expressed together in *E. coli* cells, do not spontaneously reassemble into a fluorescence

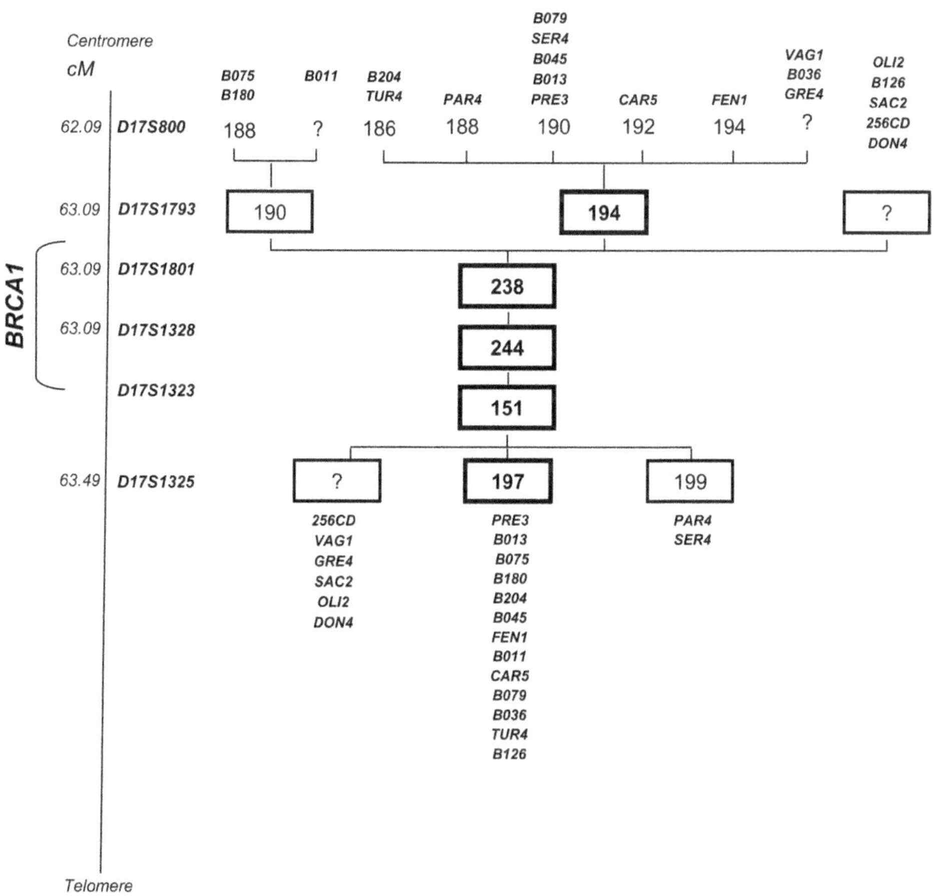

Figure 2. Haplotype branching trees in families segregating the *BRCA1* c.190T>C (p.Cys64Arg). The six short tandem repeat markers analyzed are shown together with their position in the Marshfield genetic map. Family haplotypes are indicated with the corresponding family ID codes. The most common haplotype is indicated in bold numbers.

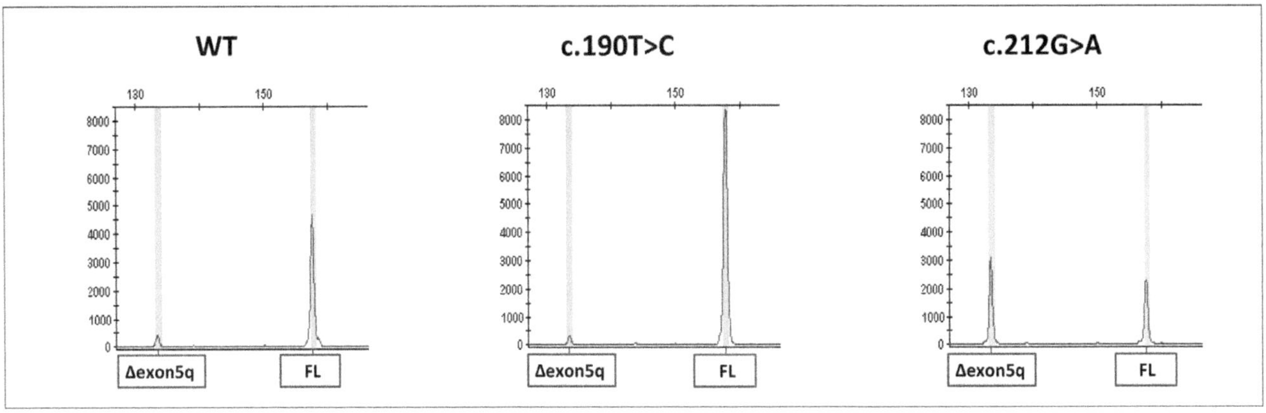

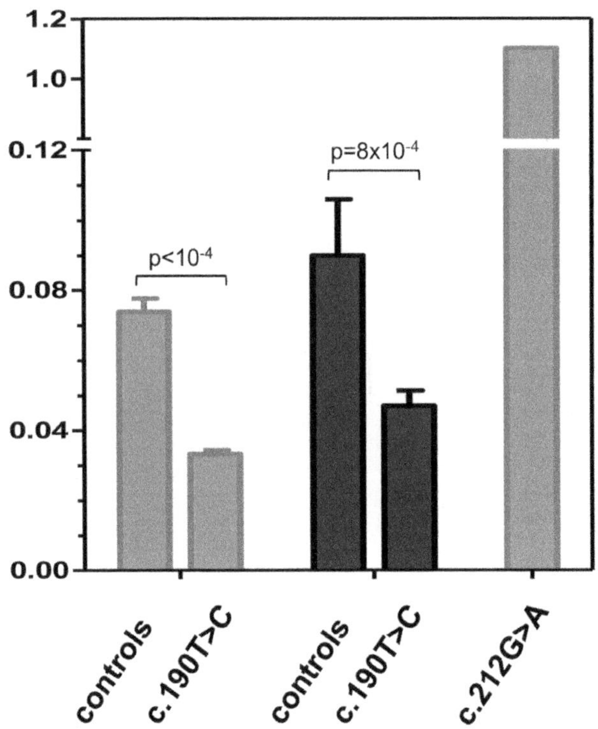

Figure 3. Semi-quantitative fragment analysis of the Δexon5q isoform. The upper panel shows the capillary electrophoresis patterns of the cDNA fragments spanning *BRCA1* exons 5 and 6 observed in LCLs from a *BRCA1* wild type individual, and from carriers of the c.190T>C and c.212G>A, which causes the up-regulation of the Δexon5q transcript, mutations. The Δexon5q and full-length (FL) isoforms are indicated. The lower panel shows the ratio between the peak areas of the Δexon5q and full-length isoforms. The LCLs were cultured in the presence (dark grey bars) and in the absence (light grey bar) of cycloheximide. Control bars represent the average value observed in six wild-type LCLs. c.190T>C bars represent the average value observed in four mutant LCLs. The error bars represent standard deviation.

protein. However, if the two fragments of GFP are each individually fused to two interacting proteins, this interaction can mediate reassembly of the GFP in co-transformed bacteria with consequent cellular fluorescence [22].

Under inducing conditions (0.2% L-arabinose and 20 µM IPTG; Fig. 4A, left column), bright fluorescence was observed in bacterial cells co-expressing BARD1-NfrGFP together with BRCA1-wild type/CfrGFP or BRCA1-D67Y/CfrGFP carrying the variant p.Asp67Tyr, previously classified as clinically neutral [3] and the strong interacting anti-parallel Z-NfrGFP/Z-CfrGFP fusion peptides. No fluorescence was observed in bacteria co-expressing the following fusion peptides: non cognate BARD1 NfrGFP/CfrGFP-Z, BARD1-NfrGFP/BRCA1-C61G-CfrGFP carrying the p.Cys61Gly disease-causing mutation [23], and BARD1-NfrGFP/BRCA1-C64R-CfrGFP carrying the p.Cys64Arg mutation. In addition, IMAC purified reassembled complexes from the soluble fraction of co-transformed cells *E. coli* BL21-(DE3) were analyzed by Western blotting (Figure 4B). Using a polyclonal anti-GFP antibody, two strong bands corresponding to the components of the GFP reassembled complexes were detected in lysates of bacterial cells co-expressing Z-NfrGFP/CfrGFP-Z and BARD1-NfrGFP together with BRCA1-wild type/CfrGFP or BRCA1-Asp67Tyr. Much more reduced bands were observed in cell lysates co-expressing BARD1-NfrGFP and BRCA1-Cys61Gly/CfrGFP or BRCA1-Cys64Arg/CfrGFP. Since unassembled GFP fusion fragments are unfolded and less soluble [24], these results indicate GFP reassembly and, therefore, BRCA1/BARD1 binding for the BRCA1-wt and BRCA1-Asp67Tyr constructs, but not for the BRCA1-Cys61Gly and BRCA1-Cys64Arg constructs. These observations are consistent with those obtained by fluorescence complementation assay. Unpurified cell lysates from co-transformed *E. coli* BL21-(DE3) bacteria, were visualized by Western blotting with a polyclonal anti-GFP antibody, revealing that all the fusion peptides were expressed to a similar extent (Figure 4C). This demonstrates that the lack of co-purification of CfrGFP-BRCA1-HA fragments for the Cys61Gly and Cys64Arg constructs is attributable to the lack of binding to BARD1 and not to poor expression of the BRCA1 mutants.

Clinical and pathological features of *BRCA1* c.190T>C carriers

Overall, a total of 86 ascertained mutation carriers and of 7 obligate carriers were identified in the families recruited in the study, including 83 females and 10 males. Among female carriers, 55 (66%) reported a diagnosis of breast carcinoma (n = 38), ovarian carcinoma (n = 12) or both breast and ovarian carcinomas (n = 5).

Available clinical and pathological features of the affected female carriers are reported in Table 2 and 3. The median ages of breast cancer and ovarian cancer diagnosis were 39.6 and 48.2 years, respectively. The large majority of breast cancers were of high grade (23/28 = 82.1%). The prevalent histological type was ductal (32/38 = 84.2%), being the remaining cases mostly of the medullary type (4/38 = 10.5%). The frequencies of cancers positive for estrogen receptor (ER), progesterone receptor (PR) and human epidermal growth factor receptor 2 (HER2/Neu) were 4/31 (12.9%), 6/31 (19.4%) and 3/22 (13.6%), respectively. The information for all the above tumor markers was available in 23

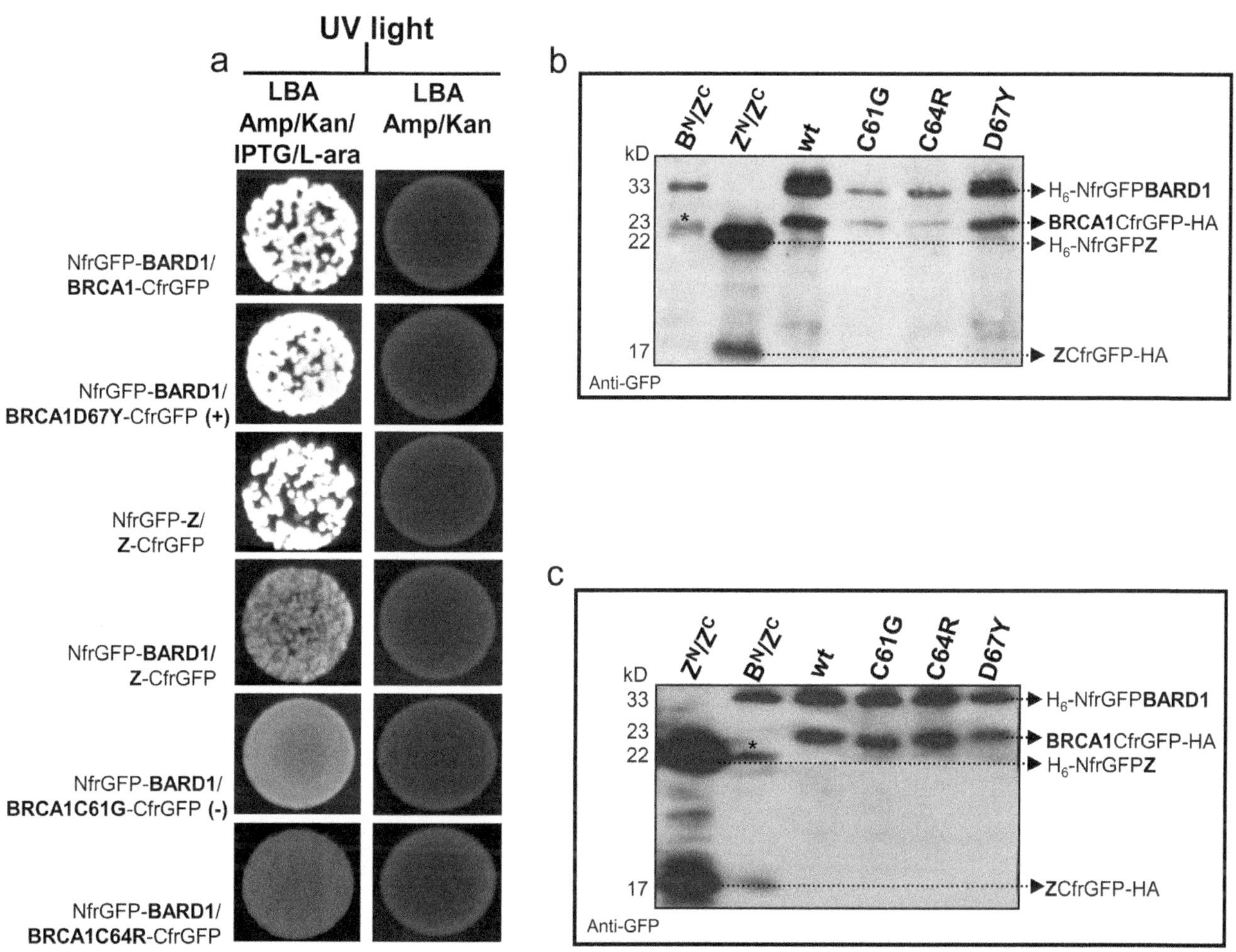

Figure 4. Detection of BRCA1/BARD1 interaction by GFP-fragment reassembly screening. (a) Fluorescence was observed after 24 h of growth at 30°C followed by 2 days of incubation at RT. No fluorescence is observed under non-inducing condition (right column). [L-ara, L-arabinose; IPTG, Isopropyl β-D-1-tiogalattopiranoside, IPTG]. (b) SDS-PAGE of purified, reassembled complexes by IMAC methods. The expected molecular masses are indicated on the left. [*Non-specific band. B^N, H_6-NfrGFPBARD1; Z^N, H_6-ZNfrGFP; Z^C, ZCfrGFP-HA]. (c) Expression of NfrGFP-BARD1 and CfrGFP-BRCA1 wild-type and mutant forms.

cases, and the majority (15 = 65.2%) displayed a triple-negative (TN) phenotype (lack of the expression of ER, PR and HER2/Neu). The frequencies of contralateral breast cancer were 8/18 (44.4%) and 12/15 (80%) 5 and 10 years after the first diagnosis of breast cancer, respectively. Three patients were diagnosed with additional cancers, including one malignant mixed mullerian tumor (MMMT) of the endometrium, one endometrial carcinoma, and one basal cell carcinoma. As for ovarian cancers, the large majority were of high grade (10/11 = 90.9%) and of the serous type (9/11 = 81.8%). Of the remaining female carriers, one reported a pheochromocytoma at 27 years, and 27 were cancer-free at the time of last contact (mean age = 41 years).

Three cancer diagnoses were reported in male carriers, one prostate carcinoma, one tumor of the central nervous system and one leukemia.

LOH at *BRCA1* locus was investigated in two tumors, one breast carcinoma and the MMMT. In both cases, the loss of the constitutional wild-type allele was observed (data not shown).

Discussion

The *BRCA1* c.190T>C mutation was firstly described in a large Polish cancer family [25]. Subsequently, it was reported in an Italian family characterized by high prevalence of ovarian and breast cancer cases by Willems and co-authors [26]. These authors showed by molecular modeling that the mutation may induce profound modifications in the structure of the BRCA1 RING finger motif, without affecting the normal splicing pattern of the transcripts.

A total of 43 apparently unrelated Italian families carrying the same mutations were referred by four different Italian clinical and university centers. The observation that a large part (23/43 = 53%) were from the same geographic area, the province of Bergamo in Northern Italy, strongly suggested an origin of the mutation from a common ancestor. Consistently, the frequencies of c.190T>C families on the total number of those that underwent BRCA gene testing and of those carrying pathogenic *BRCA1* and *BRCA2* mutations were approximately 10-fold higher in cases recruited in Bergamo, around 85% of whom referred to be born in the local area, compared to those observed in families recruited in two large cancer centers in Milan, which attract patients from all over Italy. The analysis of microsatellite marker loci revealed a shared haplotype in 21 typed families, confirming the founder effect hypothesis. In addition, we estimated the origin of this mutation within a time interval ranging from 3100 to 3350 years ago.

Interestingly, the c.190T>C affects the same nucleotide of another mutation (c.190T>G) that strengthen an alternatively used donor splice site in exon 5 and also disrupts a putative exonic splicing enhancer motif. This leads the loss of the natural donor splice site, resulting in the lack of full length expression and the up-regulation of the naturally occurring Δexon5q isoform, predicted to lead to the synthesis of a truncated protein [17,18]. In agreement with previous observations [26], no such effect was observed for the c.190T>C. Conversely, in the LCL carrying this mutation a reduction in the relative amount of Δexon5q compared to full length was observed. This finding and the detection of the c.190T>C in the full-length cDNA is consistent with a stable expression of the Cys64Arg protein in mutation carriers.

The BRCA1 p.Cys64Arg mutation is located to the gene region coding for the RING-finger motif of the protein. The RING-finger motif is defined by a conserved pattern of seven cysteine and one histidine residues arranged in an interleaved fashion forming two distinct Zn^{2+}-binding sites termed Site I and Site II [27].

Table 2. Clinical and pathological features of *BRCA1* c.190T>C related breast cancer cases.

Breast Cancers (n = 43)	n	%
Age at first diagnosis (years)		
<36	15	34.9
36	22	51.2
>50	6	14.0
Median	39.6	
Behaviour		
Invasive	40	100
In situ	-	-
Not available	3	
Histological types		
Ductal	32	84.2
Lobular	-	-
Medullary	4	10.5
Combined[a]	1	2.6
Other	1	2.6
Not available	5	
Histological grade		
1	2	7.1
2	3	10.7
3	23	82.1
Not available	15	
ER		
Positive	4	12.9
Negative	27	87.1
Not available	12	
PR		
Positive	6	19.4
Negative	25	80.6
Not available	12	
Her2/Neu		
Positive	3	13.6
Negative	19	86.4
Not available	21	
Triple Negative		
Yes	15	65.2
Not	8	34.8
Not available	20	

[a]Ductal and lobular type.

Approximately 10% of the clinically relevant mutations of BRCA1 currently reported in the Breast Cancer Information Core (BIC) database (URL: http://research.nhgri.nih.gov/bic/) map within the N-terminal 100 residues-RING domain, which contain the RING motif (residues 23–76). Functional analyses have shown that these mutations abrogate the ubiquitin-ligase activity of BRCA1 by interfering with both the heterodimerization between BRCA1 and BARD1 and the binding of E2 protein UbcH5c to the BRCA1/BARD1 complex [28,29].

Table 3. Clinical and pathological features of *BRCA1* c.190T>C related ovarian cancer cases.

Ovarian cancers (n = 17)	n	%
Age at first diagnosis (years)		
<36	-	-
36	12	70.6
>50	5	29.4
Median	48.2	
Behaviour		
Invasive	13	100
In situ	-	-
Not available	4	
Histological types		
Serous	9	81.8
Mucinous	-	-
Endometroid	2	18.2
Clear Cell	-	-
Other	-	-
Not available	6	
Histological grade		
1	-	-
2	1	9.1
3	10	90.9
Not available	6	

Presently, the BRCA1 p.Cys64Arg mutation is reported in the BIC database as a variant of unknown clinical relevance. However, *in silico* analysis using SIFT (URL: http://sift.jcvi.org/), Polyphen-2 (URL: http://genetics.bwh.harvard.edu/pph2/) and Align-GVGD (URL: http://agvgd.iarc.fr/) bioinformatics tools unanimously predicted the BRCA1 p.Cys64Arg to be deleterious. This is consistent with the notion that Cys64Arg disrupts a critical cysteine residue required for the ubiquitin-ligase activity of BRCA1, through its binding to BARD1 [30]. In fact, the analysis of the three-dimensional Nuclear Magnetic Resonance (NMR) structure of the BRCA1/BARD1 heterodimer showed that p.Cys64Arg substitution determines a profound rearrangement of the BRCA1 39–41 amino acid residues, predicted to result into the impairment of the BRCA1/BARD1 interaction [26].

The result of our GFP-fragment reassembly assay provided experimental evidence that the p.Cys64Arg actually abrogates BRCA1/BARD1 binding as the proven disease causing mutation p.Cys61Gly [31], thus further supporting the pathogenic role of this variant. Interestingly, another mutation affecting the same amino acid residue (p.Cys64Gly) was previously reported to have a similar effect [32]. In addition, our study indicates that this functional approach might be applied to the assessment of the clinical significance of a number of variants in cancer-predisposing genes, implementing currently used strategies.

The median age of breast cancer diagnosis in carriers of the c.190T>C mutation (39.7 years) was similar to that observed in 425 breast cancer patients with other pathogenic *BRCA1* mutations ascertained at the institutions participating in this study (40.1 years). Conversely, among c.190T>C carriers the median age of ovarian cancer onset (48.2 years) was lower than that observed in 192 *BRCA1*-positive ovarian cancer patients from the same institutions (51.9 years), suggesting a possible higher risk of ovarian cancer in carriers of the c.190T>C compared to carriers of other *BRCA1* mutations.

Breast cancers arising in *BRCA1* c.190T>C mutation carriers showed the peculiar histopathological features of the *BRCA1*-related breast tumor [33,34], with a propensity to be high grade invasive ductal or medullary carcinomas. In addition, the majority displayed a TN phenotype. The clinical relevance of the TN breast cancers is highlighted by the distinctive poor prognosis and no clear options for receptor targeted treatment [35,36]. In agreement with other reports on *BRCA1* associated ovarian carcinomas [37,38], invasive epithelial cancer of serous histology was found to be the most common histological subtype among *BRCA1* c.190T>C mutation carriers. Although these observations might be biased by the relative small number of ascertained individuals and by the preferential selection of high risk subjects referred to genetic testing, they are consistent (together with the findings that in two examined tumors the wild type *BRCA1* allele was lost) with the c.190T>C behaving as other *BRCA1* pathogenic variants.

In conclusion, our data show that the *BRCA1* c.190 T>C missense mutation (p.Cys64Arg) is a founder mutation of clinical relevance recurrent in high-risk families from the province of Bergamo, accounting for a significant fraction (ca. 9%) of those ascertained at the local city hospital. Additional studies are needed to assess the actual proportion of carriers of this mutation in this district and its frequency in unselected breast/ovarian cancer patients. This will allow evaluating whether screening for the c.190T>C mutation can be suggested as a cost-effective strategy for the rapid identification of at-risk individuals in the Bergamo area. In addition, they will provide a measure of associated cancer risks, thus improving decision-making regarding clinical management of mutation carriers.

Acknowledgments

We thank Giulietta Scuvera, Donata Penso, Maria Teresa Radice, Massimo Moro, Antonio Fiorino of INT and the personnel of the Cogentech Cancer Genetic Testing laboratory.

Author Contributions

Conceived and designed the experiments: LC ALP MC CBR LP PR. Performed the experiments: LC ALP MC CC CBR. Analyzed the data: LC ALP MC CBR LP PR. Contributed reagents/materials/analysis tools: MS TJM CF BP DZ SM CT MB. Wrote the paper: LC MC LP PR. Contributed to case selection by performing BRCA testing: VP LB. Provided genetic, pathological, clinical and pedigrees of enrolled cases: SM BP DZ CT MB.

References

1. Peto J, Collins R, Barfoot R, Seal S, Warren W, et al. (1991) Prevalence of BRCA1 and BRCA2 Gene Mutations in Patients with Early-Onset Breast Cancer. J Natl Cancer I 91: 943–949.
2. Fackenthal JD, Olopade OI (2007) Breast cancer risk associated with *BRCA1* and *BRCA2* in diverse populations. Nat Rev 7: 937–948.
3. Easton DF, Deffenbaugh AM, Pruss D, Frye C, Wenstrup RJ, et al. (2007) A Systematic Genetic Assessment of 1,433 Sequence Variants of Unknown Clinical Significance in the *BRCA1* and *BRCA2* Breast Cancer–Predisposition Genes. Am J Hum Genet 81: 873–883.
4. Janavičius R (2010) Founder *BRCA1/2* mutations in the Europe: implications for hereditary breast-ovarian cancer prevention and control. EPMA J 1: 397–412.

5. Tonin P, Weber B, Offit K, Couch F, Rebbeck TR, et al. (1996) Frequency of recurrent BRCA1 and BRCA2 mutations in Ashkenazi Jewish breast cancer families. Nat Med 2: 1179–1183.
6. Johannesdottir G, Gudmundsson J, Bergthorsson JT, Arason A, Agnarsson AB, et al. (1996) High Prevalence of the 999del5 Mutation in Icelandic Breast and Ovarian Cancer Patients. Cancer Res 56: 3663–3665.
7. Struewing JP, Hartge P, Wacholder S, Baker SM, Berlin M, et al. (1997) The risk of cancer associated with specific mutations of *BRCA1* and *BRCA2* among Ashkenazi Jews. New Engl J Med 336: 1401–1408.
8. Warner E, Foulkes W, Goodwin P, Meschino W, Blondal J, et al. (1999) Prevalence and penetrance of BRCA1 and BRCA2 gene mutations in unselected in Ashkenazi Jewish woman with breast cancer. J Natl Cancer Inst 9: 1241–1247.
9. Petrij-Bosch A, Peelen T, van Vliet M, van Eijk R, Olmer R, et al. (1997) BRCA1 genomic deletions are major founder mutations in Dutch breast cancer patients. Nat Genet 17: 341–345.
10. Puget N, Sinilnikova OM, Stoppa-Lyonnet D, Audoynaud C, Pagèes S, et al. (1999) An *Alu*-mediated 6-kb duplication in the *BRCA1* gene: a new founder mutation? Am J Hum Genet 64: 300–302.
11. Neuhausen SL (2000) Founder populations and their uses for breast cancer genetics. Breast Cancer Res 2: 77–81.
12. Papi L, Putignano AL, Congregati C, ZannaI, Sera F, et al. (2009) Founder mutations account for the majority of BRCA1-attributable hereditary breast/ovarian cancer cases in a population from Tuscany, Central Italy. Breast Cancer Res Treat 117: 497–504.
13. Reeve JP, Rannala B (2002) DMLE+ Bayesan linkage disequilibrum gene mapping. Bioinforma Appl Note 18: 894–895.
14. Colombo M, De Vecchi G, Caleca L, Foglia C, Ripamonti CB, et al. (2013) Comparative *In Vitro* and *In Silico* Analyses of Variants in Splicing Regions of BRCA1 and BRCA2 Genes and Characterization of Novel Pathogenic Mutations. PLOS ONE 8(2): e57173. doi: 10.1371/journal.pone.0057173.
15. Sarkar M, Magliery TJ (2008) Re-engineering a split-GFP reassembly screen to examine RING-domain interactions between BARD1 and BRCA1 mutants observed in cancer patients. Mol Biosyst 4: 599–605.
16. Ripamonti CB, Colombo M, Mondini P, Siranoush M, Peissel B, et al. (2013) First description of an acinic cell carcinoma of the breast in a BRCA1 mutation carrier: a case report. BMC Cancer 13 (1): 46. doi: 10.1186/1471-2407-13-46.
17. Claes K, Vandesompele J, Poppe B, Dahan K, Coene I, et al. (2002) Pathological splice mutations outside the invariant AG/GT splice sites of BRCA1 exon 5 increase alternative transcript levels in the 5′ end of the BRCA1 gene. Oncogene 21: 4171–5.
18. Yang Y, Swaminathan S, Martin BK, Sharan SK (2003) Aberrant splicing induced by missense mutations in BRCA1: Clues from a humanized mouse model. Hum Mol Genet 12: 2121–2131.
19. Hashizume R, Fukuda M, Maeda I, Nishikawa H, Oyake D et al. (2001) The RING Heterodimer BRCA1-BARD1 Is a Ubiquitin Ligase Inactivated by a Breast Cancer-derived Mutation. J Biol Chem 276: 14537–14540.
20. Brzovic PS, Keeffe JR, Nishikawa H, Miyamoto K, Fox III D, et al. (2003) Binding and recognition in the assembly of an active BRCA1/BARD1 ubiquitin-ligase complex. Proc Natl Acad Sci U S A 2003; 100: 5646–5651.
21. Ghosh I, Hamilton AD, Regan L (2000) Antiparallel leucine zipper-directed protein reassembly: application to the green fluorescent protein. J Am Chem Soc 122: 5658–5659.
22. Magliery TJ, Regan L (2006) Reassembled GFP: detecting protein-protein interactions and protein expression patterns. Methods Biochem Anal 47: 391–405.
23. Brzovic PS, Meza J, King MC, Klevit RE (1998) The Cancer-predisposing Mutation C61G Disrupts Homodimer Formation in the NH2-terminal BRCA1 RING Finger Domain. J Biol Chem 273: 7795–7799.
24. Magliery TJ, Wilson CGM, Pan W, Mishler D, Ghosh I, et al. (2005) Detecting protein-protein interactions with a green fluorescent protein fragment reassembly trap: scope and mechanism. J Am Chem Soc 127: 146–157.
25. Jakubowska A, Gòrski B, Byrski T, Huzarski T, Gronwald J, et al. (2001) Detection of germline mutations in the BRCA1 gene by RNA-based sequencing. Hum Mutat 18:943–949.
26. Willems P, Magri V, Cretnik M, Fasano M, Jakubowska, et al. (2009) Characterization of the c190T>C missense mutation in BRCA1 codon 64 (Cys64Arg). Int J Oncol 34: 1005–1015.
27. Xia Y, Pao GM, Chen HW, Verma IM, Hunter T (2003) Enhancement of BRCA1 E3 Ubiquitin Ligase Activity through Direct Interaction with the BARD1 Protein. J Biol Chem 278: 5255–5263.
28. Ruffner H, Joazeiro CAP, Hemmati D, Hunter T, Verma IM (2001) Cancer-predisposing mutations within the RING domain of BRCA1: Loss of ubiquitin protein ligase activity and protection from radiation hypersensitivity. PNAS 98: 5134–5139.
29. Morris JR, Pangon L, Boutell C, Katagiri T, Keep NH et al. (2006) Genetic analysis of BRCA1 ubiquitin ligase activity and its relationship to breast cancer susceptibility. Hum Mol Genet 15: 599–606. doi: 10.1093/hmg/ddi476.
30. Brzovic PS, Meza JE, King MC, Klevit RE (2001) BRCA1 RING Domain Cancer-predisposing mutations structural consequences and effects on protein-protein interactions. J Biol Chem 276: 41399–41406.
31. Spearman AD, Sweet K, Zhou XP, McLennan J, Couch FJ et al. (2008) Clinically Applicable Models to Characterize *BRCA1* and *BRCA2* Variants of Uncertain Significance. J Clin Oncol 26: 5393–5400.
32. Wu LC, Wang ZW, Tsan TJ, Spillman MA, Phung A, et al. (1996) Identification of a RING protein that can interact *in vivo* with the *BRCA1* gene product. Nat Genet 14: 430–440.
33. Lakhani SR, van de Vijver MJ, Jacquemier J, Anderson TJ, Osin PP, et al. (2002) The Pathology of Familial Breast Cancer: Predictive Value of Immunohistochemical Markers Estrogen Receptor, Progesterone Receptor, HER-2, and p53 in Patients With Mutations in BRCA1 and BRCA2. J Clin Oncol 20: 2310–2318. doi: 10.1200/JCO.2002.09.023.
34. Mavaddat N, Barrowdale D, Andrulis IL, Domchek SM, Eccles D, et al. (2012) Pathology of Breast and Ovarian Cancers among *BRCA1* and *BRCA2* Mutation Carriers: Results from the Consortium of Investigators of Modifiers of *BRCA1/2* (CIMBA). Cancer Epidemiol Biomarkers Prev 21: 134–147. doi: 10.1158/1055-9965.EPI-11-0775.
35. Kennecke H, Yerushalmi R, Woods R, Cheang MCU, Voduc D, et al. (2010) Metastatic Behavior of Breast Cancer Subtypes. J Clin Oncol 20: 3271–3277.
36. Carey LA. (2011) Directed Therapy of Subtypes of Triple-Negative Breast Cancer. The Oncologist 16 (suppl 1): 71–78.
37. Shaw PA, McLaughlin JR, Zweemer RP, Narod SA, Risch H, et al. (2002) Histopathologic Features of Genetically Determined Ovarian Cancer. Int J Gynecol Pathol 21: 407–411.
38. Manoukian S, Peissel B, Pensotti V, Barile M, Cortesi L, et al. (2007) Germline mutations of TP53 and BRCA2 genes in breast cancer/sarcoma families. Eur J Cancer 43: 601–606.

Increased Sensitivity to Chemotherapy Induced by CpG-ODN Treatment Is Mediated by microRNA Modulation

Loris De Cecco[1]☯, Martina Berardi[2]☯, Michele Sommariva[2,3], Alessandra Cataldo[3], Silvana Canevari[4], Delia Mezzanzanica[4], Marilena V. Iorio[5], Elda Tagliabue[2], Andrea Balsari[2,3]*

1 Functional Genomics Core Facility, Fondazione Istituto Di Ricovero e Cura a Carattere Scientifico Istituto Nazionale dei Tumori, Milan, Italy, **2** Molecular Targeting Unit, Fondazione Istituto Di Ricovero e Cura a Carattere Scientifico Istituto Nazionale dei Tumori, Milan, Italy, **3** Department of Biomedical Sciences for Health, University of Milan, Milan, Italy, **4** Molecular Therapies Unit, Fondazione Istituto Di Ricovero e Cura a Carattere Scientifico Istituto Nazionale dei Tumori, Milan, Italy, **5** Start Up Unit, Fondazione Istituto Di Ricovero e Cura a Carattere Scientifico Istituto Nazionale dei Tumori, Milan, Italy

Abstract

We recently reported that peritumoral CpG-ODN treatment, activating TLR-9 expressing cells in tumor microenvironment, induces modulation of genes involved in DNA repair and sensitizes cancer cells to DNA-damaging cisplatin treatment. Here, we investigated whether this treatment induces modulation of miRNAs in tumor cells and their relevance to chemotherapy response. Array analysis identified 20 differentially expressed miRNAs in human IGROV-1 ovarian tumor cells from CpG-ODN-treated mice versus controls (16 down- and 4 up-regulated). Evaluation of the role of the 3 most differentially expressed miRNAs on sensitivity to cisplatin of IGROV-1 cells revealed significantly increased cisplatin cytotoxicity upon ectopic expression of hsa-miR-302b (up-modulated in our array), but no increased effect upon reduced expression of hsa-miR-424 or hsa-miR-340 (down-modulated in our array). Accordingly, hsa-miR-302b expression was significantly associated with time to relapse or overall survival in two data sets of platinum-treated ovarian cancer patients. Use of bio-informatics tools identified 19 mRNAs potentially targeted by hsa-miR-302b, including HDAC4 gene, which has been reported to mediate cisplatin sensitivity in ovarian cancer. Both HDAC4 mRNA and protein levels were significantly reduced in IGROV-1 cells overexpressing hsa-miR-302b. Altogether, these findings indicate that hsa-miR-302b acts as a "chemosensitizer" in human ovarian carcinoma cells and may represent a biomarker able to predict response to cisplatin treatment. Moreover, the identification of miRNAs that improve sensitivity to chemotherapy provides the experimental underpinning for their possible future clinical use.

Editor: Ramiro Garzon, The Ohio State University, United States of America

Funding: This work was supported by Associazione Italiana per la Ricerca sul Cancro (AIRC). MS was supported by "Dote ricerca": FSE, Regione Lombardia. MVI is supported by Start Up AIRC Grant. The funders had no role in study design, data collection and analysis, decision to publish, or preparation of the manuscript.

Competing Interests: The authors have declared that no competing interests exist.

* E-mail: andrea.balsari@unimi.it

☯ These authors contributed equally to this work.

Introduction

Oligodeoxynucleotides (ODN) containing dinucleotides with unmethylated CpG motifs (CpG-ODN) are potent activators of both the innate and adaptive immune systems [1;2]. Recognition of CpG-ODN is mediated by Toll-like receptor 9 (TLR9), an endosomal member of the TLR family, which is critically important in detecting microbial pathogens. In a xenograft model of human IGROV-1 ovarian cancer, we recently showed that treatment with CpG-ODN induced down-modulation of DNA repair genes in tumor cells and that peritumoral injection of CpG-ODN in the peritoneal cavity was for inducing this down-modulation [3] and for the antitumor activity of CpG-ODN [4]. Considering the CpG-ODN species specificity and to the lack of TLR9 expression on IGROV1 cells, the effect cannot be mediated by a direct interaction between the oligonucleotide and tumor cells, instead it is likely that peritumoral TLR9-expressing cells, such as innate immune cells and/or endothelial cells, fibroblasts and epithelial cells, directly respond to CpG-ODN and down-regulate DNA repair in tumor cells through a direct cell-cell interaction and/or by secreting soluble factors.

MicroRNAs (miRNAs) are short (~22 nucleotide), non-coding RNAs known to alter gene expression at the post-transcriptional level [5;6]. More than 1,200 human miRNAs have been identified and validated to date (www.mirbase.org), and are predicted to regulate about one-third of the human genome, with involvement in development and progression of many diseases [7–9]. Presumably, miRNAs evolved to allow organisms and cells to effectively deal with stress [10]. Recent studies demonstrating that a single miRNA can impact hundreds of targets [11] and that multiple miRNAs can affect a single target [12] point to broad implications of miRNAs, able to affect all most important cellular processes. Indeed, several experimental and clinical findings have also implicated miRNAs in the response to chemotherapy [13], demonstrating a role for miRNAs in the modulation of genes involved in DNA repair [14;15].

The CpG-ODN-induced down-modulation of DNA repair genes in tumor cells might represent a physiologic phenomenon that occurs locally in the presence of an infectious event. Upon detection of an infectious agent via endosomal TLRs, cells involved in the immune response might induce modulation of DNA repair genes in infected (or transformed) cells to facilitate their death [16]. Identification of miRNAs that are used "physiologically" to modulate DNA repair genes may have therapeutic implications.

In the present study, we analyzed the effect of CpG-ODN on modulation of miRNAs in tumor cells, the integration of miRNA with mRNA expression modulation induced by CpG-ODN, and the relevance of the identified miRNAs for the response to chemotherapy.

Materials and Methods

Ethical Commitee

The *in vivo* experiment was approved by the Ethics Committee for Animal Experimentation of the Fondazione IRCCS Istituto Nazionale Tumori of Milan according to institutional guidelines.

Drugs and Antibodies

Purified phosphorothioated ODN1826 (5′-TCCAT-GACGTTCCTGACGTT-3′) containing CpG motifs was synthesized by TriLink Biotechnologies (San Diego, CA, USA). Phosphorothioate modification was used to reduce susceptibility of the ODN to DNase digestion, thereby significantly prolonging its *in vivo* half-life. Cisplatin was purchased from Teva Italia (Milan, Italy). Anti-HDAC4 (D15C3), anti-p21 (sc-397) and anti-GAPDH (GAPDH-71.1) antibodies were purchased from Cell Signaling Technology (Danvers, MA, USA), Santa Cruz Biotechnology (Santa Cruz, CA, USA) and Sigma (St. Louis, MO, USA), respectively.

Cells

Human IGROV-1 ovarian tumor cells (gift from Dr. J. Benard, Institute Gustave Roussy, Villejuif, France) were adapted to growth i.p. and maintained by serial i.p. passage of ascitic cells into healthy mice as described [3,17]. Every 6 months, cells were authenticated by morphologic inspection and by FACS analysis for the presence of specific markers. For *in vitro* experiments, IGROV-1 cells were maintained in RPMI medium 1640 supplemented with 10% FCS (Sigma) and 2 mM glutamine (Cambrex, East Rutherford, NJ, USA) at 37°C in a 5% CO_2 air atmosphere.

miRNA Extraction from Tumor Samples

miRNAs were extracted from the IGROV-1 xenograft tumors used for gene expression analysis or from a replica of the *in vivo* experiment [3]. Briefly, solid i.p. masses were mechanically disrupted and homogenized in the presence of QIAzol Lysis reagent (Qiagen, Valencia, CA, USA) using a Mikrodismembrator (Braun Biotech International, Melsungen, Germany). RNA was extracted using the miRNeasy Mini kit (Qiagen) according to the manufacturer's instructions. RNA concentrations were measured with the NanoDrop ND-100 Spectrophotometer (NanoDrop Technologies, Wilmington, DE, USA), while RNA quality was assessed with the Agilent 2100 Bioanalyzer (Agilent Technologies, Palo Alto, CA USA) using the RNA 6000 Nano kit (Agilent). Samples included in the present analysis had a RIN (RNA Integrity Number) score >7 and a 28S:18S rRNA ratio ~2:1.

miRNA Expression Profiling

Mature miRNAs were detected with the Illumina Human_v2 MicroRNA expression profiling kit, based on the DASL (cDNA-mediated Annealing, Selection, Extension, and Ligation) assay, according to the manufacturer's instructions (Illumina Inc., San Diego, CA, USA). Briefly, 600 ng/sample total RNA was converted to cDNA followed by annealing of a miRNA-specific oligonucleotide pool consisting of: i) a universal PCR priming site at the 5′ end; ii) an address sequence complementary to a capture sequence on the BeadArray; and iii) a miRNA-specific sequence at the 3′ end. After PCR amplification and fluorescent labeling, probes were hybridized on Illumina miRNA BeadChips, washed, and fluorescent signals were detected by the Illumina BeadArrayTM Reader. Data were collected using BeadStudio V3.0

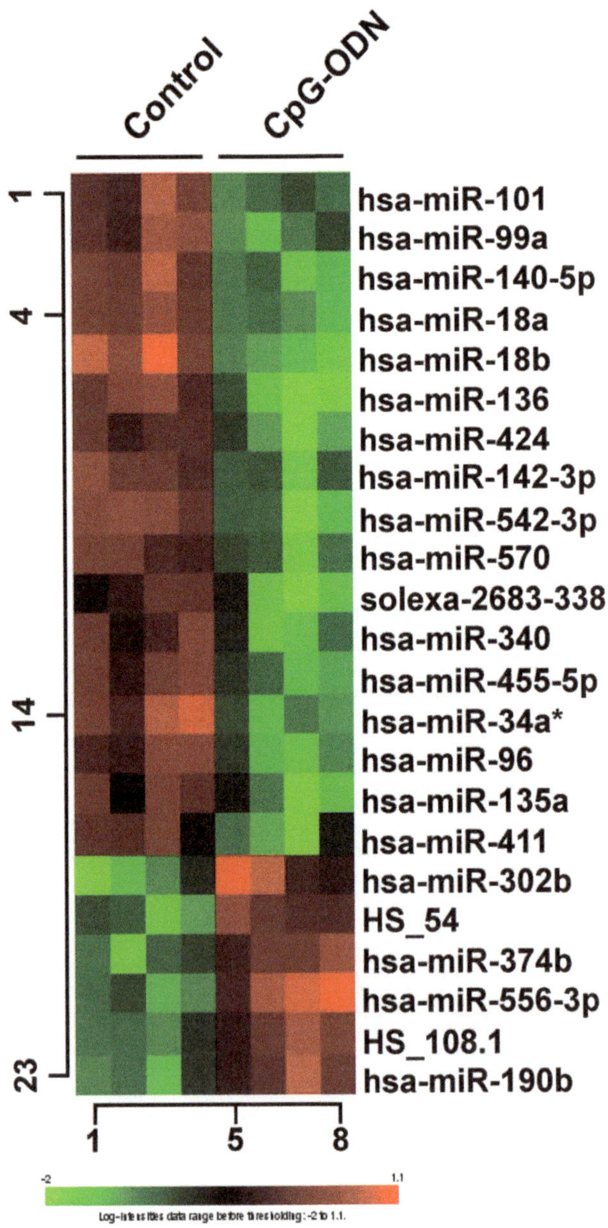

Figure 1. miRNA expression profiling in IGROV-1 ovarian tumors from CpG-ODN-treated athymic mice. Heat-map of 23 modulated miRNAs with FDR <0.1 and fold change >1.8 in CpG-ODN-versus saline-treated mice. Among the 20 miRNAs belonging to miRBase12.0, 16 were down- and 4 up-modulated in CpG-ODN-treated mice (red: up-regulated miRNAs; green: down-modulated miRNAs). Columns and rows represent samples and miRNAs, respectively.

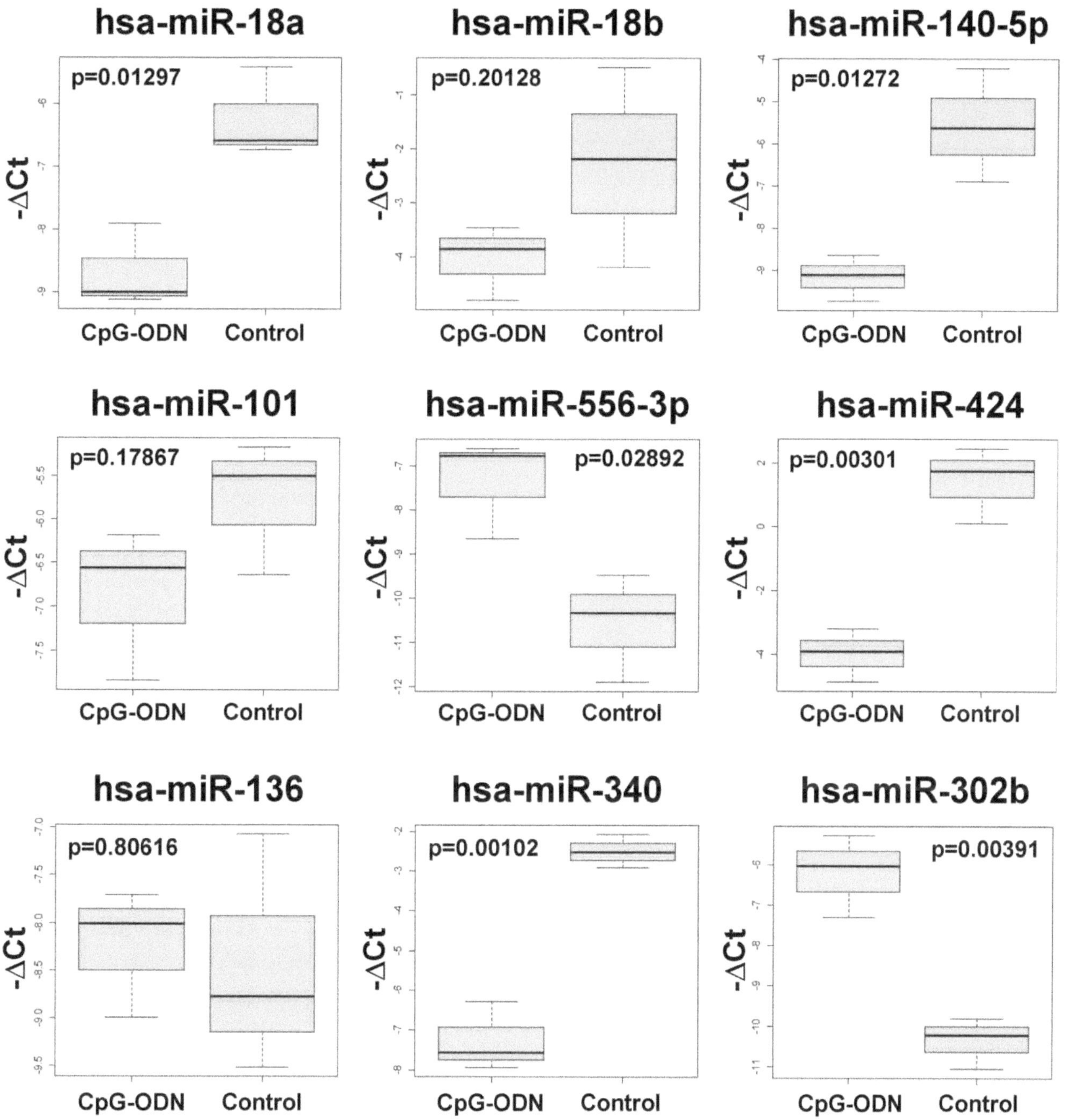

Figure 2. Independent biological validation of CpG-ODN miRNA profile. miRNA expression was assessed by RT-qPCR on IGROV-1 xenografts collected from a replica of a previous experiment [3]. RT-qPCR data are plotted as $-\Delta Ct$. P-values were calculated using two-tailed Student's t-test.

software. Raw and normalized data are available on the Gene Expression Omnibus website with accession numbers GSE41783 and GSE23441 for miRNA and gene expression profiling, respectively.

Real-time Quantitative PCR (RT-qPCR)

RT-qPCR microRNA assays specific for hsa-miR-18a, hsa-miR-18b, hsa-miR-140-5p, hsa-miR-101, hsa-miR-556-3p, hsa-miR-424, hsa-miR-136, hsa-miR-340, hsa-miR-302b were purchased from Exiqon (Vedbaek, Denmark). RT-qPCR was performed using the miRCURY LNA Universal RT microRNA PCR system (Exiqon) according to the manufacturer's instructions. Total RNA (20 ng) was polyadenylated and reverse-transcribed at 42°C (60 min), followed by heat-inactivation at 85°C (5 min) using a poly-T primer containing a 5′ universal tag. The resulting cDNA was diluted 80-fold and 8 µl used in 20-µl PCR amplification reactions at 95°C for 10 min, 40 cycles of 95°C for 10 sec, and 60°C for 60 sec. Results were normalized with snord48 (Assay ID:203903). P-values were calculated using two-tailed Student's t-test.

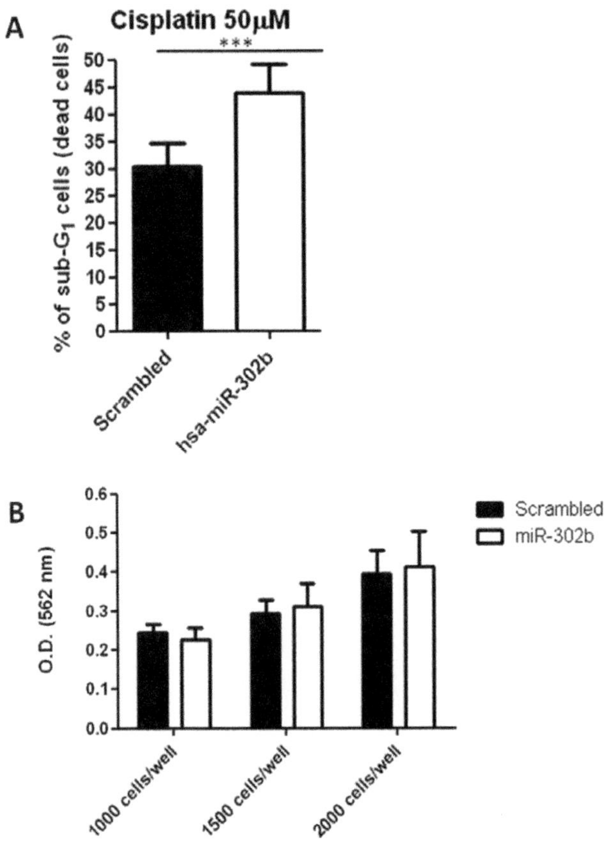

Figure 3. Forced expression of hsa-miR-302b increased cisplatin sensitivity in IGROV-1 cells without affecting cell proliferation. (A) Percent cell death of hsa-miR-302b- and scrambled-transfected cells after cisplatin treatment. IGROV-1 cells were transfected with 50 nmol/l hsa-miR-302b precursor molecule or scrambled control, and 72 h later, exposed to cisplatin (50 μM) for 1 h. Cell viability was assessed 24 h after cisplatin treatment by propidium iodide staining and flow cytometry. Data represent mean ± SEM of 6 independent experiments. ***$p<0.0001$ by paired t-test. (B) Evaluation of cell proliferation by SRB assay. Transfected cells were seeded in a 96-well plate at a density of 10^3, 1.5×10^3, and 2×10^3 cells/well. Cell growth was assessed by optical density (OD) determination 72 h after transfection. Data represent mean ± SEM of 3 independent experiments.

Bioinformatics Analysis

Analyses were performed using BRB-Array Tools v4.0 stable release developed by Dr. Richard Simon (NCI) and the BRB-Array Tools development team (EMMES Corp.) and the R package (http://www.bioconductor.org/). The same data-processing was used in both miRNA and gene expression profiling to improve data integration. Quantile normalization was used to correct experimental distortions. A detection threshold of $p<0.05$ was set for each gene and miRNA. Probes detected in less than 50% of the samples were eliminated from the analysis. Genes and miRNAs differentially expressed were identified using a random-variance t-test, which allows computation of a t-test statistic for each detected miRNA and genes between the classes of samples under investigation without assuming that all miRNAs have the same variance [18]. To limit the number of false-positive findings, miRNAs and genes were considered statistically significant at a false-discovery rate (FDR) <0.1. To identify the most likely targets, mRNA and miRNA expression data were integrated using the MAGIA web tool [19]. A parametric linear correlation measure (Pearson's correlation coefficient, recommended for normally distributed data and a sample size >5) was used to assess the degree of anti-correlation between miRNA and gene expression data.

In silico Bioinformatics Analyses

Two publicly available datasets GSE27290 [20] and GSE25204 [21] reporting miRNA expression and clinical annotated data were downloaded from the Gene Expression Omnibus (GEO) database. The former dataset consists of 62 diagnosed patients with stage III or IV serous ovarian cancer profiled on a pre-commercial version of miRNA chips (GPL7341) designed on miRBase 9.1. Raw array data were processed using GeneSpring software (Agilent) and quantile-normalized. The latter dataset reports profiling of 85 stage III or IV epithelial ovarian cancers, divided into a training set (55 cases) and test set (30 cases), profiled with Illumina human_v2 MicroRNA chips. Raw data were processed and quantile-normalized using BeadStudio V3.0 software. Non-biological experimental variations between training and test sets were adjusted using ComBat [22].

Statistical Analysis

The clinical impact on overall survival (OS) and time to relapse (TTR) in GSE27290 and GSE25204, respectively, was assessed by the Kaplan-Meier method, and differences between curves were compared using a non-parametric (log-rank) test, with hazard ratios and 95% confidence intervals also computed. GraphPadPrism v5 (GraphPad software, La Jolla, CA, USA) was used for statistical analyses.

miRNA Transfection and Cell Viability Analysis

IGROV-1 cells seeded in 6-well plates at 2×10^5 cells/well were transfected with miRCURY LNA inhibitors of hsa-miR-424 or hsa-miR-340 or negative control A (Exiqon; final concentration, 100 nmol/L) using SiPort Neo-FX (Ambion) according to the manufacturer's instructions, or with hsa-miR-302b precursor or negative control #1 pre-miR (Ambion; final concentration, 50 nmol/l). Transfections were verified by qRT-PCR as described above. Cell viability after cisplatin treatment were assessed by propidium iodide staining and flow cytometry as described [3].

Cell Growth Assay

IGROV-1 cells were transfected with 50 nmol/l pre-hsa-miR-302b or scrambled oligonucleotide using SiPort Neo-FX transfection reagent according to the manufacturer's protocol (Ambion) and seeded in a 96-well plate at a density of 10^3, 1.5×10^3, and 2×10^3 cells/well. After 72 h of culture, cells were fixed with 10% trichloroacetic acid for 1 h at 4°C, washed 5 times with distilled and de-ionized water, air-dried, and incubated with 100 μl sulforodamine (SRB) 0.4% (w/v) for 30 min. Cells were then washed 4 times with 1% acetic acid, air-dried, and 10 mM Tris solution (pH 10.5) added to dissolve the bound dye. Cell growth was assessed based on optical density (OD) at 550 nm using an ELISA microplate reader (Bio-Rad Lab, Inc., Hercules, CA, USA).

Immunoblotting

Transfected cells were lysed in lysis buffer containing 50 mM Tris-HCl (pH 7.5), 150 mM NaCl, 1% Triton X-100 (Sigma), 10% (vol/vol) glycerol, 2 mM Na-orthovanadate, 10 mM leupeptin, 10 mM aprotinin, 1 mM phenylmethylsulfonyl-fluoride, 100 mM Na-fluoride, and 10 mM Na-pyrophosphate for 30 min

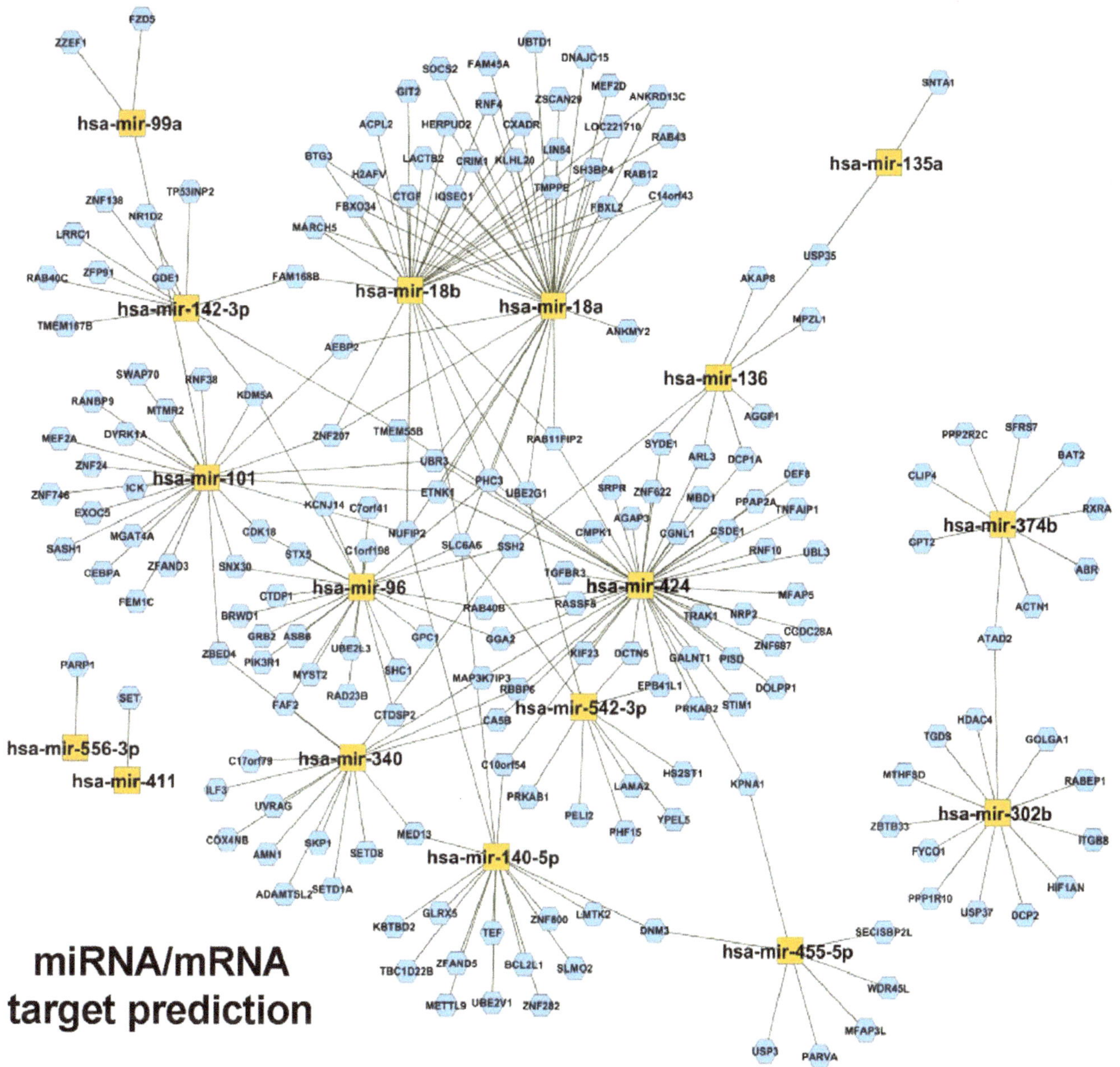

Figure 4. Computational integration of miRNA and gene expression profiles of tumor samples from CpG-ODN- and saline-treated mice. Network between 15 of 20 differentially expressed miRNAs and their anti-correlated target genes. The top 250 interactions were used to generate the network using the MAGIA tool.

at 4°C. Insoluble material was removed by 10-min centrifugation at 15,500 × g at 4°C. Protein concentrations were determined using the Coomassie technique. Equal amounts of total lysates (20 µg) were loaded and separated on 10% precast NuPage SDS-Bis-Tris gels (Invitrogen) and transferred to PVDF membranes (Millipore, Billerica, MA, USA). Western blots were performed with the indicated antibodies, and binding was detected with peroxidase-conjugated secondary antibodies and chemiluminescence ECL (GE Healthcare, Little Chalfont, UK) according to the manufacturer's instructions. Quantitation of p21 protein levels reportedly regulated post-transcriptionally by miRNAs of the hsa-miR-302 family [23] revealed the expected down-regulation of this protein in IGROV-1 cells transfected with hsa-miR-302b precursor (data not shown), suggesting that hsa-miR-302b exerts biological effects in IGROV-1 cells similar to those observed in other cellular models.

Plasmid Construction

For luciferase reporter experiments, a 1017-bp region of the HDAC4 3′ untranslated region including the binding site for hsa-miR-302b was amplified from IGROV-1 cells. The PCR product was digested with XbaI and cloned into the reporter plasmid pGL3 control (Promega, Madison, WI, USA) downstream of the luciferase gene. Mutations into the hsa-miR-302b binding site of the HDAC4-3′UTR were introduced using Quik-Change II Site-Directed Mutagenesis kit (Agilent Technologies, Santa Clara, CA).

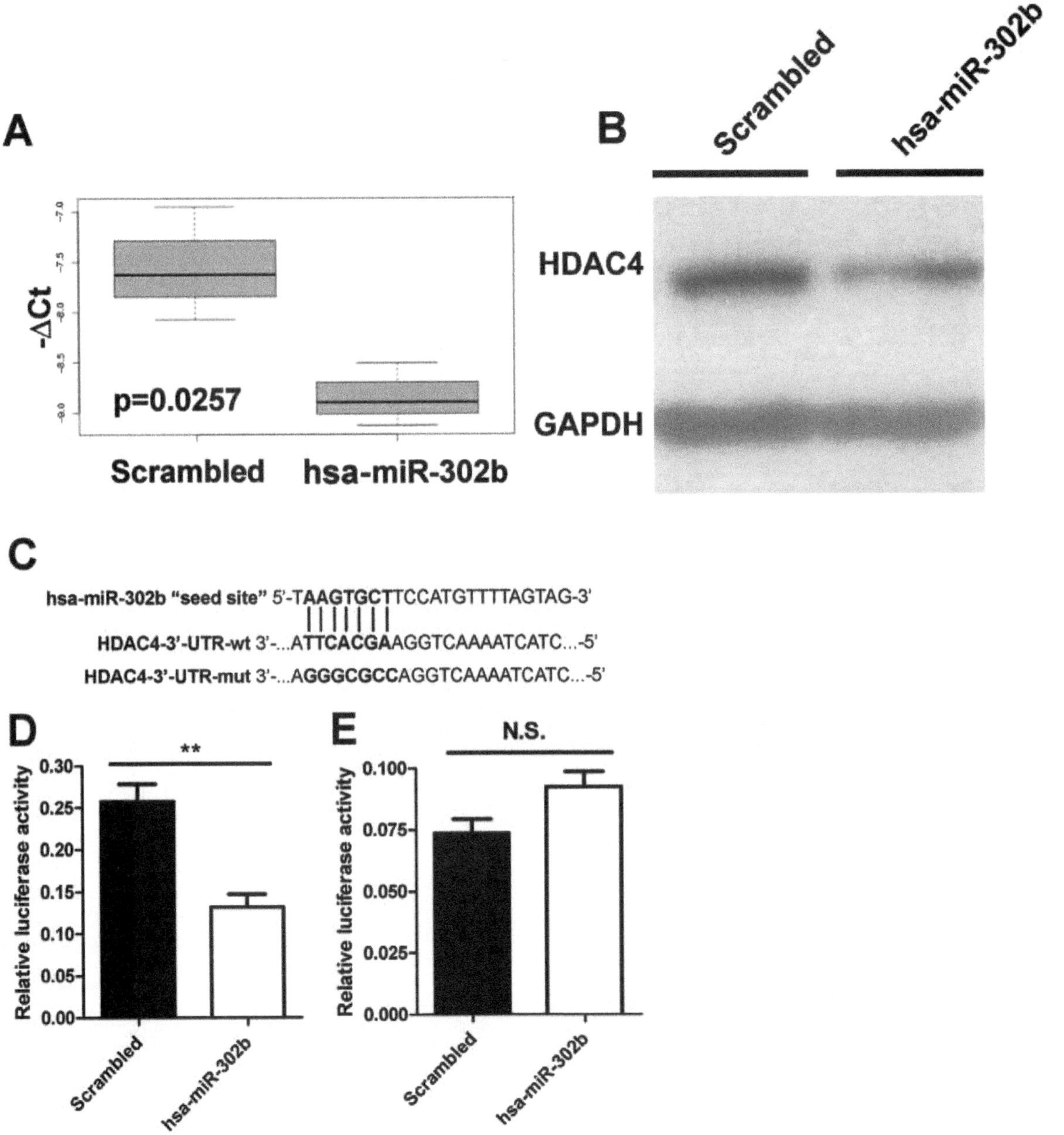

Figure 5. Targeting of HDAC4 in IGROV-1 cells by hsa-miR-302b. IGROV-1 cells were transfected with 50 nmol/l hsa-miR-302b or a scrambled oligonucleotide and RNA and proteins were collected after 72 h. HDAC4 mRNA levels were evaluated by RT-qPCR (A) and protein expression was evaluated by Western blot (B). GAPDH was used to normalize protein loading per lane. Data are representative of 6 independent experiments with superimposable results. (C) Schematic representation of the interaction between hsa-miR-302b and the binding site on the wild-type HDAC4-3′UTR and the mutated control. (D) Relative luciferase activity in IGROV-1 cells for HDAC4-3′UTR-wt co-transfected with reporter vector and with hsa-miR-302b precursor molecule or negative scrambled control for 48 h. (E) Relative luciferase activity in IGROV-1 cells for HDAC4-3′UTR mut co-transfected with reporter vector and with hsa-miR-302b precursor molecule or negative scrambled control for 48 h.

Primers for plasmid construction were:

HDAC4-wt-Fw: 5′-AATTTCTAGAGGGGGACTTAATTC-TAATCTCATT-3′.

HDAC4-wt-Rw: 5′-AATTTCTAGATTTTGTGTCAGAC-CATTACGAA-3′.

HDAC4-Mut-Fw: 5′-GCACTGGCTGGGAGTCAG-CAAGCGCCGCGGGTATATCCCTTTGACG-GAAACCCTG-3′.

HDAC4-Mut-Rw: 5′-CAGGGTTTCCCTCAAAGGGATA-TACCCGCGGCGCTTGCTGACTCCCAGCCAGTGC-3′.

Luciferase Assays for Target and Promoter Identification

pGL3 reporter vector (200 ng) containing the hsa-miR-302b binding site, 40 ng of the phRL-SV40 control vector (Promega), and 50 nmol/l miRNA precursors or scrambled sequence miRNA control (Ambion Inc, Austin, TX. USA) were co-transfected into IGROV-1 cells in 48-well plates. Cells were transfected with Lipofectamine 2000 (Invitrogen) according to the manufacturer's instructions. Firefly luciferase activity was measured with a Dual Luciferase Assay Kit (Promega) 48 h after transfection and normalized with a Renilla luciferase reference plasmid. Reporter

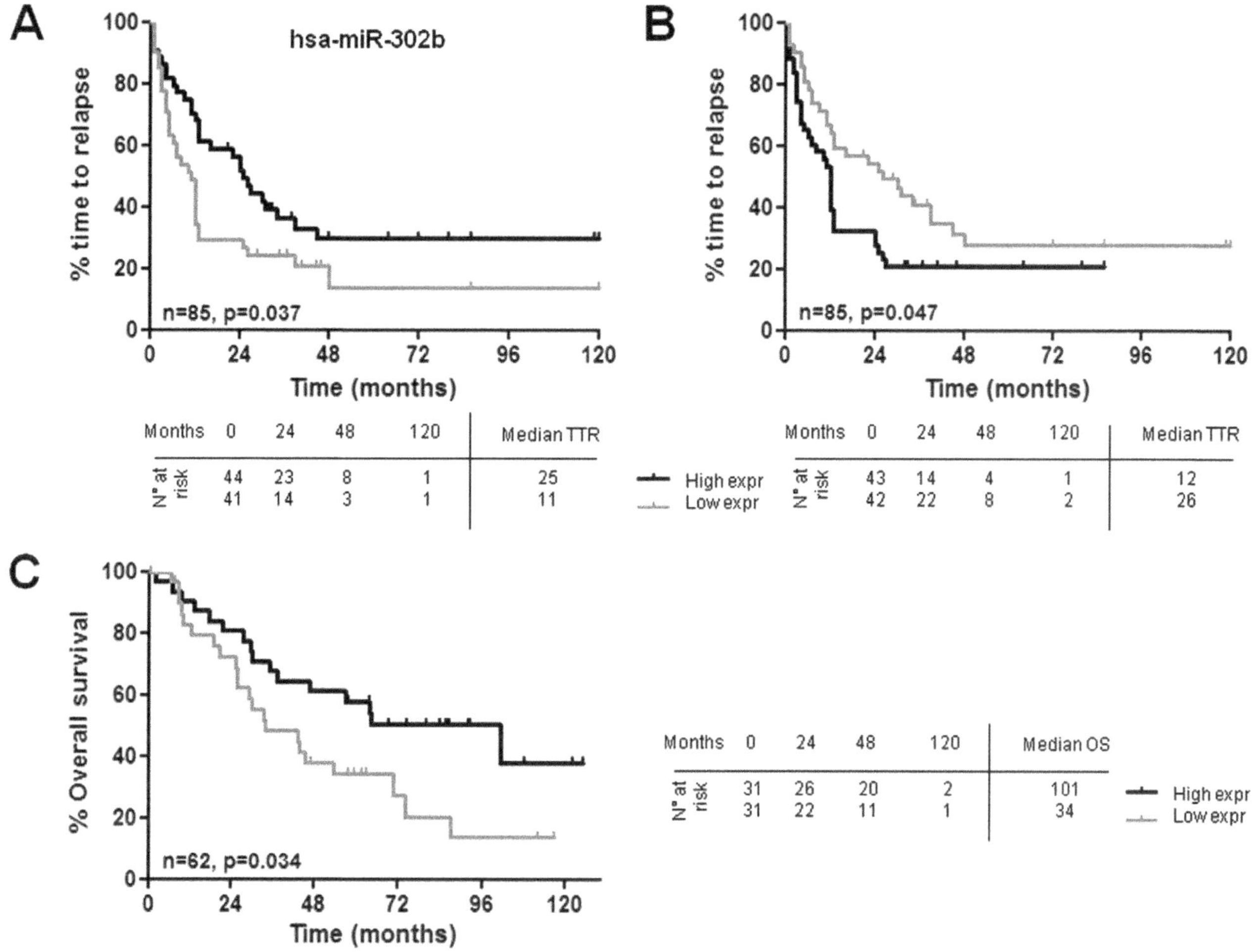

Figure 6. In silico evaluation of ovarian cancer patients' clinical course according to hsa-miR-302b and hsa-miR-340 expression levels. Kaplan-Meier survival curves of patients stratified according to hsa-miR-302b expression (A) and has-miR-340 expression (B) on GSE25204 and referred to TTR. (C) Kaplan-Meier survival curves for hsa-miR-302b expression on GSE27290 and referred to OS. Patients were dichotomized using median expression as threshold.

assays were carried out in quadruplicate. Data (mean±S.E.M.) were analyzed using unpaired Student's t-test.

Results

Differentially Expressed miRNAs in IGROV-1 Ovarian Tumors from CpG-ODN-Treated Mice

RNA extracted from omentum-adherent tumors of human IGROV-1 ovarian carcinoma-bearing mice treated i.p. with CpG-ODN or saline (control group) as described [3] was analyzed for miRNA expression using Illumina human miRNA_v2 array. Out of 1145 miRNAs represented on the Illumina chips, 567 mature miRNAs annotated on miRBase12.0, along with 150 putative miRNAs, were consistently detected. Class comparison identified 23 miRNAs showing a FDR<0.1 and a fold-change >1.8 between CpG-ODN- and saline-treated mice (Fig. 1). Among them, 20 miRNAs (16 up-regulated in saline- and 4 in CpG-ODN-treated mice) were annotated on miRBase12.0, whereas 3 miRNAs were putative miRNA sequences derived from deep- sequencing approaches as referred by Berezikov et al. [24] and Solexa (Illumina), which were excluded from further analysis due to the lack of information.

To validate the microarray data, 9 differentially expressed miRNAs were analyzed by RT-qPCR using both the RNA profiled in microarray analysis and the RNA extracted from tumor samples obtained from a replica of the IGROV-1 tumor-bearing mice treated as described [3]. Of the 9 miRNAs, hsa-miR-18a and hsa-miR-18b were selected based on their reported role in the pathogenesis of ovarian cancer [25;26], and hsa-miR-101 and hsa-miR-302b for their described involvement in DNA repair processes and sensitivity to chemotherapy [20]; the remaining 5 miRNAs were randomly selected. RT-qPCR using the RNA profiled in microarray analysis validated all 9 miRNAs (Fig. S1), whereas RT-qPCR using the RNA of the replica confirmed 6 of 9 miRNAs ($p<0.05$), with a trend observed for hsa-miR-18b and hsa-miR-101 but not for hsa-miR-136 (Fig. 2).

Increased Expression of hsa-miR-302b in IGROV-1 Cells Significantly Improved Cisplatin Activity

We previously showed that TLR9-expressing cells in the tumor microenvironment can sensitize cancer cells to DNA-damaging cisplatin treatment by down-modulating genes involved in DNA repair [3]. To determine whether miRNAs modulated by CpG-ODN treatment are able to modify the sensitivity to DNA-damaging agents, the 3 most significantly differentially expressed miRNAs in tumor samples obtained from the replica of the *in vivo* experiment (hsa-miR-424, hsa-miR-340 and hsa-miR-302b) were examined applying a gain- or loss-of-function phenotype in order to mimic the up- or down-modulation observed in miRNA profiling (see Fig. 1). To reduce expression of hsa-miR-424 and hsa-miR-340 (down-modulated in our miRNA expression profile), IGROV-1 cells were transiently transfected for 72 h with the respective LNA inhibitors or with a LNA negative control, whereas cells were transfected with hsa-miR-302b precursor molecule (or a scrambledoligonucleotide) to increase expression of hsa-miR-302b. Cells were then treated with 50 μM of cisplatin for 1 h and after 24 h the percentage of sub-G_1 cells (as an indicator of cell death) was determined by flow cytometry. Reduced expression of hsa-miR-424 or hsa-miR-340 did not significantly improve cisplatin cytotoxicity (data not shown), whereas increased expression of hsa-miR-302b significantly enhanced cisplatin cytotoxicity, with an increase of cell death ranging from 26.5 to 43.9% in 6 independent experiments as compared to negative scrambled-transfected cells ($p<0.0001$; Fig. 3A). No significant differences in cell growth were observed between IGROV-1 cells transiently transfected with hsa-miR-302b precursor molecule and control cells (Fig. 3B), ruling out the possibility that hsa-miR-302b sensitized cancer cells to cisplatin by stimulating cell proliferation.

HDAC4 is Directly Targeted by hsa-miR-302b in IGROV-1 Cells

Because the effects of miRNAs might lead to expression changes in their predicted target genes, we searched for expression patterns deregulated following CpG-ODN treatment by integrating the miRNA and mRNA expression profiles. Class comparison of whole gene expression, previously identified by Illumina HumanHT12_v3 beadchips using the same RNA samples assessed for miRNA profile [3], revealed 215 genes differentially expressed (141 up-regulated in saline- and 74 in CpG-ODN treated mice; FDR<0.1 and fold change >1.8).

To identify functional miRNA-mRNA relationships, miRNA and mRNA data were integrated using the freely available tool MAGIA [19]. Given the frequent miRNA-miRNA interactions, the 20 miRBase-annotated miRNAs were altogether compared to the gene expression profile dataset using the union of Pita, miRanda and TargetScan prediction target algorithms available on MAGIA. The Pearson's correlation between each miRNA and its predicted target was then computed. The first 250 most significantly negatively correlated miRNA-mRNA interactions were visualized as a network using Cytoscope. Evidence of the concerted interplay of miRNAs regulated by CpG-ODN and their potential target mRNAs was observed (Fig. 4) for 2 miRNAs upregulated (hsa-miR-302b and hsa-miR-374b) and for 13 miRNAs downregulated in CpG-ODN-treated mice (hsa-miR-135a, hsa-miR-136, hsa-miR-340, hsa-miR-445-5p, hsa-miR-424, hsa-miR-96, hsa-miR-142-3p, hsa-miR-140-5p, hsa-miR-542-3p, hsa-miR-18a, hsa-miR-18b, hsa-miR-101, and hsa-miR-99a). The latter 13 form a highly interconnected cluster where different miRNAs exert their biological functions targeting the same genes.

Focusing on the 19 genes potentially targeted by hsa-miR-302b as identified using MAGIA (q value <0.1, Table S1), we evaluated HDAC4, one of the top anti-correlated mRNAs, as a potential molecular target of hsa-miR-302b associated with response to chemotherapy. HDAC4, a member of the histone deacetylase family, encodes a protein that reportedly mediates cisplatin sensitivity in ovarian cancer [27]. Forced hsa-miR-302b expression in IGROV-1 cells decreased HDAC4 mRNA and protein levels (Fig. 5A and B), supporting the interaction analysis data. To determine whether the down-modulation of HDAC4 after hsa-miR-302b overexpression was due to a direct interaction between the miRNA and the mRNA of HDAC4, a luciferase reporter assay was performed. Briefly, the target site of hsa-miR-302b was identified within the HDAC4 3′UTR according to the Target Scan database (Fig. 5C), and the region including this site was cloned downstream of the luciferase gene into the reporter plasmid pGL3 control. Analysis of IGROV-1 cells co-transfected with hsa-miR-302b precursor or a scrambled oligonucleotide and the reporter vector, containing HDAC4 3′UTR, revealed a significant decrease in luciferase activity in hsa-miR-302b transfected cells as compared to scrambled transfected cells (~50% reduction, $p=0.0088$, Fig. 5D), whereas mutated HDAC4-3′UTR escaped this inhibition (Fig. 5E). These data indicate the direct effect of hsa-miR-302b on HDAC4 gene expression.

CpG-ODN-modulated miRNAs and Ovarian Cancer Patients' Clinical Course

The impact of expression levels of all 20 differentially expressed miRNAs, including those for which validation was not carried out, on the clinical course of ovarian cancer patients undergoing chemotherapy was evaluated *in silico*. The time to relapse (TTR) and overall survival (OS) with respect to each miRNA on two public datasets (GSE25204 and GSE27290) [21;22] were analyzed. Patients were stratified according to miRNA expression below (low expression) or above (high expression) the median expression value. In Bagnoli's dataset [22], Kaplan-Meier analysis showed that patients with low expression of hsa-miR-302b or with high expression of hsa-miR-340 had a shorter TTR (log-rank, $P=0.037$; $HR=1.75$, 95% CI: 1.03–2.95 and $P=0.047$; $HR=1.7$, 95% CI: 1.01–2.86, respectively) (Fig. 6A and 6B). Median TTR was 11 and 25 months for low and high expression of hsa-miR-302b (Fig. 6A), and 26 and 12 months for low and high expression of hsa-miR-340, respectively (Fig. 6B). In Shih's dataset [21], only the expression of hsa-miR-302b was significantly associated to OS (log-rank, $P=0.034$; $HR=2.02$, 95%CI: 1.05–3.88), with a median OS of 33.7 and 101.2 months for low and high expression, respectively (Fig. 6C). In both datasets, the impact of the other 18 miRNAs expression was not significantly associated to TTR or OS (data not shown).

Discussion

miRNAs are a ubiquitous feature of all cells, and functional studies prompted by the growing number of miRNA targets identified have demonstrated the involvement of miRNAs in the regulation of almost every cellular process investigated, including development, proliferation, differentiation, apoptosis, and tumorigenesis [28]. Moreover, emerging evidence suggests that miRNAs play important roles in the regulation of immunological functions, including innate immune responses of macrophages and the development, differentiation, and function of T and B cells [29;30].

Changes in miRNA expression induced by TLR ligand stimulation have been broadly investigated for their impact on development and function of innate immune cells, the primary expressors of TLRs [31]. Here, we show that *in vivo* treatment with TLR9 agonist CpG-ODNs also induces modulation of several miRNAs in tumor cells. This modulation is unlikely to reflect a direct action of CpG-ODN on IGROV-1 cells, which do not express TLR9 and do not respond to murine CpG-ODN, and instead is likely mediated by TLR9-positive cells in the tumor microenvironment directly and/or through soluble factors. Moreover, several studies indicating that miRNAs can also be transferred between cells, e.g., through exosomes [32], as a mechanism to interact and exchange information raises the intriguing possibility that the immune system responds to CpG-ODN treatment by boosting miRNA modulation and interaction with tumor cells.

Our analysis of 3 miRNAs (hsa-miR-424, hsa-miR-340 and hsa-miR-302b) for their relevance to chemotherapy response showed that the enforced expression of hsa-miR-302b on IGROV-1 cells significantly enhanced cisplatin cytotoxicity. Consistent with *in vitro* data, hsa-miR-302b expression was significantly associated to TTR or OS in two datasets of ovarian cancer patients treated with platinum-based therapy. These findings indicate that hsa-miR-302b acts as a "chemosensitizer" in human ovarian carcinoma cells and may represent a biomarker able to predict response to cisplatin treatment, leading to a more accurate selection of patients potentially responsive to a specific therapy.

Moreover, the correlation between miRNA expression and response to specific therapies also suggests the potential usefulness of miRNAs as therapeutic adjuvants. Notably, whereas to date this hypothesis mainly derives from *in vitro* gain- or loss-of-function studies, where candidate miRNAs are identified in tumor cell lines with different degrees of sensitivity to specific therapeutic drugs and then targeted in order to overcome drug resistance, by contrast our study starts using an *in vivo* model to select a candidate miRNA, then validated *in vitro* as adjuvant tool and in human samples as predictive biomarker.

The integration of miRNA and mRNA expression profiles upon CpG-ODN treatment revealed a broad concerted interplay of miRNAs with their predicted target mRNAs, suggesting a relevant role for miRNAs in CpG-ODN-induced expression of genes involved in different cellular pathways. Concerning genes involved in DNA repair, miRNA-mRNA interaction analysis identified HDAC4 as a gene potentially targeted by hsa-miR-302b, as then validated by the decreased HDAC4 mRNA and protein levels upon enforced hsa-miR-302b expression in IGROV-1 cells. Inhibition of HDAC has been reported to induce hyperacetylation of core histones and consequent relaxation of chromatin structure; such an open chromatin configuration would be expected to increase accessibility of genomic DNA to drugs targeting DNA [33;34]. These data have led to clinical studies using HDAC inhibitors in combination with current DNA damaging agents, such as topoisomerase inhibitors, DNA synthesis inhibitors, DNA intercalators and agents that covalently modify DNA, as treatment of several types of cancer [34;35]. However, whereas clinical studies have shown efficacy against human hematologic malignancies, results in solid tumor trials have been unsatisfactory because of some HDAC inhibitor limitations such as cardiac toxicity [36;37]. The observation that overexpression of miR-302b increased the sensitivity of ovarian tumor cells to cisplatin, together with the reported tissue specificity of miRNAs [38], raises the possibility of using this miRNA to modulate DNA-damaging drug sensitivity and avoiding HDAC inhibitor toxicity. Moreover, a very recent study reports direct regulation of p21 protein by members of the miR-302 family activated following DNA damage in human embryonic stem cells [20], further suggesting that miR-302 can impact the response to DNA-damaging agents by modulating different target molecules.

Overall, miRNA modulators are no longer merely theoretical, as evidenced by the recent demonstration that inhibition of hsa-miR-122 reduces viral load in hepatitis C patients [39], and instead are strong candidates as therapeutic agents [39].

Supporting Information

Figure S1 qRT-PCR validation of CpG-ODN miRNA profile. Comparison of hsa-miR-18a, hsa-miR-18b, hsa-miR-140-5p, hsa-miR-101, hsa-miR-556-3p, hsa-miR-424, hsa-miR-136, hsa-miR-340, hsa-miR-302b expression obtained by miRNA expression profile and qRT-PCR on tumors collected from human IGROV-1 ovarian tumor-bearing mice treated daily i.p. with CpG-ODN or saline (control group). *P* values of differential expression between control and CpG-ODN-treated IGROV-1 xenografts are reported. qRT-PCR data are plotted as $-\Delta Ct$ and array data are plotted as $\log_2$ (expression).

Table S1 MAGIA output representing 699 interactions between miRNA and mRNA of CpG-ODN-treated tumors with q value<0.1.

Materials & Methods S1 Supporting materials and methods.

Author Contributions

Conceived and designed the experiments: LDC AB DM. Performed the experiments: MB MS AC. Analyzed the data: LDC MVI. Contributed reagents/materials/analysis tools: SC DM. Wrote the paper: AB ET.

References

1. Krieg AM (2007) Antiinfective applications of toll-like receptor 9 agonists. Proc Am Thorac Soc 4: 289–94.
2. Abreu MT, Fukata M, Arditi M (2005) TLR signaling in the gut in health and disease. J Immunol 174: 4453–60.
3. Sommariva M, De Cecco L, De Cesare M, Sfondrini L, Ménard S, et al. (2011) TLR9-agonists oppositely modulate DNA-repair genes in tumor vesus immune cells and ehance chemotherapy effects. Cancer Res 71: 6382–90.
4. De Cesare M, Calcaterra C, Pratesi G, Gatti L, Zunino F, et al. (2008) Eradication of ovarian tumor xenografts by locoregional administration of targeted immunotherapy. Clin Cancer Res 14: 5512–8.
5. Filipowicz W, Bhattacharyya SN, Sonenberg N (2008) Mechanisms of post-transcriptional regulation by microRNAs: are the answers in sight? Nat Rev Genet 9: 102–14.
6. Bartel DP (2009) MicroRNAs: target recognition and regulatory functions. Cell 136: 215–33.
7. Griffiths-Jones S, Saini HK, van DS, Enright AJ (2008) miRBase: tools for microRNA genomics. Nucleic Acids Res 36: D154–D158.
8. Griffiths-Jones S, Grocock RJ, van DS, Bateman A, Enright AJ (2006) miRBase: microRNA sequences, targets and gene nomenclature. Nucleic Acids Res 34: D140–D144.
9. Griffiths-Jones S (2004) The microRNA Registry. Nucleic Acids Res 32: D109–D111.
10. Hermeking H (2012) MicroRNAs in the p53 network: micromanagement of tumour suppression. Nat Rev Cancer 12: 613–26.
11. Selbach M, Schwanhausser B, Thierfelder N, Fang Z, Khanin R, et al. (2008) Widespread changes in protein synthesis induced by microRNAs. Nature 455: 58–63.
12. Wu S, Huang S, Ding J, Zhao Y, Liang L, et al. (2010) Multiple microRNAs modulate p21Cip1/Waf1 expression by directly targeting its 3′ untranslated region. Oncogene 29: 2302–8.
13. Allen KE, Weiss GJ (2010) Resistance may not be futile: microRNA biomarkers for chemoresistance and potential therapeutics. Mol Cancer Ther 9: 3126–36.
14. Landau DA, Slack FJ (2011) MicroRNAs in mutagenesis, genomic instability, and DNA repair. Semin Oncol 38: 743–51.
15. Hu H, Gatti RA (2011) MicroRNAs: new players in the DNA damage response. J Mol Cell Biol 3: 151–8.
16. Sommariva M, De Cecco L, Tagliabue E, Balsari A (2012) Modulation of DNA repair genes induced by TLR9 agonists. A strategy to elimate "altered" cells? OncoImmunology 1: 258–9.
17. Benard J, Da Silva J, De Blois MC, Boyer P, Duvillard P, et al. (1985) Characterization of a human ovarian adenocarcinoma line, IGROV1, in tissue culture and in nude mice. Cancer Res 45: 4970–9.

18. Wright GW, Simon RM (2003) A random variance model for detection of differential gene expression in small microarray experiments. Bioinformatics 19: 2448–55.
19. Sales G, Coppe A, Bisognin A, Biasiolo M, Bortoluzzi S, et al. (2010) MAGIA, a web-based tool for miRNA and Genes Integrated Analysis. Nucleic Acids Res 38: W352–W359.
20. Shih KK, Qin LX, Tanner EJ, Zhou Q, Bisogna M, et al. (2011) A microRNA survival signature (MiSS) for advanced ovarian cancer. Gynecol Oncol 121: 444–50.
21. Bagnoli M, De CL, Granata A, Nicoletti R, Marchesi E, et al. (2011) Identification of a chrXq27.3 microRNA cluster associated with early relapse in advanced stage ovarian cancer patients. Oncotarget 2: 1265–78.
22. Johnson WE, Li C, Rabinovic A (2007) Adjusting batch effects in microarray expression data using empirical Bayes methods. Biostatistics 8: 118–27.
23. Dolezalova D, Mraz M, Barta T, Plevova K, Vinarsky V, et al. (2012) MicroRNAs regulate p21(Waf1/Cip1) protein expression and the DNA damage response in human embryonic stem cells. Stem Cells 30: 1362–72.
24. Berezikov E, Thuemmler F, van Laake LW, Kondova I, Bontrop R, et al. (2006) Diversity of microRNAs in human and chimpanzee brain. Nat Genet 38: 1375–7.
25. Nam EJ, Yoon H, Kim SW, Kim H, Kim YT, et al. (2008) MicroRNA expression profiles in serous ovarian carcinoma. Clin Cancer Res 14: 2690–5.
26. Kim TH, Kim YK, Kwon Y, Heo JH, Kang H, et al. (2010) Deregulation of miR-519a, 153, and 485-5p and its clinicopathological relevance in ovarian epithelial tumours. Histopathology 57: 734–43.
27. Stronach EA, Alfraidi A, Rama N, Datler C, Studd JB, et al. (2011) HDAC4-regulated STAT1 activation mediates platinum resistance in ovarian cancer. Cancer Res 71: 4412–22.
28. Baltimore D, Boldin MP, O'Connell RM, Rao DS, Taganov KD (2008) MicroRNAs: new regulators of immune cell development and function. Nat Immunol 9: 839–45.
29. Lodish HF, Zhou B, Liu G, Chen CZ (2008) Micromanagement of the immune system by microRNAs. Nat Rev Immunol 8: 120–30.
30. O'Connell RM, Rao DS, Chaudhuri AA, Baltimore D (2010) Physiological and pathological roles for microRNAs in the immune system. Nat Rev Immunol 10: 111–22.
31. Nahid MA, Satoh M, Chan EK (2011) MicroRNA in TLR signaling and endotoxin tolerance. Cell Mol Immunol 8: 388–403.
32. Valadi H, Ekstrom K, Bossios A, Sjostrand M, Lee JJ, et al. (2007) Exosome-mediated transfer of mRNAs and microRNAs is a novel mechanism of genetic exchange between cells. Nat Cell Biol 9: 654–9.
33. Jin KL, Park JY, Noh EJ, Hoe KL, Lee JH, et al. (2010) The effect of combined treatment with cisplatin and histone deacetylase inhibitors on HeLa cells. J Gynecol Oncol 21: 262–8.
34. Ozaki K, Kishikawa F, Tanaka M, Sakamoto T, Tanimura S, et al. (2008) Histone deacetylase inhibitors enhance the chemosensitivity of tumor cells with cross-resistance to a wide range of DNA-damaging drugs. Cancer Sci 99: 376–84.
35. Stiborova M, Eckschlager T, Poljakova J, Hrabeta J, Adam V, et al. (2012) The synergistic effects of DNA-targeted chemotherapeutics and histone deacetylase inhibitors as therapeutic strategies for cancer treatment. Curr Med Chem.
36. Thurn KT, Thomas S, Moore A, Munster PN (2011) Rational therapeutic combinations with histone deacetylase inhibitors for the treatment of cancer. Future Oncol 7: 263–83.
37. Gryder BE, Sodji QH, Oyelere AK (2012) Targeted cancer therapy: giving histone deacetylase inhibitors all they need to succeed. Future Med Chem 4: 505–24.
38. Miska EA (2005) How microRNAs control cell division, differentiation and death. Curr Opin Genet Dev 15: 563–8.
39. Jackson AL, Levin AA (2012) Developing microRNA Therapeutics: Approaching the Unique Complexities. Nucleic Acid Ther 22: 213–25.

Discovery of Specific Metastasis-Related *N*-Glycan Alterations in Epithelial Ovarian Cancer Based on Quantitative Glycomics

Xingwang Zhang[1]¶, Yisheng Wang[2]¶, Yifan Qian[1], Xin Wu[2], Zejian Zhang[1], Xijun Liu[1], Ran Zhao[4], Lei Zhou[1], Yuanyuan Ruan[1], Jiejie Xu[1], Haiou Liu[1], Shifang Ren[1]*, Congjian Xu[2,3,4,5]*, Jianxin Gu[1]

1 Key Laboratory of Glycoconjugate Research Ministry of Public Health, Department of Biochemistry and Molecular Biology, School of Basic Medical Sciences, Fudan University, Shanghai, China, **2** Obstetrics and Gynecology Hospital, Fudan University, Shanghai, China, **3** Department of Obstetrics and Gynecology of Shanghai Medical School, Fudan University, Shanghai, China, **4** Institute of Biomedical Sciences, Fudan University, Shanghai, China, **5** Shanghai Key Laboratory of Female Reproductive Endocrine Related Diseases, Shanghai, China

Abstract

Generally, most of ovarian cancer cannot be detected until large scale and remote metastasis occurs, which is the major cause of high mortality in ovarian cancer. Therefore, it is urgent to discover metastasis-related biomarkers for the detection of ovarian cancer in its occult metastasis stage. Altered glycosylation is a universal feature of malignancy and certain types of glycan structures are well-known markers for tumor progressions. Thus, this study aimed to reveal specific changes of *N*-glycans in the secretome of the metastatic ovarian cancer. We employed a quantitative glycomics approach based on metabolic stable isotope labeling to compare the differential *N*-glycosylation of secretome between an ovarian cancer cell line SKOV3 and its high metastatic derivative SKOV3-ip. Intriguingly, among total 17 *N*-glycans identified, the *N*-glycans with bisecting GlcNAc were all significantly decreased in SKOV3-ip in comparison to SKOV3. This alteration in bisecting GlcNAc glycoforms as well as its corresponding association with ovarian cancer metastatic behavior was further validated at the glycotransferase level with multiple techniques including real-time PCR, western blotting, transwell assay, lectin blotting and immunohistochemistry analysis. This study illustrated metastasis-related *N*-glycan alterations in ovarian cancer secretome *in vitro* for the first time, which is a valuable source for biomarker discovery as well. Moreover, *N*-glycans with bisecting GlcNAc shed light on the detection of ovarian cancer in early peritoneal metastasis stage which may accordingly improve the prognosis of ovarian cancer patients.

Editor: Rajeev Samant, University of Alabama at Birmingham, United States of America

Funding: This work was supported by grants from National Basic Research Program of China (973 Program) (2012CB8221004, 2013CB910503), National High-tech R&D Program (863 Program) (2012AA020203) and National natural science fund (31100586, 31010103906, 30930025, 31170766, 81272879, 81302258), the Shanghai Leading Academic Discipline Project (B117), and Shanghai fundamental research emphasis project (11JC1401502). The funders had no role in study design, data collection and analysis, decision to publish, or preparation of the manuscript.

Competing Interests: The authors have declared that no competing interests exist.

* E-mail: renshifang@fudan.edu.cn (SR); xucongjian@gmail.com (CX)

¶ These authors contributed equally to this work.

Introduction

Epithelial ovarian cancer is the most lethal gynecological malignancy worldwide [1,2]. According to a recent report of the American Cancer Society, approximately 22,240 new cases will be diagnosed with ovarian cancer in 2013 while nearly 14,030 will succumb to this disease [3]. Currently, pelvic ultrasonography and serum CA125 test serve as main detection routines [4,5,6,7], which are effective in some cases. However, the majority of ovarian cancer may still not be diagnosed until the tumor has progressed to an advanced stage, presenting with large-scale or remote metastasis. In the clinic, the most common metastatic pattern of ovarian cancer is recognized as peritoneal implantation [8]. Due to the fact that early peritoneal metastasis sites are usually too small to be detected macroscopically [4,9], the five-year survival rate always suffers this poor terminal diagnosis and witnesses a dramatical decrease when large-scale peritoneal metastasis occurs, from about 90% at stage I to 2–80% at stage II-IV [4,10,11]. Therefore, it is necessary to discover metastasis-related biomarker which could aid in the detection of ovarian cancer as early as possible rather than until the wide spread of tumor outside the ovaries.

Glycosylation is one of the most prevalent post-translational modifications which produces various types of glycans that are frequently attached to proteins. Glycans participate in major pathophysiology events during tumor progressions [12,13,14]. Altered glycosylation is a universal feature of malignancy, and some of these alterations contribute to metastatic processes [12,15]. For instance, increased activity or expression of *N*-acetylglucosaminyltransferase V (MGAT5) and β-1, 6 GlcNAc-branched *N*-glycans has been found in highly metastatic tumors, such as colon, hepatic and breast cancers [16,17,18,19,20]. Additionally, the alteration in sialylation has been reported contributing to the metastasis in these tumor cells as well [21,22,23,24,25,26,27]. Moreover, other aberrant glycosylation patterns including core-fucose, bisecting GlcNAc *N*-glycans have been known to be associated with metastasis of many malignant cells [28,29,30,31,32]. Accordingly, cancer-associated aberrations in glycan structures provide a compelling rationale for new biomarkers discovery [33].

In the case of ovarian cancer, aberrant glycosylation has been described in multiple studies, mainly including increased silylaiton and fucosylation of *O*-linked glycans, higher levels of biantennary *N*-linked glycans, elevated core fucosylation, and bisecting *N*-linked glycosylation [34]. Currently, the role of glycosylation modification playing in ovarian cancer metastasis has also been indicated in several studies. For example, mesothelin-MUC16 binding that facilitates peritoneal metastasis of ovarian cancers has been shown *N*-glycan dependent [35]. The cell ability of adhesion to hyaluronan in ovarian carcinoma cell lines could be altered by removing carbohydrate moieties from the cell surfaces [36]. These studies suggested the involvement of glycans in the metastasis processes, whereas exact *N*-glycan changes associated with metastasis in ovarian cancer remained unclear, such as those on cell surface and cell secreted glycoproteins. Given that specific glycan structure changes in cancer cell secretome may be potential biomarkers for non-invasive diagnosis [37], in this study, we focused on revealing the metastasis-associated *N*-glycosylation alteration in glycoproteins secreted by ovarian cancer cells.

Quantitative glycomics based on mass spectrometry (MS) has been proved to be a promising and powerful tool to identify global alterations of glycans between different biological samples [38,39,40], which includes label free strategies and stable isotope labeling strategies. The former one is much simpler while the latter one is more robust. One quantitative glycomics method based on metabolic incorporation of stable isotope labels (Isotopic Detection of Aminosugars With Glutamine, IDAWG) has been reported recently [41]. In this method, differentially labeled cells can be mixed together early in the work flow, which minimize any potential bias introduced during sample processing and offer a reliable quantification method [39,42]. In our study, different from quantitative glycomics analysis of cell surface glycoproteins using IDAWG reported previously, quantitative glycomics method based on metabolic incorporation of stable isotope labels was employed to differential *N*-glycosylation analysis of secretome between two ovarian cancer cell lines, SKOV3 and its high metastatic derivative SKOV3-ip. Subsequently, metastasis-associated *N*-glycan changes in ovarian cancer discovered by this glycomics method were further validated at glycotransferase level with different molecular biological techniques, including real-time PCR, western blotting, lectin blotting, transwell assay and immunohistochemistry analysis. The total work flow in our study was shown in Figure 1. To our knowledge, this is the first attempt to reveal global picture of the metastasis-related *N*-glycan alterations in ovarian cancer cell secretome. Moreover, among these changes, decrease in bisecting GlcNAc modification and its corresponding glycotransferase (Mannosyl (Beta-1,4-)-Glycoprotein Beta-1,4-N-Acetylglucosaminyltransferase, MGAT3) expression were demonstrated to be related to higher metastatic potential. This study provided insights into discovery of metastasis-associated biomarker, which could aid in detecting early peritoneal metastasis of ovarian cancer, and finally improving diagnosis of ovarian cancer.

Materials and Methods

Cell Culture and Metabolic Stable Isotope Labeling

Serous ovarian cancer cell line SKOV3 and its high metastatic derivative SKOV3-ip were obtained from the American Type Culture Collection (ATCC). These two ovarian cancer cell lines were grown in RPMI1640 cell media (Invitrogen, Carlsbad, CA, USA) supplemented with 10% fetal bovine serum (Invitrogen). 293T cell line was obtained from the Institute of Cell Biology Academic Sinica (Shanghai, China). 293T cells were maintained in Dulbecco's modified Eagle's medium (DMEM) containing 10% fetal bovine serum. All cells were cultured with 1% penicillin/streptomycin at 37°C in a humidified 5% CO_2 incubator. For stable isotope labeling experiments, cells were cultured for at least six doublings in the RPMI1640 medium with 10% fetal bovine serum, containing 20 mM L-glutamine (either ^{14}N or amide-^{15}N-Gln) to achieve complete incorporation of labeled *N*-glycans [41]. Amide-^{15}N-Gln (98% purity) was purchased from Cambridge Isotopes, Inc. (Andover, MA, USA).

Supernatant Acquisition

Six million labeled cells were seeded in 55-cm^2 cell culture dishes and maintained overnight for cell attachment in the RPMI1640 medium supplemented with 10% fetal bovine serum, 20 mM L-glutamine (either ^{14}N or amide-^{15}N-Gln). After 12 h, the culture medium was removed, and the cells were washed for 3 times with phosphate-buffered saline. And then 10 mL of serum-free, phenol red-free RPMI1640 medium with 20 mM L-glutamine (either ^{14}N or amide-^{15}N) was added to each dish. After incubation for 48 h, the conditioned medium was collected and filtered through a 0.22 μm Durapore PVDF Membrane (Millipore, Billerica, MA, USA). Before, during and after serum starvation, viability of cancer cells was assessed using the trypan blue dye exclusion assay. The protein concentrations of conditioned media were determined using a BCA protein assay kit (Pierce,Rockford, IL). The conditioned medium with equal protein amount obtained from SKOV3 and SKOV3-ip were mixed. Subsequently, the mixtures were concentrated by Amicon Ultra-15, 3,000 molecular weight cut off (MWCO) centrifugal filter units (Millipore, Billerica, MA, USA) with excessive salt removing for quantitative glycomics. All samples were stored at −80°C until further use.

Release and Purification of N-Glycans from Secreted Proteome

The *N*-linked glycan release and purification were performed as previously described with minor modifications [43]. Aliquots of mixed protein solution (100 μL) were diluted with equal volume of denaturing buffer composed of 200 mM NH_4HCO_3 (Sigma-Aldrich, Germany) containing 20 mM mdithiothreitol (Sigma-Aldrich, Germany). The samples were heated for 10 min in 95°C water bath. After the denatured samples cooled to the ambient room temperature, 1 μL of PNGase F (New England Biolabs, Inc., USA) was added to each sample followed by overnight incubation at 37°C. Subsequently, the deglycosylated proteins were precipitated by adding 600 μL of chilled ethanol stored at −80°C for 2 h. After centrifugation at 14,000×g, for 30 min at 4°C, the supernatant was collected and dried through vacuum centrifugation. The released glycans were further purified and desalted using a Porous Graphic Carbon Solid-Phase Extraction (PGC-SPE). To this end, the PGC microcolumns were packed with porous graphic carbon powder and prepared using GELoader tips as described before [44]. The microcolumns were preconditioned with 6 column volumes of 0.1% (v/v) trifluoroacetic acid (TFA) in 80% acetonitrile (ACN)/H_2O (v/v) and equilibrated with equal volume of water. Afterwards, the samples were applied to the columns repeatedly for 5 times to achieve complete glycans adsorption. Subsequently, the microcolumns were washed with approximately 10 column volumes of water to remove salts and buffer. Glycans

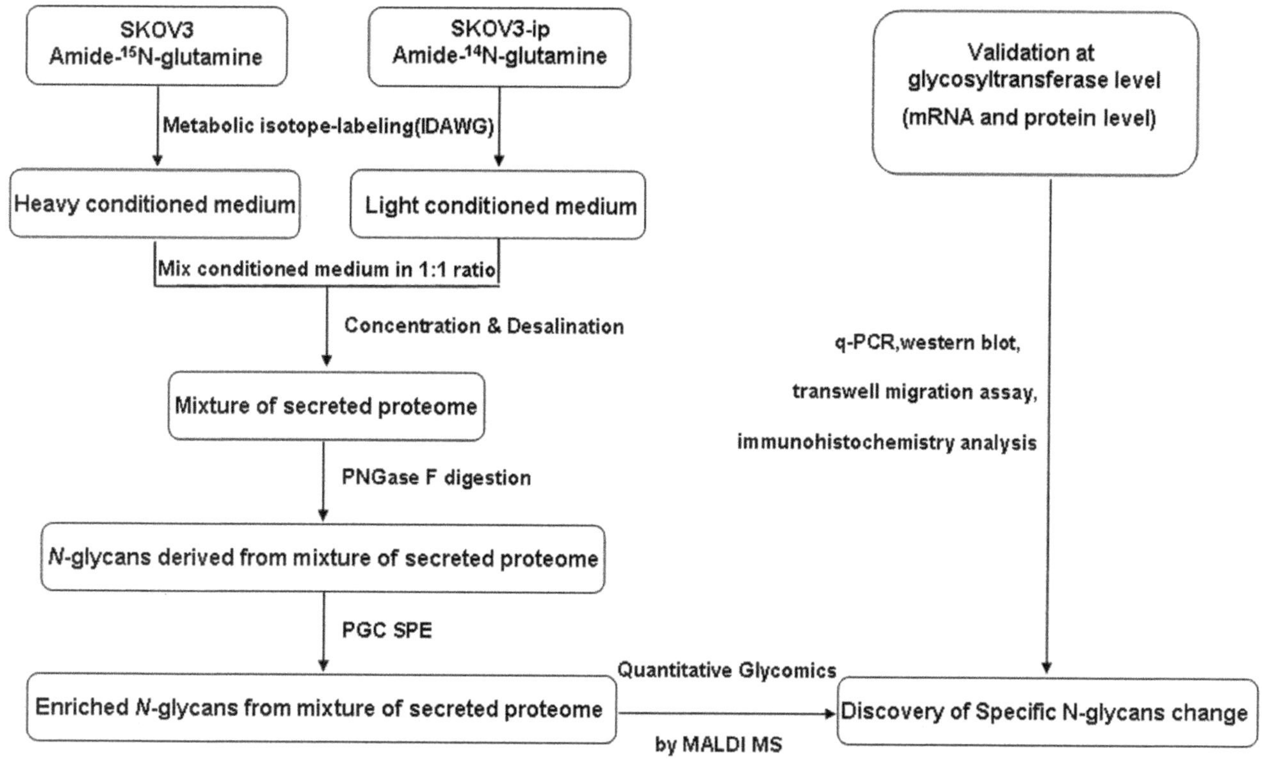

Figure 1. The total experimental workflow in this study.

were eluted with 25% (v/v) ACN containing 0.05% (v/v) TFA. Each sample was then divided into two equal aliquots and lyophilized in a vacuum freeze dryer (Martin Christ GmbH, Osterode,Germany). One equal aliquot of each sample was stored at −80°C until further analysis. Another equal aliquot of each sample was permethylated.

Permethylation of *N*-glycans

N-glycans were permethylated using a previously published procedure with minor modifications [45]. Briefly, dried *N*-glycans were suspended in 200 μL of dimethyl sulfoxide (DMSO), and approximately 20 mg NaOH powder was added. After the slurry was mixed vigorously, 100 μL of CH_3I was added and the following incubation was conducted in an ultrasonic bath for 30 min. The reaction was quenched by addition of 1 mL of water, and the excess CH_3I was removed under a stream of nitrogen. Subsequently, 1 mL of chloroform was added with strong mixing. After phase separation, the aqueous phase was discarded while the lower chloroform phase was washed 10 times with 1 mL of H_2O and dried down under a stream of nitrogen in a hood for matrix-assisted laser desorption/ionization mass spectrometry (MALDI MS) analysis.

MALDI MS Analysis

MALDI mass spectrometric analysis was performed on AXIMA Resonance MALDI QIT TOF MS (Shimadzu Corp., Kyoto, Japan) with a 337 nm nitrogen laser. All samples were analyzed at a 20-kV accelerating voltage in the positive ion and reflectron mode. CID was performed at a collision energy of 4 keV using argon as the collision gas. The instrument was externally calibrated by TOFMix™ (LaserBio Labs, France) containing eight peptides calibration standard. Prior to MS analysis, unpermethylated glycans were reconstituted in a 5-μL aliquot of 0.1% (volume/volume, v/v) TFA in 50% ACN/H_2O (v/v) and permethylated glycans were reconstituted in a 5-μL aliquot of 50% methanol. Each sample (1 μL) was spotted onto a MALDI target and allowed to dry in air at ambient temperature. Afterwards, 1 μL of 2,5-dihydroxybenzoic acid matrix (DHB, Sigma-Aldrich, Germany) at the concentration of 12.5 mg mL^{-1} in 50% ACN in water (v/v) containing 0.1% TFA was added onto the sample layer and dried under ambient conditions. Each sample was spotted in triplicate. Two laser shots were set to generate a profile and 200 profiles were accumulated from different points of laser irradiation into one file for each sample spot. For comparison of *N*-glycans from secretomes of the two ovarian cancer cells, a 1:1 mixture of ^{14}N- and ^{15}N-labeled samples was initially obtained through mixing equal starting proteins amount. And the mixture was analyzed (three replicates) to determine relative changes in the abundances of *N*-glycans between ovarian cancer cell line SKOV3 and its high metastatic derivative SKOV3-ip. All the proposed structures of identified glycans were interpreted manually based on their m/z values according to serveral previously published literatures [46,47], GlycoWorkbench [48], Glycan Mass Spectral Database [49] as well as GlycoBase (Version 2, http://glycobase.nibrt.ie/glycobase.html).

Quantitative Real-time PCR for mRNA Expression Analysis

Total RNAs were extracted from ovarian cancer cell lines with the TRIzol™ reagent (Invitrogen) and 2 μg of total RNA was reverse transcribed using RT Master Mix kit (Takara) according to the manufacturer's instruction. Real-time PCR was performed on ABI 7500 Fast Real-time PCR system (Applied Biosystems). The PCR cycling conditions consisted of a single incubation step at 95°C for 30 s, followed by 40 cycles of 5 s at 95°C, and 34 s at

60°C. All PCR reactions were performed with SYBR-green Premix Real-time PCR kit (Takara) according to the manufacturer's protocol. Primers sequences used in PCR analysis were as follows: human MGAT3 forward (5′-CAGGGCACAGGATT-GAAGAGTT-3′) and human MGAT3 reverse (5′-AGCTTGGTTTCCCTTCATATTGAG-3′); human MGAT5 forward (5′- GACCTGCAGTTCCTTCTTCG-3′) and human MGAT5 reverse (5′- CCATGGCAGAAGTCCTGTTT-3′); human Glyceraldehyde-3-phosphate dehydrogenase (GADPH) forward (5′-CTCTCTGCTCCTCCTGTTCGAC-3′) and human GAPDH reverse (5′-TGAGCGATGTGGCTCGGCT-3′). Human GADPH mRNA served as an endogenous control for normalization. Real-time PCR analysis was carried out in triplicate.

Plasmids and Gene Overexpression

SKOV3-ip and SKOV3 cells were transfected using X-tremeGENE HP DNATransfection Reagent (Roche Applied Science, Mannheim, Germany) with pcDNA3.1-MGAT3 or pcDNA3.1-MGAT5 plasmids, respectively (provided by a researcher in our laboratory), according to the manufacturer's instructions. And pcDNA3.1 vector was used as the negative control. At 48 h after transfection, the overexpression of MGAT3 and MGAT5 were confirmed by western blot analysis.

Small Interfering RNA and Knockdown of MGAT3

SKOV3 cells were transfected with MGAT3 specific siRNA Transfection Reagent Complex, (Santa Cruz Biotech, Inc., sc-44469), which was prepared according to the manufacturer's protocol. Scrambled siRNA was used as the negative control. At 48 h after transfection, cell lysates were prepared for western blot analysis to determine gene knockdown efficacy.

Western Blot and Lectin Blot Analysis

In order to obtain whole cell proteins, the cells were collected, washed with phosphate buffer solution (PBS) and then lysed in SDS lysis buffer [50]. Total protein concentrations were determined by BCA assay (Pierce,Rockford, IL). Equal amounts of total protein lysates from each cell line were separated by 10% sodium dodecyl sulfate polyacrylamide gel electrophoresis (SDS-PAGE) and then transferred to PVDF membranes (Roche Applied Science). i. Western blot analysis: After blocking with 5% skimmed milk in Tris-buffered saline containing 0.1% Tween 20 (TBST) for 2 h at room temperature, the membranes were incubated overnight at 4°C with mouse monoclonal antibody against MGAT3 (1/1000 diluted, sigma) or MGAT5 (1/1000 diluted, sigma) and then a secondary antibody at room temperature for 1 h. After washing, the membranes were detected by enhanced chemiluminescent (ECL) assay kit. ii. Lectin blot analysis: After blocking with 5% BSA in TBST, the membranes were incubated overnight at 4°C with biotinylated *Phaseolus vulgaris erythroagglutinin* (E-PHA) (1/5000 diluted,Vector Labs) or *Phaseolus vulgaris leucoagglutinin* (L-PHA) (1/5000 diluted,Vector Labs). Next, membranes were washed four times with TBST, followed by incubation with horseradish peroxidase streptavidin (Vector Labs) for 30 min at room temperature. Subsequently, the membranes were washed four times with TBST and detected by ECL assay kit.

Transwell Migration Assay

To evaluate the migratory ability, cell migration was performed using 24-well format transwell chambers (8 μm pore filter, Corning, Canton, NY). Briefly, SKOV3 cells were transfected with MGAT3 specific siRNA or MGAT5 plasmid, and SKOV3-ip cells were transfected with MGAT3 plasmid for 36 h, respectively. After that, cells were trypsinized, collected, counted, and then suspended in serum-free RPMI1640 medium. 2×10^4 cells in 100 μL of serum-free RPMI1640 medium were platted to each insert of the upper chamber. Meanwhile, 600 μL of RPMI1640 medium containing 10% FBS was added to each lower chamber. Subsequently, the cells were incubated for 12 h at 37°C. After removing the cells on the upper membrane surface, cells on the bottom surface of the membrane were fixed and stained with 0.1% crystal violet for 30 min at room temperature. Next, cells that had passed through the filter to the lower chamber were counted microscopically in 6 random regions per filter. The number of cells that traversed the membrane revealed the migratory ability of the tested cells.

Immunohistochemistry Analysis

A total of 24 ovarian cancer tissues were fixed in 4% formalin and embedded in paraffin. Tissue sections were first subjected to hematoxylin and eosin (H&E) staining for histopathological diagnosis. Then, immunohistochemical staining using anti-MGAT3 antibody (Abcam, Cambridge, MA, USA) was performed as described previously [51]. The intensity of MGAT3 staining was scaled from 0 to 3, where 0 stands for negative staining, 1, 2, 3 stand for weak, moderate, and strong staining respectively. Ovarian cancer tissues were obtained from the Obstetrics and Gynecology Hospital, Fudan University, Shanghai, China. All protocols have been approved by the Institutional Review Board of the hospital. All patients have given their written informed consent. Clinical information for these patients were shown in Table S1.

Data Processing and Statistical Analysis

MALDI MS and tandem mass spectrometry (MS/MS) data were acquired and processed in Launchpad software (Shimadzu Biotech, Kyoto, Japan). The parameters of peak processing: smoothing method: Gaussian; peak detection method: threshold-25% centroid; threshold offset: 0.500 mV. The m/z values and intensities were exported as ASCII files and peak intensities were scaled with the highest peak as 100%. The relative quantification of detected *N*-glycans was according to the protocols previously reported [42]. All statistical analyses were performed using GraphPad Prism (version 5). All the experiments were performed at least three times. The data were expressed as the means ± standard error of the mean (SEM). Student's *t*-test was used to determine the significance of differences between two groups. Wilcoxon Signed Ranks Test was used to compare immunohistochemistry data from the two groups. A *p*-value of less than 0.05 was considered to be statistically significant.

Results

Quantitative/Comparative Glycomics Analysis of Supernatant between SKOV3 and SKOV3-ip Cell

To discover the metastasis-related *N*-glycan alteration in ovarian cancer cell secretome, the total pool of *N*-glycan mixture, released by the enzyme Peptide *N*-glycosidase F from the secretome mixture of SKOV3(amide-^{15}N-Gln labeled) and SKOV3-ip cells (amide-^{14}N-Gln labeled), was analyzed by MALDI-QIT-TOF MS (Figure 2). A total of 17 *N*-glycans were identified, including high mannose, hybrid, triantennary, tetra-antennary structures and bisecting GlcNAc glycoforms. All the identified *N*-glycans with proposed structure were shown in Figure 2 and summarized in Table 1.

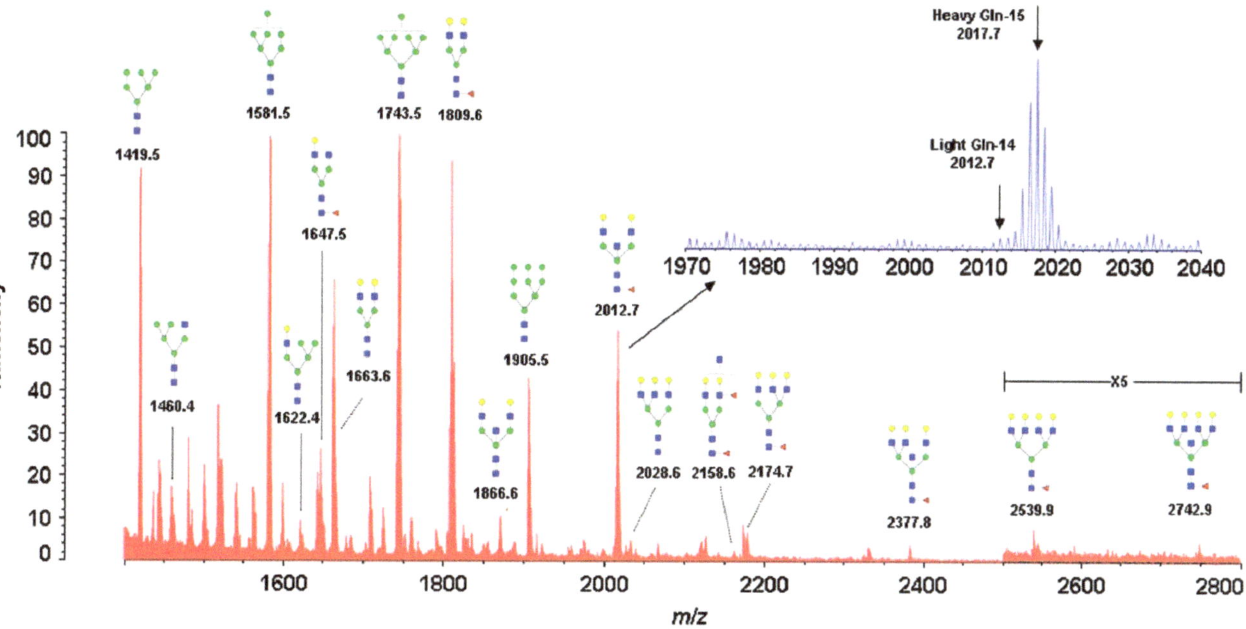

Figure 2. Quantitative analysis of *N*-linked glycans using MALDI-TOF MS. *N*-linked glycans from a 1:1 mixture of SKOV3-ip (Gln-14 labeled) and SKOV3 (Gln-15 labeled) supernatant. The structures were interpreted manually based on their *m/z* values according to several previously published literatures [46,47], GlycoWorkbench [48] as well as Glycan Mass Spectral Database [49]. Gln-14 indicates amide-^{14}N-Gln; Gln-15 indicates amide-^{15}N-Gln. Green circle indicates mannose; yellow circle indicates galactose; blue square indicates *N*-acetylglucosamine; red triangle indicates fucose.

Quantitative analysis of *N*-glycans from the secretome mixture of SKOV3 and SKOV3-ip cells was based on signal intensities. Intensity ratios (SKOV3-ip/SKOV3) of 0.83 and 1.2 were set as the threshold to estimate the down- or up-regulation of the *N*-

Table 1. Relative quantitation of *N*-glycans detected in SKOV3-ip (amide-^{14}N-Gln-labeled) and SKOV3 (amide-^{15}N-Gln-labeled) supernatant.

No.	Observed *m/z* $[M+Na]^+$	Theoretical *m/z* $[M+Na]^+$	Ratio (SKOV3-ip/SKOV3)	CV (%) (n = 9)	Change[a]	Composition	Type
1	1419.5	1419.5	1.46	4.26	up	$HexNAc_2Hex_6$	High mannose
2	1460.4	1460.5	2.05	13.44	up	$HexNAc_3Hex_5$	Hybrid
3	1581.5	1581.5	0.95	3.49	no	$HexNAc_2Hex_7$	High mannose
4	1622.4	1622.6	1.63	12.61	up	$HexNAc_3Hex_6$	Hybrid
5	1647.5	1647.6	3.40	11.48	up	$HexNAc_4Hex_4$ Fuc	Complex biantennary
6	1663.6	1663.6	3.23	8.78	up	$HexNAc_4Hex_5$	Complex biantennary
7	1743.5	1743.6	1.42	4.29	up	$HexNAc_2Hex_8$	High mannose
8	1809.6	1809.6	2.21	8.87	up	$HexNAc_4Hex_5$ Fuc	Complex biantennary
9	1866.6	1866.7	0.28	2.40	down	$HexNAc_5Hex_5$	Bisecting
10	1905.5	1905.6	2.19	10.01	up	$HexNAc_2Hex_9$	High mannose
11	2012.7	2012.7	0.12	15.20	down	$HexNAc_5Hex_5$ Fuc	Bisecting
12	2028.6	2028.7	1.32	18.06	up	$HexNAc_5Hex_6$	Triantennary
13	2158.6	2158.8	0.64	17.46	down	$HexNAc_5Hex_5$ Fuc_2	Complex biantennary
14	2174.7	2174.8	2.21	15.99	up	$HexNAc_5Hex_6$ Fuc	Triantennary
15	2377.8	2377.9	0.32	9.87	down	$HexNAc_6Hex_6$ Fuc	Bisecting
16	2539.9	2539.9	1.78	15.90	up	$HexNAc_6Hex_7$ Fuc	Tetra-antennary
17	2742.9	2743.0	0.73	15.35	down	$HexNAc_7Hex_7$ Fuc	Bisecting

[a]Ratio (SKOV3-ip/SKOV3) <0.83 or >1.20 is distinguishable as a criterion to estimate the down- or up-regulation of the glycan levels. HexNAc, N-acetylhexosamine; Hex, hexose (mannose or galactose); Fuc, fucose.

glycan levels in SKOV3-ip cells, in comparison to SKOV3 cells, since the maximum coefficient of variation (CV) (n = 9) was below 20% in this study [43]. Relative quantitation of all detected *N*-glycans between SKOV3-ip and SKOV3 cells were summarized in Table 1. The results demonstrated that three out of four high mannose structures were up-regulated in SKOV3-ip cells. *N*-glycans containing hybrid, triantennary, and tetra-antennary structures with or without fucose were elevated in SKOV3-ip cells. The similar trend was observed in three glycans with complex biantennary structures. Among all the alteration in *N*-glycans, all the *N*-glycans with bisecting GlcNAc were found to be apparently decreased in the SKOV3-ip cells, with their SKOV3-ip/SKOV3 ratios ranging from 0.73 to 0.12, while all the β-1,6 GlcNAc-branched *N*-glycans were elevated in SKOV3-ip cells. Among these altered *N*-glycans, we focused on the *N*-glycans with bisecting GlcNAc, partly because all of them decreased and they were the most obviously altered *N*-glycans. Furthermore, an increasing body of evidence has indicated that the bisecting glycans may affect tumor progression and metastasis [52].The structures containing bisecting GlcNAc were further confirmed by tandem mass spectrometry (MS/MS). Representative tandem MS spectra of m/z 2012.7 $[M+Na]^+$, and m/z 2377.8 $[M+Na]^+$ were shown in Figures S1A–B.

It is noteworthy that sialic acids, typically presented as terminal monosaccharides in the glycan moiety of many glycoproteins, play essential roles in many physiological and pathological processes. Sialylated glycans are labile and easy to be lost during direct mass spectrometric analysis of underivatized *N*-glycans. As permethylation can stabilize the sialic acid residues by converting highly polar -OH and $-COO^-$ groups of the different monosaccharides into nonpolar [38], *N*-glycans after permethylation were also analyzed. The results demonstrated that more *N*-glycans with different degree of sialylation were observed comparing to the analysis results without permethylation. Although signal of one *N*-glycan with bisecting GlcNAc could be decentralized to several signals of *N*-glycans with different degree of sialylation, the trend of alteration in all the bisecting GlcNAc structures were the same no matter permethylated or not (see Figure S2). The signal intensity of the bisecting *N*-glycan without permethylation (Figure S2A, m/z 2012.6 for example) was higher than that of permethylated *N*-glycans at m/z 2489.4, m/z 2850.3 and m/z 3211.4 containing 0, 1 and 2 sialic acids respectively (Figure S2B). It is possibly because part of the original bisecting signal intensity (Figure S2A) was contributed to the corresponding fragments of the glycans with same structure while containing additional 1 and 2 sialic acids (Figure S2B). Furthermore, the glycan profiles with permethylation were more complex (i.e.,have more peaks). Thereby, it is suggested that the permethylation step probably could be omitted in quantitative glycomics analysis of those neutral *N*-glycans which is irrelative to sialic acids, such as bisecting GlcNAc glycoform in this study.

Differential Expression of MGAT3 in SKOV3-ip and SKOV3 Cell Lines

As bisecting GlcNAc residue was synthesized by specific glycosytransferase (MGAT3), the change in *N*-glycans with bisecting GlcNAc could be correlated with the corresponding alteration in MGAT3. Therefore, real-time PCR analysis was carried out to compare the mRNA expression levels of MGAT3 between SKOV3 and SKOV3-ip cell lines. The results demonstrated that MGAT3 was differentially expressed between the two cell lines. The mRNA level of MGAT3 was significantly higher in SKOV3 cells than that in SKOV3-ip cells (61-fold, $p<0.001$, Figure 3A). Then the expression of MGAT3 in this two cell lines was further assessed at protein level by western blot analysis. The lower abundance of MGAT3 was observed for SKOV3-ip cells in contrast with SKOV3 cells (Figure 3B). Therefore, decreased MGAT3 expression in both mRNA and protein levels in SKOV3-ip cells were in accordance with decreased bisecting GluNAc modification in SKOV3-ip cell supernatant manifested by quantitative glycomics analysis.

Effects of MGAT3 on Migration Ability of Ovarian Cancer Cells

The data above showed that the levels of MGAT3 and its catalysate, *N*-glycans containing bisecting GlcNAc, were significantly lower in SKOV3-ip cells compared with that in SKOV3 cells. Since SKOV3-ip cells are the highly metastatic derivatives of SKOV3 cells, these results suggested a potential role of MGAT3 and its catalysate, bisecting glycans, on ovarian cancer cell motility. In order to test this, MGAT3 gene was overexpressed in SKOV3-ip cells by transfection. Western blot analysis demonstrated a significant increase in MGAT3 expression after transfection, compared with SKOV3-ip-control cells (Figure 4A). The level of bisecting glycans were also elevated accordingly (Figure 4B). To confirm whether overexpression of MGAT3 affect the migration ability, trans-well migration assays were performed. As shown in Figure 4C and 4D, migration ability in MGAT3 transfected cells was significantly decreased to 52% of that in control cells. Meanwhile, knockdown of MGAT3 in SKOV3 cells was performed by MGAT3-targeting siRNA transfection. Western blot analysis demonstrated efficient depression of MGAT3 expression in SKOV3 after transfection (Figure 5A). The level of bisecting glycans were down-regulated accordingly (Figure 5B). Trans-well migration assays (Figure 5C and 5D) showed 64% enhancement in migration ability in MGAT3-targeting siRNA transfected SKOV3 cells as compared with control cells. These results suggested that MGAT3 was involved in the migration ability of ovarian cancer cells, and may play a role in suppressing ovarian cancer cell metastasis.

Immunohistochemical Analysis of MGAT3 Expression in Ovarian Cancer Tissues

We further assessed MGAT3 expression in 24 ovarian cancer tissues employing immunohistochemical analysis. As shown in Figure 6, the expression levels of MGAT3 displayed a decreasing pattern, going from low grade ovarian cancer to high grade ovarian cancer. While only 14.29% of high grade ovarian cancer, 76.47% of low grade ovarian cancer specimens displayed moderate to strong staining of MGAT3. Immunohistochemical analysis indicated that lower MGAT3 expression correlated to ovarian cancers with higher malignant potential, which was in accordance with the results obtained from the SKOV3 cell line and its high metastatic derivative, SKOV3-ip cell lines.

Discussion

In the present study, a comprehensive strategy was developed to facilitate the identification and validation of specific *N*-glycan changes associated with ovarian cancer metastasis. Accordingly, SKOV3 and its high metastatic derivative SKOV3-ip cells, which were isolated from ascites in the mouse given i.p. injections of SKOV3 cells [53], were chosen as experiment model. Notably, we aimed not only to discover the corresponding *N*-glycan alterations, but to confirm the featured change through multiple molecular biology approaches, including real-time PCR, western blot, lectin blot, transwell assay and immunohistochemistry analysis, as well.

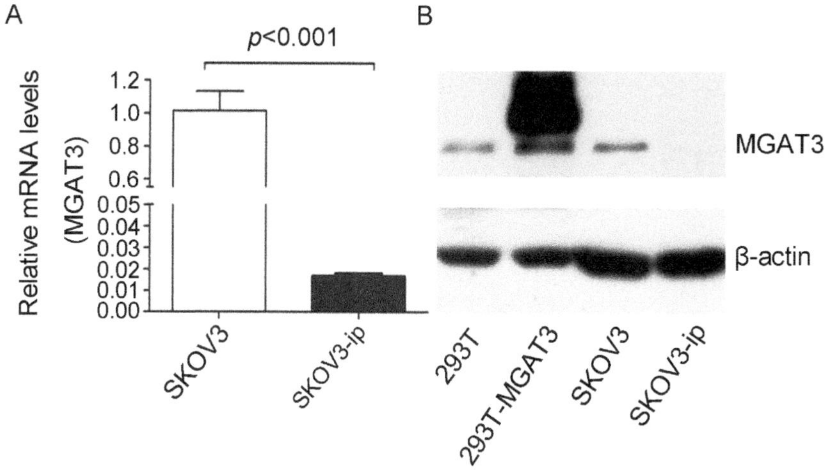

Figure 3. Differential expression of MGAT3 in SKOV3-ip and SKOV3 cell lines. (A) The mRNA expression levels of MGAT3 in SKOV3-ip and SKOV3 cell lines. The mRNA levels of MGAT3 were normalized with GAPDH levels. Mean fold changes were calculated with the $2^{-\Delta\Delta Ct}$ method. (B) The protein expression levels of MGAT3 in SKOV3-ip and SKOV3 cell lines. Cell lysates were isolated by 10% SDS-PAGE for western blotting using antibody against MGAT3. Human beta-actin served as an endogenous control. 293T cell line was used as positive control. Data are expressed as the means ± SEM. Each assay was performed at least three times. A *p*-value of less than 0.05 indicates statistical significance using Student's *t*-test.

From a clinical perspective, focusing on the glycosylation alteration of glycoproteins secreted by cancer cells is very appealing for diagnostic purposes, as they may filtrate into the peripheral blood [54,55]. Discovery of biomarkers by direct analysis of blood plasma has been very difficult so far [55,56], because plasma is a very complex fluid in which concentration of proteins are in high dynamic range. Therefore, the analysis of proteins secreted by homogeneous cancer cell populations has been reported as a more straightforward approach [57,58,59,60]. Consequently, the conditioned medium of cell lines has widely been used for the analysis of cancer secretome [55,61]. In this study, the differential *N*-glycosylation of secretome between SKOV3 and SKOV3-ip cells was investigated through global quantitative glycomic profiling of supernatant of these two cell lines based on metabolic incorporation of stable isotope labels [41]. In order to assess the changes of *N*-glycans in a reliable and sensitive manner, metabolic stable isotope labels were employed for MS-based quantitative glycomics analysis, which was reported capable of monitoring the glycan alterations associated with different biological conditions and diseases [40,45,62]. According to a recent research, a cell culture metabolic labeling strategy, IDAWG, was introduced, applying the principle of SILAC specialized for proteomic quantification to the glycomic quantification [41]. To be more specific, culture media containing amide-^{15}N-Gln was used to metabolically label cellular aminosugars with heavy nitrogen, which was proved to be a simple implementation of quantitative tool for glycomic analysis [41]. Notably, in our study, this strategy was first utilized for the quantitative glycomics analysis of cell-secreted proteomes of ovarian cancer cells. Base on this method, changes in the structures and relative abundance of *N*-glycans of secreted glycoproteins from two ovarian cancer cells with different metastasis potential were obtained in a relatively reliable way. The results demonstrated that all the *N*-glycans with bisecting GlcNAc apparently decreased, while GlcNAc-branched *N*-glycans, high mannose structures increased in SKOV3-ip cell sceretome compared with that in SKOV3 cell secretome.

Bisecting GlcNAc residue is synthesized by a specific glycotransferase, *N*-acetylglucosaminyltransferase III (MGAT3) [63], which transfers GlcNAc in β1,4-linkage to the core Man of complex or hybrid *N*-glycans. MGAT3 is considered a key glycosyltransferase in *N*-glycan biosynthetic pathways and was reported playing an important role in tumor progression [52]. Knockdown of MGAT3 expression promoted MHCC97-L cells (human hepatocarcinoma cell line) invasion and increased resistance to 5-fluorouracil *in vitro* [64]. Transfection of MGAT3 in B16 melanoma cells resulted in suppressed tumor invasion and lung metastasis [65]. Song *et al.* reported that the bisecting GlcNAc on *N*-glycans inhibited growth factor signaling and retarded mammary tumor progression [32]. However, MGAT3 was reported upregulated in high metastatic human hepatocarcinoma cell line HCCLM3 in comparison with cell line with low metastatic potential [66]. Overexpression of MGAT3 in HeLaS3 cells enhanced the epidermal growth factor (EGF) mediated cell signaling [67], and transfecting myelogenous leukemia cell line K562 with MGAT3 protected it from natural killer cytotoxicity and increased spleen colonization [68]. The combined data indicates that effects of MGAT3 on tumor progression may vary with cell type.

In the case of ovarian cancer, relationship between bisecting glycan modification as well as MGAT3 and metastatic potential remains unclear. Abbott, K. L. *et al* reported increased expression of E-PHA binding proteins in endometrioid ovarian cancer tissue compared to normal ovarian tissue [69]. However, endometrioid ovarian cancer has been demonstrated to transform from endometriosis or ovarian epithelial cells [70]. Normal ovarian tissue, which is largely composed of ovarian stoma cells, could not be used as normal counterpart of ovarian cancer tissues. Our data from quantitative glycomics analysis suggested significantly decreased bisecting glycan modification in highly metastatic ovarian cancer cell line (SKOV3-ip). This finding was further supported by decreased expression of MGAT3 on both mRNA and protein levels observed in SKOV3-ip cells. Trans-well migration assays indicated that MGAT3 behaves as a suppressor in ovarian cancer cell migration. Immunhistochemistry analysis of MGAT3 expression in ovarian cancer tissues also showed correlation of over-expression of MGAT3 with lower metastatic

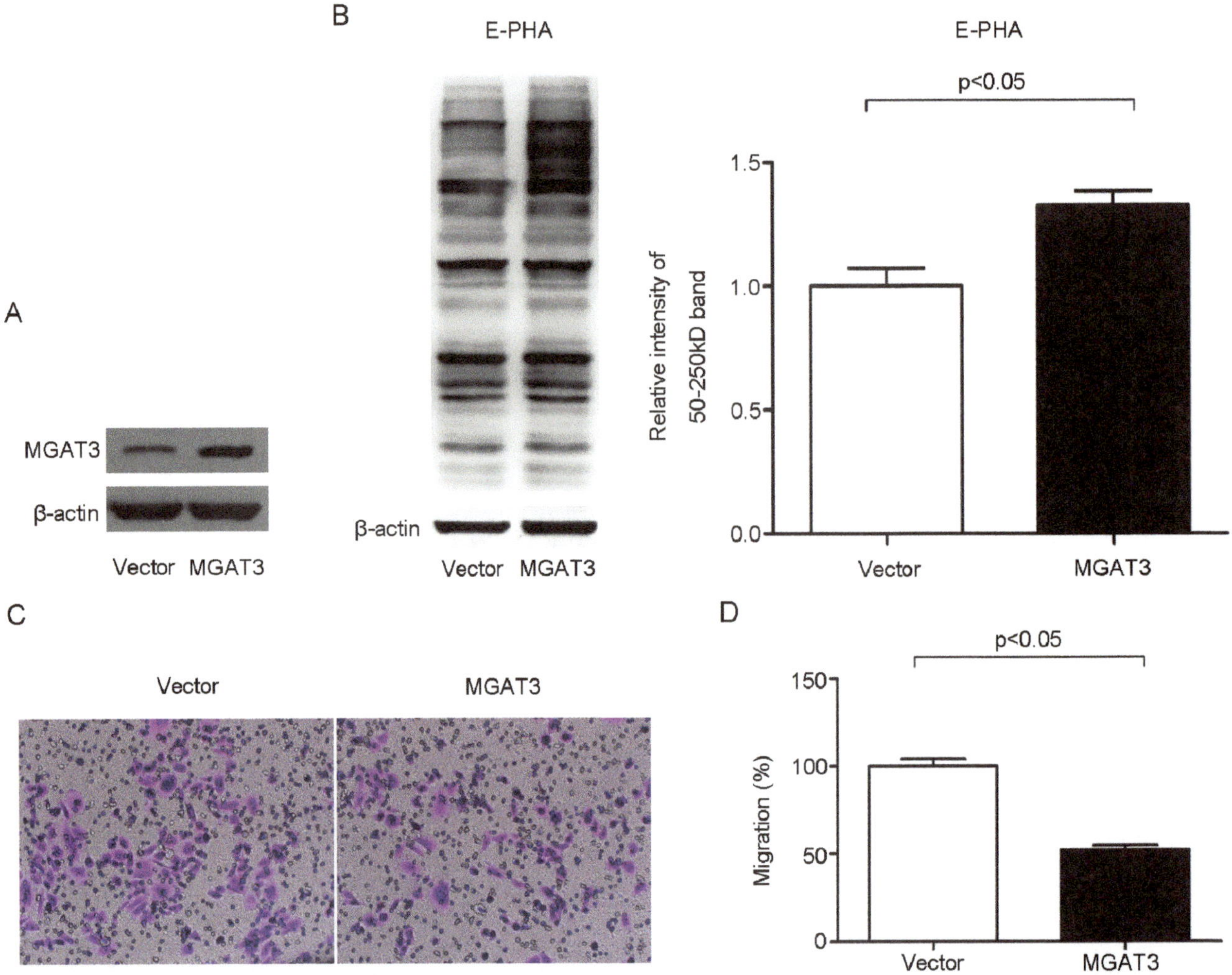

Figure 4. Overexpression of MGAT3 inhibits the migration ability of epithelial ovarian cancer cells. SKOV3-ip cells were transfected with pcDNA3.1 empty or MGAT3/pcDNA3.1 vectors. At 48 h after transfection, amounts of MGAT3 protein and its catalysate, *N*-glycans containing bisecting GlcNAc were detected by Western blotting (A) and Lectin blotting (B) in SKOV3-ip cells, respectively. Human beta-actin served as an endogenous control. All the relative expression levels of *N*-glycans containing bisecting GlcNAc were normalized to beta-actin. The left column of (B) represents the densitometry result for glycoproteins 50–250 kDa relative to control set at 1.0. It should be noted that the expression levels of MAGT3 and its catalysate, bisecting glycans were both significantly increased. Simultaneously, cells were subjected to the migration assay. Images of migrating cells from migration assay (C) and quantitative results are shown (D). Original magnification: 200x.The reported values are expressed as the means ± SEM. Each assay was performed at least three times. A *p*-value of less than 0.05 indicates statistical significance using Student's *t*-test.

potential, which was in line with the result from ovarian cancer cell lines.

One mechanism reported to be responsible for inhibitory effects of MGAT3 on cancer metastasis is that addition of bisecting GlcNAc by MGAT3 hinders β1,6 GlcNAc branching formation catalyzed by MGAT5, since MGAT5 cannot utilize the bisected oligosaccharide as an acceptor substrate [71,72]. GlcNAc-branched *N*-glycans was reported to promote cancer cell metastasis via frequent sialic acid modifications on its remote saccharides and interaction with galectins to form lattices that regulate signaling receptor endocytosis [52]. As a consequence, increased expression of MGAT3 deceased β1,6 GlcNAc branching and metastatic potential of cancer cells. In this study, the antagonistic result of bisecting GlcNAc structures and GlcNAc-branched *N*-glycans was observed (Figures S3,S4). Increasing in β1,6 GlcNAc branching and MGAT5 expression in the highly metastatic SKOV3-ip cells were also manifested (Table 1, Figure S5), which were in accordance with findings reported in other cancers. Overexpression of MGAT5 in SKOV3 cells led to increased β1,6 GlcNAc branching and cell migration (Figure S6). These data suggested competitive effects of MGAT3 and MGAT5 on *N*-glycan processing in ovarian cancer. Notably, decreased MGAT3 expression and increased MGAT5 expression may be concurrent phenomenon that both contribute to increasedβ1,6 GlcNAc branching in highly metastatic ovarian cancer.

An important approach by which bisecting GlcNAc affects tumor cell behaviors is its modification of membrane or secreted glycoproteins that mediate cell-cell and cell-matrix interaction. E-cadherin is the main epithelial cell-cell adhesion molecule. In melanoma, MGAT3 upregulation, which in turn increased bisecting GlcNAc modification of E-cadherin [65], led to an enhancement of E-cadherin-mediated cell-cell interactions owing to prolonged turnover of E-cadherin on the cell surface [29,73]. Introduction of bisecting *N*-glycan into integrin alpha(5)beta(1) inhibited cell migration on fibronectin [31]. Epidermal growth factor receptor (EGFR), a key signaling receptor for cell

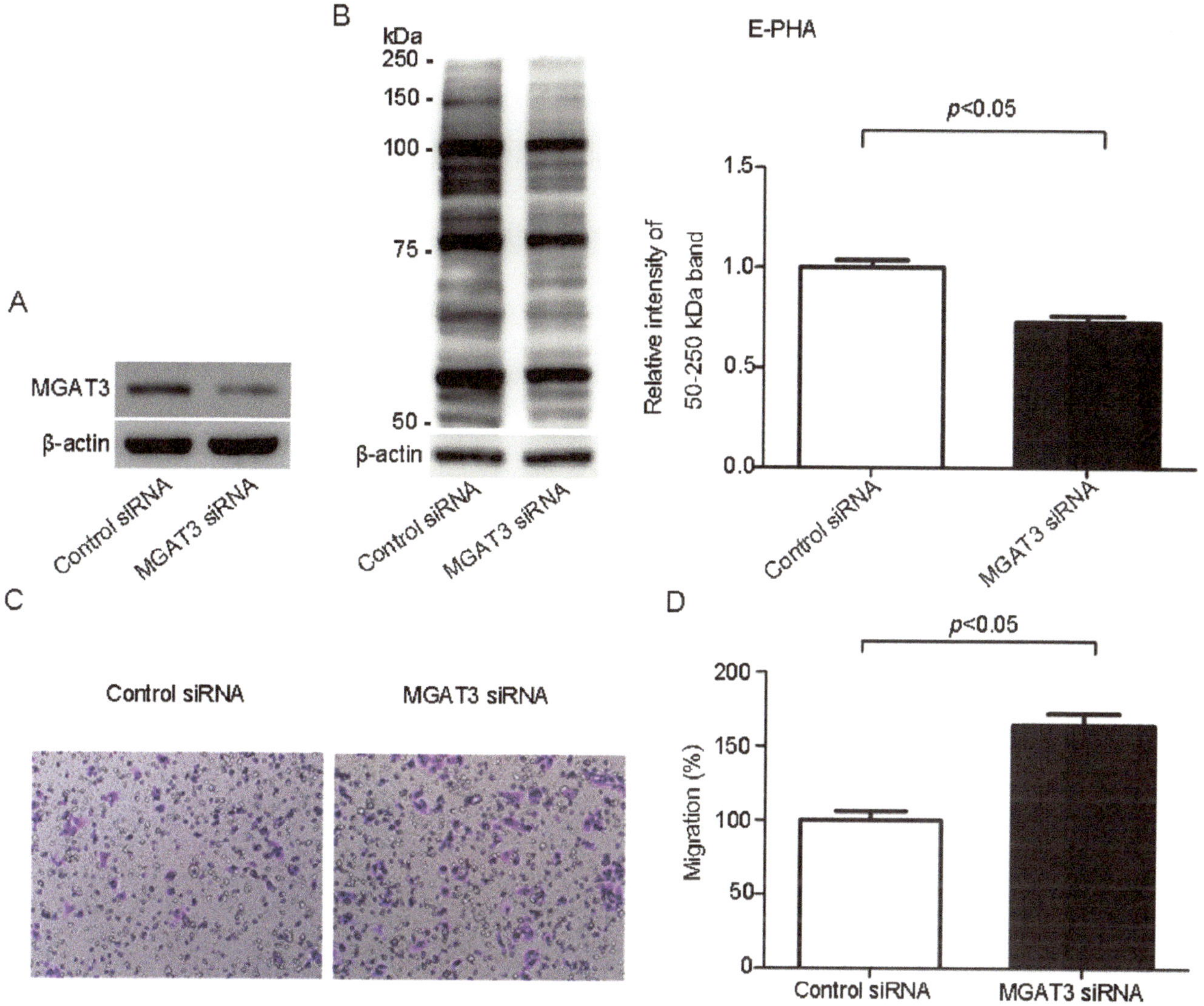

Figure 5. Knockdown of MGAT3 enhances the migration ability of epithelial ovarian cancer cells. SKOV3 cells were transfected with control siRNA and MGAT3-specific siRNA, respectively. At 48 h after transfection, amounts of MGAT3 protein and its catalysate, *N*-glycans containing bisecting GlcNAc were detected by Western blotting (A) and Lectin blotting (B) in SKOV3 cells, respectively. Human beta-actin served as an endogenous control. All the relative expression levels of *N*-glycans containing bisecting GlcNAc were normalized to beta-actin. The left column of (B) represents the densitometry result for glycoproteins 50–250 kDa relative to control set at 1.0. It should be noted that the expression levels of MAGT3 and its catalysate, bisecting glycans were both significantly decreased. Simultaneously, cells were subjected to the migration assay. Images of migrating cells from migration assay (C) and quantitative results are shown (D). Original magnification: 200x.The reported values are expressed as the means ± SEM. Each assay was performed at least three times. A *p*-value of less than 0.05 indicates statistical significance using Student's *t*-test.

proliferation and migration, showed reduced binding with EGF and autophosphorylation after bisecting *N*-glycan modification in human U373 MG glioma cells [74] and neuronal cells [75]. Moreover, it has been reported that EGFR endocytosis enhanced in LEC10B CHO cells carrying bisected *N*-glycans, which led to downregulated EGFR signaling [32,52]. Song *et al.* demonstrated that tumors and tumor-derived cells lacking Mgat3 exhibit enhanced signaling through the Ras pathway and reduced amounts of functionally glycosylated α-dystroglycan. Constitutive overexpression of an MMTV/Mgat3 transgene inhibits early mammary tumor development and tumor cell migration [32]. Interruption of lattice formation via branched *N*-glycans and galectin interaction was responsible for increased EGFR endocytosis [76,77]. In the current study, inhibition of cell migration after MGAT3 transfection was also observed. E-cadherin, EGFR, and integrins, which are all important molecules for cell malignant transformation in ovarian cancer [78,79], may also be modified by bisecting *N*-glycans. Change in their biological function or localization after bisecting *N*-glycan modification may contribute to ovarian cancer metastasis. Besides, molecules such as CA125 and CD44, which have been manifested to take part in adhesion of ovarian cancer cells to peritoneal membrane in a *N*-glycan dependent manner [35,80], may also be the target of bisecting *N*-glycan modification. Further investigations employing lectin affinity chromatography and mass spectrometry are needed to fully uncover bisecting GlcNAc modified glycoproteins that are the effecting molecules in ovarian cancer metastasis.

Conclusion

In this study, quantitative glycomics based on metablic stable isotopic labeling revealed a comprehensive picture of the

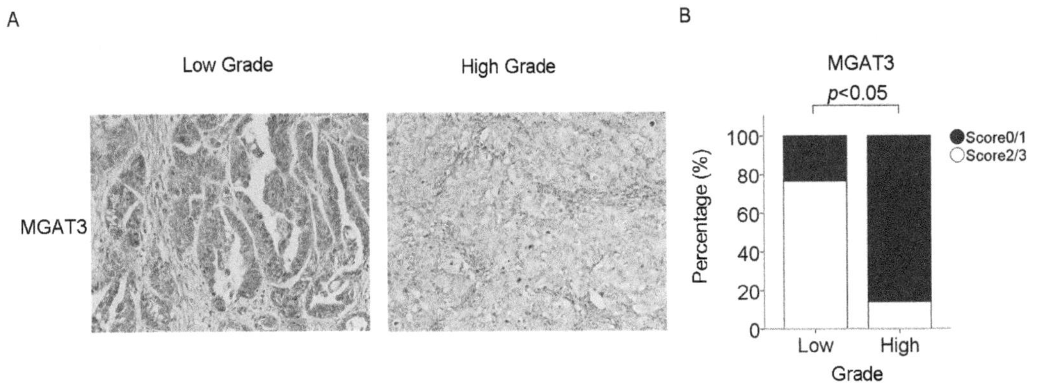

Figure 6. Expression of MGAT3 in human ovarian cancer tissues of varying grade (n = 24). (A) Representative immunohistochemistry photographs of MGAT3 expression in low grade and high grade ovarian cancer tissues. Original magnification: 200x. The immunostaining levels were scored as 0 (negative), 1 (weakly positive), 2 (moderately positive), or 3 (strongly positive). (B) Immunohistochemical staining was quantified using the scoring scale described above, as blindly determined by two pathologists. P value was calculated by Wilcoxon Signed Ranks Test and $p<0.05$ indicates statistical significance.

metastasis-related *N*-glycans alteration in cell secreted proteome of epithelial ovarian cancer for the first time. Specifically, decrease in bisecting GlcNAc structure was found to be related to higher metastatic potential. Future studies will focus on discovery of specific ovarian cancer derived glycoproteins carring these metastasis-associated bisecting *N*-glycans to promote biomarker development for early detection of ovarian cancer.

Supporting Information

Figure S1 Representative tandem MS spectra of *N*-glycans containing bisecting GlcNAc. (A) Tandem MS spectra of m/z 2012.7 $[M+Na]^+$. (B) Tandem MS spectra of m/z 2377.8 $[M+Na]^+$. N-glycans containning a bisecting GlcNAc residue were identified based on the Green circle indicates mannose; yellow circle indicates galactose; blue square indicates *N*-acetylglucosamine; red triangle indicates fucose. Asterisks (*) indicate signals of fragment ions losing water molecules.

Figure S2 Representative MALDI mass spectrum profiles of quantitative analysis of *N*-glycans mixture. (A) Unpermethylated *N*-glycans from a 1:1 mixture of SKOV3-ip (amide-^{14}N-Gln-labeled) and SKOV3 (amide-^{15}N-Gln-labeled) supernatant. (B) Permethylated *N*-glycans from a 1:1 mixture of SKOV3-ip (amide-^{14}N-Gln-labeled) and SKOV3 (amide-^{15}N-Gln-labeled) supernatant. The trend of alteration in all bisecting *N*-glycans are same whatever permethylation or not. While signal intensities were weakened and the profiles of *N*-glycans were more complex after permethylation. For instance, signal intensity of the unpermethylated *N*-glycan at an m/z value of 2012.7 was stronger than that of permethylated *N*-glycans at m/z values 2489.4, 2850.4, 3211.6 containing 0,1,2 sialic acids respectively. Green circle indicates mannose; yellow circle indicates galactose; blue square indicates *N*-acetylglucosamine; red triangle indicates fucose.

Figure S3 Expression level of β1,6 GlcNAc branching *N*-glycans after MGAT3 overexpression in SKOV3-ip cell line. SKOV3-ip cells were transfected with pcDNA3.1 empty or MGAT3/pcDNA3.1 vectors. At 48 h after transfection, amounts of MGAT3 protein and β1,6 GlcNAc branching *N*-glycans were detected by Western blotting (A) and Lectin blotting (B) in SKOV3-ip cells, respectively. Human beta-actin served as an endogenous control. All the relative expression levels ofβ1,6 GlcNAc branching *N*-glycans were normalized to beta-actin. The left column of (B) represents the densitometry result for glycoproteins 50–250 kDa relative to control set at 1.0. Each assay was performed at least three times. A *p*-value of less than 0.05 indicates statistical significance using Student's t-test.

Figure S4 Expression level of β1,6 GlcNAc branching *N*-glycans after MGAT3 knockdown in SKOV3 cell line. SKOV3 cells were transfected with control siRNA and MGAT3-specific siRNA, respectively. At 48 h after transfection, amounts of MGAT3 protein andβ1,6 GlcNAc branching *N*-glycans were detected by Western blotting (A) and Lectin blotting (B) in SKOV3 cells, respectively. Human beta-actin served as an endogenous control. All the relative expression levels of β1,6 GlcNAc branching *N*-glycans were normalized to beta-actin. The left column of (B) represents the densitometry result for glycoproteins 50–250 kDa relative to control set at 1.0. Each assay was performed at least three times. A *p*-value of less than 0.05 indicates statistical significance using Student's *t*-test.

Figure S5 Differential expression of MGAT5 in SKOV3-ip and SKOV3 cell lines. (A) The mRNA expression levels of MGAT5 in SKOV3-ip and SKOV3 cell lines. The mRNA levels of MGAT3 were normalized with GAPDH levels. Mean fold changes were calculated with the $2^{-\Delta\Delta Ct}$ method. (B) The protein expression levels of MGAT5 in SKOV3-ip and SKOV3 cell lines. Cell lysates were isolated by 10% SDS-PAGE for western blotting using antibody against MGAT5. Human beta-actin served as an endogenous control. Data are expressed as the means ± SEM. Each assay was performed at least three times. A *p*-value of less than 0.05 indicates statistical significance using Student's *t*-test.

Figure S6 Overexpression of MGAT5 enhances the migration ability of epithelial ovarian cancer cells. SKOV3 cells were transfected with pcDNA3.1 empty or MGAT5/pcDNA3.1 vectors. At 48 h after transfection, amounts of MGAT5 protein and its catalysate, β1,6 GlcNAc branching *N*-glycans were detected by Western blotting (A) and Lectin blotting (B) in SKOV3 cells, respectively. Human beta-actin served as an endogenous control. All the relative expression levels ofβ1,6 GlcNAc branching *N*-glycans were normalized to beta-actin. The left column of (B) represents the densitometry result for glycoproteins 50–250 kDa relative to control set at 1.0. It should be noted that the expression levels of MAGT5 and its catalysate, β1,6 GlcNAc branching *N*-glycans were both significantly increased. Simultaneously, cells were subjected to the migration assay. Images of migrating cells from migration assay (C) and quantitative results are shown (D). Original magnification: 200x. The reported values are expressed as the means ± SEM. Each assay was performed at least three times. A *p*-value of less than 0.05 indicates statistical significance using Student's *t*-test.

Table S1 Clinical patient information for immunohistochemistry analysis.

Author Contributions

Conceived and designed the experiments: XZ YW CX SR. Performed the experiments: XZ YW. Analyzed the data: XZ YW SR CX JG. Contributed reagents/materials/analysis tools: YQ XW ZZ XL RZ LZ YR JX HL. Wrote the paper: XZ SR.

References

1. Ozols RF, Bookman MA, Connolly DC, Daly MB, Godwin AK, et al. (2004) Focus on epithelial ovarian cancer. Cancer Cell 5: 19–24.
2. Bowtell DD (2010) The genesis and evolution of high-grade serous ovarian cancer. Nat Rev Cancer 10: 803–808.
3. Siegel R, Naishadham D, Jemal A (2013) Cancer statistics, 2013. CA Cancer J Clin 63: 11–30.
4. He Y, Wu X, Liu X, Yan G, Xu C (2010) LC-MS/MS analysis of ovarian cancer metastasis-related proteins using a nude mouse model: 14-3-3 zeta as a candidate biomarker. J Proteome Res 9: 6180–6190.
5. Woodward ER, Sleightholme HV, Considine AM, Williamson S, McHugo JM, et al. (2007) Annual surveillance by CA125 and transvaginal ultrasound for ovarian cancer in both high-risk and population risk women is ineffective. BJOG 114: 1500–1509.
6. Ma S, Shen K, Lang J (2003) A risk of malignancy index in preoperative diagnosis of ovarian cancer. Chin Med J (Engl) 116: 396–399.
7. Torres JC, Derchain SF, Faundes A, Gontijo RC, Martinez EZ, et al. (2002) Risk-of-malignancy index in preoperative evaluation of clinically restricted ovarian cancer. Sao Paulo Med J 120: 72–76.
8. Doig T, Monaghan H (2006) Sampling the omentum in ovarian neoplasia: when one block is enough. Int J Gynecol Cancer 16: 36–40.
9. Kenny HA, Kaur S, Coussens LM, Lengyel E (2008) The initial steps of ovarian cancer cell metastasis are mediated by MMP-2 cleavage of vitronectin and fibronectin. J Clin Invest 118: 1367–1379.
10. Tetsche MS, Dethlefsen C, Pedersen L, Sorensen HT, Norgaard M (2008) The impact of comorbidity and stage on ovarian cancer mortality: a nationwide Danish cohort study. BMC Cancer 8: 31.
11. Aletti GD, Gallenberg MM, Cliby WA, Jatoi A, Hartmann LC (2007) Current management strategies for ovarian cancer. Mayo Clin Proc 82: 751–770.
12. Fuster MM, Esko JD (2005) The sweet and sour of cancer: glycans as novel therapeutic targets. Nat Rev Cancer 5: 526–542.
13. Hart GW, Copeland RJ (2010) Glycomics hits the big time. Cell 143: 672–676.
14. Hakomori SI, Cummings RD (2012) Glycosylation effects on cancer development. Glycoconj J 29: 565–566.
15. Ohtsubo K, Marth JD (2006) Glycosylation in cellular mechanisms of health and disease. Cell 126: 855–867.
16. Granovsky M, Fata J, Pawling J, Muller WJ, Khokha R, et al. (2000) Suppression of tumor growth and metastasis in Mgat5-deficient mice. Nat Med 6: 306–312.
17. Pochec E, Litynska A, Amoresano A, Casbarra A (2003) Glycosylation profile of integrin alpha 3 beta 1 changes with melanoma progression. Biochim Biophys Acta 1643: 113–123.
18. Guo HB, Lee I, Kamar M, Pierce M (2003) N-acetylglucosaminyltransferase V expression levels regulate cadherin-associated homotypic cell-cell adhesion and intracellular signaling pathways. J Biol Chem 278: 52412–52424.
19. Pinho SS, Reis CA, Paredes J, Magalhaes AM, Ferreira AC, et al. (2009) The role of N-acetylglucosaminyltransferase III and V in the post-transcriptional modifications of E-cadherin. Hum Mol Genet 18: 2599–2608.
20. Handerson T, Camp R, Harigopal M, Rimm D, Pawelek J (2005) Beta1,6-branched oligosaccharides are increased in lymph node metastases and predict poor outcome in breast carcinoma. Clin Cancer Res 11: 2969–2973.
21. Dall'Olio F, Chiricolo M (2001) Sialyltransferases in cancer. Glycoconj J 18: 841–850.
22. Varki NM, Varki A (2007) Diversity in cell surface sialic acid presentations: implications for biology and disease. Lab Invest 87: 851–857.
23. Schultz MJ, Swindall AF, Bellis SL (2012) Regulation of the metastatic cell phenotype by sialylated glycans. Cancer Metastasis Rev 31: 501–518.
24. Lin S, Kemmner W, Grigull S, Schlag PM (2002) Cell surface alpha 2,6 sialylation affects adhesion of breast carcinoma cells. Exp Cell Res 276: 101–110.
25. Seales EC, Jurado GA, Brunson BA, Wakefield JK, Frost AR, et al. (2005) Hypersialylation of beta1 integrins, observed in colon adenocarcinoma, may contribute to cancer progression by up-regulating cell motility. Cancer Res 65: 4645–4652.
26. Christie DR, Shaikh FM, Lucas JAt, Lucas JA 3rd, Bellis SL (2008) ST6Gal-I expression in ovarian cancer cells promotes an invasive phenotype by altering integrin glycosylation and function. J Ovarian Res 1: 3.
27. Zhu Y, Srivatana U, Ullah A, Gagneja H, Berenson CS, et al. (2001) Suppression of a sialyltransferase by antisense DNA reduces invasiveness of human colon cancer cells in vitro. Biochim Biophys Acta 1536: 148–160.
28. Takahashi M, Kuroki Y, Ohtsubo K, Taniguchi N (2009) Core fucose and bisecting GlcNAc, the direct modifiers of the N-glycan core: their functions and target proteins. Carbohydr Res 344: 1387–1390.
29. Gu J, Sato Y, Kariya Y, Isaji T, Taniguchi N, et al. (2009) A mutual regulation between cell-cell adhesion and N-glycosylation: implication of the bisecting GlcNAc for biological functions. J Proteome Res 8: 431–435.
30. Zhao Y, Nakagawa T, Itoh S, Inamori K, Isaji T, et al. (2006) N-acetylglucosaminyltransferase III antagonizes the effect of N-acetylglucosaminyltransferase V on alpha3beta1 integrin-mediated cell migration. J Biol Chem 281: 32122–32130.
31. Isaji T, Gu J, Nishiuchi R, Zhao Y, Takahashi M, et al. (2004) Introduction of bisecting GlcNAc into integrin alpha5beta1 reduces ligand binding and down-regulates cell adhesion and cell migration. J Biol Chem 279: 19747–19754.
32. Song Y, Aglipay JA, Bernstein JD, Goswami S, Stanley P (2010) The bisecting GlcNAc on N-glycans inhibits growth factor signaling and retards mammary tumor progression. Cancer Res 70: 3361–3371.
33. Meany DL, Chan DW (2011) Aberrant glycosylation associated with enzymes as cancer biomarkers. Clin Proteomics 8: 7.
34. Abbott KL (2010) Glycomic analysis of ovarian cancer: past, present, and future. Cancer Biomark 8: 273–280.
35. Gubbels JA, Belisle J, Onda M, Rancourt C, Migneault M, et al. (2006) Mesothelin-MUC16 binding is a high affinity, N-glycan dependent interaction that facilitates peritoneal metastasis of ovarian tumors. Mol Cancer 5: 50.
36. Casey RC, Oegema TR Jr, Skubitz KM, Pambuccian SE, Grindle SM, et al. (2003) Cell membrane glycosylation mediates the adhesion, migration, and invasion of ovarian carcinoma cells. Clin Exp Metastasis 20: 143–152.
37. Yue T, Goldstein IJ, Hollingsworth MA, Kaul K, Brand RE, et al. (2009) The prevalence and nature of glycan alterations on specific proteins in pancreatic cancer patients revealed using antibody-lectin sandwich arrays. Mol Cell Proteomics 8: 1697–1707.
38. Wada Y, Azadi P, Costello CE, Dell A, Dwek RA, et al. (2007) Comparison of the methods for profiling glycoprotein glycans–HUPO Human Disease Glycomics/Proteome Initiative multi-institutional study. Glycobiology 17: 411–422.
39. Orlando R (2013) Quantitative analysis of glycoprotein glycans. Methods Mol Biol 951: 197–215.
40. Mechref Y, Hu Y, Desantos-Garcia JL, Hussein A, Tang H (2013) Quantitative glycomics strategies. Mol Cell Proteomics 12: 874–884.
41. Orlando R, Lim JM, Atwood JA 3rd, Angel PM, Fang M, et al. (2009) IDAWG: Metabolic incorporation of stable isotope labels for quantitative glycomics of cultured cells. J Proteome Res 8: 3816–3823.
42. Fang M, Lim JM, Wells L (2010) Quantitative Glycomics of Cultured Cells Using Isotopic Detection of Aminosugars with Glutamine (IDAWG). Curr Protoc Chem Biol 2: 55–69.
43. Zhang W, Wang H, Tang H, Yang P (2011) Endoglycosidase-mediated incorporation of 18O into glycans for relative glycan quantitation. Anal Chem 83: 4975–4981.
44. Qian Y, Zhang X, Zhou L, Yun X, Xie J, et al. (2012) Site-specific N-glycosylation identification of recombinant human lectin-like oxidized low density lipoprotein receptor-1 (LOX-1). Glycoconj J 29: 399–409.
45. Atwood JA 3rd, Cheng L, Alvarez-Manilla G, Warren NL, York WS, et al. (2008) Quantitation by isobaric labeling: applications to glycomics. J Proteome Res 7: 367–374.
46. Machado E, Kandzia S, Carilho R, Altevogt P, Conradt HS, et al. (2011) N-Glycosylation of total cellular glycoproteins from the human ovarian carcinoma SKOV3 cell line and of recombinantly expressed human erythropoietin. Glycobiology 21: 376–386.

47. Alley WR Jr, Vasseur JA, Goetz JA, Svoboda M, Mann BF, et al. (2012) N-linked glycan structures and their expressions change in the blood sera of ovarian cancer patients. J Proteome Res 11: 2282–2300.
48. Ceroni A, Maass K, Geyer H, Geyer R, Dell A, et al. (2008) GlycoWorkbench: a tool for the computer-assisted annotation of mass spectra of glycans. J Proteome Res 7: 1650–1659.
49. Kameyama A, Kikuchi N, Nakaya S, Ito H, Sato T, et al. (2005) A strategy for identification of oligosaccharide structures using observational multistage mass spectral library. Anal Chem 77: 4719–4725.
50. Wu W, Sun Z, Wu J, Peng X, Gan H, et al. (2012) Trihydrophobin 1 phosphorylation by c-Src regulates MAPK/ERK signaling and cell migration. PLoS One 7: e29920.
51. Liu H, Xu J, Zhou L, Yun X, Chen L, et al. (2011) Hepatitis B virus large surface antigen promotes liver carcinogenesis by activating the Src/PI3K/Akt pathway. Cancer Res 71: 7547–7557.
52. Miwa HE, Song Y, Alvarez R, Cummings RD, Stanley P (2012) The bisecting GlcNAc in cell growth control and tumor progression. Glycoconj J 29: 609–618.
53. Yu D, Wolf JK, Scanlon M, Price JE, Hung MC (1993) Enhanced c-erbB-2/neu expression in human ovarian cancer cells correlates with more severe malignancy that can be suppressed by E1A. Cancer Res 53: 891–898.
54. Clark HF, Gurney AL, Abaya E, Baker K, Baldwin D, et al. (2003) The secreted protein discovery initiative (SPDI), a large-scale effort to identify novel human secreted and transmembrane proteins: a bioinformatics assessment. Genome Res 13: 2265–2270.
55. Boersema PJ, Geiger T, Wisniewski JR, Mann M (2013) Quantification of the N-glycosylated secretome by super-SILAC during breast cancer progression and in human blood samples. Mol Cell Proteomics 12: 158–171.
56. Zhang Q, Faca V, Hanash S (2011) Mining the plasma proteome for disease applications across seven logs of protein abundance. J Proteome Res 10: 46–50.
57. Wu CC, Hsu CW, Chen CD, Yu CJ, Chang KP, et al. (2010) Candidate serological biomarkers for cancer identified from the secretomes of 23 cancer cell lines and the human protein atlas. Mol Cell Proteomics 9: 1100–1117.
58. Dowling P, Clynes M (2011) Conditioned media from cell lines: a complementary model to clinical specimens for the discovery of disease-specific biomarkers. Proteomics 11: 794–804.
59. Karagiannis GS, Pavlou MP, Diamandis EP (2010) Cancer secretomics reveal pathophysiological pathways in cancer molecular oncology. Mol Oncol 4: 496–510.
60. Makridakis M, Vlahou A (2010) Secretome proteomics for discovery of cancer biomarkers. J Proteomics 73: 2291–2305.
61. Pavlou MP, Diamandis EP (2010) The cancer cell secretome: a good source for discovering biomarkers? J Proteomics 73: 1896–1906.
62. Hu Y, Desantos-Garcia JL, Mechref Y (2013) Comparative glycomic profiling of isotopically permethylated N-glycans by liquid chromatography/electrospray ionization mass spectrometry. Rapid Commun Mass Spectrom 27: 865–877.
63. Dennis JW, Granovsky M, Warren CE (1999) Protein glycosylation in development and disease. Bioessays 21: 412–421.
64. Guo R, Cheng L, Zhao Y, Zhang J, Liu C, et al. (2013) Glycogenes mediate the invasive properties and chemosensitivity of human hepatocarcinoma cells. Int J Biochem Cell Biol 45: 347–358.
65. Yoshimura M, Nishikawa A, Ihara Y, Taniguchi S, Taniguchi N (1995) Suppression of lung metastasis of B16 mouse melanoma by N-acetylglucosaminyltransferase III gene transfection. Proc Natl Acad Sci U S A 92: 8754–8758.
66. Kang X, Wang N, Pei C, Sun L, Sun R, et al. (2012) Glycan-related gene expression signatures in human metastatic hepatocellular carcinoma cells. Exp Ther Med 3: 415–422.
67. Sato Y, Takahashi M, Shibukawa Y, Jain SK, Hamaoka R, et al. (2001) Overexpression of N-acetylglucosaminyltransferase III enhances the epidermal growth factor-induced phosphorylation of ERK in HeLaS3 cells by up-regulation of the internalization rate of the receptors. J Biol Chem 276: 11956–11962.
68. Yoshimura M, Ihara Y, Ohnishi A, Ijuhin N, Nishiura T, et al. (1996) Bisecting N-acetylglucosamine on K562 cells suppresses natural killer cytotoxicity and promotes spleen colonization. Cancer Res 56: 412–418.
69. Abbott KL, Lim JM, Wells L, Benigno BB, McDonald JF, et al. (2010) Identification of candidate biomarkers with cancer-specific glycosylation in the tissue and serum of endometrioid ovarian cancer patients by glycoproteomic analysis. Proteomics 10: 470–481.
70. Wiegand KC, Shah SP, Al-Agha OM, Zhao Y, Tse K, et al. (2010) ARID1A mutations in endometriosis-associated ovarian carcinomas. N Engl J Med 363: 1532–1543.
71. Gu J, Nishikawa A, Tsuruoka N, Ohno M, Yamaguchi N, et al. (1993) Purification and characterization of UDP-N-acetylglucosamine: alpha-6-D-mannoside beta 1–6N-acetylglucosaminyltransferase (N-acetylglucosaminyl-transferase V) from a human lung cancer cell line. J Biochem 113: 614–619.
72. Schachter H (1986) Biosynthetic controls that determine the branching and microheterogeneity of protein-bound oligosaccharides. Adv Exp Med Biol 205: 53–85.
73. Yoshimura M, Ihara Y, Matsuzawa Y, Taniguchi N (1996) Aberrant glycosylation of E-cadherin enhances cell-cell binding to suppress metastasis. J Biol Chem 271: 13811–13815.
74. Rebbaa A, Yamamoto H, Saito T, Meuillet E, Kim P, et al. (1997) Gene transfection-mediated overexpression of beta1,4-N-acetylglucosamine bisecting oligosaccharides in glioma cell line U373 MG inhibits epidermal growth factor receptor function. J Biol Chem 272: 9275–9279.
75. Gu J, Zhao Y, Isaji T, Shibukawa Y, Ihara H, et al. (2004) Beta1,4-N-Acetylglucosaminyltransferase III down-regulates neurite outgrowth induced by costimulation of epidermal growth factor and integrins through the Ras/ERK signaling pathway in PC12 cells. Glycobiology 14: 177–186.
76. North SJ, Huang HH, Sundaram S, Jang-Lee J, Etienne AT, et al. (2010) Glycomics profiling of Chinese hamster ovary cell glycosylation mutants reveals N-glycans of a novel size and complexity. J Biol Chem 285: 5759–5775.
77. Dennis JW, Lau KS, Demetriou M, Nabi IR (2009) Adaptive regulation at the cell surface by N-glycosylation. Traffic 10: 1569–1578.
78. Wilken JA, Badri T, Cross S, Raji R, Santin AD, et al. (2012) EGFR/HER-targeted therapeutics in ovarian cancer. Future Med Chem 4: 447–469.
79. Sawada K, Mitra AK, Radjabi AR, Bhaskar V, Kistner EO, et al. (2008) Loss of E-cadherin promotes ovarian cancer metastasis via alpha 5-integrin, which is a therapeutic target. Cancer Res 68: 2329–2339.
80. Kannagi R, Goto Y, Fukui F (2004) In search of the carbohydrate structures on CD44 critical for hyaluronic acid binding - Roles of sialylation and sulfation. Trends in Glycoscience and Glycotechnology 16: 211–23.

YAP Promotes Ovarian Cancer Cell Tumorigenesis and Is Indicative of a Poor Prognosis for Ovarian Cancer Patients

Yan Xia[1], Ting Chang[2], Yingmei Wang[3], Yixiong Liu[3], Wenhui Li[4], Ming Li[5], Heng-Yu Fan[1]*

1 Life Sciences Institute and Innovation Center for Cell Biology, Zhejiang University, Hangzhou, China, 2 Department of Neurology, Tangdu Hospital, the Fourth Military Medical University, Xi'an, China, 3 Department of Pathology, Xijing Hospital, the Fourth Military Medical University, Xi'an, China, 4 Department of Obstetrics and Gynecology, Xijing Hospital, the Fourth Military Medical University, Xi'an, China, 5 The Affiliated Guangren Hospital, Xi'an Jiaotong University, Xi'an, China

Abstract

YAP is a key component of the Hippo signaling pathway and plays a critical role in the development and progression of multiple cancer types, including ovarian cancer. However, the effects of YAP on ovarian cancer development *in vivo* and its downstream effectors remain uncertain. In this study we found that strong YAP expression was associated with poor ovarian cancer patient survival. Specifically, we showed for the first time that high YAP expression levels were positively correlated with TEAD4 gene expression, and their co-expression was a prognostic marker for poor ovarian cancer survival. Hyperactivation of YAP by mutating its five inhibitory phosphorylation sites (YAP-5SA) increased ovarian cancer cell proliferation, resistance to chemotherapeutic drugs, cell migration, and anchorage-independent growth. In contrast, expression of a dominant negative YAP mutant reversed these phenotypes in ovarian cancer cells both *in vitro* and *in vivo*. Our results suggested that YAP caused these effects by promoting an epithelial-to-mesenchymal transition. Thus, YAP promotes ovarian cancer cell growth and tumorigenesis both *in vitro* and *in vivo*. Further, high YAP and TEAD4 expression is a prognostic marker for ovarian cancer progression and a potential target for ovarian cancer treatment.

Editor: Hongmei Wang, Institute of Zoology, Chinese Academy of Sciences, China

Funding: This study was supported by the National Natural Science Foundation of China (81172473), the National Basic Research Program of China (2011CB944504, 2012CB944403), and Basic Scientific Research Funding of Zhejiang University (2011QN81001). The funders had no role in study design, data collection and analysis, decision to publish, or preparation of the manuscript.

Competing Interests: The authors have declared that no competing interests exist.

* E-mail: hyfan@zju.edu.cn

These authors contributed equally to this work.

Introduction

Epithelial ovarian cancers (EOCs) comprise the majority of malignant ovarian tumors in adult women and have the worst prognosis among female cancers based on their 5-year survival rates. These patients often present with non-specific pelvic or abdominal symptoms. Conventional treatments usually include surgery, platinum and Taxol-based chemotherapies, and radiation therapy. Due to the lack of specific symptoms and effective screening methods, patients are often diagnosed when at an advanced stage and their prognosis is even worse than with other cancers.

The Hippo pathway is a recently discovered signal transduction pathway. The core components of the Hippo pathway, including MST1/2, LATS, Sav1, and YAP, are highly conserved from the fruit fly (*Drosophila*) to mammals [1–6]. MST1/2 activation results in the phosphorylation and activation of their direct substrates LATS1/2. Activated LATS1/2, in turn, phosphorylate and inhibit YAP and TAZ transcription co-activator [7,8]. YAP promotes cell proliferation, inhibits cellular apoptosis, and also promotes an epidermal-mesenchymal transition (EMT) [9–12]. YAP is closely associated with tumorigenesis as a critical transcription co-activator in the Hippo pathway.

Several transcription factors, including ErbB4, RUNX2, TEAD family members, and p73, have been found to be YAP downstream target genes [13–16]. Because it lacks a DNA binding domain, YAP binds to the C-terminal region of TEAD in order to regulate downstream genes' transcription and translation. Zhao *et al* identified TEAD family transcription factors as the most potent YAP targets and TEAD family members were important for the growth-promoting function of YAP [14,17–21].

Previous studies showed that YAP was highly expressed in human ovarian cancer tissues and that high YAP activity promoted the proliferation and survival of cultured ovarian cancer cells[9,22]. However, the role of YAP in ovarian cancer development *in vivo* and the association of YAP/TEAD with ovarian cancer patient survival have not been thoroughly investigated.

In this study we show that continuous YAP activation induces increased ovarian cancer cell proliferation, resistance to cisplatin-induced cellular apoptosis, loss of contact inhibition, increased cell migration, and anchorage-independent growth both *in vitro* and *in vivo*. Consistent with these results, we also found that high YAP expression was associated with poor ovarian cancer patient survival. Further, TEAD family members were also expressed in ovarian cancer tissues. Interestingly, YAP expression was positively correlated with TEAD4 expression and their co-expression was closely associated with poor ovarian cancer patient survival. Taken together, these findings indicate that YAP is a key ovarian cancer oncogene and that YAP/TEAD4 co-expression may be a predictor of a poor prognosis for human ovarian cancer.

Materials and Methods

Nude mice xenografts and *In Vivo* treatments

Nude mice were obtained from the Center of Experimental Animals, Zhejiang University.

Mice were treated in accordance with the NIH Guide for the Care and Use of Laboratory Animals, approved by ethics committee of Zhejiang University. Mice were housed in a temperature-controlled room with proper darkness-light cycles, fed with a regular diet, and maintained under the care of the Laboratory Animal Unit, Zhejiang University, China. The ovarian cancer cell-transplanted mice were examinined daily, and were euthanized using CO2 inhalation method before being sacrificed. To examine the effects of YAP activity on tumors *in vivo*, stable cell lines that expressed YAP-5SA or dominant negative YAP were cultured and used to induce tumors by implanting 2×10^6 cells in 100 µl of PBS subcutaneously into the right abdominal flanks of 4–6 week old female nude mice. To determine if YAP has effect on the chemo-resistance, A2780CP YAP-5SA-ΔC cells and control cells (2×10^6 cells per mouse in each group) were separately inoculated (s.c.) into nude mice. After tumors grew to about 5 mm in diameter, 3.5 mg/body weight (kg)/day of CDDP was administered (i.p.) to the nude mice once a week for 4 weeks. Tumor sizes (both longitudinal and transverse widths) were measured with a caliper.

Tissue array and IHC Analysis

Formalin-fixed and paraffin-embedded ovarian cancer tissue array was obtained from US Biomax, Inc. (Rockville, MD). The tissue microarray was immunohistochemically stained for YAP (#4912, Cell Signaling), S127 phosphorylated-YAP (#4911S, Cell Signaling), TEAD1 (5178-1, Epitomics), TEAD2 (LS-C119063, Lifespan Biosciences),TEAD3 (LS-C30406, Lifespan Bioscience-s),and TEAD4 (ab97460, Abcam). In addition, 45 human ovarian cancer specimens for patient follow-up are from the Department of Pathology, Xijing Hospital of Fourth Military Medical University. The ovarian cancer specimen use and the study protocol were approved by the Ethics Committee of Xijing Hospital, and written informed consent was obtained from each patient.

All the final score of each sample (negative or positive) was scored independently by two pathologists and assessed by adding the scores for the intensity and extent of staining. The intensity of staining was scored as 0 (negative), 1 (weak), or 2 (strong). The extent of staining was scored based on the percentage of positive tumor cells: 0 (negative), 1 (1%–30%), 2 (30%–60%), and 3 (61%–100%). Each case was finally considered negative if the final score was 0 (negative) or 1 (weak positive) and positive if the final score was 2 to 3 (+) or 4 to 5 (strong positive).

Cell lines

All the cell lines used in this study were originally purchased from ATCC. All the cell culture media were from Invitrogen. SKOV-3 cells were cultured in McCoy's 5A medium with 10% FBS. A2780 cells were grown in DMEM High Glucose medium supplemented with 10% FBS and a 1% penicillin-streptomycin solution. OVCAR3 cells were cultured in DMEM medium with 0.01 mg/ml of insulin and 15% FBS. OVCAR8 cells were grown in RPMI 1640 medium with 10% FBS. All cell lines were cultured with 10 units/ml of penicillin and 10 ng/ml of streptomycin. Stable cell lines were grown in culture medium and selected using different concentrations of puromycin.

Cell proliferation assay

For each condition described above, cells were cultured in triplicate wells in 96 well plates at 2000 cells/well. Cell growth was determined by measuring the absorbance with a plate reader (Bio-Rad) after culture for 24 hours. Three independent experiments were done for each treatment.

Western Blot analysis

Cell extracts containing 30 µg of protein were resolved by SDS-PAGE and transferred to PVDF membranes (Millipore Corp., Bedford, MA). After probing with primary antibodies, the membranes were incubated with horseradish peroxidase-linked anti-rabbit antibodies (Cell Signaling Technologies, Danvers, MA) and then washed. Bound antibodies were visualized using an Enhanced Chemiluminescence Detection Kit (Amersham). The primary antibodies were: YAP (#4912), S127 phosphorylated-YAP (#4911S), PARP (#9542), cleaved caspase-3 (#9664), β-actin (#AC40), E-cadherin (#3195), Slug (#3195), and Snail (#3895) from Cell Signaling. A TEAD1 (5178-1) antibody was from Epitomics. TEAD2 (LS-C119063) and TEAD3 (LS-C30406) antibodies were from Lifespan Biosciences. A TEAD4 (ab97460) antibody was from Abcam.

Flat colony and soft agar colony forming assays

Cells were plated in triplicate wells in 6-well plates for 14 days for a flat colony formation assay. For a soft agar assay, 2,000 cells were plated in complete medium plus 0.6% agar in triplicate wells in 6-well plates. Medium was replaced every 48 hours and visible colonies were counted by light microscopy after 21 days.

Scratch assay

Cells were plated in 6-well plates and cultured in serum-free medium to block proliferation. After 12 hours, cells were scratched using a 200 µl pipette tip. Then, images of 10 scratches per cell line were acquired at 0 h, 12 h, and 24 h.

Apoptosis assay

Cells were cultured in medium with different concentrations of cisplatin for 48 hours. Then, cells were harvested with an apoptosis detection kit (BD Biosciences, 559763) by flow cytometry and for Western blot analysis.

In vitro and *in vivo* metastatic model and bioluminescent imaging

A 24-well transwell plate (8-µm pore size, Corning, USA) was used to determine the migration and invasive capability of each cell line. For transwell migration assays, 5×10^4 cells were seeded in the top chamber that was lined with a non-coated membrane. The lower chambers were all added into 500 ul culture medium with 20% FBS. The mean values of triplicate assays for each experimental condition were determined.

For *in vivo* metastasis assays, HO8910 PM-YAP ΔC stable cells was infected with a lusiferase reporter plasmid and injected into the caudal veins of 4 week female null mice. After two weeks, the animals were imaged weekly by the animal imaging machine using an intensified charge coupled device (CCD) camera system. For *in vivo* bioluminescence imaging, mice were anesthetized using a 1–2% isofluorane/air mixture and injected with a single (i.p.) dose of

100 mg/kg of Luciferin (Promega, WI) and bioluminescence was detected with an IVIS 100 Imaging System (Xenogen).

Besides the bioluminescence imaging, mice were executed at 60 days after ovarian cancer cell-injection for investigating the post-inoculation organ metastases.

Statistical analysis

For the 45 subjects with complete immunohistochemical and outcome data, disease-specific 5-year survival was estimated using the Kaplan-Meier method and compared between groups using log-rank tests. Correlation analysis was completed by Chi-square test. Student's t test was used to compare the results of each measured variable with control results. P-values of <0.05 were considered significant. All analyses were done using SPSS software (version 11.0).

Results

YAP is significantly upregulated in human ovarian cancer tissues and high YAP expression predicts poor patient prognosis

To investigate if YAP was upregulated in human ovarian cancer, total and phosphorylated YAP (pYAP) were detected by immunohistochemistry (IHC) and slides were evaluated based on cytoplasmic and nuclear YAP staining levels. These IHC sections were categorized as having either negative, low, or high staining. As a control, 10 normal ovarian tissue sections were immunohistochemically stained with YAP. However, YAP expression was not detected in these sections (Figure 1A).

YAP expression and subcellular localization varied for different tumor types (Figure 1A). High nuclear YAP levels were observed for 22.64% of the 106 ovarian tumor samples analyzed, which included 9 metastatic ovarian cancer samples, whereas pYAP was observed in 11.88% of tumor samples. Of 24 samples with strong YAP IHC signals, 13 were also strongly positive for pYAP. Among the four major types of ovarian cancers, YAP was strongly expressed in serous and endometrioid cancinoma samples (86.67%; $N = 15$).

To determine if YAP and pYAP distributions were associated with ovarian cancer patient survival, YAP and pYAP localization and expression levels were evaluated in 45 ovarian cancer pathological sections. These results were used for Kaplan-Meier analysis to estimate disease-specific survival. Both cytoplasmic YAP (cYAP) and pYAP alone were not associated with a poor prognosis for human ovarian cancer. However, when total YAP expression levels were taken into account, these were significantly associated with a poor prognosis (Figure 1B). These results suggested that high YAP expression levels rather than its subcellular distributions were associated with ovarian cancer patient survival.

YAP promotes ovarian cancer cell proliferation and tumorigenesis

In addition to human ovarian cancer samples, we also determined endogenous YAP expression in 11 cultured ovarian cancer cell lines. Western blotting results showed that YAP was highly expressed in most of these cell lines, with the weakest expression in A2780 cells and the highest expression in OVCAR8 cells (Figure 2A). Thus, these two cell lines were used for the following experiments.

To investigate a role for YAP in ovarian cancer cell proliferation and metastasis, we generated A2780 and OVCAR8 stable cell lines that overexpressed constitutively active YAP (YAP with five LATS1/2 phosphorylation site mutations; YAP-5SA) and dominant negative YAP (YAP-5SA with a C-terminal transactivation domain deletion; YAP-5SA-ΔC; Figure 2B-C). Cell growth curves showed that YAP-5SA expressing cells had greater proliferative activity than the controls (Figure 2D, upper panel). In contrast, YAP-5SA-ΔC expressing OVCAR8 cells had a decreased proliferation rate relative to control cells (Figure 2D, lower panel).

Next, we investigated if YAP activity affected cell transformation and migration in ovarian cancer cells using a plate colony formation assay. These results showed that constitutively active YAP-5SA promoted clone formation, but that dominant negative YAP-5SA-ΔC suppressed clone formation (Figure 2E). In addition, we used a soft agar assay to determine anchorage-independent growth, another indicator of tumourigenicity. As shown in Figure 2F, YAP activity was positively correlated with ovarian cancer cells' colony formation capability in soft agar.

YAP promotes ovarian cancer cells proliferation and tumorigenesis *in vivo*

Previous studies did not investigate if YAP could enhance tumorigenesis *in vivo*. Thus, we subcutaneously injected YAP-5SA and YAP-5SA-ΔC expressing cells, as well as their respective control cells, into 4-week-old nude mice. After 3 weeks, the tumors derived from YAP-5SA stable cells were significantly larger than those of controls (Figure 2G). These results were consistent with our *in vitro* assays.

YAP enhances ovarian cancer cell lines' resistance to Cisplatin and Taxol

Cisplatin and Taxol are the primary anti-cancer drugs used for ovarian cancer therapy. Thus, we sought to determine if YAP activity affected ovarian cancer cells' sensitivities to Cisplatin and Taxol. As shown in Figure 3A, YAP-5SA expressing cells were more resistant to both of these drugs than were control cells at different doses. In contrast, YAP-5SA-ΔC expressing cells were more susceptible to both drugs than were control cells. The apoptotic cell markers cleaved PARP and cleaved caspase 3 were detected in A2780 control cells after Cisplatin treatment in a dose-dependent manner (0–100 μM). However, the increased expressions of these apoptosis markers were less significant in similarly treated YAP-5SA expressing cells (Figure 3B).

Flow cytometry results showed that a previously reported cisplatin-resistant ovarian cancer cell line (A2780CP) was indeed resistant to cisplatin treatment at low doses (10–40 μM). However, YAP-5SA-ΔC expression in these cells caused an increase in cellular apoptosis after cisplatin treatment at all of the doses tested (Figure 3C–D). Moreover, YAP-5SA-ΔC expressing A2780CP cells showed remarkably increased expression of cleaved PARP and caspase 3 than did control cells after cisplatin treatment (Figure 3E).

To determine whether YAP conferred drug resistance to ovarian cancer cells *in vivo*, we subcutaneously injected nude mice with A2780CP cells that stably expressed YAP-5SA-ΔC and with control cells. At 1 week after cell injections, mice were treated with cisplatin by caudal vain injection every three days. Tumor sizes were measured at 5 weeks after ovarian cancer cell injections. Compared with controls, tumors that were derived from YAP-5SA-ΔC expressing cells were smaller in size compared to those derived from control cells (Figure 3F-G). Cell proliferation marker Ki67 expression was weaker in YAP-5SA-ΔC expressing cells than in control cells (Figure 3H).

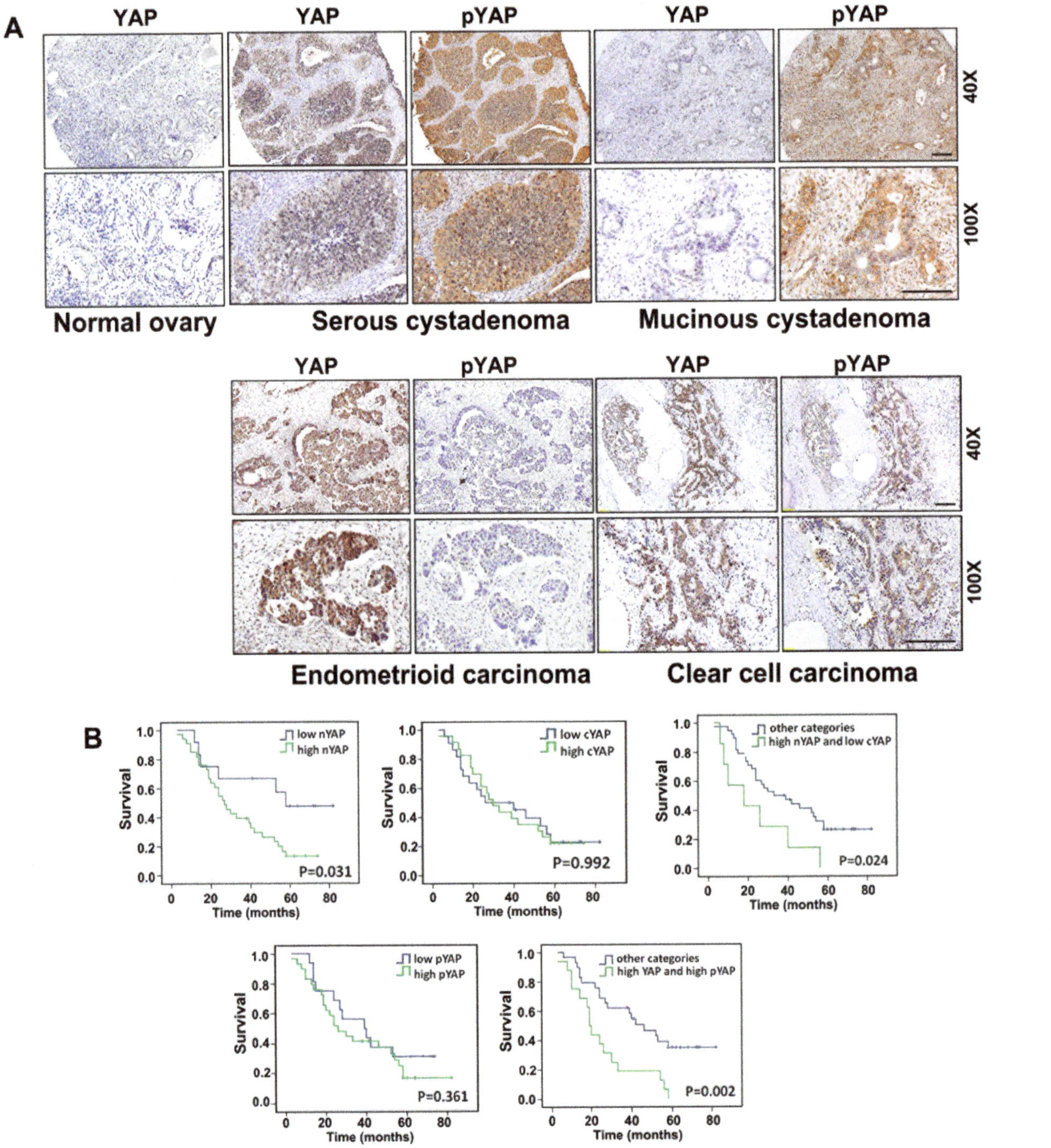

Figure 1. YAP is significantly upregulated in human ovarian cancer tissues and is associated with patient prognosis. A: Immunohistochemistry results for YAP and pYAP expression in normal human ovary tissues and four subtypes of ovarian cancer tissue. Sections were counterstained with hematoxylin. Magnifications at 40× and 100× are shown. Scale bar = 100 μM for all panels. **B**: Kaplan-Meier analysis for associations between YAP expression, localization, and phosphorylation and ovarian cancer patient survival. P-values are from log-rank tests.

YAP enhances the migration and anchorage-independent growth of ovarian cancer cells

We next investigated the effects of YAP activity on ovarian cancer cell migration. In both scratch assays (Figure 4A) and transwell assays (Figure 4B), YAP-5SA expressing cells migrated faster, whereas YAP-5SA-ΔC expressing cells migrated slower than the control cells.

In addition, we did *in vivo* experiments to test if YAP activity was required for ovarian cancer metastasis. We established YAP-5SA-ΔC- and luciferase-expressing stable cell lines using HO8910-PM cells, a human ovarian cancer cell line with a high metastatic capacity, and injected these cells into nude mice through their caudal veins (5×10^6 cells/mouse). At two weeks after injection, mice were imaged for metastasis using an animal imaging system.

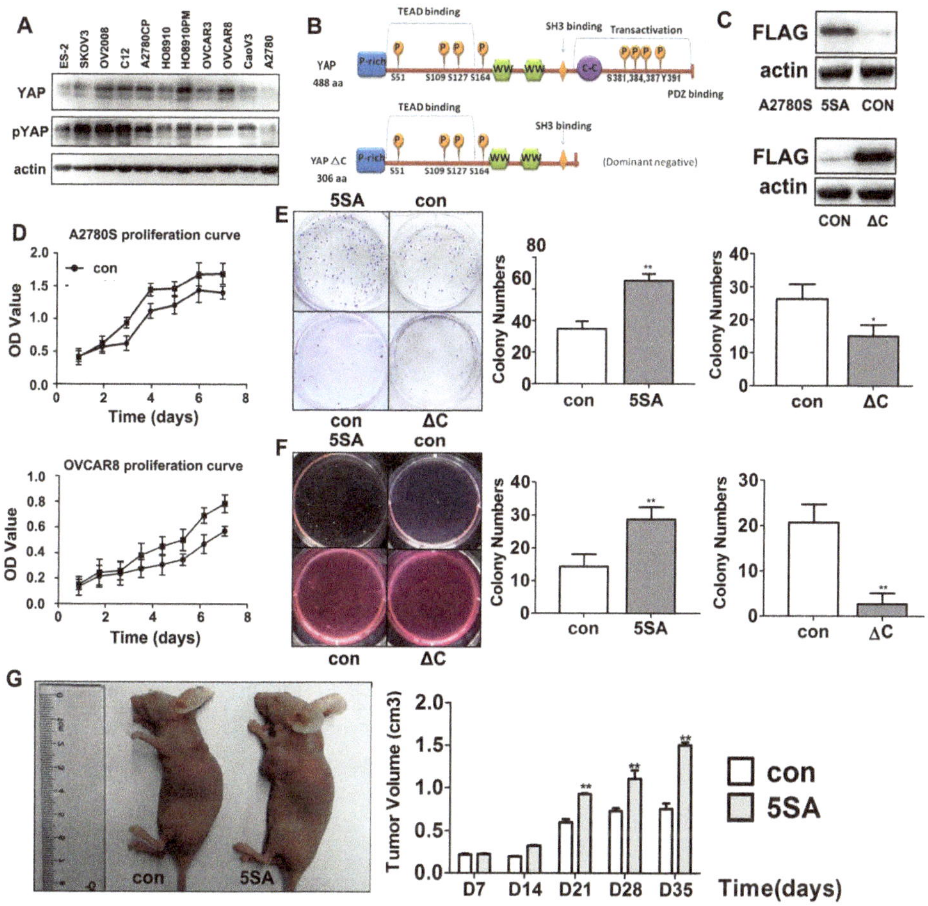

Figure 2. YAP promotes human ovarian cancer cell proliferation and tumorigenesis. A: Western blotting results for endogenous YAP expression in 11 ovarian cancer cell lines. **B**: Diagram of the main functional structural domains and phosphorylation sites in human YAP (full length and C-terminal deleted, YAP-ΔC, forms). **C**: Western blotting results for the expression of FLAG-tagged YAP-5SA and YAP-5SA-ΔC in established stable cell lines. **D**: Growth curves for cells that stably expressed YAP-5SA (upper panel) and YAP-5SA-ΔC (lower panel) and their control cells during a 7-day culture period. **E**: Images and quantitative results for flat plate colony formation assays. Cells that expressed YAP-5SA or YAP-5SA-ΔC and their control cells were cultured in 6-well plates for 2 weeks. **F**: Images and quantitative results for colonies grown in soft agar. Cells that expressed YAP-5SA or YAP-5SA-ΔC and their control cells were seeded in soft agar for 3 weeks. **G**: Images and quantitative results for xenografts grown in nude mice. Mice were subcutaneously injected with YAP-5SA expressing and control cells. Each point is the mean of 3 experiments. Error bars represent s.d. 's; n = 5. Statistically significant differences as compared with a control as determined by Student's t-test are denoted by *($P<0.05$) or **($P<0.01$).

As shown in Figure 4C–D, those xenografts derived from YAP-5SA-ΔC-expressing cells were smaller than those derived from control cells. IHC results showed that the xenografts were positive for CA125 and YAP, which confirmed their origins from the injected ovarian cancer cells. Significantly, post-inoculation metastases were detected in the livers of all 10 mice that were injected with control HO8910 cells, but only in 2 of 10 mice injected with YAP-5SA-ΔC-expressing cells (Figure 4E). In addition, YAP-5SA-ΔC-expressing cells formed far fewer metastatic nodules (YAP-positive) than control cells in the livers of injected mice (Figure 4F–G). These results suggested that decreased YAP activity retarded ovarian cancer cells metastasis *in vivo*.

An epithelial-to-mesenchymal transition (EMT) is thought to be an important process during the acquisition of those properties required for tumor metastasis. In both cultured ovarian cancer cells and in those isolated from *in vivo*, YAP-5SA promoted the expression of the EMT marker Snail and inhibited the expression of the epithelial marker E-cadherin. However, YAP-5SA-ΔC had the opposite effects (Figure 4H).

High nuclear YAP and TAED4 levels are associated with a poor human ovarian cancer prognosis

YAP does not have a DNA binding domain. It functions as a transcription co-activator by binding with TEAD family transcription factors (TEAD1-4). However, it has not been investigated if TEADs play any role in ovarian cancer prognosis. Thus, we investigated TEAD1-4 expression in human ovarian cancer samples. The expressions of the 4 subtypes of TEAD family proteins were investigated individually in an ovarian cancer tissue microarray by IHC (Figure 5A). Correlation analysis results showed that YAP and pYAP were positively correlated with TEAD1-4 expression, and were most closely correlated with TEAD4 expression (Figure 5B).An association analysis using 45 ovarian cancer patient samples was done in which we ranked Kaplan-Meier survival estimates. These results showed that YAP expression was positively correlated with TEAD4 expression (Figure 5C, $P = 0.0284$).

We further investigated if TEAD4 alone might be associated with ovarian cancer patient survival. Kaplan-Meier estimates and comparisons of disease-specific survival showed that high TEAD4

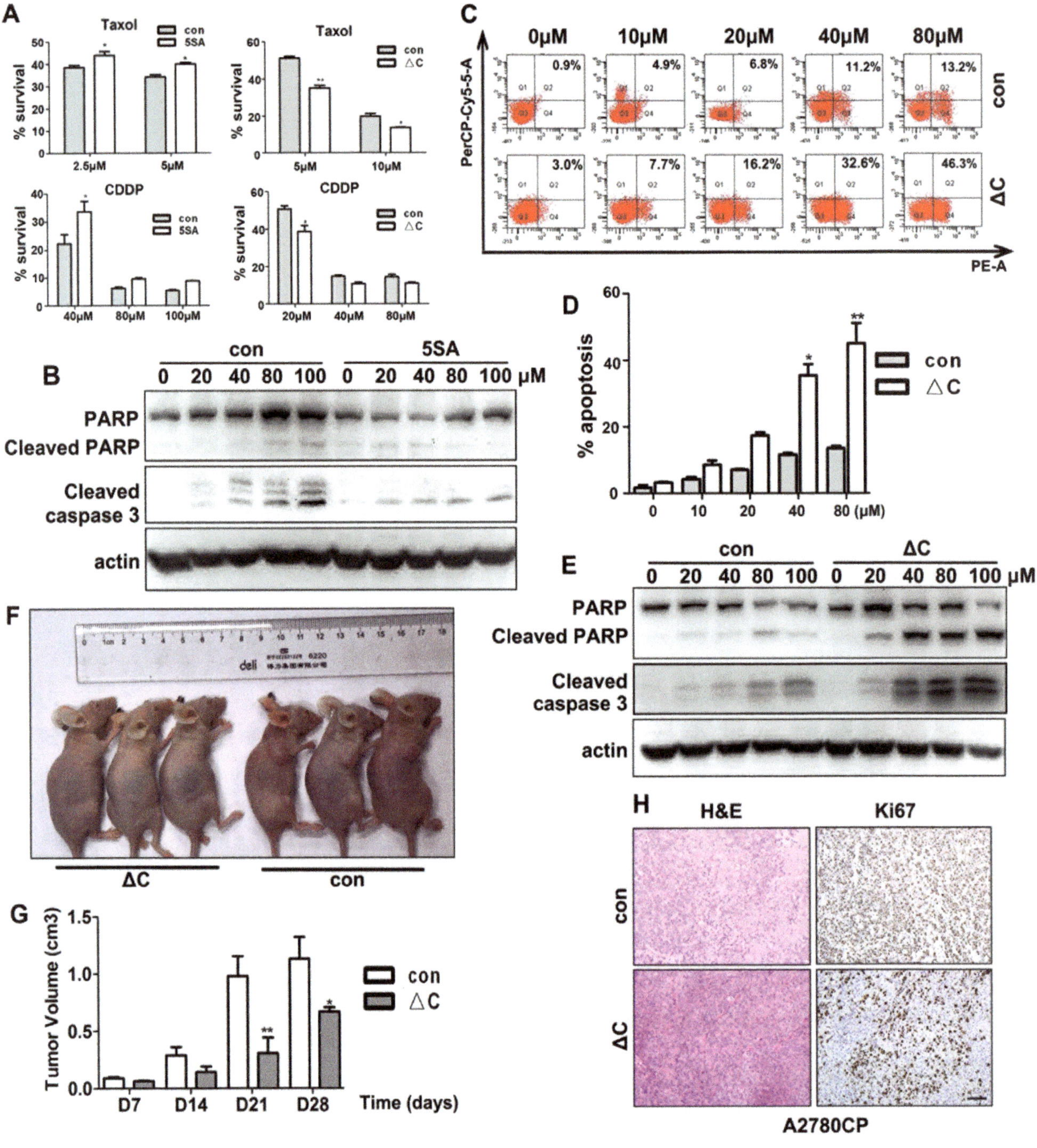

Figure 3. YAP enhances chemotherapeutic drug resistance by ovarian cancer cells. A: Viability of YAP-5SA and YAP-5SA-ΔC expressing cells after treatment with Taxol or CDDP, as assessed by MTT assay. **B**: Western blotting results for the apoptosis markers cleaved caspase 3 and PARP in YAP-5SA expressing and control cells after treatment with the indicated doses of CDDP for 48 h. **C**: Flow cytometry results for apoptosis of A2780CP cells with or without YAP-5SA-ΔC transfection and after treatment with different doses of CDDP for 48 h. **D**: Western blotting results for cleaved caspase 3 and PARP in YAP-5SA-ΔC expressing and control cells after treatment with the indicated doses of CDDP for 48 h. **F-G**: Images and quantitative results for *in vivo* tumorigenic capacity of A2780CP cells with or without YAP-5SA-ΔC expression. Nude mice were injected with CDDP through a caudal vein once each week for four weeks after tumor xenografts reached 5 mm in diameter. **H**: IHC results for the proliferation marker Ki67 on the indicated tumor tissue sections. Scale bar = 100 μM.

staining intensity was associated with poor patient survival (Figure 5D, left panel). The survival of patients with both high YAP and high TEAD4 expression was significantly worse than for the other categories (Figure 5D, middle panel; P = 0.002). In addition, the Kaplan-Meier estimate for combined high YAP/TEAD4 and the EMT marker β-catanin expression was also statistically significant (Figure 5D, right panel). Taken together, these results indicated that YAP and TEAD4 were two significant

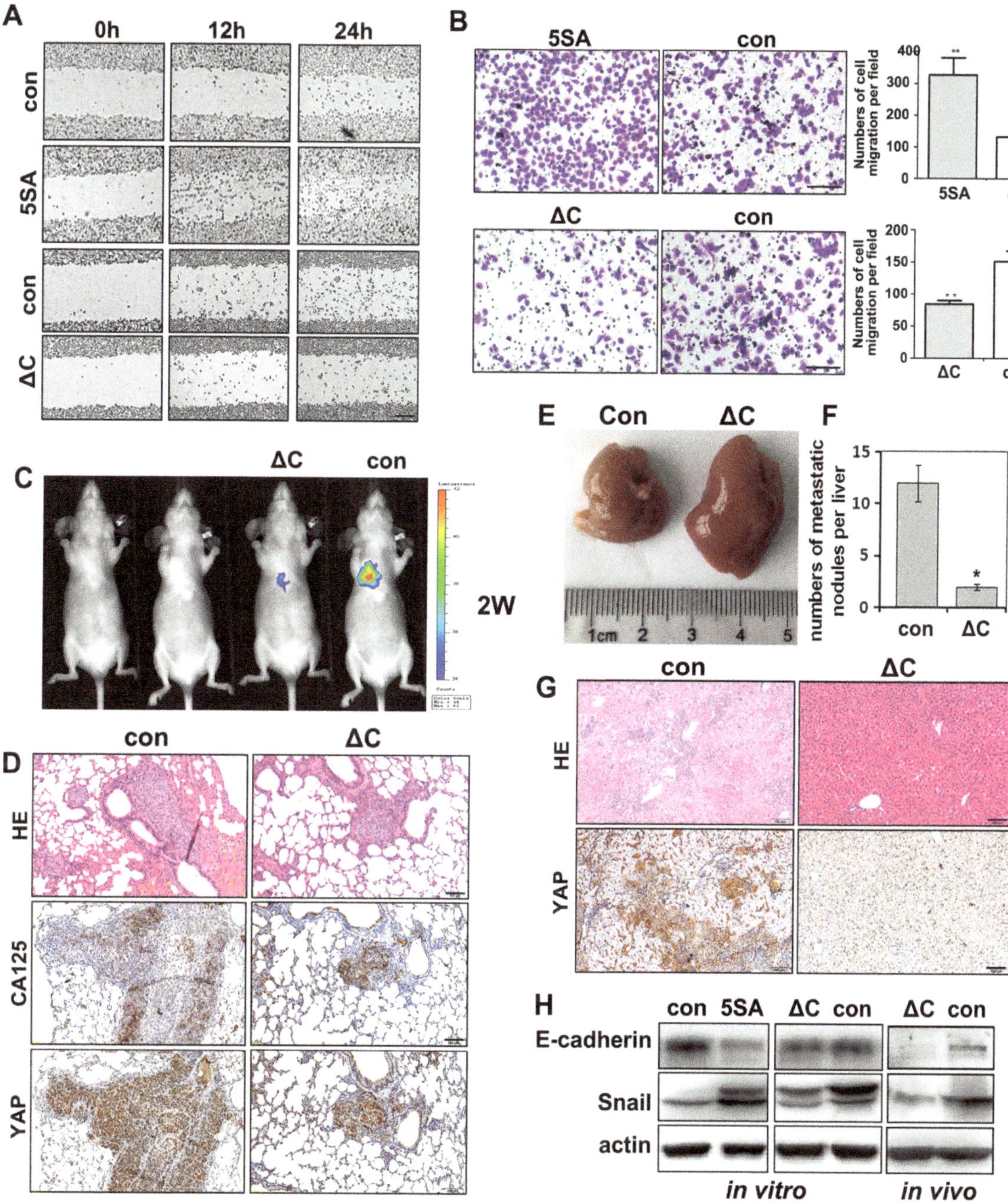

Figure 4. YAP promotes ovarian cancer cells migration and distant metastasis *in vitro* and *in vivo*. **A**. Wound-healing assay for the migration of YAP-5SA and YAP-5SA-ΔC expressing cells after culture for 12 and 24 hours. Scale bar = 100 μM for all panels. **B**. Transwell assays for the migration of YAP-5SA and YAP-5SA-ΔC expressing cells. **, P<0.01. **C**. Bioluminescence imaging assays showing lung metastasis of control and YAP-5SA-ΔC expressing HO8910PM cells after they were injected into the caudal veins of nude mice. **D**. HE and IHC staining of lung metastasis sites shown in C. **E-F**: Images and statistical analysis results of liver metastasis by caudal vein injected HO8910 PM cells. **G**: HE and YAP IHC results of liver metastasis sites shown in E. **H**. Western blot results for EMT marker expressions in cultured YAP-5SA and YAP-5SA-ΔC expressing cells and *in vivo* xenografts derived from these cells.

independent markers for poor patient survival and their combined evaluation might be a strong independent predictor of disease-specific survival for ovarian cancer patients.

Discussion

YAP has been implicated as a possible oncogene with different subcellular localizations regulated by its upstream genes in the Hippo pathway. Increased YAP expression and a nuclear localization have been observed in multiple human cancers, including liver, colon, ovarian, and lung cancers [23–30]. In the present study, we showed that YAP protein levels were high in multiple ovarian cancer cell lines. More importantly, YAP was highly expressed in ovarian cancer samples but not in normal ovarian tissue, which suggested that YAP expression was directly related to ovarian cancer development or progression.

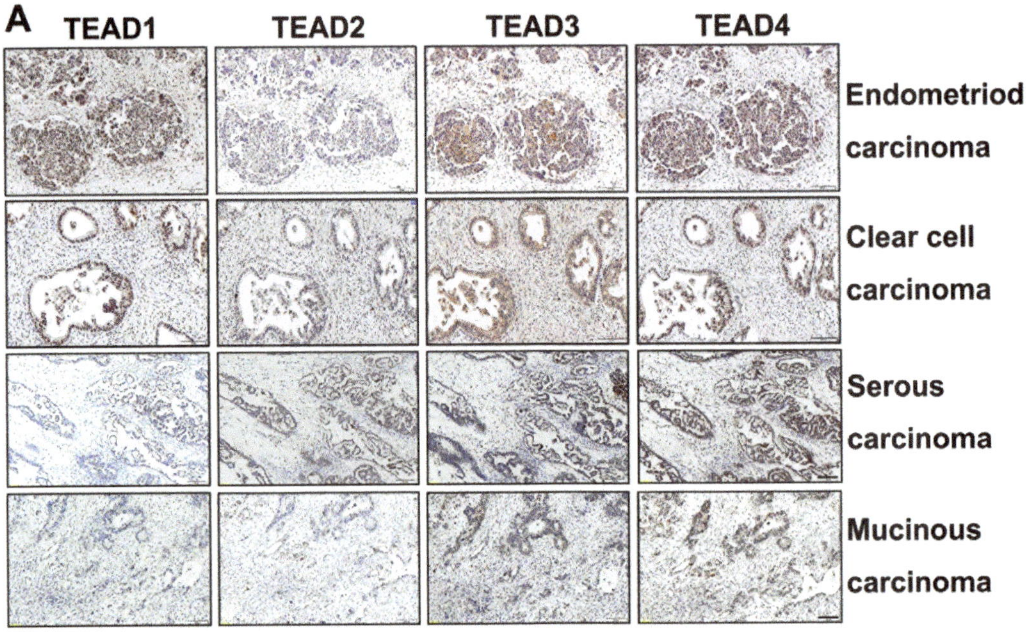

B

		YAP			pYAP		
		Positive (n=55)	Negative (n=37)	P value	Positive (n=67)	Negative (n=25)	P value
TEAD1	positive	47	25	0.012*	35	15	0.744
	negative	8	12		32	10	
TEAD2	positive	44	18	0.004*	50	12	0.002*
	negative	11	19		17	13	
TEAD3	positive	35	35	0.313	46	14	0.001*
	negative	20	12		21	11	
TEAD4	positive	37	13	0.001*	58	16	<0.001*
	negative	18	24		9	9	

C

		YAP		P value
		Negative(12)	Positive(33)	
TEAD4	Negative(10)	5	5	0.0284*
	Positive(35)	7	28	

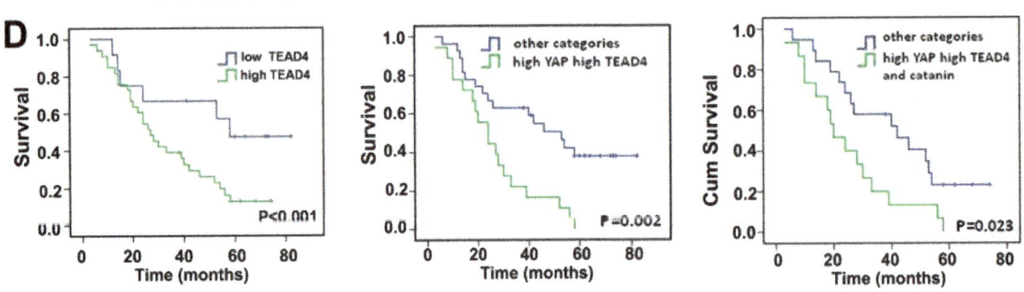

Figure 5. High YAP and TEAD4 co-expression levels are associated with a poor prognosis with primary human ovarian cancers. A. IHC results for TEADs expression in human ovarian cancer tissues. Scale bar = 100 μM. **B.** Associations between YAP/pYAP expressions and TEAD expressions in an ovarian cancer tissue array. **C.** Associations between YAP and TEAD4 expressions in 45 ovarian cancer samples ranked by Kaplan-Meier survival estimates. **D.** YAP and TEAD4 co-expression is associated with a poor prognosis with human ovarian cancer. High TEAD expression versus low TEAD4 expression (left), high YAP expression combined with high TEAD4 expression versus other categories (middle), high YAP expression and high TEAD4 expression combined with high β-catanin versus other categories (right).

Previous studies also suggested that YAP might function as an oncogene in ovarian cancer [31]. However, none of these studies investigated possible associations between YAP/TEAD expression levels and ovarian cancer patient survival. In this study, we showed that high YAP expression in ovarian tumors was associated with shorter disease-specific survival for ovarian cancer patients, and that low YAP expression in ovarian tumors was associated with a longer disease-specific survival for these patients. Further, we found for the first time that TEAD4, a direct binding partner of YAP, was also closely associated with patient survival. The co-expression of YAP and TEAD4 in ovarian cancer tissues was even more dramatically associated with poor patient survival. Thus, high YAP/TEAD4 levels could be a predictor for determining ovarian cancer malignancy levels and for estimating the prognosis of these patients.

Primary epithelial ovarian cancers are usually treated with platinum-based drugs, such as cisplatin coupled with taxol. These drugs are administered either intravenously or intraperitoneally. Apoptotic and anti-apoptotic signals are the two aspects of cell cross-talk between cell survival and cell death pathways that determine the fates of cells in their reactions to exogenous circumstances. For tumors, drug-induced apoptosis is governed not only by the upregulation of apoptotic factors or tumor suppressors, but also by the modulation of cell survival factors. In the present study, we showed that up- and down-regulation of YAP activity could modulate the proliferation, colony formation and migration capabilities, and the resistance to chemotherapeutic agents by ovarian cancer cell lines. A constitutively active YAP mutant increased the resistance to drug-induced apoptosis by ovarian cancer cells, whereas dominant negative YAP restored drug sensitivity in Cisplatin-resistant ovarian cancer cells.

The precise mechanisms by which YAP enhances drug resistance remain unclear. Several studies focused on the PI3K/Akt pathway for chemo-resistance in ovarian cancers and showed that Cisplatin could upregulate p53 and induce apoptosis in these cancer cells after expression of dominant negative AKT, which suggested that cisplatin-mediated p53 upregulation was opposed by AKT. The PI3K/AKT pathway might also participate in YAP-mediated drug resistance, as it has been clearly shown that YAP was involved in cross-talk with PI3K pathways and facilitated AKT activation in other cell types [32,33]. Previous studies also showed that hyperactivation of the PI3K pathway initiated ovarian cancer development in mouse models. The interaction of these two pathways needs to be further investigated in ovarian cancer cells.

It has been hypothesized that cancer cells lose their epithelial characteristics and acquire certain mesenchymal properties that promote extracellular environment invasion and distant metastasis in an EMT-like process. Epithelial markers that are down-regulated during this transition include E-cadherin, cytokeratins, ZO-1 and others. Hippo signaling pathway components are required for E-cadherin-dependent contact inhibition of proliferation. Knockdown of Hippo signaling components or YAP overexpression inhibits the decreased cell proliferation caused by E-cadherin homophilic binding at the cell surface [34].

In our study, we found that YAP could enhance the migration of ovarian cancer cell lines. We also found that the expression of EMT markers was modulated by YAP activity in tumor tissues of nude mice and confirmed that YAP enhanced ovarian cancer cell metastasis *in vivo*. Although YAP expression combined with EMT marker expressions was associated with patient prognosis, E-cadherin and other EMT genes alone were not associated with patient survival (data not shown). Thus, E-cadherin and other EMT genes were not independent predictors for ovarian cancer risk prediction. If YAP is taken into account, then EMT markers might be a predictor of ovarian cancer risk.

Previous studies suggested that YAP was an independent prognostic marker for poor survival with ovarian cancer and other carcinomas [9,30]. Our study also confirmed this using survival analysis. In our data set, YAP was positively associated with patient prognosis, whereas its cytoplasmic distribution and pYAP were not indicators of survival. Patients with high nuclear YAP (nYAP) expression and low cytoplasmic YAP (cYAP) expression had a nearly eight times greater risk of death from this disease than other patients. The nYAP/cYAP pattern might reflect YAP activity in a tumor: YAP has transcription-promoting activity only when it is localized in the nucleus and is presumably transcriptionally inactive when it is retained in the cytoplasm and is phosphorylated at S127 by LATS1/2.

Several studies found that increased YAP activity could promote TEAD-dependent transcription in a manner that depended on the TEAD-interaction domain of YAP [14,35–38]. Thus, we investigated whether increased YAP activity was associated with increased TEAD expression in ovarian cancer and its relationship with patient survival. Our immunostaining results showed that YAP was positively correlated with TEAD family proteins' expression, except for TEAD3. The correlation with TEAD4 was the highest among the four TEAD family genes.

We categorized TEAD4-expressing ovarian cancer samples into those with weak and strong expressions and compared these with patient prognosis. These results showed that strong YAP and TEAD4 expression was a predictor of reduced ovarian cancer survival. Thus, YAP and TEAD4 might biochemically function together in ovarian cancer progression, and YAP-TEAD4 co-expression may be important for assessing ovarian cancer patient outcomes.

Acknowledgments

We thank Dr. Kaichun Wu and Dr. Nie Yongzhan of the Fourth Military Medical University for their help with this work.

Author Contributions

Conceived and designed the experiments: YX HYF. Performed the experiments: YX TC YL WL ML. Analyzed the data: YX YW HYF. Wrote the paper: YX HYF.

References

1. Jia J, Zhang W, Wang B, Trinko R, Jiang J (2003) The Drosophila Ste20 family kinase dMST functions as a tumor suppressor by restricting cell proliferation and promoting apoptosis. Genes Dev 17: 2514–2519.
2. Wu S, Huang J, Dong J, Pan D (2003) hippo encodes a Ste-20 family protein kinase that restricts cell proliferation and promotes apoptosis in conjunction with salvador and warts. Cell 114: 445–456.
3. Huang J, Wu S, Barrera J, Matthews K, Pan D (2005) The Hippo signaling pathway coordinately regulates cell proliferation and apoptosis by inactivating Yorkie, the Drosophila Homolog of YAP. Cell 122: 421–434.
4. Pantalacci S, Tapon N, Leopold P (2003) The Salvador partner Hippo promotes apoptosis and cell-cycle exit in Drosophila. Nat Cell Biol 5: 921–927.
5. Harvey KF, Pfleger CM, Hariharan IK (2003) The Drosophila Mst ortholog, hippo, restricts growth and cell proliferation and promotes apoptosis. Cell 114: 457–467.
6. Camargo FD, Gokhale S, Johnnidis JB, Fu D, Bell GW, et al. (2007) YAP1 increases organ size and expands undifferentiated progenitor cells. Curr Biol 17: 2054–2060.
7. Zhao B, Li L, Tumaneng K, Wang CY, Guan KL (2010) A coordinated phosphorylation by Lats and CK1 regulates YAP stability through SCF(beta-TRCP). Genes Dev 24: 72–85.
8. Lei QY, Zhang H, Zhao B, Zha ZY, Bai F, et al. (2008) TAZ promotes cell proliferation and epithelial-esenchymal

9. transition and is inhibited by the hippo pathway. Mol Cell Biol 28: 2426–2436.
10. Hall CA, Wang R, Miao J, Oliva E, Shen X, et al. (2010) Hippo pathway effector Yap is an ovarian cancer oncogene. Cancer Res 70: 8517–8525.
11. Zhang X, George J, Deb S, Degoutin JL, Takano EA, et al. (2011) The Hippo pathway transcriptional co-activator, YAP, is an ovarian cancer oncogene. Oncogene 30: 2810–2822.
12. Udan RS, Kango-Singh M, Nolo R, Tao C, Halder G (2003) Hippo promotes proliferation arrest and apoptosis in the Salvador/Warts pathway. Nat Cell Biol 5: 914–920.
13. Zhao B, Wei X, Li W, Udan RS, Yang Q, et al. (2007) Inactivation of YAP oncoprotein by the Hippo pathway is involved in cell contact inhibition and tissue growth control. Genes Dev 21: 2747–2761.
14. Yagi R, Chen LF, Shigesada K, Murakami Y, Ito Y (1999) A WW domain-containing yes-associated protein (YAP) is a novel transcriptional co-activator. EMBO J 18: 2551–2562.
15. Vassilev A, Kaneko KJ, Shu H, Zhao Y, DePamphilis ML (2001) TEAD/TEF transcription factors utilize the activation domain of YAP65, a Src/Yes-associated protein localized in the cytoplasm. Genes Dev 15: 1229–1241.
16. Basu S, Totty NF, Irwin MS, Sudol M, Downward J (2003) Akt phosphorylates the Yes-associated protein, YAP, to induce interaction with 14-3-3 and attenuation of p73-mediated apoptosis. Mol Cell 11: 11–23.
17. Komuro A, Nagai M, Navin NE, Sudol M (2003) WW domain-containing protein YAP associates with ErbB-4 and acts as a co-transcriptional activator for the carboxyl-terminal fragment of ErbB-4 that translocates to the nucleus. J Biol Chem 278: 33334–33341.
18. Zhao B, Ye X, Yu J, Li L, Li W, et al. (2008) TEAD mediates YAP-dependent gene induction and growth control. Genes Dev 22: 1962–1971.
19. Nishioka N, Inoue K, Adachi K, Kiyonari H, Ota M, et al. (2009) The Hippo signaling pathway components Lats and Yap pattern Tead4 activity to distinguish mouse trophectoderm from inner cell mass. Dev Cell 16: 398–410.
20. Liu-Chittenden Y, Huang B, Shim JS, Chen Q, Lee SJ, et al. (2012) Genetic and pharmacological disruption of the TEAD-YAP complex suppresses the oncogenic activity of YAP. Genes Dev 26: 1300–1305.
21. Xie Q, Chen J, Feng H, Peng S, Adams U, et al. (2013) YAP/TEAD-mediated transcription controls cellular senescence. Cancer Res 73: 3615–3624.
22. Ota M, Sasaki H (2008) Mammalian Tead proteins regulate cell proliferation and contact inhibition as transcriptional mediators of Hippo signaling. Development 135: 4059–4069.
23. Steinhardt AA, Gayyed MF, Klein AP, Dong J, Maitra A, et al. (2008) Expression of Yes-associated protein in common solid tumors. Hum Pathol 39: 1582–1589.
24. Zhang X, George J, Deb S, Degoutin JL, Takano EA, et al. (2011) The Hippo pathway transcriptional co-activator, YAP, is an ovarian cancer oncogene. Oncogene 30: 2810–2822.
25. Wang J, Ma L, Weng W, Qiao Y, Zhang Y, et al. (2013) Mutual interaction between YAP and CREB promotes tumorigenesis in liver cancer. Hepatology 58: 1011–1020.
26. Zhou D, Zhang Y, Wu H, Barry E, Yin Y, et al. (2011) Mst1 and Mst2 protein kinases restrain intestinal stem cell proliferation and colonic tumorigenesis by inhibition of Yes-associated protein (Yap) overabundance. Proc Natl Acad Sci USA 108: E1312–1320.
27. Konsavage WM, Jr., Kyler SL, Rennoll SA, Jin G, Yochum GS (2012) Wnt/beta-catenin signaling regulates Yes-associated protein (YAP) gene expression in colorectal carcinoma cells. J Biol Chem 287: 11730–11739.
28. Yi C, Shen Z, Stemmer-Rachamimov A, Dawany N, Troutman S, et al. (2013) The p130 isoform of angiomotin is required for Yap-mediated hepatic epithelial cell proliferation and tumorigenesis. Sci Signal 6: 1–12.
29. Wang J, Park JS, Wei Y, Rajurkar M, Cotton JL, et al. (2013) TRIB2 acts downstream of Wnt/TCF in liver cancer cells to regulate YAP and C/EBPalpha function. Mol Cell 51: 211–225.
30. Wang Y, Dong Q, Zhang Q, Li Z, Wang E, et al. (2010) Overexpression of yes-associated protein contributes to progression and poor prognosis of non-small-cell lung cancer. Cancer Sci 101: 1279–1285.
31. Xu MZ, Yao TJ, Lee NP, Ng IO, Chan YT, et al. (2009) Yes-associated protein is an independent prognostic marker in hepatocellular carcinoma. Cancer 115: 4576–4585.
32. Cai H, Xu Y (2013) The role of LPA and YAP signaling in long-term migration of human ovarian cancer cells. Cell Commun Signal 11: 31.
33. Qin LF, Ng IO (2002) Induction of apoptosis by cisplatin and its effect on cell cycle-related proteins and cell cycle changes in hepatoma cells. Cancer Lett 175: 27–38.
34. Buttitta F, Marchetti A, Gadducci A, Pellegrini S, Morganti M, et al. (1997) p53 alterations are predictive of chemoresistance and aggressiveness in ovarian carcinomas: a molecular and immunohistochemical study. Br J Cancer 75: 230–235.
35. Kim NG, Koh E, Chen X, Gumbiner BM (2011) E-cadherin mediates contact inhibition of proliferation through Hippo signaling-pathway components. Proc Natl Acad Sci U S A 108: 11930–11935.
36. Hau JC, Erdmann D, Mesrouze Y, Furet P, Fontana P, et al. (2013) The TEAD4-YAP/TAZ protein-protein interaction: expected similarities and unexpected differences. Chembiochem 14: 1218–1225.
37. Cao X, Pfaff SL, Gage FH (2008) YAP regulates neural progenitor cell number via the TEA domain transcription factor. Genes Dev 22: 3320–3334.
38. Chen L, Chan SW, Zhang X, Walsh M, Lim CJ, et al. (2010) Structural basis of YAP recognition by TEAD4 in the hippo pathway. Genes Dev 24: 290–300.
39. Lamar JM, Stern P, Liu H, Schindler JW, Jiang ZG, et al. (2012) The Hippo pathway target, YAP, promotes metastasis through its TEAD-interaction domain. Proc Natl Acad Sci U S A 109: E2441–2450.

19

Polymorphisms of *MUC16* (CA125) and *MUC1* (CA15.3) in Relation to Ovarian Cancer Risk and Survival

Kristina A. Williams[1,2], Kathryn L. Terry[1,2,3], Shelley S. Tworoger[3,4], Allison F. Vitonis[1], Linda J. Titus[5], Daniel W. Cramer[1,2,3]*

1 Obstetrics and Gynecology Epidemiology Center, Department of Obstetrics and Gynecology, Brigham and Women's Hospital, Boston, Massachusetts, United States of America, **2** Harvard Medical School, Boston, Massachusetts, United States of America, **3** Department of Epidemiology, Harvard School of Public Health, Boston, Massachusetts, United States of America, **4** Channing Division of Network Medicine, Department of Medicine, Brigham and Women's Hospital and Harvard Medical School, Boston, Massachusetts, United States of America, **5** Department of Community & Family Medicine, Department of Pediatrics, Dartmouth-Hitchcock Medical Center Lebanon, New Hampshire, United States of America

Abstract

Objective: To examine single nucleotide polymorphism (SNPs) in *MUC16* (CA125) and *MUC1* (CA15.3) in relation to ovarian cancer risk and survival.

Methods: We genotyped germline variants of *MUC16* (rs2547065, rs1559168, rs12984471, rs2121133) and *MUC1* (rs2070803, rs4072037, rs1045253) using samples collected from 758 ovarian cancer cases and 788 controls enrolled in the New England Case-Control Study between 2003 and 2008. We calculated age-adjusted odds ratios (OR) and 95% confidence intervals (CIs) for disease risk using unconditional and polytomous logistic regression and hazard ratios (HR) for survival using Cox proportional hazard ratios. In a subset of cases, we compared log-normalized CA125 values by genotype using generalized linear models.

Results: Cases homozygous for the variant allele of *MUC16* SNP, rs12984471, had poorer overall survival (log-rank $p = 0.03$) and higher CA125 levels, especially cases over age 65 ($p = 0.01$). For *MUC1* SNP, rs4072037, women homozygous for the G variant had a non-significantly decreased risk for serous invasive types but elevated risk for serous borderline tumors, mucinous borderline and invasive tumors, and endometrioid tumors. Women with the variant allele of *MUC16* SNP, rs2547065, especially those who were homozygous had an elevated risk for ovarian cancer; but this association was not confirmed in an independent dataset.

Conclusion: This targeted screen of seven polymorphisms of *MUC16* and *MUC1* genes failed to identify and confirm effects on ovarian cancer risk overall. However, there may be effects of *MUC16* rs12984471 on survival and *MUC1* rs4072037 on risk for histologic types of ovarian cancer other than invasive serous. Further study is warranted.

Editor: Surinder K. Batra, University of Nebraska Medical Center, United States of America

Funding: Work was supported by NIH grant numbers R01CA054419, P50CA105009, R01CA49449, R01CA67272, R01CA50383, UM1 CA176726, and P01CA87969; Department of Defense grant number W81XWH-10-1-0280 and the Scholars in Medicine Office at Harvard Medical School and the Department of Obstetrics and Gynecology at Brigham and Women's Hospital. The funders had no role in study design, data collection and analysis, decision to publish or preparation of the manuscript.

Competing Interests: The authors have declared that no competing interests exist.

* E-mail: dcramer@partners.org

Introduction

The tethered human mucins (MUC) are a family of large, heavily glycosylated transmembrane proteins that have a diverse range of functions [1]. CA125, or MUC16, is the largest glycoprotein of the mucin family, and is normally expressed in the epithelial lining of various tissues, especially that of the female reproductive tract [1]. CA125 is elevated in the serum of about 82% of ovarian cancer patients and is used to predict recurrence [2,3]. CA15.3, or MUC1, also is expressed in the epithelial lining of various tissues, exhibiting strong expression in the mammary gland and the female reproductive tract during pregnancy and lactation. CA15.3 is over-expressed in a wide variety of cancers, including breast and ovarian [1,4]. Although these two mucins are best known as tumor markers, evidence suggests that they may play a role in cancer metastasis, tumor growth and survival, inhibition of immune response, and prognosis [1,5,6].

Several studies have examined genetic variation in genes involved in glycosylation of CA125 and CA15.3 and ovarian cancer risk, observing overall null associations [7,8,9,10]; however, there are few studies of genetic variation specifically in *MUC16* or *MUC1* and their association with ovarian cancer risk or survival. Therefore, we examined the association between a targeted set of single nucleotide polymorphisms (SNPs) in *MUC16* (rs2547065, rs1559168, rs12914471, rs2121133) and *MUC1* (rs2070803, rs4072037, rs1045253) in relation to ovarian cancer risk and survival.

Methods

Ethics Statement

Institutional Review Boards at Brigham and Women's Hospital, Dana Farber Cancer Institute, and Dartmouth Medical School approved the studies and all study participants signed informed consent.

Study Population and Design

Data and specimens come from the last enrollment phase of the New England Case Control Study of ovarian cancer from 2003–2008 (NECC). Details regarding case and control enrollment for this study are described elsewhere [11,12]. Briefly, of 1610 incident cases of ovarian cancer identified through hospital tumor boards and statewide cancer registries between 2003 and 2008, 897 of 1238 eligible agreed to participate. Controls were identified through town books in eastern Massachusetts and drivers' license lists in New Hampshire. Exclusion criteria for controls included inability to be contacted, history of bilateral oophorectomy, language barriers, or relocation outside of the study area. Of 2522 controls identified, 1673 were eligible and 857 agreed to participate.

After written informed consent, demographic information, reproductive and medical history, and lifestyle factors were assessed by in-person interviews and heparinized blood samples were collected.

Genotyping

DNA was extracted and genotyping was performed at the Dana-Farber/Harvard Cancer Center (DF/HCC) High Throughput Polymorphism Core, an affiliate of the Partners Healthcare Center for Personalized Genetic Medicine. DNA was extracted from buffy coat samples using QIAmp (Qiagen, Chatworth, CA). Genotyping of *MUC16* (rs2547065, rs1559168, rs12914471, rs2121133) and *MUC1* (rs2070803, rs4072037, rs1045253) was performed using 5′ nuclease assays (Taqman®) on the Applied Biosystems Prism 7900HT Sequence Detection System (Applied Biosystems, Foster City, California). Primers, probes, and conditions for genotyping assays are available upon request. Replicates of 10% of the samples were included for quality control. Laboratory personnel were blinded to case control status and the location of quality controls.

Based on preliminary data, we sought to validate one of the SNPs in an independent dataset. We used samples from 534 cases and 1513 controls from the Nurses' Health Study cohorts (NHS/NHSII) [13]. The NHS includes 121,700 participants, 32,826 of whom provided blood samples in 1990 and 33,040 who gave buccal cells specimens from 2001–2004. The NHSII includes 116,430 participants, of whom 29,611 provided blood from 1996–1999 and 29,859 provided buccal cells from 2004–2006. Cases were identified after sample collection and before June 1, 2010 (NHS) or June 1, 2009 (NHSII). Demographic information on NHS and NHSII participants have been described previously [13]. Briefly, participants in both cohorts are predominantly white (> 96%), but NHS is an older cohort than NHSII which is reflected in participants' mean age (NHS:65years, NHSII:49years), ever a child birth (95% NHS, 76% NHSII), and ever oral contraceptive use (45% NHS, 81% NHSII).

Preoperative CA125 Levels

We reviewed all medical records and computerized laboratory reports for cases who received care at Brigham and Women's Hospital or Massachusetts General Hospital (n = 809) [14]. CA125 values were abstracted for women whose levels had been measured prior to surgery and/or neoadjuvant chemotherapy. We were able to retrieve CA125 values on 353 of the cases genotyped in this study. Data on CA15.3 were not available.

Statistical Analysis

We used chi-square tests to assess Hardy–Weinberg Equilibrium (HWE) for each SNP among controls. Unconditional logistic regression was used to calculate overall odds ratios (OR) and 95% confidence intervals (95% CI) of ovarian cancer risk adjusted for age (continuous), study center (Massachusetts or New Hampshire), and race (white or non-white). The more common allele for each SNP served as the reference group in the regression models. Co-dominant (heterozygous vs. wild type or homozygous variant vs. wild type), recessive (homozygous variant vs. heterozygous and wild type), and per allele (trend test) models were computed. Multivariate regression models were additionally adjusted for family history of ovarian or early onset breast cancer and a personal history of breast cancer.

Polytomous logistic regression was used to calculate OR (95%CI) for risk of various histological subtypes adjusted for age, study center, and race. Likelihood ratio tests were used to test for heterogeneity across histologic categories (serous borderline, serous invasive [includes high grade transitional cell and mixed serous], mucinous [borderline and invasive], endometrioid or mixed endometrioid/clear cell, clear cell, undifferentiated [includes unspecified and Brenner tumours]) comparing a model that allows the estimate of the association to vary by histologic type to a model that restricts to one estimate of the association for all histologic types.

Cox proportional hazard models (HR) were used to examine the association between each polymorphism and survival, adjusting for study center and race and in a secondary model for stage (I-IV) and histology (serous, non-serous). Co-dominant, recessive, and per allele models were used as described in supplemental methods (Methods S1). The Kaplan–Meier method was used to estimate survival curves and calculate log-rank statistics.

Geometric mean CA125 values by genotype were calculated for each *MUC16* polymorphism. Statistical analyses used general linear regression, adjusted for age, race, and time between CA125 measurement and diagnosis (≤30 days, >30days, missing), using continuous log transformed CA125 levels and a variable that represents increasing variant alleles for each polymorphism (0, 1, 2). CA125 levels can vary during the menstrual cycle, and levels vary between pre and postmenopausal women [15,16], so we stratified these analyses into three age/menopausal categories (premenopausal, "midlife" postmenopausal (age<65), and "elderly" postmenopausal (age> = 65)). All analyses were performed using SAS v 9.1 (SAS, Cary, North Carolina) and Intercooled Stata 9 (StataCorp LP, College Station, Texas).

Results

A total of 758 women with ovarian cancer and 788 controls were included in the final analytic sample (Table 1). For both cases and controls, mean age was 54. Our study population consisted primarily of Caucasian women (>95%) and white ethnicity was more common among controls. On average, controls had higher parity, longer duration of oral contraceptive use, and a higher frequency of tubal ligation, endometriosis or painful periods, and a personal history of breast cancer. Family history of ovarian or early onset breast cancer, smoking status, and menopausal status did not differ significantly between cases and controls. Serous invasive (49.7%) was the most frequent histologic subtype among cases followed by endometrioid (17.8%).

Table 1. Descriptive characteristics of ovarian cancer cases and controls, New England-based ovarian cancer case-control study 2003–2008.

	Controls		Cases		
Variable	**N = 788**		**N = 758**		**p[b]**
Age, mean (SD)	54.4	(11.8)	54.2	(11.3)	0.77
Study Center					
Massachusetts	670	(85.0)	609	(80.3)	0.01
New Hampshire	118	(15.0)	149	(19.7)	
White Ethnicity, n (%)	774	(98.2)	715	(94.3)	<0.0001
Parous, n (%)	652	(82.7)	522	(68.9)	<0.0001
Mean Pregnancies Among Parous (SD)	2.6	(1.2)	2.4	(1.2)	0.01
Oral Contraceptive Use, n (%)	541	(68.7)	439	(57.9)	<0.0001
Mean Years Among Users (SD)	6.3	(5.3)	5.1	(5.0)	0.0003
Tubal Ligation, n (%)	176	(22.3)	92	(12.1)	<0.0001
Ever Smoker, n (%)	405	(51.4)	398	(52.5)	0.66
Menopausal Status, n (%)					
Premenopausal	294	(37.3)	278	(36.7)	0.90
Postmenopausal, Age <65	346	(43.9)	333	(43.7)	
Postmenopausal, Age ≥65	148	(18.8)	149	(19.7)	
Endometrioses/Painful Periods, n (%)	279	(35.5)	347	(45.8)	<0.0001
Family History,[a] n (%)	62	(7.9)	74	(9.8)	0.19
Personal History of Breast Cancer, n (%)	35	(4.4)	67	(8.8)	0.0005
Histologic Subtype, n (%)					
Serous Borderline			62	(8.2)	
Serous Invasive			385	(50.8)	
Mucinous			75	(9.9)	
Endometrioid			134	(17.7)	
Clear Cell			50	(6.6)	
Other/Undifferentiated			52	(6.9)	

Cases and controls are frequency matched by age.
[a]Includes ovarian and early onset (before age 50) breast cancers.
[b]p value from chi square or t-test.

All seven polymorphisms were in Hardy-Weinberg equilibrium and had genotyping success greater than 95% except for rs2547065 (93%). In general the minor allele frequencies (MAF) we found for our controls were comparable to that of the Caucasian European (CEU) HapMap populations (data not shown). In the NECC study, one of the four *MUC16* polymorphisms was associated with ovarian cancer risk (Table 2). For polymorphism rs2547065, we observed an increase in ovarian cancer risk (per allele OR = 1.26, 95% CI: 1.09–1.47). Risk was most apparent for the homozygous variant genotype when compared to the wild type genotype (OR = 1.68, 95% CI: 1.23–2.29). However, polymorphism rs2547065 was not associated with ovarian cancer risk (per allele: OR = 1.05, 95% CI: 0.91–1.21) in an independent dataset including 534 cases and 1513 controls from the Nurses' Health Study cohorts (NHS/NHSII). There was no significant heterogeneity by histologic type for any of the *MUC16* polymorphisms.

For *MUC1*, none of the polymorphisms we tested were significantly associated with overall ovarian cancer risk in the per allele model. Women carrying two copies of the *MUC1* polymorphism rs2070803 variant had an increased risk of serous invasive cancer of borderline statistical significance (OR = 1.35, 95% CI 0.99–1.86) in the recessive model. Although we observed no significant risk associated with *MUC1* polymorphism rs4072037 overall, significant heterogeneity by histology was observed when evaluating the recessive model for this polymorphism (p-heterogeneity = 0.02). Women homozygous for the G variant of rs4072023 had a non-significantly decreased risk for invasive serous cancers but elevated risks for serous borderline tumors (OR = 1.91, 95% CI 1.08–3.36), mucinous borderline and invasive (OR = 1.68, 95% CI 1.00–2.83), and endometrioid tumors (OR = 1.54, 95% CI 1.01–2.33). Adjusting for family history of ovarian or early onset breast cancer and personal history of breast cancer did not change estimates for any of the *MUC1* or *MUC16* polymorphisms.

In examining the effect of mucin polymorphisms and survival, we observed poorer overall survival among women carrying the variant allele of *MUC16* polymorphism rs12984471 (log-rank p = 0.03; Figure 1A) as well as an increased mortality (age-adjusted HR = 1.23 95% CI: 1.02–1.48, Table 3). These associations were strongest in women age 65 and older (log-rank p = 0.02; age-adjusted HR = 1.53 95% CI: 1.07–2.19) (Figure 1B). Mortality was 57% greater for women who were homozygous for the variant allele of rs12984471 (age-adjusted HR = 1.57 95% CI: 1.09–2.28). Adjustment for stage and histology attenuated the association (multivariate HR = 1.32 95% CI: 0.91–1.92); stage was the strongest predictor of survival. No other associations between the remaining mucin polymorphisms and survival were observed.

Finally, we evaluated the association between *MUC16* polymorphisms and serum levels of CA125 measured preoperatively (Table 4). Among all cases, we observed no linear associations between *MUC16* polymorphisms and CA125 levels; however, rs2121133 had the highest CA125 levels for heterozygotes (319.9) and lowest for homozygous variants (110.0) (p = 0.03). Among elderly postmenopausal women, increasing variant alleles of polymorphism rs12984471 were significantly associated with increasing levels of CA125 (p = 0.02).

Discussion

The *MUC1* gene is located on 1q21–22, which is a region frequently altered in both neoplastic and non-neoplastic disorders. *MUC1* gene amplification due to increased gene copy number has been observed in ovarian, breast, papillary thyroid, and gastric cancers [17,18,19,20]. Neoplastic mammary cells have been shown to have a high frequency of altered DNA within the variable nucleotide repeat region (VNTR) of MUC1- the largest region of the this protein and the site of O-glycosylation [1,21,22]. MUC1 has been shown to be essential for ovarian cancer tumorigenesis in mouse models and is over expressed in approximately 90–100% of serous carcinomas [23,24,25]. The three *MUC1* SNPs we studied were selected based on previous publications that studied associations between *MUC1* polymorphisms and gastrointestinal cancers [26,27]. Polymorphism rs4072037 has been correlated with serum MUC1 levels and is known to play a role in alternative splicing [28,29]. Polymorphism rs2070803 is located upstream of the *MUC1* gene in a large LD block, and polymorphism rs1045253 was previously identified as a tagSNP representative of the *MUC1* region [30,31,32]. None of these three polymorphisms affected risk or survival for ovarian cancer overall. Women who were homozygous for the variant G allele of rs2070803 had a 35% elevation in risk for invasive serous ovarian cancer. Although our finding was of borderline statistical

Table 2. Association between mucin polymorphisms and risk of epithelial ovarian cancer, New England-based ovarian cancer case-control study, 2003–2008.

		Controls (N = 788)	All Cases (N = 758)		Serous Invasive Cases (N = 385)		
	MAF	N(%)	N(%)	OR(95% CI)[a]	N (%)	OR (95% CI)[b]	p_{het}[c]
MUC16							
RS12984471	33%						
GG		348 (45.2)	326 (44.7)	1.00 (ref)	158 (43.3)	1.00 (ref)	0.74[d]
CG		338 (43.9)	307 (42.1)	1.01 (0.81, 1.25)	157 (43.0)	1.05 (0.80, 1.37)	
CC		84 (10.9)	97 (13.3)	1.28 (0.92, 1.79)	50 (13.7)	1.36 (0.91, 2.02)	
Per C Allele				1.09 (0.94, 1.27)		1.13 (0.94, 1.36)	0.64[e]
CC vs. GG/GC				1.28 (0.93, 1.75)		1.32 (0.91, 1.93)	0.35[f]
RS1559168	18%						
TT		660 (85.6)	630 (86.3)	1.00 (ref)	322 (87.7)	1.00 (ref)	
AT		107 (13.9)	96 (13.2)	0.92 (0.68, 1.24)	43 (11.7)	–	
AA		4 (0.5)	4 (0.5)	1.06 (0.26, 4.26)	2 (0.5)	–	
Per A Allele				0.94 (0.71, 1.24)		0.84 (0.60, 1.21)	0.36[e]
AA vs. TT/AT				1.07 (0.26, 4.31)		–	
RS2121133	33%						
AA		377 (50.2)	393 (55.0)	1.00 (ref)	193 (53.3)	1.00 (ref)	0.65[d]
AG		318 (42.3)	277 (38.7)	0.84 (0.68, 1.05)	149 (41.2)	0.92 (0.71, 1.20)	
GG		56 (7.5)	45 (6.3)	0.78 (0.51, 1.18)	20 (5.5)	0.69 (0.40, 1.18)	
Per G Allele				0.86 (0.73, 1.02)		0.88 (0.72, 1.08)	0.48[e]
GG vs. AA/AG				0.84 (0.55, 1.26)		0.71 (0.42, 1.21)	0.69[f]
RS2547065	39%						
GG		269 (36.7)	223 (31.9)	1.00 (ref)	113 (32.4)	1.00 (ref)	0.96[d]
GC		359 (49.0)	330 (47.2)	1.11 (0.88, 1.40)	165 (47.3)	1.09 (0.82, 1.46)	
CC		104 (14.2)	146 (20.9)	1.68 (1.23, 2.29)	71 (20.3)	1.61 (1.11, 2.34)	
Per C Allele				1.26 (1.09, 1.47)		1.24 (1.03, 1.48)	0.90[e]
CC vs. GG/GC				1.58 (1.20, 2.09)		1.53 (1.09, 2.13)	0.86[f]
MUC1							
RS1045253	30%						
GG		355 (47.7)	322 (44.5)	1.00 (ref)	148 (40.9)	1.00 (ref)	0.63[d]
GA		332 (44.4)	338 (46.7)	1.09 (0.88, 1.35)	180 (49.7)	1.25 (0.96, 1.63)	
AA		58 (7.8)	63 (8.7)	1.13 (0.76, 1.67)	34 (9.4)	1.41 (0.89, 2.24)	
Per A Allele				1.07 (0.91, 1.26)		1.21 (1.00, 1.48)	0.33[e]
AA vs. GG/GA				1.08 (0.74, 1.58)		1.26 (0.82, 1.95)	0.51[f]
RS2070803	48%						
AA		253 (33.1)	228 (31.3)	1.00 (ref)	96 (26.6)	1.00 (ref)	0.30[d]
AG		386 (50.5)	346 (47.5)	0.96 (0.76, 1.21)	186 (51.5)	1.22 (0.91, 1.64)	
GG		125 (16.4)	155 (21.3)	1.27 (0.94, 1.71)	79 (21.9)	1.43 (1.07, 2.22)	
Per G Allele				1.10 (0.95, 1.28)		1.23 (1.03, 1.47)	0.46[e]
GG vs. AA/AG				1.30 (0.99, 1.69)		1.35 (0.99, 1.86)	0.84[f]
RS4072037	47%						
AA		214 (28.3)	226 (31.1)	1.00 (ref)	118 (32.9)	1.00 (ref)	0.06[d]
AG		376 (49.7)	329 (45.3)	0.87 (0.69, 1.11)	174 (48.5)	0.87 (0.65, 1.16)	
GG		167 (22.1)	172 (23.7)	1.06 (0.80, 1.41)	67 (18.7)	0.78 (0.54, 1.11)	
Per G Allele				1.02 (0.88, 1.18)		0.89 (0.74, 1.06)	0.12[e]
GG vs. AA/AG				1.15 (0.90, 1.47)		0.85 (0.62, 1.16)	0.02[f]

[a]OR (95%CI) modeled with unconditional logistic regression; adjusted for age, study center, and race (white, non-white).
[b]OR (95%CI) modeled with polytomous logistic regression adjusted for age, study center, and race.
[c]p-values for heterogeneity (het) are computed with likelihood ratio tests comparing a model that allows the estimate of the association to vary by histologic type (serous borderline, serous invasive, mucinous, endometrioid, clear cell, undifferentiated) to a model that restricts to one estimate of the association for all histologic

types.
[d]p_{het} for co-dominant model.
[e]p_{het} for per allele model.
[f]p_{het} for recessive model.

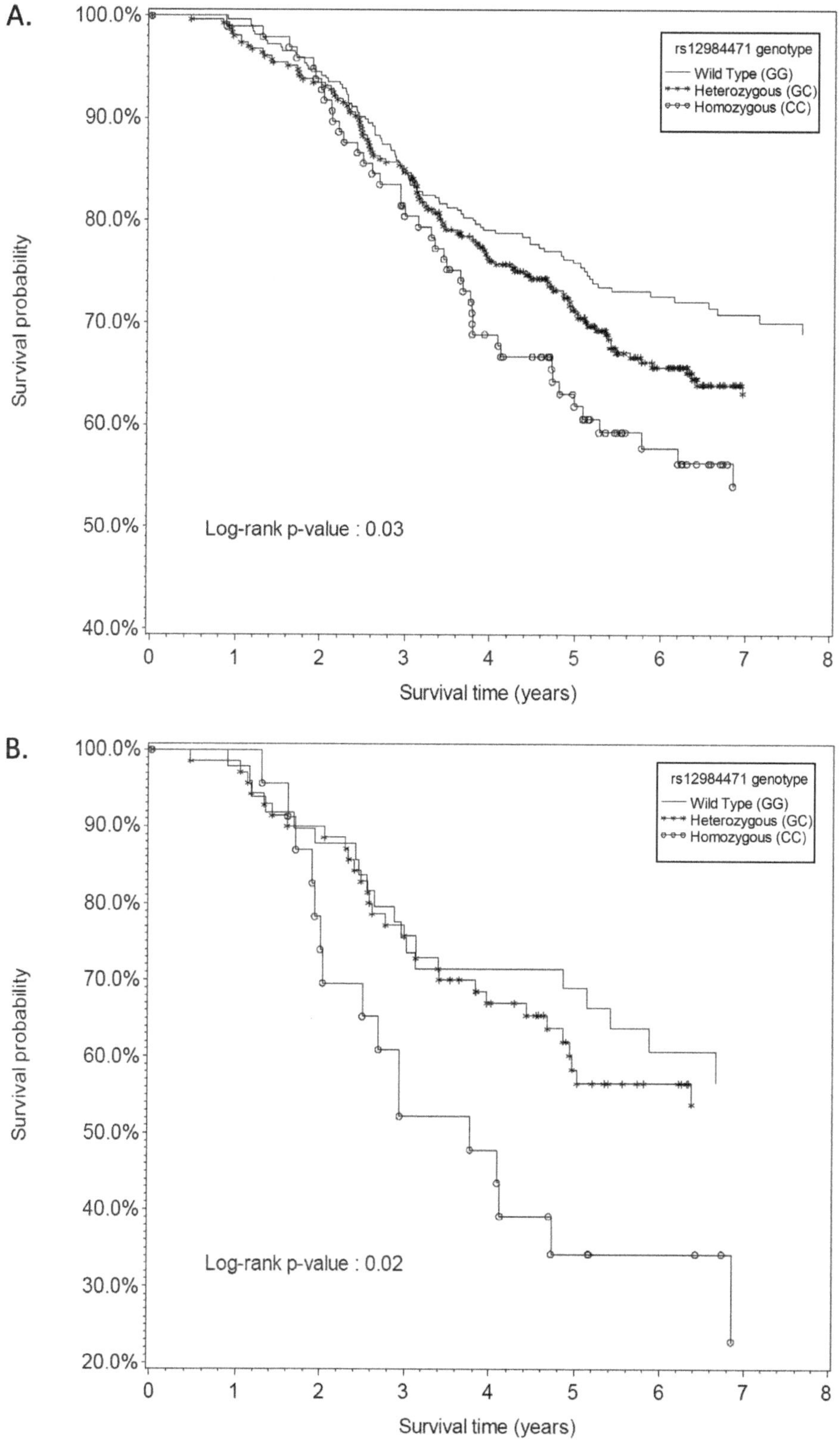

Figure 1. Kaplan–Meier estimates of survival according to rs12984471 genotype among women with epithelial ovarian cancer, New-England based case control study, 2003–2008. A. All women **B**. Postmenopausal women age 65 and older.

Table 3. Association between mucin polymorphisms and epithelial ovarian cancer survival, New England-based ovarian cancer case-control study, 2003–2008.

	Age-Adjusted	Multivariate	Age-Adjusted	Multivariate
	HR (95% CI)[a]	HR (95% CI)[b]	HR (95% CI)[a]	HR (95% CI)[b]
MUC16				
RS12984471				
GG	1.00 (ref)	1.00 (ref)	1.00 (ref)	1.00 (ref)
CG	1.13 (0.85, 1.50)	1.13 (0.85, 1.51)	1.16 (0.85, 1.58)	1.15 (0.85, 1.57)
CC	1.57 (1.09, 2.28)	1.32 (0.91, 1.92)	1.17 (0.75, 1.81)	1.11 (0.72, 1.73)
Per C Allele	1.23 (1.02, 1.48)	1.15 (0.96, 1.37)	1.10 (0.90, 1.35)	1.08 (0.88, 1.32)
CC vs. GG/GC	1.48 (1.06, 2.07)	1.25 (0.89, 1.75)	1.08 (0.72, 1.63)	1.04 (0.69, 1.56)
RS1559168				
TT	1.00 (ref)	1.00 (ref)	1.00 (ref)	1.00 (ref)
AT	1.00 (0.68, 1.47)	1.13 (0.77, 1.67)	1.15 (0.75, 1.76)	1.16 (0.76, 1.77)
AA	–	–	–	–
Per A Allele	0.89 (0.61, 1.28)	1.02 (0.70, 1.47)	1.00 (0.67, 1.48)	1.04 (0.69, 1.54)
AA vs. TT/AT	–	–	–	–
RS2121133				
AA	1.00 (ref)	1.00 (ref)	1.00 (ref)	1.00 (ref)
AG	0.86 (0.65, 1.12)	0.86 (0.65, 1.13)	0.92 (0.68, 1.24)	0.91 (0.68, 1.23)
GG	0.94 (0.54, 1.64)	0.95 (0.55, 1.65)	1.21 (0.66, 2.21)	1.11 (0.61, 2.02)
Per G Allele	0.91 (0.73, 1.13)	0.91 (0.73, 1.13)	1.00 (0.78, 1.27)	0.98 (0.77, 1.24)
GG vs. AA/AG	1.01 (0.59, 1.73)	1.01 (0.59, 1.74)	1.26 (0.70, 2.26)	1.16 (0.64, 2.08)
RS2547065				
GG	1.00 (ref)	1.00 (ref)	1.00 (ref)	1.00 (ref)
GC	1.02 (0.76, 1.39)	0.97 (0.71, 1.31)	1.03 (0.74, 1.43)	0.99 (0.71, 1.38)
CC	1.04 (0.71, 1.51)	0.93 (0.64, 1.36)	0.76 (0.49, 1.18)	0.74 (0.47, 1.15)
Per C Allele	1.02 (0.85, 1.23)	0.97 (0.80, 1.16)	0.90 (0.73, 1.10)	0.88 (0.71, 1.08)
CC vs. GG/GC	1.02 (0.74, 1.42)	0.95 (0.69, 1.32)	0.75 (0.50, 1.11)	0.74 (0.50, 1.10)
MUC1				
RS1045253				
GG	1.00 (ref)	1.00 (ref)	1.00 (ref)	1.00 (ref)
GA	1.25 (0.94, 1.65)	1.12 (0.85, 1.47)	1.03 (0.75, 1.41)	1.05 (0.77, 1.42)
AA	0.99 (0.60, 1.65)	0.89 (0.54, 1.47)	0.78 (0.45, 1.35)	0.81 (0.48, 1.37)
Per A Allele	1.07 (0.88, 1.30)	1.01 (0.82, 1.24)	0.95 (0.76, 1.19)	0.95 (0.76, 1.19)
AA vs. GG/GA	0.89 (0.55, 1.44)	0.84 (0.53, 1.35)	0.77 (0.46, 1.29)	0.79 (0.48, 1.30)
RS2070803				
AA	1.00 (ref)	1.00 (ref)	1.00 (ref)	1.00 (ref)
AG	0.90 (0.67, 1.21)	0.83 (0.62, 1.12)	0.80 (0.58, 1.12)	0.87 (0.63, 1.22)
GG	1.06 (0.74, 1.52)	1.02 (0.71, 1.47)	1.02 (0.69, 1.52)	1.05 (0.70, 1.57)
Per G Allele	1.01 (0.84, 1.22)	0.99 (0.82, 1.20)	0.99 (0.81, 1.23)	1.01 (0.82, 1.25)
GG vs. AA/AG	1.12 (0.82, 1.54)	1.15 (0.84, 1.57)	1.18 (0.84, 1.66)	1.15 (0.81, 1.61)
RS4072037				
AA	1.00 (ref)	1.00 (ref)	1.00 (ref)	1.00 (ref)
AG	1.03 (0.76, 1.38)	1.02 (0.76, 1.38)	1.10 (0.80, 1.52)	1.16 (0.85, 1.60)
GG	0.84 (0.58, 1.21)	0.89 (0.61, 1.28)	0.85 (0.56, 1.30)	0.82 (0.53, 1.25)
Per G Allele	0.93 (0.78, 1.11)	0.95 (0.79, 1.14)	0.95 (0.78, 1.16)	0.94 (0.77, 1.14)
GG vs. AA/AG	0.83 (0.60, 1.14)	0.87 (0.64, 1.20)	0.80 (0.55, 1.17)	0.74 (0.51, 1.09)

Modeled with Cox proportional hazard ratios; "–" frequencies for this SNP were too low to compute co-dominant/recessive models.
[a]Adjusted for age, study center, and race.
[b]Adjusted for age, study center, race, stage (I-IV) and histologic subtype (non-serous, serous).

Table 4. Geometric mean levels of preoperative serum CA125 levels among women with ovarian cancer by MUC16 gene polymorphisms, New England-based ovarian case-control study, 2003–2008.

	All Women			Premenopausal			Postmenopausal <65			Postmenopausal ≥65		
	N	GM	p[a]	N	GM	p[a]	N	GM	p[a]	N	GM	p[a]
RS12984471												
GG	145	193.5	0.15	58	139.9	0.94	63	265.8	0.64	24	184.0	0.02
CG	145	254.6		41	166.2		65	290.7		39	319.9	
CC	49	398.4		14	163.2		22	423.6		13	939.4	
RS1559168												
TT	303	242.1	0.68	98	161.9	0.98	133	277.5	0.40	72	325.5	0.89
AT	34	302.4		12	124.5		15	527.2		7	420.8	
AA	1	102.9		0	-		1	102.9		0	-	
RS2121133												
AA	201	226.7	0.03	62	141.9	0.06	89	288.4	0.90	50	263.8	0.07
AG	121	319.9		45	224.5		52	313.4		24	650.1	
GG	17	110.0		5	25.7		7	245.5		5	153.1	
RS2547065												
GG	98	194.2	0.16	39	192.5	0.10	41	166.5	0.06	18	281.6	0.74
GC	166	290.3		50	147.5		71	393.5		45	381.2	
CC	67	186.9		20	88.9		32	232.6		15	315.4	

Abbreviations: GM = Geometric mean.
[a]modeled with general linear regression; adjusted for age, study center, race and time between CA125 to diagnosis (≤30days, >30days, missing).

significance, a Japanese study found risk for "diffuse" type gastric cancer to be increased with possession of the G allele [31]. In tests we did for heterogeneity by histologic type of ovarian cancer, only rs4072037 varied with increased risks for types other than invasive serous including especially serous borderline, mucinous, and endometrioid. In general, all histologic types of epithelial ovarian tumors, both benign and malignant, express MUC1 on the cell surface by immunohistochemistry [33]. However a recent study using gene expression proposed that MUC1 expression is low in one subtype of invasive serous tumors [34].

The *MUC16* gene is located at 19p13, which is altered in a variety of cancers, especially ovarian. In ovarian carcinoma, 19p13 has been identified as the chromosome band most frequently involved in structural rearrangement [35,36]. This region has also been shown to be highly amplified in high grade serous carcinoma [37]. Polymorphisms rs12984471, rs1559168, rs2121133 are tagSNPs and were selected for our study because they are representative of various regions of the *MUC16* gene. The minor alleles of rs12984471 and rs1559168 introduce missense mutations while rs2121133 is within an intron [38]. Polymorphism rs2547065 was selected because it was previously studied in relation to epithelial ovarian cancer [39] and introduces a missense mutation that could potentially contribute to a functional modification of the gene product. Among the *MUC16* polymorphisms studied, we observed associations between rs2547065 and ovarian cancer risk and between rs12984471 and survival.

In a small study that examined two *MUC16* variants including rs2547065, Bouanene et al. observed that the CC genotype was more frequent in cases (49%) than in controls (34%), similar in direction to what we observed but not significant in their study which included only 41 cases and 76 controls [39]. Despite the fact that homozygous variant genotype (CC) of polymorphism rs2547065 was associated with ovarian cancer risk overall and invasive serous ovarian cancer in the NECC data, we were unable to validate this finding in independent data from the Nurses' Health Study. With positive results from our study, supportive results from the only published study related to this SNP, but null results from the NHS, validation will be necessary and is planned within the Ovarian Cancer Association Consortium.

MUC16 polymorphism rs12984471 was the only SNP associated with survival. The variant allele, which conferred poorer survival among all cases, also was correlated with high CA125 serum levels in postmenopausal women, especially those over the age of 65. The possibility that the association between rs12984471 and survival may have a biologic basis is suggested by possible functional consequences on MUC16 protein. Polymorphism rs12984471 is located in the largely uncharacterized extracellular subunit where the C variant is responsible for a conservative missense mutation changing a glutamate to an aspartate [38,40]. Conservative amino acid changes are theorized to confer 40% likelihood of gene function modification compared to a silent mutation [41]. Thus, it is plausible that the missense mutations caused by this polymorphism could influence the function of the *MUC16* gene product as suggested by its effects on CA125 levels in cases.

In conclusion, our study examined four SNPs in *MUC16* (CA125) and three SNPs in *MUC1* (CA15.3) in relation to ovarian cancer risk and survival in the New England Case-Control study.

One of four *MUC16* SNPs, rs2547065, was associated with increased risk for ovarian cancer. A different *MUC16* SNP, rs12984471, was associated with survival and also correlated with serum levels of CA125. Of the three *MUC1* SNPs studied, we found one, rs4072037, which displayed significant heterogeneity by histologic type. We had the opportunity to examine one of these findings, rs2547065 with increased risk, in data from the Nurse's Health Study. The finding was not validated raising the issue of chance in explaining our findings. However, the association of rs12984471 in *MUC16* with survival has some biologic support in that it is also correlated with CA125 levels. Since our study population is composed of primarily Caucasian women, we were not able to generalize our results to other ethnicities. Our study should not be considered definitive because we targeted SNPs as opposed to conducting a comprehensive gene or genome wide investigation. Evaluation of a broader set of tagging SNPs is planned in the Ovarian Cancer Association Consortium.

Supporting Information

Methods S1 Supplementary methods on age and histologic type classification, statistical models, and SNP selection and genotyping.

Acknowledgments

We would like to thank the participants and staff of the NHS and NHSII cohorts for their valuable contributions as well as the following state cancer registries for their help: AL, AZ, AR, CA, CO, CT, DE, FL, GA, ID, IL, IN, IA, KY, LA, ME, MD, MA, MI, NE, NH, NJ, NY, NC, ND, OH, OK, OR, PA, RI, SC, TN, TX, VA, WA, WY. In addition, this study was approved by the Connecticut Department of Public Health (DPH) Human Investigations Committee. Certain data used in this publication were obtained from the DPH. The authors assume full responsibility for analyses and interpretation of these data.

Author Contributions

Conceived and designed the experiments: DWC KLT. Analyzed the data: KAW AFV KLT. Wrote the paper: KAW KLT SST AFV LJT DWC.

References

1. Hattrup CL, Gendler SJ (2008) Structure and function of the cell surface (tethered) mucins. Annu Rev Physiol 70: 431–457.
2. Bast RC, Jr., Klug TL, St John E, Jenison E, Niloff JM, et al. (1983) A radioimmunoassay using a monoclonal antibody to monitor the course of epithelial ovarian cancer. N Engl J Med 309: 883–887.
3. Buller RE, Berman ML, Bloss JD, Manetta A, DiSaia PJ (1992) Serum CA125 regression in epithelial ovarian cancer: correlation with reassessment findings and survival. Gynecol Oncol 47: 87–92.
4. Giuntoli RL, 2nd, Rodriguez GC, Whitaker RS, Dodge R, Voynow JA (1998) Mucin gene expression in ovarian cancers. Cancer Res 58: 5546–5550.
5. Wang L, Ma J, Liu F, Yu Q, Chu G, et al. (2007) Expression of MUC1 in primary and metastatic human epithelial ovarian cancer and its therapeutic significance. Gynecol Oncol 105: 695–702.
6. Theriault C, Pinard M, Comamala M, Migneault M, Beaudin J, et al. (2011) MUC16 (CA125) regulates epithelial ovarian cancer cell growth, tumorigenesis and metastasis. Gynecol Oncol 121: 434–443.
7. Sellers TA, Huang Y, Cunningham J, Goode EL, Sutphen R, et al. (2008) Association of single nucleotide polymorphisms in glycosylation genes with risk of epithelial ovarian cancer. Cancer Epidemiol Biomarkers Prev 17: 397–404.
8. Phelan CM, Tsai YY, Goode EL, Vierkant RA, Fridley BL, et al. (2010) Polymorphism in the GALNT1 gene and epithelial ovarian cancer in non-Hispanic white women: the Ovarian Cancer Association Consortium. Cancer Epidemiol Biomarkers Prev 19: 600–604.
9. Goode EL, Maurer MJ, Sellers TA, Phelan CM, Kalli KR, et al. (2010) Inherited determinants of ovarian cancer survival. Clin Cancer Res 16: 995–1007.
10. Terry KL, Vitonis AF, Hernandez D, Lurie G, Song H, et al. (2010) A polymorphism in the GALNT2 gene and ovarian cancer risk in four population based case-control studies. Int J Mol Epidemiol Genet 1: 272–277.
11. Harris HR, Cramer DW, Vitonis AF, DePari M, Terry KL (2012) Folate, vitamin B(6), vitamin B(12), methionine and alcohol intake in relation to ovarian cancer risk. Int J Cancer 131: E518–529.
12. Vitonis AF, Titus-Ernstoff L, Cramer DW (2011) Assessing ovarian cancer risk when considering elective oophorectomy at the time of hysterectomy. Obstet Gynecol 117: 1042–1050.
13. Tworoger SS, Gates MA, Lee IM, Buring JE, Titus-Ernstoff L, et al. (2009) Polymorphisms in the vitamin D receptor and risk of ovarian cancer in four studies. Cancer Res 69: 1885–1891.
14. Cramer DW, Vitonis AF, Welch WR, Terry KL, Goodman A, et al. (2010) Correlates of the preoperative level of CA125 at presentation of ovarian cancer. Gynecol Oncol 119: 462–468.
15. Skates SJ, Mai P, Horick NK, Piedmonte M, Drescher CW, et al. (2011) Large prospective study of ovarian cancer screening in high-risk women: CA125 cut-point defined by menopausal status. Cancer Prev Res (Phila) 4: 1401–1408.
16. Bon GG, Kenemans P, Dekker JJ, Hompes PG, Verstraeten RA, et al. (1999) Fluctuations in CA 125 and CA 15-3 serum concentrations during spontaneous ovulatory cycles. Hum Reprod 14: 566–570.
17. Takano M, Fujii K, Kita T, Kikuchi Y, Uchida K (2004) Amplicon profiling reveals cytoplasmic overexpression of MUC1 protein as an indicator of resistance to platinum-based chemotherapy in patients with ovarian cancer. Oncol Rep 12: 1177–1182.
18. Wreesmann VB, Sieczka EM, Socci ND, Hezel M, Belbin TJ, et al. (2004) Genome-wide profiling of papillary thyroid cancer identifies MUC1 as an independent prognostic marker. Cancer Res 64: 3780–3789.
19. Myllykangas S, Junnila S, Kokkola A, Autio R, Scheinin I, et al. (2008) Integrated gene copy number and expression microarray analysis of gastric cancer highlights potential target genes. Int J Cancer 123: 817–825.
20. Lacunza E, Baudis M, Colussi AG, Segal-Eiras A, Croce MV, et al. (2010) MUC1 oncogene amplification correlates with protein overexpression in invasive breast carcinoma cells. Cancer Genet Cytogenet 201: 102–110.
21. Bieche I, Lidereau R (1997) A gene dosage effect is responsible for high overexpression of the MUC1 gene observed in human breast tumors. Cancer Genet Cytogenet 98: 75–80.
22. Waltz MR, Pandelidis SM, Pratt W, Barnes D, Swallow DM, et al. (1998) A microsatellite within the MUC1 locus at 1q21 is altered in the neoplastic cells of breast cancer patients. Cancer Genet Cytogenet 100: 63–67.
23. Schroeder JA, Masri AA, Adriance MC, Tessier JC, Kotlarczyk KL, et al. (2004) MUC1 overexpression results in mammary gland tumorigenesis and prolonged alveolar differentiation. Oncogene 23: 5739–5747.
24. Feng H, Ghazizadeh M, Konishi H, Araki T (2002) Expression of MUC1 and MUC2 mucin gene products in human ovarian carcinomas. Jpn J Clin Oncol 32: 525–529.
25. Tashiro Y, Yonezawa S, Kim YS, Sato E (1994) Immunohistochemical study of mucin carbohydrates and core proteins in human ovarian tumors. Hum Pathol 25: 364–372.
26. Palmer AJ, Lochhead P, Hold GL, Rabkin CS, Chow WH, et al. (2012) Genetic variation in C20orf54, PLCE1 and MUC1 and the risk of upper gastrointestinal cancers in Caucasian populations. Eur J Cancer Prev 21: 541–544.
27. Li FX, Yang XX, He XQ, Hu NY, Wu YS, et al. (2012) Association of 10q23 with colorectal cancer in a Chinese population. Mol Biol Rep 39: 9557–9562.
28. Horimasu Y, Hattori N, Ishikawa N, Kawase S, Tanaka S, et al. (2012) Different MUC1 gene polymorphisms in German and Japanese ethnicities affect serum KL-6 levels. Respir Med 106: 1756–1764.
29. Ng W, Loh AX, Teixeira AS, Pereira SP, Swallow DM (2008) Genetic regulation of MUC1 alternative splicing in human tissues. Br J Cancer 99: 978–985.
30. Marin F, Bonet C, Munoz X, Garcia N, Pardo ML, et al. (2012) Genetic variation in MUC1, MUC2 and MUC6 genes and evolution of gastric cancer precursor lesions in a long-term follow-up in a high-risk area in Spain. Carcinogenesis 33: 1072–1080.
31. Saeki N, Saito A, Choi IJ, Matsuo K, Ohnami S, et al. (2011) A functional single nucleotide polymorphism in mucin 1, at chromosome 1q22, determines susceptibility to diffuse-type gastric cancer. Gastroenterology 140: 892–902.
32. Shi Y, Hu Z, Wu C, Dai J, Li H, et al. (2011) A genome-wide association study identifies new susceptibility loci for non-cardia gastric cancer at 3q13.31 and 5p13.1. Nat Genet 43: 1215–1218.
33. Feng H, Ghazizadeh M, Konishi H, Araki T (2002) Expression of MUC1 and MUC2 mucin gene products in human ovarian carcinomas. Japanese journal of clinical oncology 32: 525–529.
34. Tothill RW, Tinker AV, George J, Brown R, Fox SB, et al. (2008) Novel molecular subtypes of serous and endometrioid ovarian cancer linked to clinical outcome. Clin Cancer Res 14: 5198–5208.

35. Pejovic T, Heim S, Mandahl N, Baldetorp B, Elmfors B, et al. (1992) Chromosome aberrations in 35 primary ovarian carcinomas. Genes Chromosomes Cancer 4: 58–68.
36. Thompson FH, Liu Y, Emerson J, Weinstein R, Makar R, et al. (1994) Simple numeric abnormalities as primary karyotype changes in ovarian carcinoma. Genes Chromosomes Cancer 10: 262–266.
37. Micci F, Weimer J, Haugom L, Skotheim RI, Grunewald R, et al. (2009) Reverse painting of microdissected chromosome 19 markers in ovarian carcinoma identifies a complex rearrangement map. Genes Chromosomes Cancer 48: 184–193.
38. Sherry ST, Ward MH, Kholodov M, Baker J, Phan L, et al. (2001) dbSNP: the NCBI database of genetic variation. Nucleic Acids Res 29: 308–311.
39. Bouanene H, Hadj Kacem H, Ben Fatma L, Ben Limem H, Ben Ahmed S, et al. (2011) Polymorphisms in the MUC16 gene: potential implication in epithelial ovarian cancer. Pathol Oncol Res 17: 295–299.
40. Carraway KL, Hull SR (1989) O-glycosylation pathway for mucin-type glycoproteins. Bioessays 10: 117–121.
41. Tabor HK, Risch NJ, Myers RM (2002) Candidate-gene approaches for studying complex genetic traits: practical considerations. Nat Rev Genet 3: 391–397.

First In-Mouse Development and Application of a Surgically Relevant Xenograft Model of Ovarian Carcinoma

Øystein Helland[1,2], Mihaela Popa[3], Olav K. Vintermyr[4,5], Anders Molven[4,5], Bjørn Tore Gjertsen[2,6], Line Bjørge[1,2], Emmet McCormack[2,6]*

1 Department of Obstetrics and Gynecology, Haukeland University Hospital, Bergen, Norway, 2 Department of Clinical Science, University of Bergen, Bergen, Norway, 3 KinN Therapeutics, Bergen, Norway, 4 The Gade Laboratory for Pathology, Department of Clinical Medicine, University of Bergen, Bergen, Norway, 5 Department of Pathology, Haukeland University Hospital, Bergen, Norway, 6 Department of Medicine, Hematology Section, Haukeland University Hospital, Bergen, Norway

Abstract

Purpose: Preclinical models of epithelial ovarian cancer have not been exploited to evaluate the clinical standard combination therapy of surgical debulking with follow-up chemotherapy. As surgery is critical to patient survival, here we establish a combined surgical/chemotherapy xenograft model of epithelial ovarian cancer and demonstrate its translational relevance.

Experimental Design: SKOV-3^{luc+} ovary cancer cells were injected topically into the ovaries of immunodeficient mice. Disease development and effect of clinical standard treatment including hysterectomy, bilateral salpingoophorectomy and removal of metastasis with follow up chemotherapy (carboplatin 12 mg/kg + paclitaxel 15 mg/kg) was evaluated by clinical parameters. Tumor burden was quantified by bioluminescence imaging (BLI).

Results: The xenograft ovarian tumors developed were poorly differentiated and multicystic and the disease disseminated into the peritoneal cavity. When compared to the controls with a mean survival time of 4.9 weeks, mice treated with surgery and chemotherapy, surgery or chemotherapy demonstrated significantly improved mean survival of 16.1 weeks ($p = 0.0008$), 12.7 weeks ($p = 0.0008$), or 10.4 weeks ($p = 0.008$), respectively.

Conclusion: Combined surgical intervention and adjuvant chemotherapy was demonstrated for the first time in an orthotopic xenograft model of ovarian cancer. Similar to observation in human studies the combined approach resulted in the longest medial survival time, advocating application of this strategy in future preclinical therapeutic development for this disease.

Editor: Viji Shridhar, Mayo Clinic College of Medicine, United States of America

Funding: This study has been supported by the Norwegian Cancer Society, Western Health Board of Norway, Bergen Research Foundation and MedViz (www.medviz.uib.no), a medical imaging and visualization R&D cluster in Western Norway founded by Haukeland University Hospital, University of Bergen, and Christian Michelsen Research. The funders had no role in study design, data collection and analysis, decision to publish, or preparation of the manuscript.

Competing Interests: Mihaela Popa is a fully paid employee of KinN Therapeutics AS, and both Emmet McCormack and Bjørn Tore Gjertsen own shares in the same company. KinN Therapeutics AS has no intellectual property rights or ownership of the model system or any of the described methodology in the paper. The work described in this paper was collaborative, with KinN Therapeutics AS gaining no financial payment or incentive for the work. At time of publication shareholders in KinN Therapeutics AS have never received payment or dividend.

* E-mail: Emmet.Mc.Cormack@med.uib.no

Introduction

Epithelial ovarian cancer (EOC) represents about 5% of all cancers in females worldwide and is the leading cause of neoplasm-related deaths among gynecological diseases in the Western world [1]. Debulking surgery is the cornerstone in EOC treatment with the aim of maximum cytoreduction [2,3]. First-line adjuvant chemotherapy, a combination of platinum-paclitaxel, yields response rates above 80%, including 40–60% complete responses, and improve both overall and progression free survival in all patient subgroups [4,5]. However, most patients will later relapse and succumb to their disease due to innate or acquired drug resistance [6]. Despite improvement of surgical techniques and chemotherapeutic regimens, the overall 5-year survival rate is still below 45% [1]. New strategies, including improvement of today's standards of care, substantiated in relevant preclinical models are critical should survival rates be improved.

Preclinical evaluation of therapy in ovarian cancer has been predominantly performed in murine experimental models [7–9]. The syngeneic, genetically engineered mouse models (GEMM) and xenograft systems described mimic different aspects of the complexity of EOC [10]. Whereas an intact immune system in syngeneic models allows evaluation of host-tumor interactions [11], GEMM have their greatest application in unravelling the molecular basis of disease. However, a caveat in the application of

GEMM relates to the relative indiscriminate nature of the genetic insertion process, which may often result in unrepresentative models of EOC. Moreover, syngeneic models are not human disease. Subsequently, results gleaned from preclinical drug screening in such systems may have questionable clinical relevance [10]. As such, xenograft EOC models of defined human cell lines are possibly a more ideal approach to study the chemo-sensitivity of both cytotoxic therapeutics and targeted agents [10,12]. Generally, xenograft models of EOC have exploited the subcutaneous and intraperitoneal routes, owing primarily to the simplicity and ease of both inoculations of cells and to monitor therapeutic intervention. Inoculation of human cells or cell lines into orthotopic sites may nevertheless be clinically more relevant as they also replicate the early stages of tumor development [8,10,13,14].

Bioluminescence imaging (BLI) has an important role in both therapeutic and molecular imaging of orthotopic xenografts of EOC [15–17]. However, despite advances in orthotopic xenograft model development and progression of preclinical imaging techniques of immunodeficient hosts [18], surgical intervention, i.e. the backbone of clinical therapeutic regimes in ovarian cancer [2,19], has not been applied in a preclinical setting. Preclinical orthotopic xenografts have thus far exclusively been used to analyze the effect of cytostatics and new therapeutics [5,20]. Therefore, the objective of this study was to evaluate surgical intervention together with a standard adjuvant chemotherapy regimen in a preclinical orthotopic xenograft model.

To achieve this we established a bioluminescent orthotopic EOC model of ovarian cancer based on the SKOV-3 cell line expressing luciferase. Xenografts disseminated into the peritoneal cavity and resulted in ascitic fluid formation analogous to what detected de novo in EOC patients. Primary tumor tissues detected by BLI were surgical removed and the effect of surgical intervention alone and/or in combination with intraperitoneal carboplatin-paclitaxel adjuvant chemotherapy in an EOC mouse model was demonstrate for the very first time.

Materials and Methods

Cell lines and reagents

The human ovarian adenocarcinoma cell line SKOV-3 (ATCC HTB-77) was obtained from American Type Culture Collection (ATCC, Manassas, VA, USA). The cells were cultivated in Dulbecco's modified Eagle's medium (DMEM; Gibco, Paisley, UK) supplemented with 10% heat-inactivated fetal calf serum (FCS; Gibco), 2 mM L-glutamine (Gibco) and penicillin 100 IU/ml and 100 µg/ml streptomycin (Gibco) at 37°C in a humidified atmosphere with 5% CO_2. Cells were grown in 75 cm^2 cell culture flasks (Costar, Cambridge, MA, USA) and subcultured twice a week. Suspensions of the cells were obtained by washing the cells twice with 10% phosphate buffered saline (PBS; Dulbecco's tablets, Oxoid Limited, Hampshire, UK) and incubating the cell cultures with Trypsin EDTA (Gibco). Thereafter, the cells were washed in growth medium, resuspended or snap-frozen for later thawing and reuse [21].

Retroviral transfection of SKOV-3 cells

SKOV-3 clones stably expressing luciferase, denoted SKOV-3^{luc+} were engineered using the luciferase expressing construct, L192, coding for the luciferase enzyme and co-transduced with the tetracycline-regulated transactivator (tTA) which has a promoter localized upstream of L192 that drive the expression of the luciferase enzyme. Retroviral infection was performed as described earlier [22]. L192 has a puromycine resistance gene, and after two passages the cells were selected with puromycine 2 µg/ml. (Sigma-Aldrich, Oslo, Norway, stock: 25 µg/µl diluted in 0.9% sterile NaCl). Before injecting the transfected cells into animals, luciferase expression was tested. 10 µl D-luciferin (Promega, Madison, WI, USA, 150 µg/µl) was added 10 minutes prior to optical imagine to 100 µl cell suspensions containing 1×10^5 cells in a 96-well plate (Costar).

DNA fingerprinting

For DNA fingerprinting, genomic DNA was isolated from primary SKOV-3 cells, the SKOV-3^{luc+} cells and xenografted SKOV-3^{luc+} by the Tissue DNA kit (EZNA OMEGA Bio-tek, Norcross, GA USA, Cat.no. D3396-02) according to the manufacturer's protocol for purification of total DNA from cells. DNA concentration was determined by a Powerwave spectrophotometer by OD readings at 260 nm. The AmpFlSTR Profiler Plus PCR Amplification Kit (Applied Biosystems, Foster City, CA, USA) was employed according to the manufacturer's protocol using 1.25 ng DNA, 25 µl reaction volume and 28 amplification cycles. This kit amplifies nine tetranucleotide short tandem repeat loci and the amelogenin locus in a single reaction. Samples were run and allele sizes interpreted on an ABI 3100 Genetic Analyzer with Gene Mapper v3.7 software (both from Applied Biosystems) [23].

Histology and immunhistochemistry

For histopathological examination, tissue sections (4 µm) were stained with hematoxylin and eosin (H&E) before they were examined by an experienced pathologist (OKM). The immunohistochemistry (IHC) staining was performed on formalin-fixed and paraffin-embedded ovarian tumor tissue sectioned at 4 µm thickness. After de-paraffination in xylene and rehydration through graded ethanol series and distilled water solution, the tissues were subjected to heat-induced epitope retrieval undertaken in TRS (Target Retrieval Solution), pH 9.9 (DakoCytomation, Copenhagen, Denmark, S3307) or citrate buffer (pH = 6.0) by the use of microwave oven at 350 W for 15 minutes. Proteinase K (Dako) endogen peroxidase activity was blocked with 0.3% peroxidase (Dako) for 5 minutes. The sections were incubated with the following primary antibodies in room temperature for 30 minutes: Monoclonal Mouse Anti-Human Cytokeratin, clone MNF116, Monoclonal Mouse Anti-Human Vimentin, clone V9, Monoclonal Mouse Anti-Human Epithelial Antigen, clone Ber-EP4, Anti-Human Wilms Tumor 1 (WT1) Protein, clone 6F-H2 (Dako, Glostrup, Denmark) and Monoclonal Mouse Anti-TAG-72, clone B72.3 (BioGenex, Fremont, USA). The staining was performed using a DAKO autostainer using the EnVision (DAKO 5007) as secondary antibody for 30 minutes for all primary antibodies. Diaminobenzine, DAB was used as chromogen for 10 minutes in development of all antibodies. Sections were counterstained with hematoxylin (Dako S3301 for 3 minutes, dehydrated and mounted in Eukitt (O. Kindler GmbH & Co, Freiburg, Germany). Negative control sections underwent the same procedure but without including primary antibody. Human tissue from high-grade serous ovarian carcinoma with known reactivity to the selected markers was used as positive control.

Animals

The protocol for animal studies was approved by the Norwegian State Commission for Laboratory Animals (ID 3417) and the experiments were performed according to the European Convention for the Protection of Vertebrates Used for Scientific Purposes. Female NSG mice (6–8 weeks old; Vivarium, University of Bergen) were maintained under defined flora conditions in individually ventilated (HEPA-filtered air) sterile microisolator

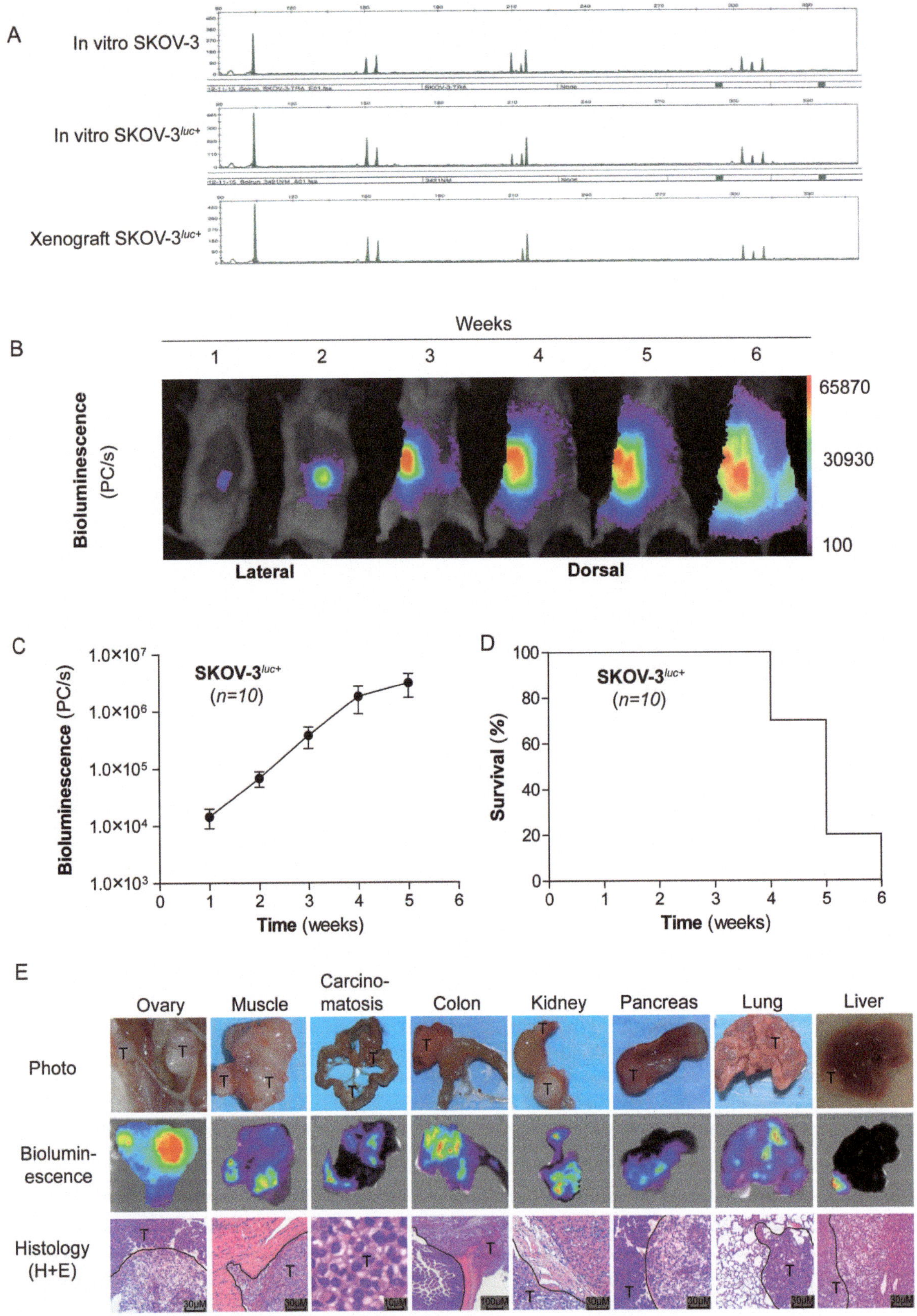

Figure 1. Characterization of the experimental *in vivo* mouse model. (**A**), DNA fingerprinting illustrating unique shared microsatellite DNAs between native SKOV-3, mutant SKOV-3^{luc+}, and *in vivo* xenografted SKOV-3^{luc+} cells. (**B**), Illustration of *in vivo* bioluminescence imaging of orthotopic SKOV-3^{luc+} cells from one representative untreated control mouse. (**C**), Relative mean tumor growth vs time as determined by bioluminescence

image analysis. (**D**), Kaplan-Meier survival curve for untreated xenografted mice (n = 10). E, Illustrations of tumor manifestations in various organs in surgical specimens (photographs), by bioluminescence imaging (BLI), and morphology (H+E). Tumors are denominated "T." Tumor delineation against normal tissue is indicated by dashed line on H-E staining.

cages (Techniplast, Buguggiate, Italy) at the University of Bergen's animal facility. No more than five mice were in each individually ventilated cage that was kept on a 12 hr dark/night schedule at a constant temperature of 21°C and at 50% relative humidity. Bedding and cages were autoclaved and changed twice per month. The mice had continuous supply of sterile water and food and were monitored daily by the same personnel for the duration of the experiment and weighed three times per week. Under depilation (shaving and depilatory cream) and imaging, mice were anesthetized with 3% isoflurane (Isoba Vet, Schering-Plough, Brussel, Belgium).

Orthotopic ovarian cancer model

Mice were anesthetized with isoflurane 3% and placed on a heating pad in lateral decubitus. The fur was clipped on the left lateral side of the abdomen, from the thoraco-lumbar junction to the iliac crest. Skin was disinfected with chlorhexidine 5 mg/ml, (Fresenius Kabi, Halden, Norway) and 70% ethanol (Kemetyl, Vestby, Norway). A 5 mm incision was made in the skin and abdominal wall, parallel and ventral to the spine, midway and between the last rib and the iliac crest. The ovarian fat pads were exteriorized and the ovaries were held in position facing the surgeon with the oviduct ventral, using a serrefine clamp. The cell suspensions (10 μL) containing 1×10^4 SKOV-3^{luc+} cells, were inoculated inserting the needle (30 gauge) at the junction between the bursa and the fat pad. Before closing muscles and skin with continuous 5-0 monofilament non-absorbable sutures (Ethilon 5-0, Johnson & Johnson, New Brunswick, NJ, USA) the ovaries were put back to the original position. After the surgery the animals received 0.1 mg/kg buprenorphine hydrochloride (Temgesic, Reckitt Benckiser, Berkshire, UK) and were placed in a warm environment until full recovery.

Table 1. Tumor engraftment and tumor progression.

	(%)
Graft take	100
Metastatic incidence	100
Pelvic metastasis	
Bladder	80
Ovary	70
Lymph nodes metastasis	
Para-aortic lumbar	70
Para aortic renal	50
Mesenteric	40
Abdominal metastasis	
Peritoneum	100
Pancreas	80
Liver	60
Kidney	80
Spleen	70
Distal metastasis	
Thoracic	50

Xenograft disease characteristics. Data is derived from 10 xenografted mice.

Surgery (hysterectomy, salpingoophorectomy and debulkment)

Mice were anesthetized in the same manner as for orthotopic injection and were placed in dorsal recumbence with the tail towards the surgeon. The abdominal area was shaved and swabbed with chlorhexidine and ethanol. A 2 cm midline incision was made through the skin, subcutaneous fat, muscles and linea alba. After opening the peritoneum with a scissor the abdomen was explored. Ascites, if present, was removed and staging of the cancer disease in each mouse was performed according to the FIGO system [24]. The ovaries and uterus were then removed. The ovary vein and artery were identified in mesometrium and cauterized close to the ovary on each side using a low temperature cautery, fine tip (Aaron Medical, St Petersburg, Russia). Thereafter, a single ligature with 5-0 silk suture Deknatel; (Silk-Fine Science Tools, Teleflex, NY, USA) was placed around cervix and cervix was cut with a scissor above the ligature before the uterine horns and ovaries were taken out. Any visible metastases in the peritoneum (omentum and mesentery) or adipose tissue were also eradicated. Skin and muscles were closed separately using non-absorbable suture material. The animals were kept under observation until they completely recovered from the anesthesia, and analgesics were administrated if needed [25].

Chemotherapy

In this study, we chose an intraperitoneal route for administration of chemotherapy because it is less demanding to administrate in mice. Moreover, in human studies intraperitoneal delivery has at least the same response rate as the intravenous route and therefore are used more and more in clinical practice [26]. To determine the maximum tolerable dosage (MTD) of carboplatin (Teva, Helsingborg, Sweden 10 mg/ml) and paclitaxel (Fresenius Kabi, Halden, Norway 6 mg/ml), the following different dosages were evaluated. Carboplatin 15, 20 or 30 mg/kg, paclitaxel 12, 16 or 20 mg/kg as monotherapy or combined ($n = 3$ mice per group, total 27 mice) twice weekly for three consecutive weeks (Q2Wx3). Body weight was monitored for 28 days. A combination consisting of carboplatin 15 mg/kg together with paclitaxel 12 mg/kg was found to be the MTD. At the end of study the mice were euthanized.

Design of trial

The mice were randomized into 4 different treatment arms with 6 mice in each group ($n = 6$): (a) control, (b) surgery alone (hysterectomy, bilateral salpingoophorectomy and removement of metastasis if present), (c) carboplatin 15 mg/kg + paclitaxel 12 mg/kg, Q2Wx3 and (d) surgery followed by carboplatin 15 mg/kg + paclitaxel 12 mg/kg Q2Wx3. Efficacy was evaluated throughout the study by BLI.

Optical imaging (In vivo and ex vivo)

10 minutes before optical imaging with an Optix MX2 Small Animal Molecular Imager (ART Inc., Saint-Laurent, QC, Canada). Optix Optiview (version 2.00.01, ART Inc.) the mice were injected i.p. with D-luciferin (150 mg/kg). Whole body

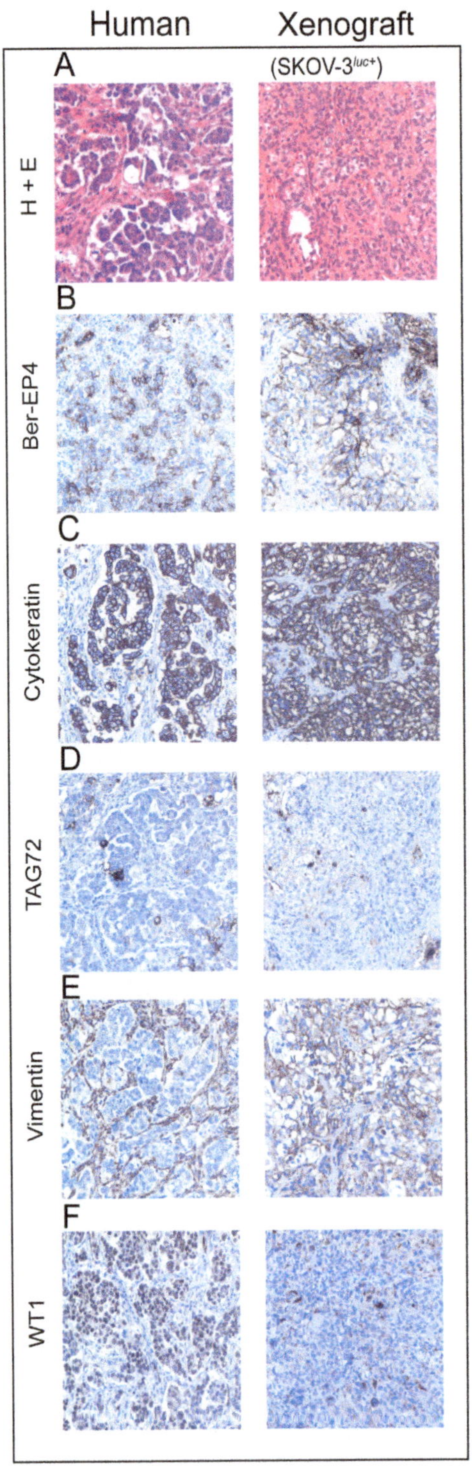

Figure 2. Morphological evaluation of human vs xenografted mice ovarian serous adenocarcinomas. The left column shows a high-grade serous adenocarcinoma from human ovary. The right column shows a mouse with a representative ovarian xenograft derived from human SKOV-3^{luc+} cells. (**A**), Formalin fixed paraffin embedded H+E stained sections of human (left) vs xenografted (right) mice (10× magnification), (**B–F**), Detection of various cancer protein biomarkers (Ber-EP4, cytokeratin, TAG72, vimentin, and WT1) by immunohistochemistry in human (left) vs xenografted (right) mice (10× magnification).

imaging in addition to imaging and examination of single organs removed after euthanasia was performed.

Necropsy

The health status and the weight of the mice were monitored daily and mice were humanely euthanized when moribund as defined by; weight loss >10–15%, lethargy or ruffled fur. The post-mortem examination included macroscopic description of the primary tumor, metastasis and ascitic fluid. All organs were imaged ex vivo to give a further description of metastasis. The tissue biopsies were fixed in 4% buffered formalin and embedded in paraffin before they were processed for histological analysis or snap-frozen in liquid nitrogen.

Statistical methods

Survival data was analyzed using the Kaplan and Meier method. The Mantel-Haenzel log-rank statistics (GraphPad Prism 5.0, GraphPad Software, La Jolla, CA) was used to analyze survival distribution. Survival times are quoted as mean ± standard error of the mean (SEM). Prior to initiation of the therapeutic study, xenografted mice were randomized into groups based on BLI and body weight (i.e. no individual mouse demonstrated >20% differences in either body weight or BLI from group counterparts) and ANOVA performed to ensure that there were no statistical differences between groups. For all statistical analysis, $p<0.05$ was regarded significant.

Results

Generation of stable, high luciferase expressing SKOV-3 cells and DNA microsatellite analysis

To develop a bioluminescent ovarian cancer cell line to permit longitudinal spatio-temporal monitoring of orthotopic xenografts, the ovarian adenocarcinoma cell line SKOV-3 was transfected with a luciferase reporter as previously described [27]. Stably transfected SKOV-3^{luc+} were selected with puromycin. The DNA microsatellite analysis of SKOV-3^{luc+} and wild-type SKOV-3 cells showed identical fingerprint patterns (Fig. 1A). Moreover, a comparison of DNA fingerprints with the data published for the SKOV-3 cell line in the ATCC database (www.atcc.org) established that the cells have the same origin.

Orthotopic xenograft model

To generate a bioluminescent xenograft model of SKOV-3^{luc+} cells, the mice underwent a laparotomy by a 5 mm incision, the ovary was exteriorized and approximately 1×10^4 SKOV-3^{luc+} cells were injected orthotopically into the left ovary of NSG mice. BLI was performed weekly (Fig. 1B). Initially, the bioluminescence was detected only at the injected ovary (week 1) and in the following two weeks disease progression, with infiltration and metastasis to the right ovary, was observed with a log increase in BLI signal (Fig. 1C). Full metastatic dissemination of the entire abdomen and thoracic cavity was observed from week 3 (Fig. 1B). Clinically, at the final week of follow-up, all mice had generated progressive volumes of ascites, defined by weight gain and pallor. The ascites were hemorrhagic and recovered volumes from peritoneal aspirates varied between 0.5 to 4 ml (data not shown). In general, mice orthotopically implanted with SKOV-3^{luc+} cells ($n=10$) exhibited a consistent disease pattern with mice succumbing to terminal disease within 4.9±0.2 weeks (Fig. 1D). Previously, primary patient ovarian cancer samples have been demonstrated to exhibit genetic instability following xenograft in NSG mice, affecting reproducibility of that xenograft system [28]. DNA fingerprinting analysis of xenografted SKOV-3^{luc+} cells from our

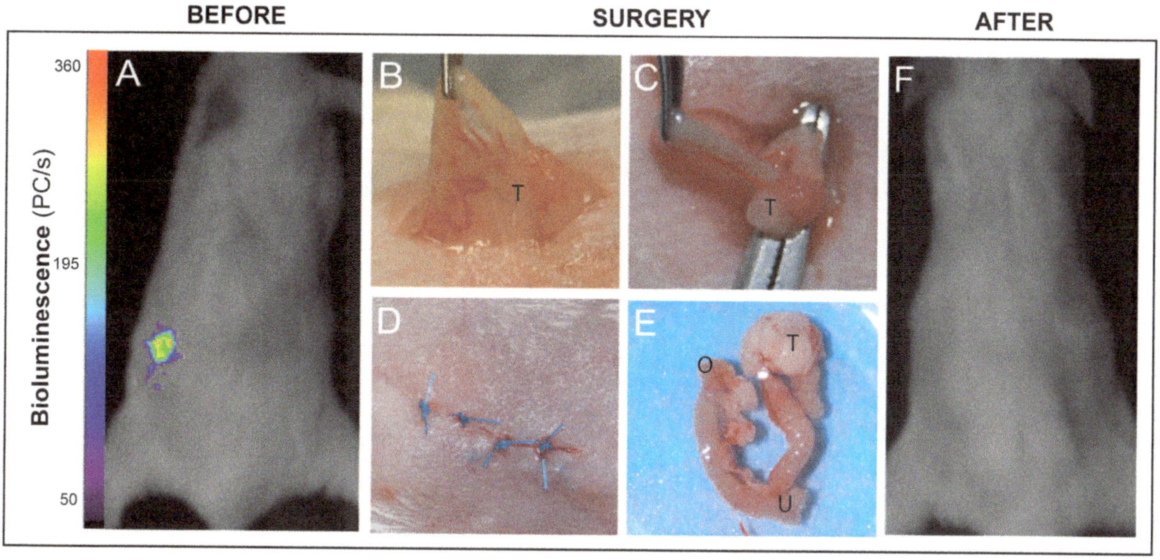

Figure 3. Surgical procedures and monitoring of tumor growth in xenografted mice by bioluminescence image analysis. (**A**), Preoperative bioluminescence imaging of a representative xenografted (SKOV-3^{luc+} cells) mouse (dorsal aspect) with colour bar illustrating photon counts per raster scan point (1 mm^2). (**B–D**), Illustrations of various routine surgical procedures with exposure of right tube (B), ovary (C) and after closure of the incision in the mouse abdominal wall (D). (**E**), Routine surgical resection specimen illustrating uterus (U), ovaries (O) and the ovarian tumor (T). (**F**), Immediate postoperative (dorsal view) bioluminescent negative view indicating apparent complete surgical removal of xenografted SKOV-3^{luc+} cells.

orthotopic model was consistent with the parental and luciferase transfected cell lines (Fig. 1A). At necropsy, a macro-anatomical description and ex vivo BLI analysis revealed not only primary ovarian tumors as anticipated but also extensive local and distal metastasis as described in Table 1 and illustrated by ex vivo bioluminescence imaging, photography and histology (Fig. 1E).

Characterization of orthotopic tumors by histopathology and immunohistochemistry analysis

Histological analysis of the tumor grafts including the metastases showed that the mice had developed a highly invasive growing tumor with markedly pleomorphic nuclei with increased nuclear to cytoplasmic ratios.

Immunohistochemistry analysis of both the xenografts as well as the human tumor tissue demonstrated an epithelial phenotype with positive staining for BerEp4, cytokeratin PAN and TAG-72 (Fig. 2). Only the stroma of the human tumor and not the one in the xenografts showed positive staining for Vimentin and WT-1 (Fig. 2).

Preclinical Surgery and combination chemotherapy in a bioluminescent orthotopic xenograft model of ovarian cancer

The main criterion in development of this novel xenograft model of ovarian carcinoma was to enable therapeutic regimes that incorporated surgical intervention and permitted comparison of chemotherapy and surgery in the same model. Thus, 24 NSG mice were orthotopically implanted in the left ovary with 1×10^4 SKOV-3^{luc+} cells and disease progression monitored by BLI. Following establishment of primary ovarian tumors and prior to identification of metastasis by BLI, mice were randomized into four groups each with six mice per group; (A) control, (B) combination chemotherapy with carboplatin (15 mg/kg) + paclitaxel (12 mg/kg) administered twice weekly and repeated for three weeks, (C) surgery (i.e. hysterectomy, salpingoophorectomy and evident metastasis; illustrated in Fig. 3) and (D) combined surgery and chemotherapy with therapeutic intervention monitored by BLI (Fig. 3 and 4A).

When operated, all mice had developed a tumor localized in the ovary. Most tumors were confined to the injected ovary, but three mice had already developed macroscopic visible tumors in the peritoneal lining in pelvis. According to the staging system of the International Federation of Gynecology and Obstetrics (FIGO) the mice had all stage IA to IIB.

As anticipated, all control mice developed progressive tumor growth and log increase in bioluminescence as previously observed (Fig. 4A). They were moribund within 4.9±0.5 weeks (Fig. 4 A–D). In comparison, mice treated with combination chemotherapy at week 0 and maintained on chemotherapy for three weeks, demonstrated stabilized disease for up to two weeks post-chemotherapy, before relapse to moribund condition within 10.4±1.2 weeks. In contrast, the surgical cohort initially demonstrated absence of bioluminescence in all mice following surgery on week 0. However the recurrence rate was 100% and all mice relapsed to moribund condition in 12.7±2.7 weeks. No significant differences between surgical and chemotherapeutic cohort ($p = 0.70$) was observed. Finally, the cohort treated with debulking surgery followed by adjuvant cytostatics replicated clinical response with the greatest debulkment of disease and therapeutic response. Indeed, overall survival was extended to 16.1±2.9 weeks with one mouse considered cured with no bioluminescence observed even after 40 weeks of follow-up (Fig. 4 A). While all the three treatment regimens showed significant improvement of survival rate ($p < 0.05$) when compared to controls (Fig. 4 C and D), significantly curative treatment was only observed following combination of surgical intervention and cytostatics, replicating the clinical picture in EOC patients.

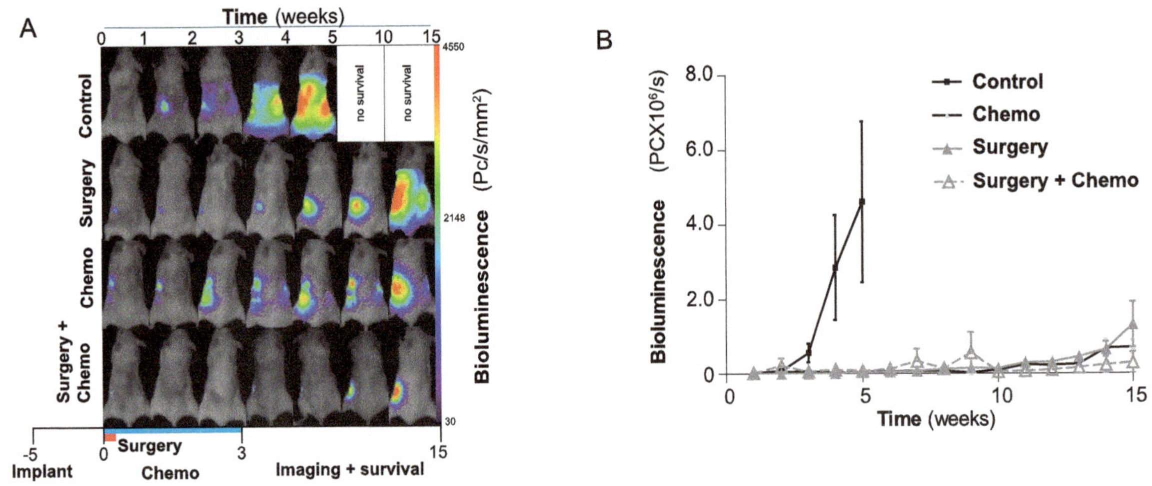

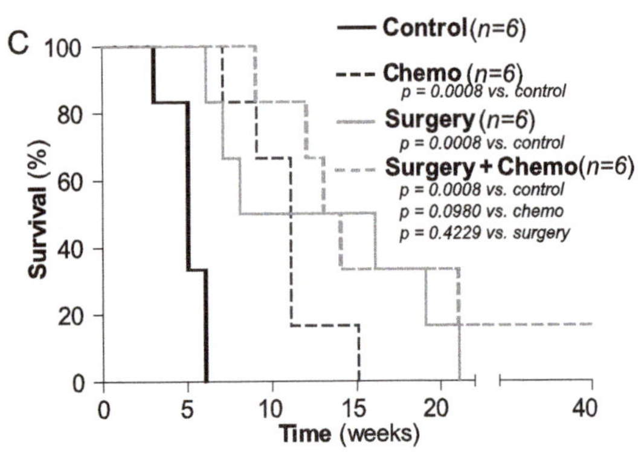

D

	MSW *	EST (%) **	Survivors (n)
Control	4.9	-	0
Surgery (S)	12.7	154	0
Chemo (C)	10.4	108	0
S + C	16.1	222	1

*MSW: Mean survival week
**EST: Extended survival time

Figure 4. Effect of surgical treatment and chemotherapy on survival in xenografted mice. (**A**), Illustration of weekly bioluminescent image analysis of representative xenografted mice in a) control treated, b) surgical treated c) chemotherapy treated (Carboplatin and Paclitaxel) and d) surgical and chemotherapy treated mice. (**B**), Bioluminescence mean signal for the different treatment regimen with time. (**C**), Kaplan-Meyer cumulative survival curves of control, surgery, chemotherapy, a combination of surgery and chemotherapy treated mice. (**D**), Mean survival week, extended survival time (%) and number of survivors (**n**) in the variously treated groups.

Discussion

Despite being the cornerstone in the treatment of ovarian cancer, the effect of surgery has not been evaluated in preclinical models of ovarian cancer and is currently not considered when designing preclinical trials of new therapies. Here we have developed a novel bioluminescent, orthotopic xenograft, surgical model and demonstrate the application and effect of surgical debulking in combination with chemotherapy for the very first time.

Primary debulking surgery is the preferred initial treatment of women with advanced ovarian cancer [29–31]. Within oncology, the aggressive surgical approaches used in metastatic ovarian cancer is unique, and no other malignancies have shown demonstrable advantages of surgery in the setting of disseminated disease [19,29]. Notably, the current preclinical EOC models have not taken this into account. Therefore, we developed an orthotopic and bioluminescent ovarian epithelial xenograft model to explore the potential of surgery in preclinical therapy development. In line with previous studies, we demonstrate that when ovarian cancer cells are injected into the unique microenvironment of the bursal membrane, a tumor xenograft was created [32]. Thereafter the tumor cells disseminated into the peritoneal cavity and a disease similar to what seen in EOC patients was established. (Fig. 1B and 1E) [8,33–35]. As the use of primary patient material in xenografts has resulted in phenotypic heterogeneity and tumour cell instability we decided to use a well-defined cell line and not primary patient material [28]. The histological and immunohistochemical comparison of the xenograft and the human sample were close to identical with the exception of reduced human vimentin staining, reflecting mouse stroma, as previously demonstrated also in primary breast cancer xenografts [36,37]. It is tempting to suggest the SKOV-3 xenograft as representative of a high-grade serous EOC (Fig. 2). However a recent study revealed the genetic profile of the SKOV-3 cells, and other frequently used cell lines, to be different from high-grade serous ovarian tumor samples. This implies that this orthotopic model has its limitations and must be evaluated in this specific context before used in preclinical studies [38]. BLI made it possible to visualise disease progression including metastatic dissemination and development of distal metastasis in liver and lungs (Fig. 1B and 4A), and the intensity of the bioluminescence signal correlated with the tumour load [27,39–41]. We subsequently developed a surgical procedure (Fig. 3) permitting maximum cytoreduction, confirmed by BLI (Fig. 3F). In order to standardise the methodology and surgical procedure used, at the time of surgery all mice were operated at a lower stage of disease than most human patients at their time of clinical presentation [42]. Analogous to what has been observed clinically, surgery was the treatment modality with the greatest impact on the outcome variables (Fig. 4C and Fig. 4D) when compared to chemotherapy [43].

The group of mice treated with debulking surgery followed by adjuvant chemotherapy was, similar to observations in human studies, found to have the longest mean survival time (Fig. 4C) [44]. After maximal cytoreductive surgery, where the primary tumor is removed, there is no evidence of either local or distant metastases in patients. This was illustrated also in our model, both by the macroscopic findings after surgery and by the BLI-analysis performed after the procedure (Fig. 3F). As all mice were macroscopic tumor free after the cytoreductive surgery it was interesting to note the rather large discrepancies in disease development in the surgical cohorts with variation of ± 2.7 weeks. Although we cannot rule out that sufficient cytoreduction was not achieved and also the presence of occult metastases not visible to the surgical team or BLI undetectable, micro-metastasis were the most likely cause of the early relapses. To circumvent this problem clinically, imaging (including MRI and PET/CT) has become an important facet of presurgical planning and postoperative follow-up. More recently, the emergence of fluorescence-based image-guided surgery incorporating a fluorescently labeled biomarker of an overexpressed membrane-bound protein or receptor has been successfully translated to clinical surgery of ovarian cancer [45,46]. Preclinical development of image-guided surgery has also been performed with human cell lines inoculated subcutaneously and within the peritoneal cavity [46,47]. While these models are not an accurate paradigm of human ovarian cancer, the application of our surgical model will now permit the realistic evaluation of image-guided surgery techniques combined with targeted drug therapy/chemotherapeutics prior to clinical translation.

Orthotopic nude mouse models have been developed for ovary carcinoma with surgical implantation of tissue [34,48] but with less infiltrative and invasive growth compared to what is seen in our model. Although inclusion of primary patient cells isolated from ascites is a natural step in the evolution of our orthotopic model, a recent study demonstrates the complications of phenotypic heterogeneity and instability of human ovarian tumour cells [28]. Therefore we suggest that application of our reproducible cell line-based model would be more conducive in therapeutic evaluation.

In summary, we have developed a surgical orthotopic ovarian cancer xenograft model of SKOV-3^{luc+} cells resulting in a clinically relevant metastatic disease of EOC, which could be monitored by BLI. We demonstrate surgical intervention and adjuvant chemotherapy for the first time in a xenograft model of ovarian cancer, advocating this combined strategy for pre-selecting drugs regiment with greatest promise of efficacy in human clinical trials.

Supporting Information

Figure S1 Weight curves generated from a maximum tolerated dose (MTD) study for the combination of Carboplatin (C) and Paclitaxel (P) in NSG mice.

Acknowledgments

The authors thank Edith Fick for immunohistochemistry, Solrun Steine for preparation of DNA fingerprints, Tereza Osdal and Siv Lise Bedringaas for assistance in generating luciferase positive cells and Lene M. Vikebø and Wenche Eilifsen for technical support with animal studies.

Author Contributions

Conceived and designed the experiments: BTG LB EMC. Performed the experiments: ØH MP. Analyzed the data: ØH MP OKV AM LB EMC. Contributed reagents/materials/analysis tools: OKV AM BTG LB EMC. Wrote the paper: ØH MP OKV AM BTG LB EMC.

References

1. Jemal A, Siegel R, Ward E, Hao Y, Xu J, et al. (2009) Cancer statistics, 2009. CA Cancer J Clin 59: 225–249.
2. Mutch DG (2002) Surgical management of ovarian cancer. Semin Oncol 29: 3–8.
3. Zivanovic O, Aldini A, Carlson JW, Chi DS (2009) Advanced cytoreductive surgery: American perspective. Gynecol Oncol 114: S3–9.
4. Ozols RF, Bundy BN, Greer BE, Fowler JM, Clarke-Pearson D, et al. (2003) Phase III trial of carboplatin and paclitaxel compared with cisplatin and paclitaxel in patients with optimally resected stage III ovarian cancer: a Gynecologic Oncology Group study. J Clin Oncol 21: 3194–3200.
5. du Bois A, Neijt JP, Thigpen JT (1999) First line chemotherapy with carboplatin plus paclitaxel in advanced ovarian cancer–a new standard of care? Ann Oncol 10 Suppl 1: 35–41.
6. Agarwal R, Kaye SB (2003) Ovarian cancer: strategies for overcoming resistance to chemotherapy. Nat Rev Cancer 3: 502–516.
7. Kerbel RS (2003) Human tumor xenografts as predictive preclinical models for anticancer drug activity in humans: better than commonly perceived-but they can be improved. Cancer Biol Ther 2: S134–139.
8. Connolly DC (2009) Animal models of ovarian cancer. Cancer Treat Res 149: 353–391.
9. Voskoglou-Nomikos T, Pater JL, Seymour L (2003) Clinical predictive value of the in vitro cell line, human xenograft, and mouse allograft preclinical cancer models. Clin Cancer Res 9: 4227–4239.
10. Ricci F, Broggini M, Damia G (2013) Revisiting ovarian cancer preclinical models: Implications for a better management of the disease. Cancer Treat Rev 39: 561–568.
11. Benencia F, Courreges MC, Conejo-Garcia JR, Mohamed-Hadley A, Zhang L, et al. (2005) HSV oncolytic therapy upregulates interferon-inducible chemokines and recruits immune effector cells in ovarian cancer. Mol Ther 12: 789–802.
12. Morelli MP, Calvo E, Ordonez E, Wick MJ, Viqueira BR, et al. (2012) Prioritizing phase I treatment options through preclinical testing on personalized tumorgraft. J Clin Oncol 30: e45–48.
13. Bibby MC (2004) Orthotopic models of cancer for preclinical drug evaluation: advantages and disadvantages. Eur J Cancer 40: 852–857.
14. Teicher BA (2006) Tumor models for efficacy determination. Mol Cancer Ther 5: 2435–2443.
15. Cordero AB, Kwon Y, Hua X, Godwin AK (2010) In vivo imaging and therapeutic treatments in an orthotopic mouse model of ovarian cancer. J Vis Exp.
16. Ray P, Lewin SA, Mihalko LA, Schmidt BT, Luker KE, et al. (2011) Noninvasive imaging reveals inhibition of ovarian cancer by targeting CXCL12-CXCR4. Neoplasia 13: 1152–1161.
17. Wu R, Hu TC, Rehemtulla A, Fearon ER, Cho KR (2011) Preclinical testing of PI3K/AKT/mTOR signaling inhibitors in a mouse model of ovarian endometrioid adenocarcinoma. Clin Cancer Res 17: 7359–7372.
18. Bankert RB, Balu-Iyer SV, Odunsi K, Shultz LD, Kelleher RJ, Jr., et al. (2011) Humanized mouse model of ovarian cancer recapitulates patient solid tumor progression, ascites formation, and metastasis. PLoS One 6: e24420.
19. Schorge JO, McCann C, Del Carmen MG (2010) Surgical debulking of ovarian cancer: what difference does it make? Rev Obstet Gynecol 3: 111–117.
20. Oliva P, Decio A, Castiglioni V, Bassi A, Pesenti E, et al. (2012) Cisplatin plus paclitaxel and maintenance of bevacizumab on tumour progression, dissemination, and survival of ovarian carcinoma xenograft models. Br J Cancer 107: 360–369.
21. Bjorge L, Hakulinen J, Vintermyr OK, Jarva H, Jensen TS, et al. (2005) Ascitic complement system in ovarian cancer. Br J Cancer 92: 895–905.
22. Lorens JB, Jang Y, Rossi AB, Payan DG, Bogenberger JM (2000) Optimization of regulated LTR-mediated expression. Virology 272: 7–15.
23. Ke XS, Li WC, Hovland R, Qu Y, Liu RH, et al. (2011) Reprogramming of cell junction modules during stepwise epithelial to mesenchymal transition and accumulation of malignant features in vitro in a prostate cell model. Exp Cell Res 317: 234–247.
24. FIGO Committee on Gynecologic Oncology (2009) Current FIGO staging for cancer of the vagina, fallopian tube, ovary, and gestational trophoblastic neoplasia. Int J Gynaecol Obstet 105: 3–4.
25. Nadeau ME, Kaartinen MJ, Lague MN, Paquet M, Huneault LM, et al. (2009) A mouse surgical model for metastatic ovarian granulosa cell tumor. Comp Med 59: 553–556.
26. Teefey P, Zgheib NB, Apte SM, Gonzalez-Bosquet J, Judson PL, et al. (2013) Factors associated with improved toxicity and tolerability of intraperitoneal chemotherapy in advanced-stage epithelial ovarian cancers. Am J Obstet Gynecol 208: 501.e501–e507.

27. McCormack E, Haaland I, Venas G, Forthun RB, Huseby S, et al. (2012) Synergistic induction of p53 mediated apoptosis by valproic acid and nutlin-3 in acute myeloid leukemia. Leukemia 26: 910–917.
28. Stewart JM, Shaw PA, Gedye C, Bernardini MQ, Neel BG, et al. (2011) Phenotypic heterogeneity and instability of human ovarian tumor-initiating cells. Proc Natl Acad Sci U S A 108: 6468–6473.
29. Griffiths CT (1975) Surgical resection of tumor bulk in the primary treatment of ovarian carcinoma. Natl Cancer Inst Monogr 42: 101–104.
30. Hacker NF, Berek JS, Lagasse LD, Nieberg RK, Elashoff RM (1983) Primary cytoreductive surgery for epithelial ovarian cancer. Obstet Gynecol 61: 413–420.
31. Wimberger P, Lehmann N, Kimmig R, Burges A, Meier W, et al. (2007) Prognostic factors for complete debulking in advanced ovarian cancer and its impact on survival. An exploratory analysis of a prospectively randomized phase III study of the Arbeitsgemeinschaft Gynaekologische Onkologie Ovarian Cancer Study Group (AGO-OVAR). Gynecol Oncol 106: 69-74.
32. Shaw TJ, Senterman MK, Dawson K, Crane CA, Vanderhyden BC (2004) Characterization of intraperitoneal, orthotopic, and metastatic xenograft models of human ovarian cancer. Mol Ther 10: 1032–1042.
33. Kiguchi K, Kubota T, Aoki D, Udagawa Y, Yamanouchi S, et al. (1998) A patient-like orthotopic implantation nude mouse model of highly metastatic human ovarian cancer. Clin Exp Metastasis 16: 751–756.
34. Fu X, Hoffman RM (1993) Human ovarian carcinoma metastatic models constructed in nude mice by orthotopic transplantation of histologically-intact patient specimens. Anticancer Res 13: 283–286.
35. Singer G, Stohr R, Cope L, Dehari R, Hartmann A, et al. (2005) Patterns of p53 mutations separate ovarian serous borderline tumors and low- and high-grade carcinomas and provide support for a new model of ovarian carcinogenesis: a mutational analysis with immunohistochemical correlation. Am J Surg Pathol 29: 218–224.
36. Czernobilsky B, Moll R, Levy R, Franke WW (1985) Co-expression of cytokeratin and vimentin filaments in mesothelial, granulosa and rete ovarii cells of the human ovary. Eur J Cell Biol 37: 175–190.
37. DeRose YS, Wang G, Lin YC, Bernard PS, Buys SS, et al. (2011) Tumor grafts derived from women with breast cancer authentically reflect tumor pathology, growth, metastasis and disease outcomes. Nat Med 17: 1514–1520.
38. Domcke S, Sinha R, Levine DA, Sander C, Schultz N (2013) Evaluating cell lines as tumour models by comparison of genomic profiles. Nat Commun 4: 2126.
39. Kotopoulis S, Delalande A, Popa M, Mamaeva V, Dimcevski G, et al. (2013) Sonoporation-Enhanced Chemotherapy Significantly Reduces Primary Tumour Burden in an Orthotopic Pancreatic Cancer Xenograft. Mol Imaging Biol.
40. Jarzabek MA, Huszthy PC, Skaftnesmo KO, McCormack E, Dicker P, et al. (2013) In vivo bioluminescence imaging validation of a human biopsy-derived orthotopic mouse model of glioblastoma multiforme. Mol Imaging 12: 161–172.
41. Wang J, Daphu I, Pedersen PH, Miletic H, Hovland R, et al. (2011) A novel brain metastases model developed in immunodeficient rats closely mimics the growth of metastatic brain tumours in patients. Neuropathol Appl Neurobiol 37: 189–205.
42. Yancik R (1993) Ovarian cancer. Age contrasts in incidence, histology, disease stage at diagnosis, and mortality. Cancer 71: 517–523.
43. Bristow RE, Tomacruz RS, Armstrong DK, Trimble EL, Montz FJ (2002) Survival effect of maximal cytoreductive surgery for advanced ovarian carcinoma during the platinum era: a meta-analysis. J Clin Oncol 20: 1248–1259.
44. Piccart MJ, Bertelsen K, James K, Cassidy J, Mangioni C, et al. (2000) Randomized intergroup trial of cisplatin-paclitaxel versus cisplatin-cyclophosphamide in women with advanced epithelial ovarian cancer: three-year results. J Natl Cancer Inst 92: 699–708.
45. van Dam GM, Themelis G, Crane LM, Harlaar NJ, Pleijhuis RG, et al. (2011) Intraoperative tumor-specific fluorescence imaging in ovarian cancer by folate receptor-alpha targeting: first in-human results. Nat Med 17: 1315–1319.
46. Harlaar NJ, Kelder W, Sarantopoulos A, Bart J, Themelis G, et al. (2013) Real-time near infrared fluorescence (NIRF) intra-operative imaging in ovarian cancer using an alpha(v)beta(3-)integrin targeted agent. Gynecol Oncol 128: 590–595.
47. Terwisscha van Scheltinga AG, van Dam GM, Nagengast WB, Ntziachristos V, Hollema H, et al. (2011) Intraoperative near-infrared fluorescence tumor imaging with vascular endothelial growth factor and human epidermal growth factor receptor 2 targeting antibodies. J Nucl Med 52: 1778–1785.
48. Vidal A, Munoz C, Guillen MJ, Moreto J, Puertas S, et al. (2012) Lurbinectedin (PM01183), a new DNA minor groove binder, inhibits growth of orthotopic primary graft of cisplatin-resistant epithelial ovarian cancer. Clin Cancer Res 18: 5399–5411.

21

An mDia2/ROCK Signaling Axis Regulates Invasive Egress from Epithelial Ovarian Cancer Spheroids

Krista M. Pettee[1], Kaitlyn M. Dvorak[1], Andrea L. Nestor-Kalinoski[2], Kathryn M. Eisenmann[1]*

1 Department of Biochemistry and Cancer Biology, University of Toledo Health Science Campus, Toledo, Ohio, United States of America, **2** Department of Surgery, University of Toledo Health Science Campus, Toledo, Ohio, United States of America

Abstract

Multi-cellular spheroids are enriched in ascites of epithelial ovarian cancer (OvCa) patients. They represent an invasive and chemoresistant cellular population fundamental to metastatic dissemination. The molecular mechanisms triggering single cell invasive egress from spheroids remain enigmatic. mDia formins are Rho GTPase effectors that are key regulators of F-actin cytoskeletal dynamics. We hypothesized that mDia2-driven F-actin dynamics promote single cell invasive transitions in clinically relevant three-dimensional (3D) OvCa spheroids. The current study is a dissection of the contribution of the F-actin assembly factor mDia2 formin in invasive transitions and using a clinically relevant ovarian cancer spheroid model. We show that RhoA-directed mDia2 activity is required for tight spheroid organization, and enrichment of mDia2 in the invasive cellular protrusions of collagen-embedded OVCA429 spheroids. Depleting mDia2 in ES-2 spheroids enhanced invasive dissemination of single amoeboid-shaped cells. This contrasts with spheroids treated with control siRNA, where a mesenchymal invasion program predominated. Inhibition of another RhoA effector, ROCK, had no impact on ES-2 spheroid formation but dramatically inhibited spheroid invasion through induction of a highly elongated morphology. Concurrent inhibition of ROCK and mDia2 blocked single cell invasion from ES-2 spheroids more effectively than inhibition of either protein alone, indicating that invasive egress of amoeboid cells from mDia2-depleted spheroids is ROCK-dependent. Our findings indicate that multiple GTPase effectors must be suppressed in order to fully block invasive egress from ovarian cancer spheroids. Furthermore, tightly regulated interplay between ROCK and mDia2 signaling pathways dictates the invasive capacities and the type of invasion program utilized by motile spheroid-derived ovarian cancer cells. As loss of the gene encoding mDia2, *DRF3,* has been linked to cancer progression and metastasis, our results set the stage for understanding molecular mechanisms involved in mDia2-dependent egress of invasive cells from primary epithelial tumors.

Editor: Pontus Aspenstrom, Karolinska Institutet, Sweden

Funding: This work was supported by the University of Toledo Foundation (KME, ALNK), the Department of Defense Ovarian Cancer Concept Award (KME, OC073269), the DeArce Memorial Endowment Fund in Support for Medical Research and Development (KME), and the National Cancer Institute (KME, ALNK R01CA151632). The funders had no role in study design, data collection and analysis, decision to publish, or preparation of the manuscript.

Competing Interests: The authors have declared that no competing interests exist.

* E-mail: Kathryn.Eisenmann@utoledo.edu

Introduction

Ovarian cancer (OvCa) is the 5th leading cause of cancer-related deaths in American women. The American Cancer Society predicts 22,000 new diagnoses and 15,000 deaths from epithelial ovarian cancer (EOC) in 2012. Cells derived from the ovarian surface epithelium account for >90% of primary OvCa and metastatic lesions [1]. Exfoliated OvCa cells are detected in peritoneal ascites as single cells, small aggregates or highly-ordered and compacted multi-cellular spheroids [1–5]. Compacted spheroids are poorly understood invasive and chemoresistant structures. Cell-cell adhesions, supported in part by N- and E-cadherin drive the formation and compaction of OvCa spheroids [6]. It is unclear what specific molecular or environmental cues contribute to invasive transitions in the spheroids.

A growing body of evidence suggests that compact spheroids promote OvCa metastasis within the peritoneal cavity. *In vitro,* cells within OvCa spheroids undergo anchorage-independent growth, disaggregate upon adhering to three-dimensional (3D) collagen-I gels and invade underlying mesothelial cells [7–9]. Importantly, spheroid formation and compaction directly correlate with invasion [3,4]. Human OvCa cells with the capacity to form compact spheroids *in vitro* can generate robust tumors when injected intraperitoneally into immunodeficient mice. In contrast, non-spheroid forming cells fail to form tumors in mice [10]. The apparent connection between the formation of compact spheroids and dissemination of invasive OvCa cells underscores the need for better understanding of molecular mechanisms supporting these processes [11].

In response to extracellular cues, epithelial-derived cancer cells can convert to a mesenchymal-like phenotype. This can be achieved via dissociation of tight and adherens junctions (AJ), detachment of single cells from epithelial sheets or 3D structures, and migration into adjacent tissues (reviewed in [12–15]). Hallmark cellular and molecular changes associated with the epithelial-mesenchymal transition (EMT) and invasion into the surrounding stroma include loss of E-cadherin expression, upregulation of matrix metalloprotease (MMP), activation of transcriptional regulators and adoption of a spindle-like, polarized fibroblastic morphology. During mesenchymal migration, expansion of the leading edge and retraction of the trailing edge of the motile cells involves coordinate regulation of cortical F-actin polymerization and actomyosin contraction. F-actin assembly precedes contraction to promote extension of actin-rich protrusions, and ROCK-mediated phosphorylation of myosin light chain (pMLC) regulates actomyosin contraction [16].

Formins have emerged as key regulators of F-actin and microtubule cytoskeletal dynamics. Formin family proteins are Rho GTPase effectors. The mammalian Diaphanous (mDia)-related formins (mDia1-3) have critical roles in diverse cellular activities, including gene transcription, cell cycle progression, and membrane trafficking. mDia proteins also regulate F-actin networks critical for maintaining the integrity of multi-cellular epithelial structures [17–22]. For example, depletion of mDia inhibits the formation of cell-cell junctions in MDCK cells [23], and disrupts MCF-7 monolayers by mislocalizing E-cadherin away from cell-cell contacts [24]. Furthermore, suppressing Diaphanous, the mDia homologue in *D. melanogaster*, decreased pMLC at AJs and destabilizes normal tissue boundaries and increased cell protrusiveness [25]. Collectively, these data implicate the mDia-Rho signaling axis in the organization of complex 3D structures important for morphogenesis, and potentially, for tumor progression.

Several lines of evidence suggest that formins play conserved roles in regulating cancer cell motility, invasion and metastasis. mDia2 influences the invasive behavior of breast cancer cells, which ultimately depends on MMP and formation of actin-rich protrusions called invadopodia [26]. Interaction of mDia2 with its negative regulator, DIP [27], promotes the transition of mesenchymal MDA-MB-231 cells into highly motile and invasive ROCK-dependent amoeboid cells [28]. Similarly, modulation of mDia2 also affects amoeboid invasion and migration in DU145 prostate cancer cells [29,30]. A related formin, mDia1 directs neutrophil chemotaxis [31,32], cell invasion [33], and T-cell migration and trafficking into peripheral lymphoid organs [34,35]. Other formin family members, including isoforms of FRL, FHOD and Formin1, have also been implicated in regulating migratory plasticity and interconversion between mesenchymal and amoeboid motility in breast and other tumor cells[36–41].

The genes encoding mDia or FMNL/FRL are frequently lost in breast, prostate, colorectal, hepatic carcinomas, and hematopoetic cancers [29,30,41,42]. mDia proteins also function in the normal ovary as well as ovarian cancers. Disruption of *Diaphanous* is associated with premature ovarian failure [43]. Loss of *DIAPH1/DRF1*, the gene encoding mDia1, was shown in a model of OvCa progression [10]. Furthermore, the genes encoding mDia2 (*DIAPH3/DRF3*) and formin 1 (*FMN1*) were downregulated in early to late stage OvCa cells. This was accompanied by disruption in F-actin accumulation and increases in cell deformability [44,45]. Taken together, the foregoing observations suggest a role for mDia-controlled actin dynamics in progression of ovarian disease. It is unclear if changes in the activation state of mDia influence cell-cell adhesions to maintain OvCa spheroid integrity, or if modulation of mDia directs the transitions that underlie cell invasion into the underlying mesothelium.

To explore these questions, we examined the role of Rho/mDia signaling in OvCa migration and invasion. Our results show that a RhoA/mDia2/ROCK signaling axis drives invasive transitions in ES-2 OvCa cells in 2D cultures and a 3D spheroid invasion model. Activation of RhoA was increased during spheroid formation, while suppression of mDia2 disrupted spheroid architecture. In contrast to the effects of mDia2, depletion of mDia1 had no effect on the formation or integrity of spheroids. When mDia2-depleted spheroids were embedded into collagen-I gels, it was possible to enhance single cell invasion through a ROCK-dependent amoeboid transition. These findings demonstrate the interdependence of mDia2 and ROCK for the promotion of invasive transitions in OvCa spheroids.

Results

Spatial localization of mDia proteins in migrating human OVCA cells

We obtained a panel of human OvCa cell lines representing several clinical subtypes, including serous and clear cell adenocarcinomas. Some of these cell lines form compact spheroids (OVCA429 and ES-2) while others form looser honeycomb structures (SKOV3) (Figure S1 and [4]). All of the cell types expressed mDia1 and mDia2, regardless of spheroid-forming ability (Figure 1A).

The OVCA panel was screened for adhesive, migratory and invasive properties (Figure 1, B–D, respectively) to identify a highly invasive, spheroid-forming cell line. SKOV3, OVCA429 and ES-2 cells were equally adhesive on collagen 2D substrates. However, the OVCA429 and ES-2 cells were more migratory and invasive than the SKOV-3 line in response to FBS gradients. Therefore, our remaining studies were conducted with either OVCA429 or ES-2 cells.

The spatial localization of endogenous mDia proteins was evaluated in migrating OVCA429 cells using a Dunn chamber to maintain a stable FBS gradient. Immunofluorescence (IF) was performed after 5 h migration (Figure 1E). Both mDia1 and mDia2 exhibited a polarized distribution oriented toward the FBS gradient within migrating OVCA429 cells (arrow indicates gradient location). mDia1 and mDia2 localized predominantly to the lamellae, as opposed to the F-actin rich lamellapodia, as previously seen in migrating epithelial cells [46]. These results suggest a possible role for mDia1 and/or mDia2 in stabilizing cortical actin pools during OvCa chemotaxis.

Requirement for mDia2 in chemotactic migration in OVCA429 cells

We next asked if mDia protein activity and/or expression were required for chemotactic migration. The distance migrated by transfected OVCA429 cells in a Dunn chamber was quantified by live-cell tracking. Cells were engineered to express either mDia-YFP-fusion proteins alone, or various combinations of control YFP vector and FLAG-tagged proteins. mDia overexpression was validated by Western blotting (Figure 2A). Cells expressing dominant-negative YFP-mDia-FH2ΔN, which interferes with both mDia1 and mDia2-driven F-actin assembly, [34,47,48] migrated poorly relative to YFP controls. Conversely, cells expressing the constitutively-activated mDia2 M1041A [49], in which the autoinhibited state is relieved, exhibited increased migration relative to YFP+3XFLAG empty vector controls. mDia1 overexpression did not alter cell migration relative to empty vector controls. These data suggest that mDia2 autoinhibition must be released in order for effective cell migration to occur. In the next series of studies, the role of mDia2 in chemotactic migration was assessed by seeding mDia2-depleted OVCA429 cells into transwells. While lipid and control siRNA-treated cells robustly migrated toward FBS (relative to serum-free control wells), migration was significantly reduced in the mDia2-depleted cells (Figure 2C). Collectively, these data indicate that mDia2 expression and/or activity is required for optimal chemotactic migration of OVCA429 cells.

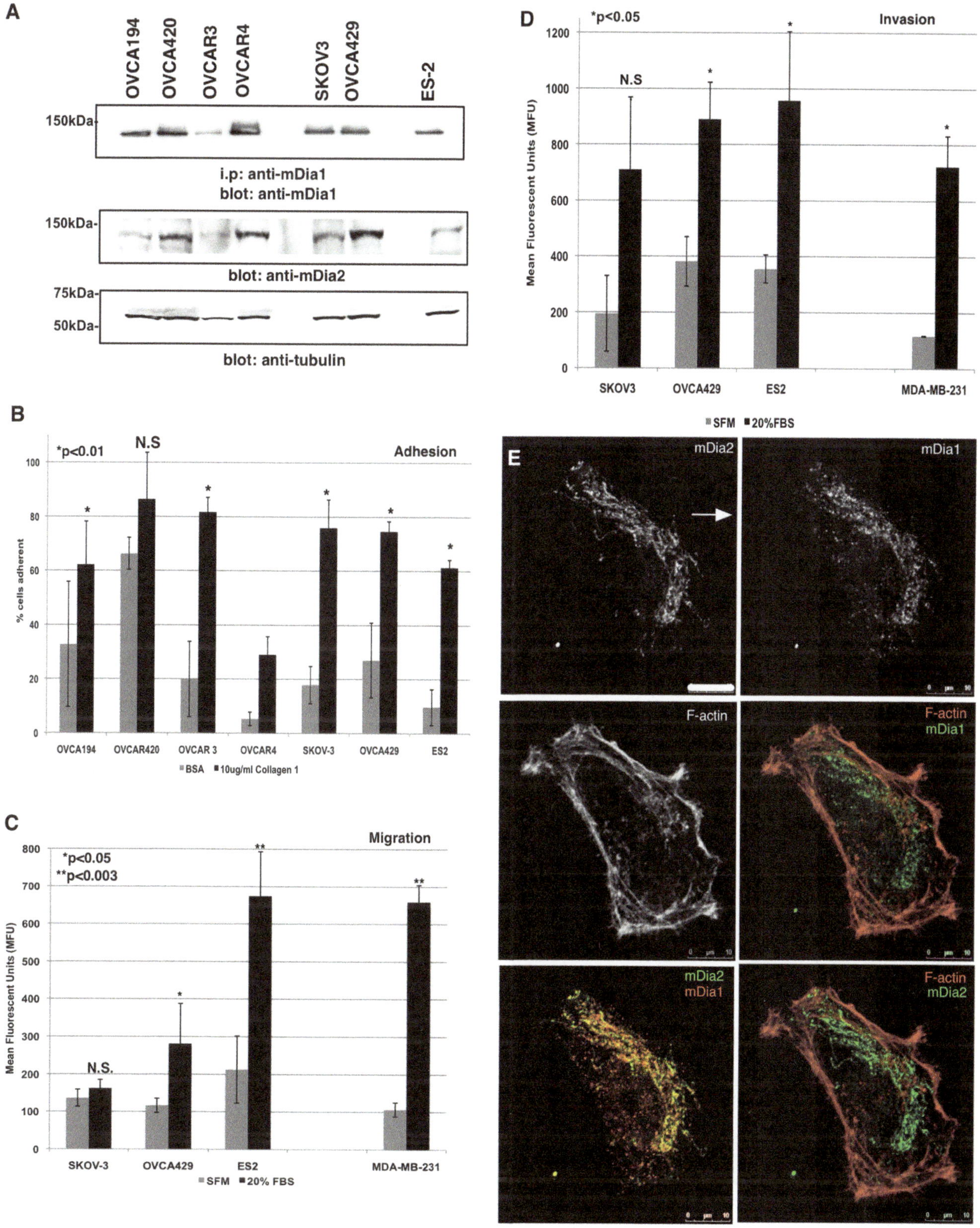

Figure 1. Polarized mDia expression in migrating OvCa cells. A. mDia1 and mDia2 were assessed by immunoprecipitation and/or Western blotting in a panel of human OvCa cells. Tubulin was blotted as a loading control. B. Cell adhesion to BSA- or Collagen-I-coated wells. The experiment was performed in triplicate wells and the experiment was repeated thrice. p values are BSA vs. collagen-I for each cell line. C. Transwell migration assays were performed in triplicate wells and the experiment was repeated thrice for 5 h towards SFM or 20% FBS. MDA-MB-231 human breast cancer cells are a positive migration control. p values are for SFM vs. 20% FBS for each cell line. D. Transwell invasion assays were performed in triplicate wells and the experiment was repeated thrice for 24 h through 2 mg/ml Collagen-I gels towards either SFM or 20% FBS. MDA-MB-231 cells are a positive invasion control. p values are SFM vs. 20% FBS for each cell line. E. OVCA429 cells migrated towards 20% FBS for 5 h in a Dunn chamber. mDia1,

mDia2 and the F-actin architecture were visualized by IF. Arrow denotes direction of the gradient. N.S. = not significant. All error bars correspond to SDs Shown are representative experiments from each assay.

The RhoA/mDia2 signaling axis in formation of compact OvCa spheroids

Rho-responsive mDia proteins can regulate cell-cell contacts and promote single cell motility [18,26–28,49]. We next determined whether the RhoA/mDia2 signaling axis was involved in OvCa spheroid formation. ES-2 cells rapidly formed highly compacted spheroids (Figure S1) and were used for the remaining studies. The requirement for Rho GTPase activity in spheroid formation was tested by exposing ES-2 cells to increasing concentrations (0.5–2.0 μg/ml) of C3 transferase, an inhibitor of RhoA-C. As shown in Figure S2A, C3-treated spheroids were more loosely organized and less compacted relative to vehicle-treated controls. Since previous work has shown that total levels of RhoA are increased in spheroids derived from hepatocarcinoma [50], we next asked if changes in RhoA activity occur in conjunction with formation of ES-2 spheroids. Spheroids were formed from 500 cells within 24 h (Figure 3A). RhoA and expression of its downstream effectors, mDia1 and mDia2 was then evaluated in lysates from cell monolayers and pooled spheroids harvested between 24–120 h. Overall, mDia2 levels declined in spheroids relative to monolayers. Within the spheroid populations, time-dependent differences in mDia2 expression were observed, with slightly lower levels noted in 72 and 96 h spheroids, relative to 24, 48 and 120 h spheroids (Figures 3B and S3A). In contrast to mDia2, the levels of mDia1

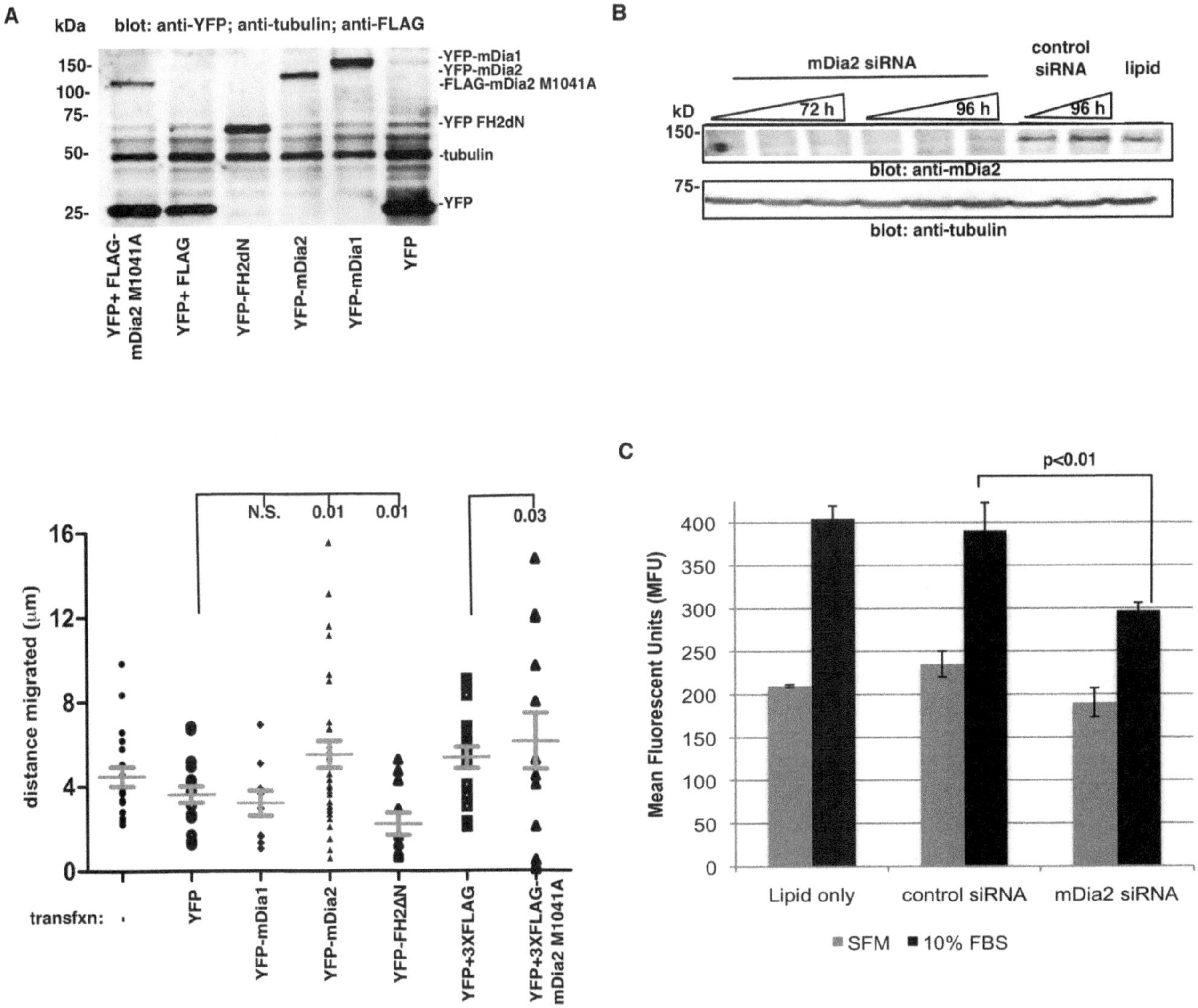

Figure 2. A role for mDia2 in chemotactic migration in OVCA429 cells. A. Transfected OVCA429 migrated for 5 h in a Dunn chamber towards 20% FBS. Live single-cell tracking of transfected cells was performed, and total distance migrated calculated. At least 10 cells were tracked per condition. p values listed are calculated relative to respective empty vector controls. B. OVCA429 cells were transfected with lipid only, control siRNA or siRNA directed against mDia2 at increasing concentrations (25, 50, 100 nM, denoted by wedges) for either 72 or 96 h. mDia2 depletion was confirmed by Western blot. C. OVCA429 cells were transfected with 100 nM siRNA for 72 h, and transwell migration assays performed for 5 h towards a SFM or 10% FBS. The assay was performed in triplicate wells and the experiment was repeated thrice. A representative experiment is shown. p value shown are 10% FBS treated control vs. mDia2-depleted cells. All error bars correspond to SDs for that representative experiment.

were increased in spheroids relative to monolayers. In the spheroids mDia1 declined slightly from 24 h through 120 h (Figures 3B and S3B). Total RhoA levels also declined in spheroids, relative to monolayers. Yet, RhoA levels dramatically recovered at 120 h of spheroid formation (Figure 3B and S3C). Since, the interaction of RhoA with its downstream effectors (such as mDia or ROCK) is dependent on activation by GTP-binding, we next quantified the levels of active GTP-bound RhoA in spheroids by G-LISA. The amount of RhoA-GTP was significantly increased in spheroids formed for 48–120 h compared to unstimulated ES-2 cell monolayers, approaching that observed in monolayers treated with a known RhoA activator, lysophosphatidic acid (LPA) (Figure 3C). Therefore, overall levels of RhoA activation are enhanced upon spheroid maturation.

As a first step toward determining if RhoA-dependent activation of mDia2 might affect the formation of cell-cell junctions, we next asked if mDia2 and F-actin are co-localized in spheroids at cell-cell junctions (Figure 3D). Spheroids formed for 72 h revealed distinct F-actin-enriched cell-cell junctions, with punctate mDia2 underlying/proximal to these junctions (filled arrowhead). In some junctions, mDia2 appeared to co-localize with F-actin (unfilled arrowhead). This suggests a potential role for mDia2 in regulating F-actin dynamics necessary for development or maintenance of cell-cell junctions.

mDia2 depletion leads to the formation of smaller, disorganized spheroids

To further evaluate the role of mDia proteins in ovarian spheroid formation/integrity, we employed an RNA interference strategy. Robust siRNA-mediated knockdown of either mDia2 or mDia1 was validated through 120 h in monolayer cultures, with slight recovery by 144 h (Figure 4A and S4). Spheroids were formed from monolayer cells 72 h post-siRNA treatment. Spheroid diameters were then measured 24–48 h later (96–120 h total siRNA treatment). mDia2 depletion at 48 h resulted in a modest, yet statistically significant decrease (10–20%) in spheroid diameter relative to control siRNA treatment. Similar results were obtained when mDia2 was depleted with siRNA pools or individual siRNA directed against mDia2 (Figure S4), although the suppression of mDia2 expression with pooled siRNA was more consistent and sustained. Therefore, all subsequent studies were performed using pooled siRNA. In addition to the slight decrease in spheroid diameter, mDia2-depleted ES-2 spheroids were visibly less-organized with ragged edges and some single cells loosely attached to the edges. A similar disorganized spheroid phenotype resulted from addition of an mDia1/mDia2 FH2 inhibitor, SMIFH2 (Figure S5) [51]. There results were attributable to mDia2 depletion, as mDia1 depletion had no effect upon spheroid size (Figure 4B,C).

Possible explanations for the slightly smaller size of ES-2 spheroids could include diminished cell proliferation, decreased average cell size, cell detachment or greater spheroid compaction via increased RhoA-directed pMLC2 activity. We therefore determined if RhoA-GTP levels were altered in mDia2-depleted spheroids. mDia2 depletion was validated in spheroids formed for 24–48 h (siRNA treatment for 72–96 h) (Figure 4D). At 96 hrs post-siRNA treatment, RhoA-GTP activity was unaffected in control and mDia2-depleted spheroids (Figure 4E). Consistent with this observation, pMLC2 remained unchanged in cell monolayers (Figure 4F). Furthermore, mDia2 depletion did not change the cellular numbers within disaggregated spheroids (Figure 4G). This indicates that neither cell proliferation nor loss of de-adhered cells was solely responsible for the smaller spheroid size. It also suggests that while the siRNA-mediated depletion of mDia2 causes a more disorganized and irregular spheroid assembly, the remaining mDia2 protein is likely sufficient to sustain both RhoA-mediated contractility and cellular proliferation. The latter concept is consistent with a previous study of mDia1 in T cell activation, where low levels of mDia proteins appeared to be sufficient to sustain some cellular processes (*e.g.*, F-actin accumulation vs. microtubule dynamics), while concurrently impairing other functions [52].

mDia2 depletion enhances ES-2 spheroid invasion via an amoeboid transition

To evaluate whether the RhoA/mDia2 axis functions in spheroid invasion, ES-2 spheroids were embedded in collagen at (T0) and allowed to invade through 168 h (Figure 5A). A rapidly advancing front of invasive cells appeared by 24 h, and gel contraction was extensive enough to rip the gels within 72 h. Spheroid invasion was measured by drawing a region of interest around the perimeter of the invasive front, which encompassed at least 95% of invasive cells (as determined by fluorescence labeling). Invasion depended upon Rho GTPases, as the invasive front was markedly reduced in ES-2 spheroids that were grown and embedded in the presence of C3 transferase, relative to vehicle control-treated spheroids (Figure S2, B and C). Since Rho-directed mDia proteins drive invasion in a variety of epithelial-derived cancer cells [26,29,30], we visualized the spatial localization of mDia proteins in fixed invasive ES-2 spheroids. mDia2 was distributed in a polarized pattern, with enrichment at the spheroid edges where invasive cells emanated into the collagen (Figure 5B). At higher magnification of the invasive front, mDia2 was dramatically localized to elongated structures resembling tubulated endosomes [53], which extended throughout the long protrusions of the mesenchymal cells. Interestingly, mDia1 was mostly nuclear in invading cells, consistent with previous reports for nuclear activated mDia1 directing SRF-mediated F-actin dynamics within the nucleus [54]. We observed multiple cellular morphologies in invasive cells in collagen, including spherical amoeboid cells (~40% invading cells), and elongated, polarized mesenchymal cells (~60% invading cells) migrating in strands (data not shown). Interestingly, invasive spheroids reproducibly (using several primary antibodies of different host and commercial derivations) showed distinct, punctate mDia2 staining within the matrix (Figure 5C, and data not shown). Previously, mDia proteins were detected in pro-migratory OvCa-derived microparticles [55] and mDia2 directed pro-migratory oncosome formation in prostate cancer cells [29]. Biochemical studies are currently underway to characterize the mDia2-enriched extracellular particles present in invading OvCa spheroids.

To evaluate the role of mDia in single cell invasion, we measured the invasive area of embedded mDia1 or mDia2-depleted ES2 spheroids after 0 h (104 h post-knockdown) and 18 h (122 h post-knockdown). Untreated and control siRNA-treated spheroids robustly invaded the collagen matrix within 20 h. However, mDia2-depleted spheroids revealed significantly enhanced invasion relative to controls (Figure 5D and Figure S4C), despite their modestly smaller size upon embedding (Figure 4C). Conversely, mDia1-depleted spheroids invaded to the same extent as control spheroids (Figure S6), indicating that mDia1 does not play a significant role in OvCa spheroid invasion. Because changes in mDia2 expression and/or function associated with amoeboid transitions [27–29], we calculated elongation indices (EI) in the invasive cells derived from the spheroids by dividing the long axis of the cell by the short axis; An EI of 2 or more indicates an elongated mesenchymal shape, while an EI of less than 2 indicates a more prominent rounded, amoeboid

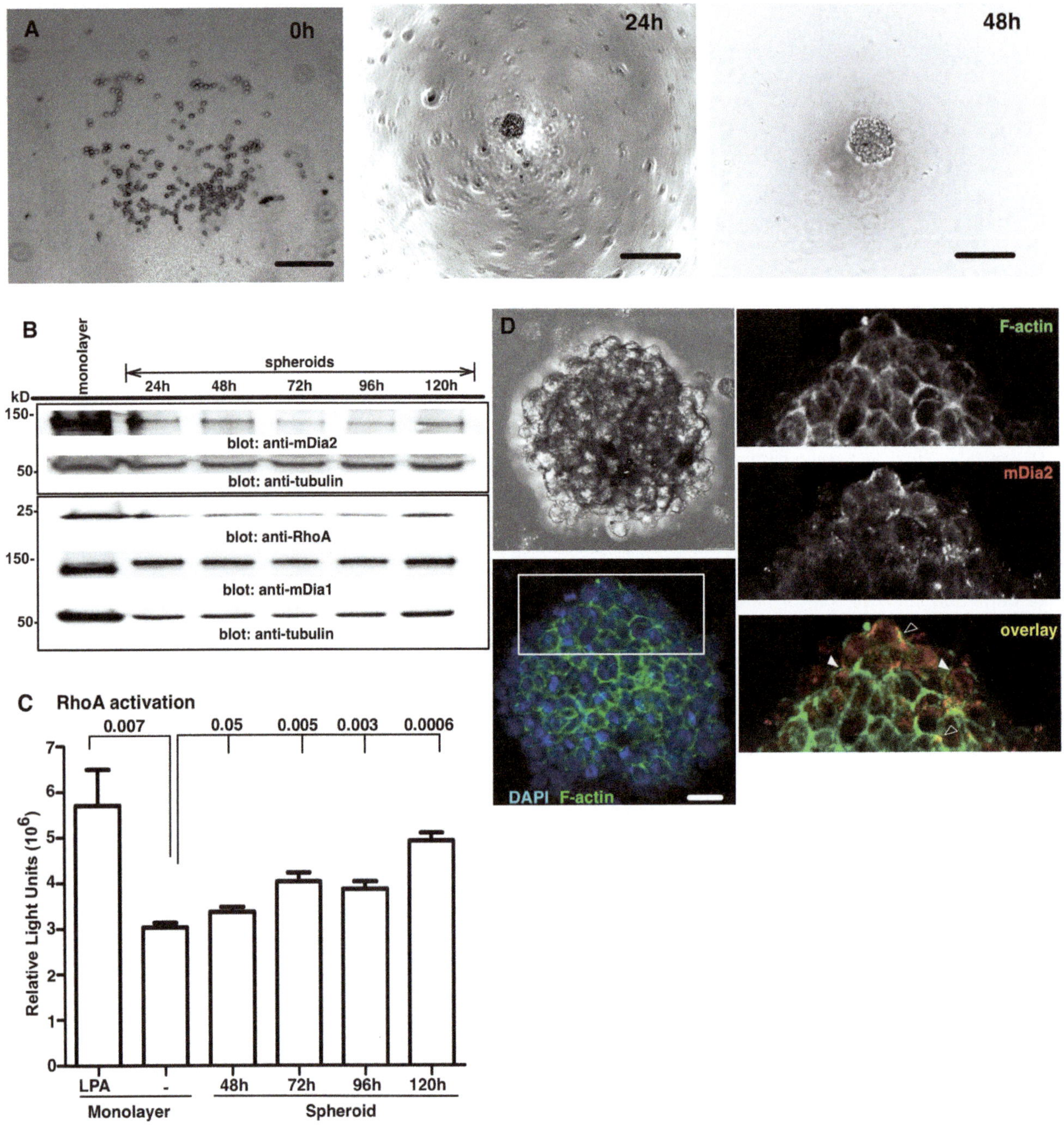

Figure 3. Expression of the RhoA:mDia axis in compacted ES-2 spheroids. A. ES-2 spheroids imaged by brightfield microscopy. Scale bar = 250 μm. (Note: out of focus plate-coating imaging artifact and/or condensation within irregular plastic plates seen here is common to BF imaging). B. Lysates from ES-2 monolayers or spheroids were Western-blotted after the designated times. C. RhoA G-LISAs were performed upon untreated or LPA-treated ES-2 monolayers, or spheroids. p values are relative to untreated monolayer. The experiment was performed in quadruplicate wells and the experiment was then repeated thrice. Data combined from 3 experiments are shown. p values are shown above bars and are relative to untreated monolayer controls. D. Spheroids formed for 72 h were embedded, fixed and mDia2 visualized by confocal microscopy. Images were obtained using a 20× objective with 3D-rendering of serial slices. Bar = 25 μm. Open arrows indicate areas of overlap, while closed arrows indicate a juxtaposition of F-actin and mDia2. All error bars correspond to SDs for that representative experiment, unless noted.

phenotype. The results indicate that in the spheroids where mDia2 depletion enhanced invasion, the invasive cells were predominantly amoeboid in shape relative to untreated and control siRNA-treated spheroids (Figure 5E).

ROCK supports both mesenchymal and amoeboid 3D motility programs in invasive ES-2 spheroids

Amoeboid transitions can involve Rho-directed ROCK signaling to direct contractility [56,57]. ROCK also antagonizes mDia proteins with respect to maintaining cell-cell junctions in 2D monolayers [18]. However, the interplay between ROCK and

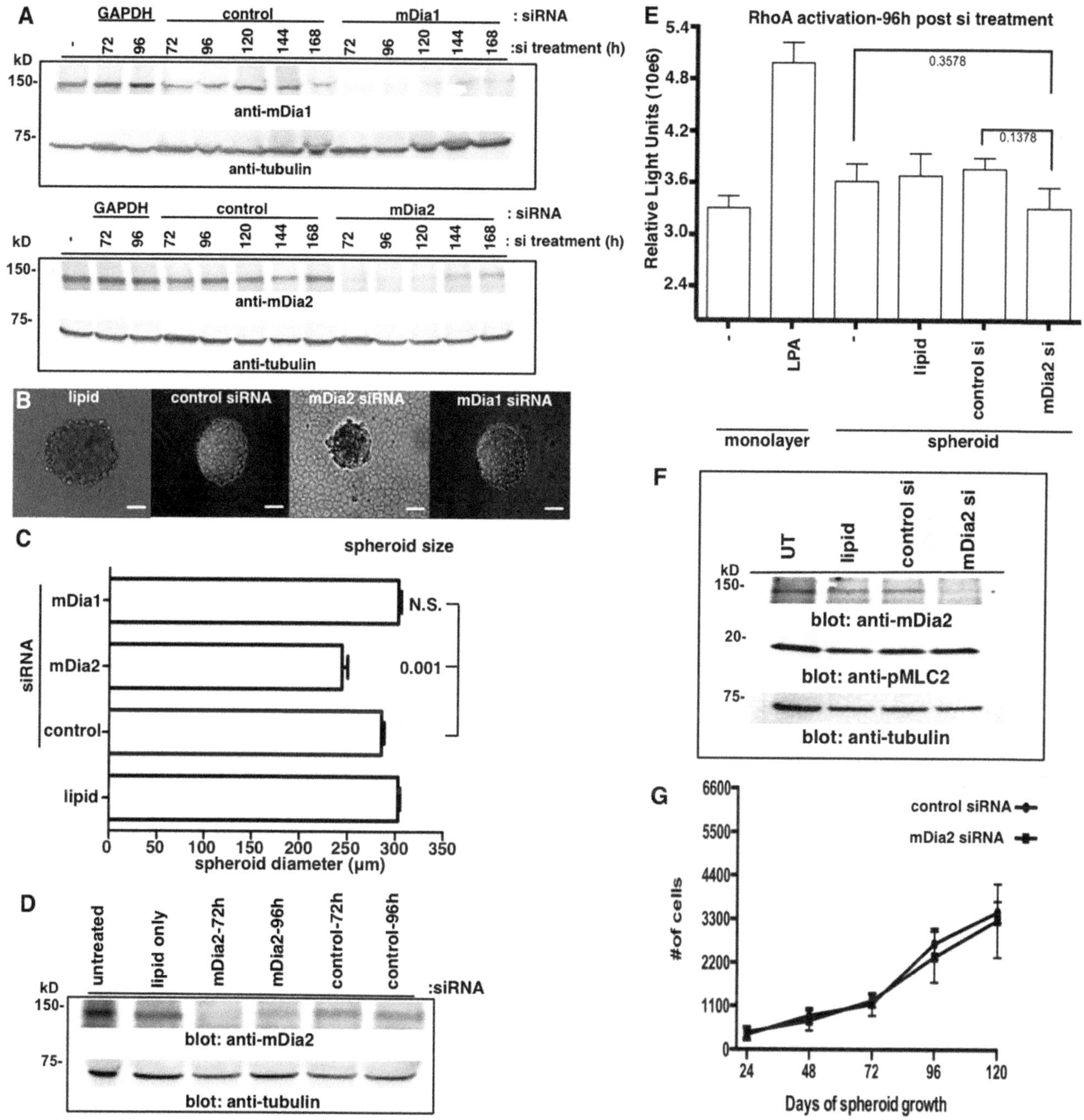

Figure 4. mDia2 depletion induces formation of small, disorganized spheroids. A. siRNA-mediated mDia1 (upper) or mDia2 (lower) knockdowns were performed upon ES-2 monolayers (Note: out of focus plate-coating imaging artifact/condensation within irregular plastic plates seen here is common to BF imaging). B–C. After 72 h post-siRNA or control treatment, spheroids were formed and diameters measured under brightfield microscopy 48 h later (120 h post-siRNA treatment). Bar = 100 μm. At least 30 spheroids were measured for each condition. p values are listed above bars and are relative to control siRNA spheroids. D–E. ES-2 monolayers were untreated or treated with the designated siRNAs for 48 h, spheroids formed for an additional 48 h, and Western blots or RhoA G-LISAs performed upon lysates. LPA is a positive control for RhoA activation. The G-LISA experiment was performed twice, in quadruplicate, and combined data is shown with p values listed to the side of bars. P values are relative to either untreated or control siRNA-treated spheroids, as noted. F. Untreated (UT), lipid only or siRNA-mediated control and mDia2 knockdowns were performed upon ES-2 monolayers for 72 h and pMLC2 levels assessed by Western blotting. G. Control and mDia2 knockdowns were performed for 72 h, and spheroids formed. Spheroids were disaggregated at the indicated times after formation and cells counted. The experiment was repeated 5 times. A representative experiment is shown. Error bars correspond to SDs from a representative experiment.

mDia proteins for maintaining cell-cell junctions in 3D structures such as OvCa spheroids is unclear. We therefore assessed the role of ROCK activity in spheroid formation. We blocked ROCK activity by treating spheroids with the specific inhibitor, Y27632. Spheroid size was slightly reduced through 48 h of treatment (Figure 6A), suggesting that ROCK/myosin-mediated crosslinking of mDia-regulated F-actin may play a role in spheroid formation. Inhibition of ROCK dramatically suppressed spheroid invasion

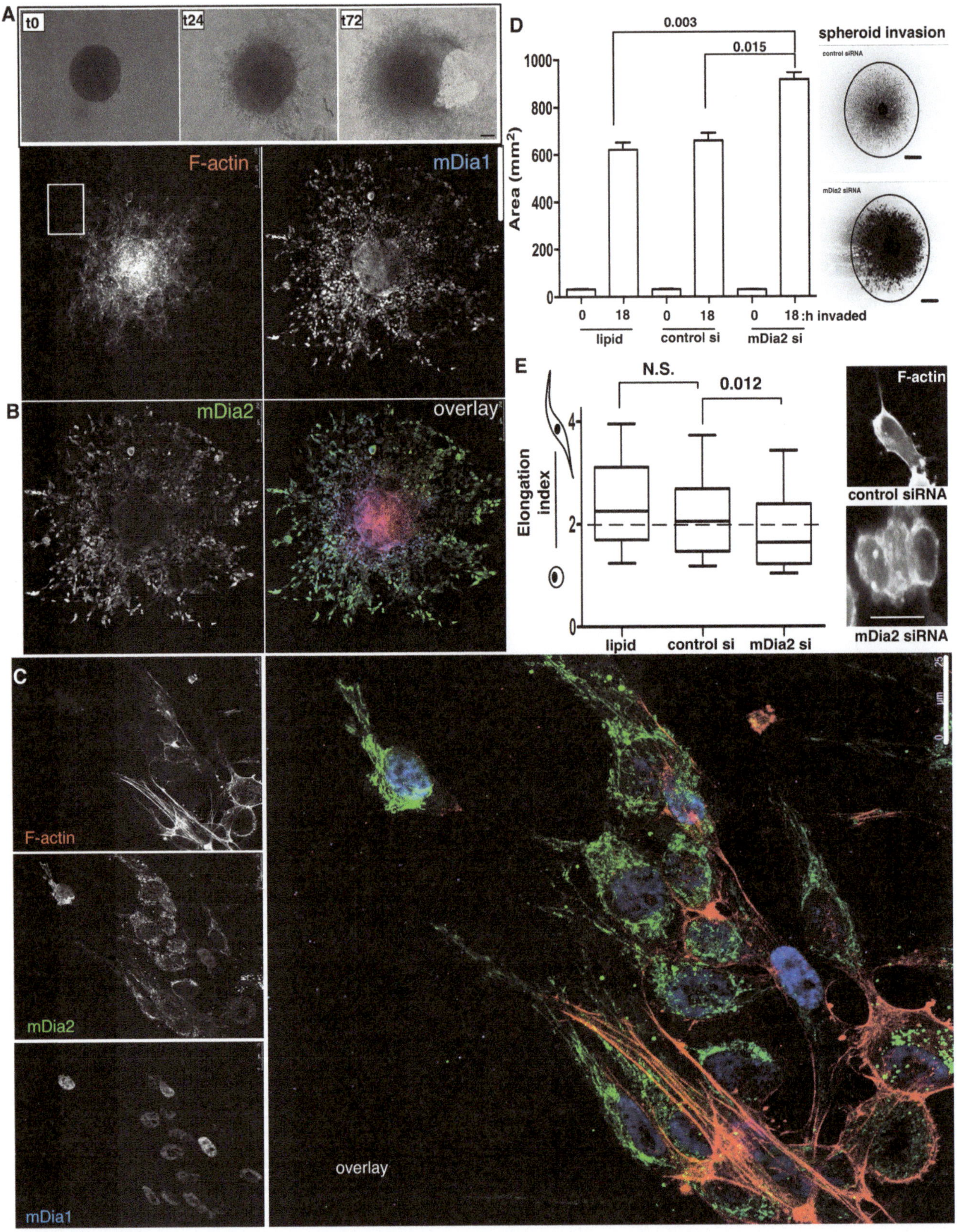

Figure 5. mDia2 depletion drives ES-2 spheroid invasion via amoeboid transitions. A. Spheroids were formed first for 48 h, embedded in collagen-I gels, and imaged by brightfield microscopy after the designated times. Bar = 150 μm. B. Spheroids were formed for 72 h, embedded in collagen I gels and allowed to invade for 24 h. Spheroids were fixed and IF performed for mDia1, mDia2 and F-actin. Bar = 100 μm. C. Higher magnification image (63×) of invading cells from the designated ROI in B. mDia1, mDia2, and F-actin were visualized by confocal microscopy. Bar =

25 μm. D. After 56 h post-siRNA treatment, spheroids were formed and embedded in collagen at 104 h post-siRNA treatment. The area for ROI drawn corresponding to 95% of invasive cells was calculated for 0 and 18 h post invasion (122 h post-siRNA treatment). Representative spheroids at 4X are shown stained for phalloidin and images contrast enhanced. Bar = 100 μm. At least 30 spheroids were measured for each condition. p values are shown above the histogram and are relative to invasion at 18 h for either lipid or control treated spheroids. E. Elongation indices were calculated for invasive cells from D. At least 30 invasive cells were measured per condition. Representative phalloidin staining is shown. Bar = 25 μm. EI> 2 (dashed line) is considered mesenchymal cell type. p values are shown above the plot and are relative to invasion at 18 h for either lipid or control treated spheroids. All error bars correspond to SDs from a representative experiment.

relative to controls (Figure 6B), consistent with prior studies implicating ROCK in blebbing of colorectal [58] and Caov3 ovarian cancer monolayer cells [59]. A strikingly exaggerated mesenchymal transition predominated in the few cells populating the modest invasive front in cells treated with the ROCK inhibitor (Figure 6C), indicating a requirement for ROCK to effectively direct cellular contractility in both amoeboid and mesenchymal invasion programs.

Finally, we asked whether enhanced invasion upon mDia2 depletion was due to transition from mDia2-driven mesenchymal to ROCK-driven amoeboid invasion. mDia2-depleted spheroids were treated with Y27632 and invasion evaluated after 24 h (Figure 6D–F). As before, both mDia2-kncokdown and Y27632 treatment caused the ES-2 cells to form slightly smaller spheroids relative to controls at T0 (Figure S7). mDia2 depletion also enhanced invasion, whereas ROCK inhibition suppressed invasion (Figure 6D–F). Strikingly, simultaneously inhibiting both pathways completely blocked invasion and total spheroid diameters were comparable to T0 embedded spheroids. Few invasive cells were observed upon combined ROCK and mDia2 inhibition (Figure 6D). This contrasted with the mixed morphology observed in the plethora of control invasive cells. mDia2 depletion drove a predominant amoeboid morphology (Figure 5E). Yet, ROCK inhibition Y27632 alone or combined mDia2/ROCK suppression resulted in highly elongated cells amongst the very few cells that did invade (Figure 6F). This invasive morphology was similar to that observed upon inhibition of Rho GTPase with C3 transferase treatment (Figure S2D), suggesting that RhoA directs migratory plasticity through its effectors ROCK and mDia2.

Discussion

Much of what we know about tumor cell invasion programs is derived from Boyden-chamber type experiments, in which single cell suspensions are seeded atop layers of matrigel. While informative, these results do not fully address mechanisms driving the rare invasive events initiated from a 3D tumor mass. Our current study dissects the contribution of the F-actin assembly factor mDia2 in invasive transitions using a clinically relevant OvCa spheroid model. Multi-cellular spheroids represent more invasive and tumorigenic OvCa cell populations [3,4,10]. Selection for this subset of chemotherapy-resistant OvCa cells could influence disease progression and/or recurrence. Little is known about the molecular underpinnings of OvCa spheroid formation or the cellular cues that trigger single cell invasive egress from spheroids into the underlying peritoneal mesothelium. Our data reveal that mDia2 induces highly adaptable single cell invasion from OvCa spheroids by functioning within a RhoA/ROCK-mediated cytoskeletal signaling network. While single cell invasion from spheroids utilizes both mesenchymal and amoeboid motility, mDia2 depletion specifically impacts spheroid organization/integrity so that amoeboid invasion predominates. Our results also show that suppression of ROCK inhibits spheroid single cell motility, by inducing exaggerated cellular elongation. Finally, we showed that the amoeboid program induced through mDia2 depletion is dependent upon Rho-mediated activation of ROCK, as spheroid invasion is completely abrogated upon concurrent mDia2 and ROCK inhibition. These data suggest that tightly regulated interplay and interdependence between ROCK and mDia2 signaling dictates the invasive capacities of motile spheroid-derived OvCa cells.

Studies firmly place mDia proteins in the queue of cytoskeleton reorganizing proteins driving tumor progression. Loss of *DIAPH3*, which encodes the mDia2 protein, occurs in primary and metastatic prostate cancer tumors, hepatocarcinoma, breast carcinoma, and in an OvCa progression model [10,29,30,44]. In prostate and ovarian cancer studies, *DIAPH3* was lost steadily from early through late stage disease models, and was accompanied by a disorganized cytoskeleton depleted of F-actin and a more aggressive phenotype [29,44]. We, along with others, have demonstrated that loss of mDia2 drives amoeboid motility [28–31]. mDia2 clearly directs plasticity in motility programs: That is, inhibition of mDia2 function promotes amoeboid motility through disruption of cortical F-actin assembly to induce bleb extrusion, while activation of mDia2 promotes assembly of F-actin rich pro-migratory structures such as lamellae, invadopodia and filopodia [26,46,52,60]. Therefore, when considering mDia2 as an anti-motility therapeutic target for tumor cells, inhibition is predicted to be counter-therapeutic in some disease models.

Loss of *DIAPH1,* which encodes mDia1 protein, is associated with myelodysplastic syndrome [42] and defects in T cell and neutrophil trafficking/polarization [32,34,35]. mDia1 is also significantly depleted in a cell-culture model of OvCa progression [10], although it is concentrated in pro-migratory microparticles shed from ovarian carcinomas [55]. In the present study, we show that mDia1 depletion affects neither ES-2 spheroid formation nor spheroid invasion (Figures 4 and S6). Interestingly, mDia1 loss was previously shown to slightly diminish RhoA and ROCK activity, the latter of which could favor mDia2-mediated F-actin dynamics [38,61,62]. In our system, the highly polarized localization and the temporal regulation of mDia1 may contribute to regulation of F-actin dynamics in migrating OvCa cells. In addition, mDia1 may support the nuclear actin network-as suggested by the extensive nuclear localization of mDia1 in Figure 5C and in [54]). Nevertheless, we show here that mDia2 is the predominant formin involved in mediating 3D OvCa spheroid organization and invasive transitions.

While targeting either mDia2 or ROCK led to slightly smaller spheroids, spheroid architecture was affected only upon mDia2 suppression (Figures 4, S5, respectively). This suggests that mDia2 maintains the integrity and cohesion of compacted spheroids. The individual roles of ROCK and mDia and the functional implications of their potential interplay for regulation of cell-cell junctions in epithelial cells are complex. ROCK and mDia have opposing effects in maintaining/stabilizing cell-cell junctional integrity. High RhoA-GTP levels led to ROCK-dependent junctional destabilization through generation of contractile force. However, moderate RhoA activity favors mDia-directed AJ stabilization [18]. Further, ROCK cooperates with mDia to drive migration via actinomyosin-based contractility. High levels of RhoA-GTP activated both mDia and ROCK, while lower levels preferentially targets mDia1 [63]. This effect is potentially

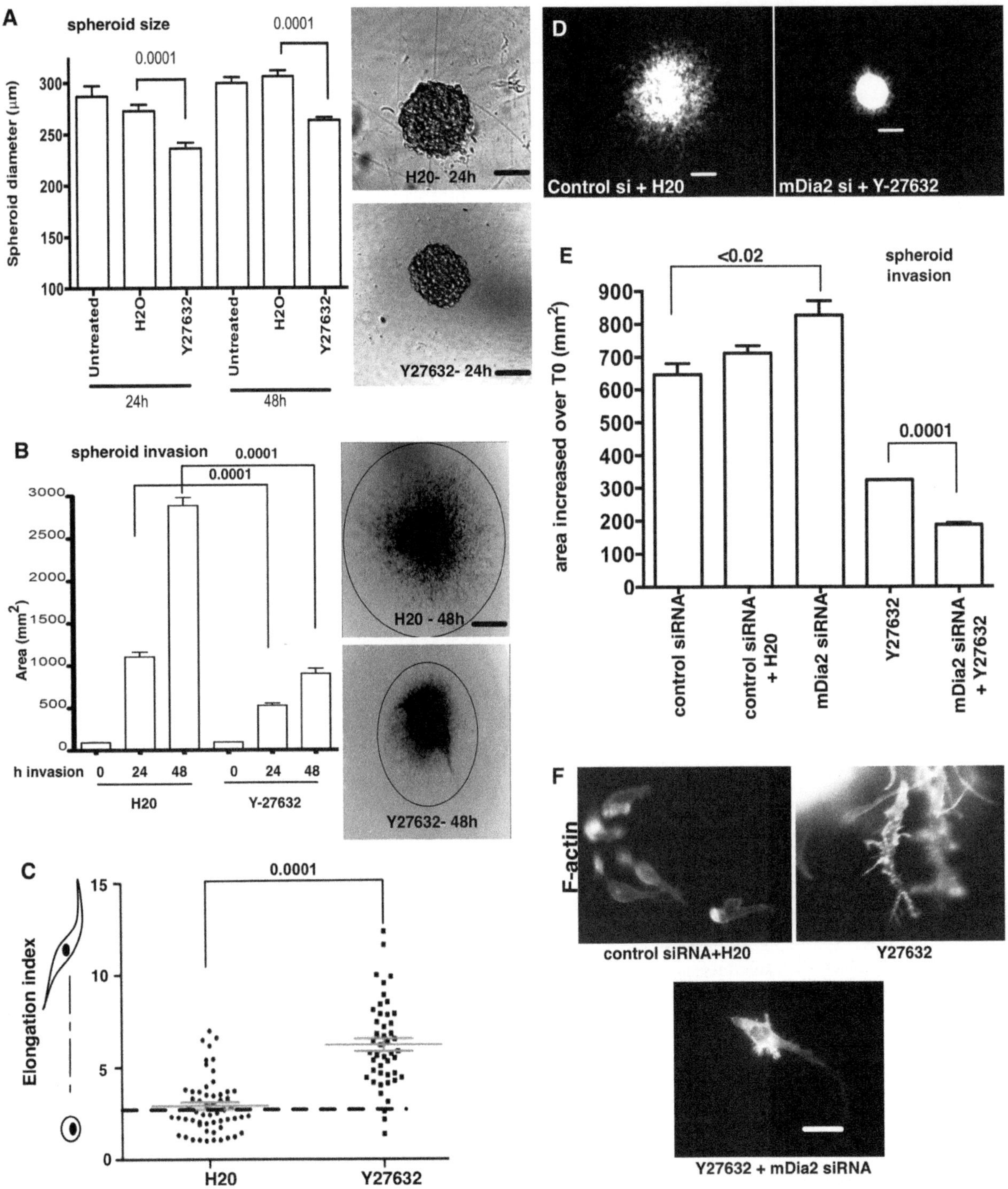

Figure 6. ROCK signaling drives ES-2 spheroid invasion. A. Spheroids were formed in the presence of vehicle or 90 μM Y27632 for the indicated times. Spheroid diameters were then measured for at least 30 spheroids at 10×. Bar = 100 μm. p values are shown above the plot and are control H_20-treated spheroids. B. Spheroids were formed for 48 h in the presence of Y27632, and then embedded in collagen-I for 0–48 h in the presence of vehicle or Y27632. Invasive fronts were measured at each time point for at least 30 spheroids per condition. Bar = 400 μm. Representative spheroids at 4× are shown stained for phalloidin and images contrast enhanced. P values are listed above the graph and are relative to control H_20-treated spheroids. C. Elongation indices were calculated for invasive cells in the collagen gels shown in B. EI> 2 (dashed line) were considered mesenchymal cell type. At least 30 cells were measured per condition. p values are listed above the chart and are relative to control H_20-treated spheroids. D–E. Spheroids were formed in the presence of Y27632; siRNA-treated spheroids were formed at 48 h post-siRNA treatment in the presence of 90 μM Y27632. Spheroids were then embedded in collagen for 24 h Y27632 was maintained in both the gel and media with spheroids through 104 h post-siRNA treatment, and upon embedding for an additional 24 h. Spheroids were fixed and stained for F-actin. Images shown in D are 4× and scale bar = 200 μm. At least 20 spheroids were measured for each condition for E. p values are listed above (E) and are relative to control siRNA-treated spheroids, or Y27632-treated spheroids, as noted. F. Representative 40× phalloidin staining of invasive cells. Bar = 40 μm. All error bars correspond to SDs from a representative experiment.

explained by the finding that the K_d for mDia1 binding to RhoA-GTP is lower than the K_d for ROCK binding to RhoA-GTP [64,65]. In invasive hepatocyte spheroids, RhoA activation is tightly regulated both spatially and temporally, and is inversely correlated with cadherin engagement within the cell-cell junctions (*i.e.*, high cadherin: low activated-RhoA) [50]. In the latter study, it was suggested that RhoA activation was a consequence of to disruptions of cadherins in cell-cell attachments. This potentially allowed RhoA to interact with effectors (*i.e.*, ROCK, mDia) that promote single cellular migration/invasion. Our data reveal increases in RhoA-GTP as spheroids mature (Figure 3C). Indeed, ES-2 spheroids caused contraction of 3D collagen-I gels, which is indicative of high actinomyosin forces and, by inference, Rho/ROCK activity [4]. Collectively these data suggest that within the spheroid a balance between mDia2 and ROCK activity exists, coordinated by levels of RhoA-GTP as well as the spatial and temporal localization of RhoA-GTP [62] and its effectors. The underlying spheroid cell-cell junctions are potentially supported by mDia2-mediated F-actin dynamics, under conditions of lower RhoA-GTP levels. As RhoA-GTP levels increase during spheroid maturation and upon engaging the extracellular matrix, ROCK signaling may ultimately prevail to disrupt AJ, and destabilize the spheroid architecture. mDia2 suppression (Figures 5–6) potentially promotes invasion transitions due to default RhoA-mediated ROCK activation (and junctional destabilization). Experiments are currently in progress to test this hypothesis.

While ROCK inhibition failed to affect spheroid formation, it dramatically reduced spheroid invasion within collagen (Figure 6). Both amoeboid and mesenchymal morphologies were present in control spheroids, yet ROCK inhibition significantly blocked spheroid invasion. The few remaining invasive cells had dramatically increased EI indicative of defects in retraction, as previously demonstrated [66–68]. Our data supports the notion that activated ROCK promotes both mesenchymal and amoeboid motility. Inhibition of ROCK therefore has a dual effect: 1., suppressing actinomyosin-based contractility required for initiation and retraction of amoeboid blebs [69–72], and 2., facilitating extension/retraction of mesenchymal cellular protrusions [73]. It is unclear from our 3D experiments whether amoeboid or mesenchymal single cell invasion represents a more efficient mode of invasion, as judged by distance travelled, velocities, etc. Experiments addressing this question are currently underway.

Our data shed light on a possible mechanism whereby modulating the RhoA/mDia/ROCK axis induces invasive transitions in OvCa spheroids. The work of Brugge and colleagues recently revealed that OVCA433 spheroids generated actinomyosin contractility to clear the underlying mesothelia and drive OvCa dissemination [74]. The activation mechanism of myosin contractility has not been explored. The enhanced RhoA-GTP levels present in mature spheroids may act as a driver for forces inducing single cell transmesothelial migration and/or clearance. It is tempting to speculate that induction of Rho/ROCK/mDia2-dependent amoeboid motility promotes efficient single cell transmesothelial migration. Similarly the Rho/ROCK axis could generate actinomyosin-based force to induce mesenchymal invasion. It will be interesting to determine if targeting ROCK in the spheroid-mesothelial invasion model inhibits mesothelial clearance, thereby disrupting both mesenchymal and amoeboid single cell invasion.

Finally, we have shown that mDia2 depletion effectively induces amoeboid invasive transitions in OvCa spheroids (Figure 5). It is unclear what physiological triggers, outside of loss of mDia2, could promote such invasive transitions *in vivo*. We previously showed that CXCL12 promotes amoeboid transitions [28] through the formation of a complex between mDia2 and its functional inhibitor, DIP, in MDA-MB-231 breast cancer cells. A role for CXCL12 and its receptor, CXCR4, in OvCa progression, peritoneal dissemination, and metastasis has also been established [75–80]. Elevated levels of mesothelium-derived CXCL12 have been detected in patient ascites and expression of CXCR4 in OvCa cells correlated with a poorer prognosis and reduced survival [76]. A potential role for CXCR4 in driving OvCa metastasis is further supported by the finding that treatment of xenografted ES-2 cells with a CXCR4 antagonist reduced peritoneal dissemination of the tumor cells[75]. In light of these and our current studies, it would be interesting to evaluate whether CXCL12 promotes invasive transitions and peritoneal dissemination through functional inhibition of mDia2 in OvCa spheroids.

Conclusions

Our findings indicate that multiple Rho GTPase effectors must be suppressed to fully block egress of invasive cells from 3D ovarian cancer spheroids. Furthermore, tightly regulated interplay and interdependence between ROCK and mDia2 signaling pathways dictates the invasive capacities and the type of invasion program utilized by motile spheroid-derived ovarian cancer cells. Loss of the gene encoding mDia2, *DRF3,* has been linked to cancer progression and metastasis. Our results set the stage for a broader understanding of the molecular mechanisms involved in mDia2-dependent dissemination of invasive cells tumor cell from primary tumor lesions, potentially in a variety of epithelial cancers.

Methods

Cell lines, chemicals, plasmids and transfections

ES-2, SKOV3, OVCAR3 cells were from ATCC. OVCAR4 was from the National Cancer Institute's Tumor Repository. OVCA cell lines OVCA 420 and OVCA 429 are cell lines previously established and derived from patients with late-stage serous ovarian adenocarcinomas [81]. The OVCA194 cell line was were previously described [82]. The OVCAR4, OVCA429, OVCA420 and OVCA194 were kind gifts from Drs. Deborah Vestal and William Maltese. OVCA429, SKOV3, OVCAR4, OVCA420, OVCA194, and ES-2 cells were grown in RPMI-1640 containing 10% (v/v) FBS and 100 μg streptomycin in a 37°C incubator with 5% CO_2. OVCAR3 cells were grown in RPMI-1640 containing 20% FBS and 100 μg streptomycin. The constructs encoding EYFP, EYFP-mDia2, EYFP-mDia1, EYFP-FH2ΔN, and EYFP-mDia2 M1041A were kind gifts from Dr. Art S. Alberts. Y27632 was from Sigma. SMIFH2 was from EMD Biochemicals.

OVCA429 cells were transfected with the preceding expression constructs for 48 h using Fugene (Promega), per the manufacturer's protocol. For siRNA-mediated suppression of mDia1or mDia2, 25–100 nM smart pool or individual siRNAs targeted against the human sequences were obtained from Dharmacon and transfected into adherent cells using the Dharmafect-1 reagent (Thermoscientific). Parallel cultures were transfected with control siRNAs.

Adhesion, Migration and Invasion Assays

Cells were loaded with 4 μg/ml Calcein AM-FITC (Invitrogen) for 15 min at 37°C prior to adhesion assays. Cells (1×10^4) in serum-free media (SFM) were added to 96-well plates coated overnight with 10 μg/ml collagen-I (BD Biosciences) or BSA (Sigma). Cells were incubated for 45 min at 37°C, after which wells were aspirated and washed five times with PBS/0.5% BSA, rotating the plate 90° with each wash. Adherent cells were detected in a fluorescent plate reader (485/538 nm excitation/emission), with total adherent cells extrapolated from a standard curve derived from a known number of cells. Adhesion assays were performed in triplicate and the experiment was repeated thrice. Standard deviations (SDs) were expressed from triplicate wells from a representative experiment.

For migration, cells were serum-starved overnight and loaded with Calcein AM-FITC as above. 1×10^5 cells in SFM were added to the upper well of 8 μm pore-size Fluoroblok inserts (Falcon) coated overnight with 10 μg/ml collagen-I (BD Biosciences). SFM or 20% FBS was added to the lower well. Cells were incubated for 5 h at 37°C prior to enumerating migrating cells in a fluorescent plate reader. Migration assays were performed in triplicate and the experiment repeated thrice. SDs were expressed from triplicate wells from a representative experiment.

Invasion assays were performed as previously described [28]. Briefly, 50,000 Calcein AM-FITC labeled cells were seeded upon 2 mg/ml collagen gels previously polymerized within the upper well of 8 μm pore inserts. Invasion assays were performed in triplicate and the experiment was repeated thrice for 24 h at 37°C in response to either SFM or 20% FBS gradients. SDs were expressed from triplicate wells from a representative experiment.

Microscopy

Confocal imaging of live and fixed cells was performed using a Leica Microsystems TCS SP5 multiphoton laser-scanning confocal microscope system with a 8000 Hz resonant scanner and environmental controls for maintaining 37°C, humidity and 5% CO_2, and laser lines of 488, 514, 633 and 710–990 nm from a tunable Ti-Sapphire MP laser. Hardware is controlled from the Leica AFM acquisition/analytical software suite. MetaMorph software suite (Molecular Devices) was used for data analysis. Dunn chamber acquisition was performed using a Leica 10X HC PL APO CS Dry UV 0.40NA objective lens. Confocal spheroid imaging was performed using a Leica 20X HCX PL APO CS Dry UV 0.70NA objective lens. Spheroids processed for immunofluorescence were stored and imaged in RPMI.

Immunostained coverslips and brightfield documentation of spheroid formation were acquired using an IX81 inverted microscope (Olympus) equipped with YFP, TRITC and CY5 filters. Acquisition and analysis were performed using MetaMorph software suite. 2D cell images were acquired with an Olympus 40X UPlan Apo 1.00 oil lens; spheroid images for measuring size and invasion were acquired with either an Olympus 10X UPlanFL 0.30NA objective lens, or Olympus 4x UPlanFL 0.13NA objective lens, respectively. Coverslips and spheroids were mounted using Fluoromount-G mounting media (Southern Biological) and RPMI, respectively.

Dunn Chemotactic Migration Assay

Dunn chambers (Hawksley) were set up as described [83,84]. Coverslips were coated with 10 μg/ml collagen-I (BD Biosciences) overnight. Cells were loaded with Calcein AM-Red Orange (Invitrogen) for 15 min at 37°C. Cells (2.5×10^4) were plated and allowed to adhere overnight. The inner well of the chamber was filled with SFM. The outer well was exchanged with medium containing 20% (v/v) serum. The chamber was maintained at 37°C with humidity on the microscope stage. The cells located over the bridge were imaged every 15 min for 5 h.

Spheroid formation and collagen embedding

Spheroids were formed by centrifugation of poly-HEMA coated plates as described [85]. Briefly, 96-well plates were coated with 0.5% poly-HEMA and dried at 37°C. Cells were detached using Versene (Invitrogen) and resuspended in RPMI with 10% FBS and 2.5% of 15 μl/ml matrigel (BD Biosciences). 500 cells per well were pelleted by centrifugation at 1000×g for 10 min. Unless specified, spheroids were formed for 72 h before use. Collagen-I was prepared at 2 mg/ml; a thin layer was partially polymerized in 8-well chamberglass (Lab-Tek) before adding spheroids, and excess media removed before adding the top layer of collagen. Gels were polymerized for 45 min before adding media or fixing, as described [4].

2D Immunofluorescence (IF)

Cells imaged by IF were processed as described [28]. Briefly, cells were plated upon sterilized coverslips overnight, fixed in 4% paraformaldehyde for 20 min, permeabilized with 0.2% Triton X-100 for 20 min and stained with antibodies against mDia2 and mDia1 (Proteintech) overnight at 4°C followed by incubation with Alexa-Fluor secondary antibodies (Invitrogen) for 4 h at 37°C. Alexa-Fluor-conjugated phalloidin (Invitrogen) was used to visualize the F-actin architecture. DAPI (Invitrogen) was used for nuclear staining.

3D Immunofluorescence and Invasion of Spheroids

Embedded spheroids were stained as described, with minor changes [86]. Briefly, invasive spheroids were fixed in 4% paraformaldehyde for 20 min at RT, washed in PBS, and permeabilized with 0.5% Triton X-100 for 60 min at RT. Spheroids were washed with 100 mM glycine before blocking. Primary antibodies were incubated at 4°C overnight, and incubated with Alexa-Fluor secondary antibodies (Invitrogen) and Alexa Fluor 488 phalloidin (Invitrogen) at 37°C for 3 h or at 4°C overnight. The specimen was washed, DAPI was added for 20 min at RT, washed once in PBS then coated in Fluoromount-G (Southern Biotech). Images were collected using an Olympus IX-81 microscope. Invasive area was calculated using Metamorph software, by drawing a region of interest (ROI) upon embedding and after invasion around the spheroid invasive front. The R0I area was selected and drawn to encompass the spherical perimeter of invasive cells and validated with Metamorph software to contain at least 95% of fluorescent pixels corresponding to phalloidin staining.

RhoA G-LISA

RhoA G-LISA (Cytoskeleton, Inc) was performed according to the manufacture's specifications. Briefly, monolayer cells were grown to confluence before being stimulated with 10 μM 1-Oleoyl Lysophosphatidic acid LPA (Cayman Chemical) for 5 minutes. Cells were collected using the lysis buffer from the kit. A minimum of 200 spheroids were collected at 48, 72, 96, and 120hr. Spheroids were collected on ice, centrifuged briefly to pellet. Lysis buffer was added and the spheroids were dissociated before starting the assay. Each condition was testing in triplicate and the experiment was performed thrice. Standard deviations (SD) were expressed from at least triplicate wells for a representative experiment. Luminescence was measured on the SpectraMax5 (Molecular Devices).

Statistical Analysis

One-tailed Students t-tests were performed with a 95% confidence value. p values of 0.05 or less were considered statistically significant. All error bars are expressed as standard deviations (SDs) from representative experiments, unless otherwise noted. Graphs and statistics were generated in GraphPad Prism software.

Supporting Information

Figure S1 Spheroid formation in OvCa cells. The formation of spheroids from single cell suspensions was documented after 24 h by brightfield microscopy. Bar = 50 μm.

Figure S2 Requirement for Rho GTPases in ES-2 spheroid compaction and invasion. A. Spheroids were formed for 48 h from 500 cells in the presence of H_20 vehicle, 0.5, 1.0 or 2.0 μg/ml. Scale bar = 400 μm. B., Spheroids were then embedded in collagen gels and T0 measurements taken. Spheroids were allowed to invade for 18 h. Scale bar = 1000 μm. C., ROI were drawn to measure the invasive area, encompassing at least 95% of cells, at T0 and T18. D., After 18 h, spheroids were fixed and stained with phalloidin, and invasive edges images by fluorescent epifluorescent microscopy. Arrows indicate highly elongated cells emanating from the limited invasive edge. Images were acquired using a 10X objective. Scale bar = 1000 μm.

Figure S3 Levels of total mDia2, mDia1 and RhoA in monolayers and spheroids. Spheroids were formed for the indicated times. Cell lysates were collected from pooled spheroids or monolayers and Western blots were performed for mDia2 (A), mDia1 (B) or RhoA (C), along with tubulin as a loading control. Densitometry was performed on the resulting blots (Figure 3) and ratios of mDia1,mDia2, or RhoA:tubulin were determined. Values shown were normalized by setting monolayer values to 100 percent.

Figure S4 mDia2 depletion via both pooled and single siRNAs influence spheroid formation. A. Time course analysis of mDia2 depletion in monolayers treated with individual siRNA (mDia2 06, 08) or pooled mDia2 siRNA. Lysates were prepared at the designated times and western blotted for mDia2 or tubulin (loading control). B. ES-2 spheroids were formed from cells depleted for 72 h with individual siRNA (mDia2 06, 08) or pooled siRNA. Spheroid diameters were measured 48 h post spheroid formation. At least 12 spheroids were measured for each condition. p values are listed above the chart and are relative to control siRNA-treated spheroids. C. Spheroids from B were embedded in collagen gels and allowed to invade for 18hrs, after which spheroids were fixed, stained with phalloidin and imaged. ROI were drawn to measure the invasive area, encompassing at least 95% of cells, at T0 and T18. p values are listed above the chart and are relative to control siRNA-treated spheroids. Error bars correspond to SD for a representative experiment.

Figure S5 Functional mDia inhibition promotes disorganized spheroid formation. ES-2 spheroids were formed in the presence of 10 μM SMIFH2. Images were acquired by brightfield microscopy after 48 h formation. Bar = 50 μm.

Figure S6 mDia1 depletion does not alter spheroid single cell invasion. mDia1 or control GAPDH were depleted in ES-2 monolayers. Spheroids were formed for 48 h, embedded and invaded for 24 h. p values are shown above the chart and are relative to untreated spheroids. Error bars correspond to SD for a representative experiment

Figure S7 Spheroid diameter measurements upon embedding in response to combined ROCK/mDia2 inhibition. Spheroids were formed in the presence of Y27632; siRNA-treated spheroids were formed at 48 h post-siRNA treatment in the presence of 90 μM Y27632. Spheroids were then embedded in collagen and T0 measurements taken. At least 20 spheroids were measured for each condition. $p<0.01$, relative to control si + vehicle control spheroids. Error bars correspond to SDs for a representative experiment.

Acknowledgments

We thank members of the Eisenmann lab, Lot R. Haak, Kandace Williams, William Maltese and Ellie Petyak for critical reading of the manuscript and helpful discussion; Sarah D. Banks and Jacob Jessinger for technical assistance; the University of Toledo Advanced Microscopy and Imaging Core for imaging assistance and Dr. Art Alberts (Van Andel Research Institute, Grand Rapids, MI) for supporting the initial stages of this work. We thank the Polar Vortex of 2014 and the 900 snow days we had for accelerating the final stages of this work.

Author Contributions

Conceived and designed the experiments: KME ALNK KMP. Performed the experiments: KME ALNK KMP KMD. Analyzed the data: KME ALNK KMP KMD. Contributed reagents/materials/analysis tools: KME ALNK. Wrote the paper: KME.

References

1. Vergara D, Merlot B, Lucot JP, Collinet P, Vinatier D, et al. (2010) Epithelial-mesenchymal transition in ovarian cancer. Cancer Lett 291: 59–66.
2. Landen CN Jr, Birrer MJ, Sood AK (2008) Early events in the pathogenesis of epithelial ovarian cancer. J Clin Oncol 26: 995–1005.
3. Sodek KL, Murphy KJ, Brown TJ, Ringuette MJ (2012) Cell-cell and cell-matrix dynamics in intraperitoneal cancer metastasis. Cancer Metastasis Rev 31: 397–414.
4. Sodek KL, Ringuette MJ, Brown TJ (2009) Compact spheroid formation by ovarian cancer cells is associated with contractile behavior and an invasive phenotype. Int J Cancer 124: 2060–2070.
5. Theriault BL, Shepherd TG, Mujoomdar ML, Nachtigal MW (2007) BMP4 induces EMT and Rho GTPase activation in human ovarian cancer cells. Carcinogenesis 28: 1153–1162.
6. Patel IS, Madan P, Getsios S, Bertrand MA, MacCalman CD (2003) Cadherin switching in ovarian cancer progression. Int J Cancer 106: 172–177.
7. Burleson KM, Hansen LK, Skubitz AP (2004) Ovarian carcinoma spheroids disaggregate on type I collagen and invade live human mesothelial cell monolayers. Clin Exp Metastasis 21: 685–697.
8. Burleson KM, Casey RC, Skubitz KM, Pambuccian SE, Oegema TR Jr, et al. (2004) Ovarian carcinoma ascites spheroids adhere to extracellular matrix components and mesothelial cell monolayers. Gynecol Oncol 93: 170–181.
9. Burleson KM, Boente MP, Pambuccian SE, Skubitz AP (2006) Disaggregation and invasion of ovarian carcinoma ascites spheroids. J Transl Med 4: 6.
10. Zietarska M, Maugard CM, Filali-Mouhim A, Alam-Fahmy M, Tonin PN, et al. (2007) Molecular description of a 3D in vitro model for the study of epithelial ovarian cancer (EOC). Mol Carcinog 46: 872–885.
11. Bijman MN, van Berkel MP, van Nieuw Amerongen GP, Boven E (2008) Interference with actin dynamics is superior to disturbance of microtubule function in the inhibition of human ovarian cancer cell motility. Biochem Phamacol 76: 707–716.
12. Thiery JP, Sleeman JP (2006) Complex networks orchestrate epithelial-mesenchymal transitions. Nat Rev Mol Cell Biol 7: 131–142.
13. Guarino M (2007) Epithelial-mesenchymal transition and tumour invasion. Int J Biochem Cell Biol 39: 2153–2160.
14. Yilmaz M, Christofori G (2009) EMT, the cytoskeleton, and cancer cell invasion. Cancer Metastasis Rev 28: 15–33.
15. Klymkowsky MW, Savagner P (2009) Epithelial-mesenchymal transition: a cancer researcher's conceptual friend and foe. Am J Pathol 174: 1588–1593.

16. Rath N, Olson MF (2012) Rho-associated kinases in tumorigenesis: re-considering ROCK inhibition for cancer therapy. EMBO Rep 13: 900–908.
17. Thumkeo D, Shinohara R, Watanabe K, Takebayashi H, Toyoda Y, et al. (2011) Deficiency of mDia, an Actin Nucleator, Disrupts Integrity of Neuroepithelium and Causes Periventricular Dysplasia. PLoS One 6: e25465.
18. Sahai E, Marshall CJ (2002) ROCK and Dia have opposing effects on adherens junctions downstream of Rho. Nat Cell Biol 4: 408–415.
19. Ryu JR, Echarri A, Li R, Pendergast AM (2009) Regulation of cell-cell adhesion by Abi/Diaphanous complexes. Mol Cell Biol 29: 1735–1748.
20. Kobielak A, Pasolli HA, Fuchs E (2004) Mammalian formin-1 participates in adherens junctions and polymerization of linear actin cables. Nat Cell Biol 6: 21–30.
21. Herzog D, Loetscher P, van Hengel J, Knusel S, Brakebusch C, et al. (2011) The small GTPase RhoA is required to maintain spinal cord neuroepithelium organization and the neural stem cell pool. J Neurosci 31: 5120–5130.
22. Carramusa L, Ballestrem C, Zilberman Y, Bershadsky AD (2007) Mammalian diaphanous-related formin Dia1 controls the organization of E-cadherin-mediated cell-cell junctions. J Cell Sci 120: 3870–3882.
23. Xing H, Wang S, Weng D, Chen G, Yang X, et al. (2007) Knock-down of P-glycoprotein reverses taxol resistance in ovarian cancer multicellular spheroids. Oncol Rep 17: 117–122.
24. Frankel A, Buckman R, Kerbel RS (1997) Abrogation of taxol-induced G2-M arrest and apoptosis in human ovarian cancer cells grown as multicellular tumor spheroids. Cancer Res 57: 2388–2393.
25. Homem CC, Peifer M (2008) Diaphanous regulates myosin and adherens junctions to control cell contractility and protrusive behavior during morphogenesis. Development 135: 1005–1018.
26. Lizarraga F, Poincloux R, Romao M, Montagnac G, Le Dez G, et al. (2009) Diaphanous-related formins are required for invadopodia formation and invasion of breast tumor cells. Cancer Res 69: 2792–2800.
27. Eisenmann KM, Harris ES, Kitchen SM, Holman HA, Higgs HN, et al. (2007) Dia-interacting protein modulates formin-mediated actin assembly at the cell cortex. Curr Biol 17: 579–591.
28. Wyse MM, Lei J, Nestor-Kalinoski AL, Eisenmann KM (2012) Dia-interacting protein (DIP) imposes migratory plasticity in mDia2-dependent tumor cells in three-dimensional matrices. PLoS One 7: e45085.
29. Di Vizio D, Kim J, Hager MH, Morello M, Yang W, et al. (2009) Oncosome formation in prostate cancer: association with a region of frequent chromosomal deletion in metastatic disease. Cancer Res 69: 5601–5609.
30. Hager MH, Morley S, Bielenberg DR, Gao S, Morello M, et al. (2012) DIAPH3 governs the cellular transition to the amoeboid tumour phenotype. EMBO Mol Med 4: 743–760.
31. Shi Y, Dong B, Miliotis H, Liu J, Alberts AS, et al. (2009) Src kinase Hck association with the WASp and mDia1 cytoskeletal regulators promotes chemoattractant-induced Hck membrane targeting and activation in neutrophils. Biochem Cell Biol 87: 207–216.
32. Shi Y, Zhang J, Mullin M, Dong B, Alberts AS, et al. (2009) The mDial formin is required for neutrophil polarization, migration, and activation of the LARG/RhoA/ROCK signaling axis during chemotaxis. J Immunol 182: 3837–3845.
33. Narumiya S, Tanji M, Ishizaki T (2009) Rho signaling, ROCK and mDia1, in transformation, metastasis and invasion. Cancer Metastasis Rev 28: 65–76.
34. Eisenmann KM, West RA, Hildebrand D, Kitchen SM, Peng J, et al. (2007) T cell responses in mammalian diaphanous-related formin mDia1 knock-out mice. J Biol Chem 282: 25152–25158.
35. Sakata D, Taniguchi H, Yasuda S, Adachi-Morishima A, Hamazaki Y, et al. (2007) Impaired T lymphocyte trafficking in mice deficient in an actin-nucleating protein, mDia1. J Exp Med 204: 2031–2038.
36. Dettenhofer M, Zhou F, Leder P (2008) Formin 1-isoform IV deficient cells exhibit defects in cell spreading and focal adhesion formation. PLoS One 3: e2497.
37. Han Y, Eppinger E, Schuster IG, Weigand LU, Liang X, et al. (2009) Formin-like 1 (FMNL1) is regulated by N-terminal myristoylation and induces polarized membrane blebbing. J Biol Chem 284: 33409–33417.
38. Hannemann S, Madrid R, Stastna J, Kitzing T, Gasteier J, et al. (2008) The Diaphanous-related Formin FHOD1 associates with ROCK1 and promotes Src-dependent plasma membrane blebbing. J Biol Chem 283: 27891–27903.
39. Kitzing TM, Sahadevan AS, Brandt DT, Knieling H, Hannemann S, et al. (2007) Positive feedback between Dia1, LARG, and RhoA regulates cell morphology and invasion. Genes Dev 21: 1478–1483.
40. Kitzing TM, Wang Y, Pertz O, Copeland JW, Grosse R (2010) Formin-like 2 drives amoeboid invasive cell motility downstream of RhoC. Oncogene 29: 2441–2448.
41. Liang L, Li X, Zhang X, Lv Z, He G, et al. (2012) MicroRNA-137, a HMGA1 Target, Suppresses Colorectal Cancer Cell Invasion and Metastasis in Mice by Directly Targeting FMNL2. Gastroenterology 144: 624–635.
42. Peng J, Kitchen SM, West RA, Sigler R, Eisenmann KM, et al. (2007) Myeloproliferative defects following targeting of the Drf1 gene encoding the mammalian diaphanous related formin mDia1. Cancer Res 67: 7565–7571.
43. Bione S, Sala C, Manzini C, Arrigo G, Zuffardi O, et al. (1998) A human homologue of the Drosophila melanogaster diaphanous gene is disrupted in a patient with premature ovarian failure: evidence for conserved function in oogenesis and implications for human sterility. Am J Hum Genet 62: 533–541.
44. Creekmore AL, Silkworth WT, Cimini D, Jensen RV, Roberts PC, et al. (2011) Changes in gene expression and cellular architecture in an ovarian cancer progression model. PLoS One 6: e17676.
45. Ketene AN, Schmelz EM, Roberts PC, Agah M (2012) The effects of cancer progression on the viscoelasticity of ovarian cell cytoskeleton structures. Nanomedicine 8: 93–102.
46. Gupton SL, Eisenmann K, Alberts AS, Waterman-Storer CM (2007) mDia2 regulates actin and focal adhesion dynamics and organization in the lamella for efficient epithelial cell migration. J Cell Sci 120: 3475–3487.
47. Copeland JW, Copeland SJ, Treisman R (2004) Homo-oligomerization is essential for F-actin assembly by the formin family FH2 domain. J Biol Chem 279: 50250–50256.
48. Copeland JW, Treisman R (2002) The diaphanous-related formin mDia1 controls serum response factor activity through its effects on actin polymerization. Mol Biol Cell 13: 4088–4099.
49. Alberts AS (2001) Identification of a carboxyl-terminal diaphanous-related formin homology protein autoregulatory domain. J Biol Chem 276: 2824–2830.
50. Dohda T, Nakamura Y, Kamihira M, Iijima S (2004) Functional role of RhoA in growth regulation of primary hepatocytes. J Biochem 135: 631–637.
51. Rizvi SA, Neidt EM, Cui J, Feiger Z, Skau CT, et al. (2009) Identification and characterization of a small molecule inhibitor of formin-mediated actin assembly. Chem Biol 16: 1158–1168.
52. Chhabra ES, Higgs HN (2007) The many faces of actin: matching assembly factors with cellular structures. Nat Cell Biol 9: 1110–1121.
53. Wallar BJ, Deward AD, Resau JH, Alberts AS (2007) RhoB and the mammalian Diaphanous-related formin mDia2 in endosome trafficking. Exp Cell Res 313: 560–571.
54. Baarlink C, Wang H, Grosse R (2013) Nuclear Actin Network Assembly by Formins Regulates the SRF Coactivator MAL. Science 340: 864–867.
55. Press JZ, Reyes M, Pitteri SJ, Pennil C, Garcia R, et al. (2012) Microparticles from ovarian carcinomas are shed into ascites and promote cell migration. Int J Gynecol Cancer 22: 546–552.
56. Sahai E, Marshall CJ (2003) Differing modes of tumour cell invasion have distinct requirements for Rho/ROCK signalling and extracellular proteolysis. Nat Cell Biol 5: 711–719.
57. Wolf K, Mazo I, Leung H, Engelke K, von Andrian UH, et al. (2003) Compensation mechanism in tumor cell migration: mesenchymal-amoeboid transition after blocking of pericellular proteolysis. J Cell Biol 160: 267–277.
58. de Toledo M, Anguille C, Roger L, Roux P, Gadea G (2012) Cooperative anti-invasive effect of Cdc42/Rac1 activation and ROCK inhibition in SW620 colorectal cancer cells with elevated blebbing activity. PLoS One 7: e48344.
59. Han Z, Xu G, Zhou J, Xing H, Wang S, et al. (2005) Inhibition of motile and invasive properties of ovarian cancer cells by ASODN against Rho-associated protein kinase. Cell Commun Adhes 12: 59–69.
60. Peng J, Wallar BJ, Flanders A, Swiatek PJ, Alberts AS (2003) Disruption of the Diaphanous-related formin Drf1 gene encoding mDia1 reveals a role for Drf3 as an effector for Cdc42. Curr Biol 13: 534–545.
61. Takeya R, Taniguchi K, Narumiya S, Sumimoto H (2008) The mammalian formin FHOD1 is activated through phosphorylation by ROCK and mediates thrombin-induced stress fibre formation in endothelial cells. EMBO J 27: 618–628.
62. Terry SJ, Zihni C, Elbediwy A, Vitiello E, Leefa Chong San IV, et al. (2011) Spatially restricted activation of RhoA signalling at epithelial junctions by p114RhoGEF drives junction formation and morphogenesis. Nat Cell Biol 13: 159–166.
63. Arakawa Y, Bito H, Furuyashiki T, Tsuji T, Takemoto-Kimura S, et al. (2003) Control of axon elongation via an SDF-1alpha/Rho/mDia pathway in cultured cerebellar granule neurons. J Cell Biol 161: 381–391.
64. Blumenstein L, Ahmadian MR (2004) Models of the cooperative mechanism for Rho effector recognition: implications for RhoA-mediated effector activation. J Biol Chem 279: 53419–53426.
65. Rose R, Weyand M, Lammers M, Ishizaki T, Ahmadian MR, et al. (2005) Structural and mechanistic insights into the interaction between Rho and mammalian Dia. Nature 435: 513–518.
66. Worthylake RA, Burridge K (2003) RhoA and ROCK promote migration by limiting membrane protrusions. J Biol Chem 278: 13578–13584.
67. Worthylake RA, Lemoine S, Watson JM, Burridge K (2001) RhoA is required for monocyte tail retraction during transendothelial migration. J Cell Biol 154: 147–160.
68. Iwanicki MP, Vomastek T, Tilghman RW, Martin KH, Banerjee J, et al. (2008) FAK, PDZ-RhoGEF and ROCKII cooperate to regulate adhesion movement and trailing-edge retraction in fibroblasts. J Cell Sci 121: 895–905.
69. Charras GT (2008) A short history of blebbing. J Microsc 231: 466–478.
70. Charras GT, Hu CK, Coughlin M, Mitchison TJ (2006) Reassembly of contractile actin cortex in cell blebs. J Cell Biol 175: 477–490.
71. Fackler OT, Grosse R (2008) Cell motility through plasma membrane blebbing. J Cell Biol 181: 879–884.
72. Paluch E, Sykes C, Prost J, Bornens M (2006) Dynamic modes of the cortical actomyosin gel during cell locomotion and division. Trends Cell Biol 16: 5–10.
73. Olson MF, Sahai E (2009) The actin cytoskeleton in cancer cell motility. Clin Exp Metastasis 26: 273–287.
74. Iwanicki MP, Davidowtiza RA, Ng MR, Besser A, Muranen T, et al. (2011) Ovarian Cancer Spheroids Use Myosin-Generated Force to Clear the Mesothelium. Cancer Discovery 1: 2–14.

75. Kajiyama H, Shibata K, Terauchi M, Ino K, Nawa A, et al. (2008) Involvement of SDF-1alpha/CXCR4 axis in the enhanced peritoneal metastasis of epithelial ovarian carcinoma. Int J Cancer 122: 91–99.
76. Barbolina MV, Burkhalter RJ, Stack MS (2011) Diverse mechanisms for activation of Wnt signalling in the ovarian tumour microenvironment. Biochem J 437: 1–12.
77. Leinster DA, Kulbe H, Everitt G, Thompson R, Perretti M, et al. (2012) The peritoneal tumour microenvironment of high-grade serous ovarian cancer. J Pathol 227: 136–145.
78. Righi E, Kashiwagi S, Yuan J, Santosuosso M, Leblanc P, et al. (2011) CXCL12/CXCR4 blockade induces multimodal antitumor effects that prolong survival in an immunocompetent mouse model of ovarian cancer. Cancer Res 71: 5522–5534.
79. Popple A, Durrant LG, Spendlove I, Rolland P, Scott IV, et al. (2012) The chemokine, CXCL12, is an independent predictor of poor survival in ovarian cancer. Br J Cancer 106: 1306–1313.
80. Jiang YP, Wu XH, Shi B, Wu WX, Yin GR (2006) Expression of chemokine CXCL12 and its receptor CXCR4 in human epithelial ovarian cancer: an independent prognostic factor for tumor progression. Gynecol Oncol 103: 226–233.
81. Bast RCJ, Feeney M, Lazarus H, Nadler LM, Colvin RB, Knapp RC (1981) Reactivity of monoclonlantibody with human ovarian carcinoma. Journal of Clinical Investigation 68: 1331–1337.
82. Lee LF, Hellendall RP, Wang Y, Haskill JS, Mukaida N, et al. (2000) IL-8 Reduced Tumorigenicity of Human Ovarian Cancer Due to Neutrophil Infiltration. The Journal of Immunology 164: 2769–2775.
83. Wells CM, Ridley AJ (2005) Analysis of cell migration using the Dunn chemotaxis chamber and time-lapse microscopy. Methods Mol Biol 294: 31–41.
84. Zicha D, Dunn GA, Brown AF (1991) A new direct-viewing chemotaxis chamber. J Cell Sci 99 (Pt 4): 769–775.
85. Ivascu A, Kubbies M (2006) Rapid generation of single-tumor spheroids for high-throughput cell function and toxicity analysis. J Biomol Screen 11: 922–932.
86. Debnath J, Muthuswamy SK, Brugge JS (2003) Morphogenesis and oncogenesis of MCF-10A mammary epithelial acini grown in three-dimensional basement membrane cultures. Methods 30: 256–268.

Permissions

All chapters in this book were first published in PLOS ONE, by The Public Library of Science; hereby published with permission under the Creative Commons Attribution License or equivalent. Every chapter published in this book has been scrutinized by our experts. Their significance has been extensively debated. The topics covered herein carry significant findings which will fuel the growth of the discipline. They may even be implemented as practical applications or may be referred to as a beginning point for another development.

The contributors of this book come from diverse backgrounds, making this book a truly international effort. This book will bring forth new frontiers with its revolutionizing research information and detailed analysis of the nascent developments around the world.

We would like to thank all the contributing authors for lending their expertise to make the book truly unique. They have played a crucial role in the development of this book. Without their invaluable contributions this book wouldn't have been possible. They have made vital efforts to compile up to date information on the varied aspects of this subject to make this book a valuable addition to the collection of many professionals and students.

This book was conceptualized with the vision of imparting up-to-date information and advanced data in this field. To ensure the same, a matchless editorial board was set up. Every individual on the board went through rigorous rounds of assessment to prove their worth. After which they invested a large part of their time researching and compiling the most relevant data for our readers.

The editorial board has been involved in producing this book since its inception. They have spent rigorous hours researching and exploring the diverse topics which have resulted in the successful publishing of this book. They have passed on their knowledge of decades through this book. To expedite this challenging task, the publisher supported the team at every step. A small team of assistant editors was also appointed to further simplify the editing procedure and attain best results for the readers.

Apart from the editorial board, the designing team has also invested a significant amount of their time in understanding the subject and creating the most relevant covers. They scrutinized every image to scout for the most suitable representation of the subject and create an appropriate cover for the book.

The publishing team has been an ardent support to the editorial, designing and production team. Their endless efforts to recruit the best for this project, has resulted in the accomplishment of this book. They are a veteran in the field of academics and their pool of knowledge is as vast as their experience in printing. Their expertise and guidance has proved useful at every step. Their uncompromising quality standards have made this book an exceptional effort. Their encouragement from time to time has been an inspiration for everyone.

The publisher and the editorial board hope that this book will prove to be a valuable piece of knowledge for researchers, students, practitioners and scholars across the globe.

List of Contributors

Rosemary Braun
Robert H. Lurie Comprehensive Cancer Center, Northwestern University, Chicago, Illinois, United States of America
Center for Biomedical Informatics and Information Technology, National Cancer Institute, National Institutes of Health, Bethesda, Maryland, United States of America

Richard Finney, Chunhua Yan, Qing-Rong Chen, Ying Hu, Michael Edmonson and Daoud Meerzaman
Center for Biomedical Informatics and Information Technology, National Cancer Institute, National Institutes of Health, Bethesda, Maryland, United States of America

Kenneth Buetow
Computational Science and Informatics Program, Complex Adaptive Systems Initiative, Arizona State University, Phoenix, Arizona, United States of America
Center for Biomedical Informatics and Information Technology, National Cancer Institute, National Institutes of Health, Bethesda, Maryland, United States of America

Sébastien Baribeau, Parvesh Chaudhry, Sophie Parent and Éric Asselin
Research Group in Molecular Oncology and Endocrinology, Department of Medical Biology, Université du Québec à Trois-Rivières, Trois-Rivières, Québec, Canada

Man-Tat Lau, Wai-Kin So and Peter C. K. Leung
Department of Obstetrics and Gynecology, Child and Family Research Institute, University of British Columbia, Vancouver, British Columbia, Canada

Shashikant B. Lele
Departments of Gynecologic Oncology, Roswell Park Cancer Institute, Buffalo, New York, United States of America

Kunle Odunsi
Departments of Gynecologic Oncology, Roswell Park Cancer Institute, Buffalo, New York, United States of America
Immunology; Roswell Park Cancer Institute, Buffalo, New York, United States of America
Center for Immunotherapy; Roswell Park Cancer Institute, Buffalo, New York, United States of America

Feng Qian
Immunology; Roswell Park Cancer Institute, Buffalo, New York, United States of America
Center for Immunotherapy; Roswell Park Cancer Institute, Buffalo, New York, United States of America

Amy Beck and Zikun Qian
Center for Immunotherapy; Roswell Park Cancer Institute, Buffalo, New York, United States of America

Jianqun Liao
Departments of Gynecologic Oncology, Roswell Park Cancer Institute, Buffalo, New York, United States of America
Surgical Oncology, Roswell Park Cancer Institute, Buffalo, New York, United States of America

Wendy J. Hu
Urology Oncology, Roswell Park Cancer Institute, Buffalo, New York, United States of America
Pharmacology & Therapeutics, Roswell Park Cancer Institute, Buffalo, New York, United States of America

Carl D. Morrison and Paulette Mhawech-Fauceglia
Pathology, Roswell Park Cancer Institute, Buffalo, New York, United States of America

Xinhui Wang
Surgical Oncology, Massachusetts General Hospital, Harvard Medical School, Boston, United States of America

Nana Tchabo
Atlantic Health System Morristown/Overlook Medical Centers, Women's Cancer Center, Morristown and Summit, New Jersey, United States of America

Wenjing Shen, Tianren Li and Yanjie Hu
Department of Gynecology, The First Affiliated Hospital of China Medical University, Shenyang, China

Min Song
Department of Pathology, The First Affiliated Hospital and College of Basic Medical Sciences, China Medical University, Institute of Pathology and Pathophysiology, Shenyang, China

Jie Liu
Experimental Technology Center, China Medical University, Shenyang, China

Guangrong Qi
Department of Medical Genetics, China Medical University, Shenyang, China

Hongbo Liu
Department of Health Statistics, School of Public Health, China Medical University, Shenyang, China

Saleh M. Rachidi and Zihai Li
Department of Microbiology and Immunology, South Carolina Clinical and Translational Research Institute (SCTR), Medical University of South Carolina, Charleston, South Carolina, United States of America
Hollings Cancer Center, South Carolina Clinical and Translational Research Institute (SCTR), Medical University of South Carolina, Charleston, South Carolina, United States of America

Tingting Qin
Division of Bioinformatics, Department of Biochemistry and Molecular Biology, South Carolina Clinical and Translational Research Institute (SCTR), Medical University of South Carolina, Charleston, South Carolina, United States of America

Shaoli Sun
Department of Pathology and Laboratory Medicine, South Carolina Clinical and Translational Research Institute (SCTR), Medical University of South Carolina, Charleston, South Carolina, United States of America,

W. Jim Zheng
Division of Bioinformatics, Department of Biochemistry and Molecular Biology, South Carolina Clinical and Translational Research Institute (SCTR), Medical University of South Carolina, Charleston, South Carolina, United States of America,
Computational Biology Core Facility, South Carolina Clinical and Translational Research Institute (SCTR), Medical University of South Carolina, Charleston, South Carolina, United States of America

Ercan Cacan, Nathaniel H. Boyd and Susanna F. Greer
Division of Cellular Biology and Immunology, Center for Inflammation, Immunity and Infection, Department of Biology, Georgia State University, Atlanta, Georgia, United States of America

Mourad W. Ali and Shelley B. Hooks
Department of Pharmaceutical and Biomedical Sciences, University of Georgia, Athens, Georgia, United States of America

Rebecca R. Carter and Jiayang Sun
Department of Epidemiology and Biostatistics, School of Medicine, Case Western Reserve University, Cleveland, Ohio, United States of America

Analisa DiFeo and Guo-Qiang Zhang
Case Comprehensive Cancer Center, Case Western Reserve University, Cleveland, Ohio, United States of America

Kath Bogie
Departments of Orthopaedics and Biomedical Engineering, Case Western Reserve University, Cleveland, Ohio, United States of America

Lindsey M. Hoskins and Mark H. Greene
Clinical Genetics Branch, National Cancer Institute, Bethesda, Maryland, United States of America

Allison Werner-Lin
Social Policy and Practice, University of Pennsylvania, Philadelphia, Pennsylvania, United States of America

Lynn A. Beer, Huan Wang, Hsin-Yao Tang, Zhijun Cao, Tony Chang-Wong, Qin Liu and David W. Speicher
Center for Systems and Computational Biology, and Molecular and Cellular Oncogenesis Program, The Wistar Institute, Philadelphia, Pennsylvania, United States of America

Janos L. Tany
Ovarian Cancer Research Center, The University of Pennsylvania, Philadelphia, Pennsylvania, United States of America

Rugang Zhang
Gene Expression and Regulation Program, The Wistar Institute, Philadelphia, Pennsylvania, United States of America

Matthew Schwede
Biostatistics and Computational Biology, Dana-Farber Cancer Institute, Boston, Massachusetts, United States of America

Aedín C. Culhane and David Harrington
Biostatistics and Computational Biology, Dana-Farber Cancer Institute, Boston, Massachusetts, United States of America
Biostatistics, Harvard School of Public Health, Boston, Massachusetts, United States of America

Oliver Hofmann
Biostatistics, Harvard School of Public Health, Boston, Massachusetts, United States of America

Dimitrios Spentzos
Division of Hematology/Oncology, Department of Medicine, Beth Israel Deaconess Medical Center, Boston, Massachusetts, United States of America

Stefan Bentink
Biostatistics and Computational Biology, Dana-Farber Cancer Institute, Boston, Massachusetts, United States of America
Exosome Diagnostics GmbH, Martinsried, Germany

John Quackenbush
Biostatistics and Computational Biology, Dana-Farber Cancer Institute, Boston, Massachusetts, United States of America
Biostatistics, Harvard School of Public Health, Boston, Massachusetts, United States of America
Cancer Biology, Dana-Farber Cancer Institute, Boston, Massachusetts, United States of America

Benjamin Haibe-Kains
Biostatistics and Computational Biology, Dana-Farber Cancer Institute, Boston, Massachusetts, United States of America
Integrative Systems Biology, Institut de recherches cliniques de Montre´al, Montreal, Quebec, Canada

Claire M. Mach
Department of Obstetrics and Gynecology, Baylor College of Medicine, Houston, Texas, United States of America
College of Pharmacy, University of Houston, Houston, Texas, United States of America

Ying-Wooi Wan
Department of Pediatrics, Baylor College of Medicine, Houston, Texas, United States of America
Department of Obstetrics and Gynecology, Baylor College of Medicine, Houston, Texas, United States of America,
Department of Pathology and Immunology, Baylor College of Medicine, Houston, Texas, United States of America

Matthew L. Anderson
Department of Obstetrics and Gynecology, Baylor College of Medicine, Houston, Texas, United States of America
Department of Pathology and Immunology, Baylor College of Medicine, Houston, Texas, United States of America
Dan L. Duncan Cancer Center, Baylor College of Medicine, Houston, Texas, United States of America

Zhandong Liu
Dan L. Duncan Cancer Center, Baylor College of Medicine, Houston, Texas, United States of America
Computational and Integrative Biomedical Research (CIBR) Center, Baylor College of Medicine, Houston, Texas, United States of America
Neurological Research Institute, Texas Children's Hospital, Houston, Texas, United States of America

Genevera I. Allen
Department of Pediatrics, Baylor College of Medicine, Houston, Texas, United States of America
Neurological Research Institute, Texas Children's Hospital, Houston, Texas, United States of America,
Department of Statistics and Electrical & Computer Engineering, Rice University, Houston, Texas, United States of America

Harsh Vardhan Jain
Department of Mathematics, Florida State University, Tallahassee, Florida,United States of America,

Alan Richardson
Institute for Science and Technology in Medicine, Keele University, Stoke-on-Trent, United Kingdom

Michael Meyer-Hermann
Department of Systems Immunology, Helmholtz Centre for Infection Research, Braunschweig, Germany
Bio Centre for Life Science, Braunschweig University of Technology, Braunschweig, Germany

Helen M. Byrne
Oxford Centre for Collaborative and Applied Mathematics, Mathematical Institute, University of Oxford, Oxford, United Kingdom

Department of Computer Science, University of Oxford, Oxford, United Kingdom

Jing Yan and Jing-Ping Zhang
State Key Laboratory of Oncology in South China, Sun Yat-sen University Cancer Center, Guangzhou, P. R. China

Yi Zhang, Jing Liang and Lian Li
State Key Laboratory of Biocontrol, School of Life Sciences, Sun Yat-sen University, Guangzhou, P. R. China

Limin Zheng
State Key Laboratory of Oncology in South China, Sun Yat-sen University Cancer Center, Guangzhou, P. R. China
State Key Laboratory of Biocontrol, School of Life Sciences, Sun Yat-sen University, Guangzhou, P. R. China

Laura Calec,. Mara Colombo, Carla B. Ripamonti, Claudia Foglia and Paolo Radice
Unit of Molecular Bases of Genetic Risk and Genetic Testing, Department of Preventive and Predictive Medicine, Fondazione IRCCS Istituto Nazionale dei Tumori (INT), c/o Amadeolab, Milano, Italy

Caterina Congregati and Laura Papi
Department of Biomedical, Experimental and Clinical Sciences, University of Florence, Florence, Italy

Anna Laura Putignano
Department of Biomedical, Experimental and Clinical Sciences, University of Florence, Florence, Italy
FiorGen Foundation for Pharmacogenomics, Sesto Fiorentino, Italy

Mohosin Sarkar and Thomas J. Magliery
Department of Chemistry and Department of Biochemistry, The Ohio State University, Columbus, Ohio, United States of America

Bernard Peissel, Daniela Zaffaroni, Siranoush Manoukian
Unit of Medical Genetics, Department of Preventive and Predictive Medicine, Fondazione IRCCS Istituto Nazionale dei Tumori, Milan, Italy

Carlo Tondini
Unit of Medical Oncology, Azienda Ospedaliera Papa Giovanni XXIII, Bergamo, Italy

Monica Barile
Division of Cancer Prevention and Genetics, Istituto Europeo di Oncologia, Milan, Italy

Valeria Pensotti
COGENTECH-Cancer Genetic Testing Laboratory, Milan, Italy
Fondazione Istituto FIRC di Oncologia Molecolare, Milan, Italy

Loris Bernard
COGENTECH-Cancer Genetic Testing Laboratory, Milan, Italy
Department of Experimental Oncology, Istituto Europeo di Oncologia, Milan, Italy

Loris De Cecco
Functional Genomics Core Facility, Fondazione Istituto Di Ricovero e Cura a Carattere Scientifico Istituto Nazionale dei Tumori, Milan, Italy

Martina Berardi and Elda Tagliabue
Molecular Targeting Unit, Fondazione Istituto Di Ricovero e Cura a Carattere Scientifico Istituto Nazionale dei Tumori, Milan, Italy

Michele Sommariva, and Andrea Balsari
Molecular Targeting Unit, Fondazione Istituto Di Ricovero e Cura a Carattere Scientifico Istituto Nazionale dei Tumori, Milan, Italy
Department of Biomedical Sciences for Health, University of Milan, Milan, Italy

Alessandra Cataldo
Department of Biomedical Sciences for Health, University of Milan, Milan, Italy

Silvana Canevari and Delia Mezzanzanica
Molecular Therapies Unit, Fondazione Istituto Di Ricovero e Cura a Carattere Scientifico Istituto\ Nazionale dei Tumori, Milan, Italy

Marilena V. Iorio
Start Up Unit, Fondazione Istituto Di Ricovero e Cura a Carattere Scientifico Istituto Nazionale dei Tumori, Milan, Italy

Xingwang Zhang, Zejian Zhang, Xijun Liu, Lei Zhou, Yuanyuan Ruan, Jiejie Xu, Haiou Liu, Shifang Ren Jianxin Gu and Yifan Qian
Key Laboratory of Glycoconjugate Research Ministry of Public Health, Department of Biochemistry and Molecular Biology, School of Basic Medical Sciences, Fudan University, Shanghai, China

Yisheng Wang and Xin Wu
Obstetrics and Gynecology Hospital, Fudan University, Shanghai, China

Ran Zhao
Institute of Biomedical Sciences, Fudan University, Shanghai, China

Congjian Xu
Obstetrics and Gynecology Hospital, Fudan University, Shanghai, China
Department of Obstetrics and Gynecology of Shanghai Medical School, Fudan University, Shanghai, China
Institute of Biomedical Sciences, Fudan University, Shanghai, China
Shanghai Key Laboratory of Female Reproductive Endocrine Related Diseases, Shanghai, China

Yan Xia and Heng-Yu Fan
Life Sciences Institute and Innovation Center for Cell Biology, Zhejiang University, Hangzhou, China

Ting Chang
Department of Neurology, Tangdu Hospital, the Fourth Military Medical University, Xi'an, China

Yingmei Wang and Yixiong Liu
Department of Pathology, Xijing Hospital, the Fourth Military Medical University, Xi'an, China

Wenhui Li
Department of Obstetrics and Gynecology, Xijing Hospital, the Fourth Military Medical University, Xi'an, China

Ming Li
The Affiliated Guangren Hospital, Xi'an Jiaotong University, Xi'an, China

Kristina A. Williams
Obstetrics and Gynecology Epidemiology Center, Department of Obstetrics and Gynecology, Brigham and Women's Hospital, Boston, Massachusetts, United States of America
Harvard Medical School, Boston, Massachusetts, United States of America

Allison F. Vitonis
Obstetrics and Gynecology Epidemiology Center, Department of Obstetrics and Gynecology, Brigham and Women's Hospital, Boston, Massachusetts, United States of America

Kathryn L. Terry and Daniel W. Cramer
Obstetrics and Gynecology Epidemiology Center, Department of Obstetrics and Gynecology, Brigham and Women's Hospital, Boston, Massachusetts, United States of America
Harvard Medical School, Boston, Massachusetts, United States of America
Department of Epidemiology, Harvard School of Public Health, Boston, Massachusetts, United States of America

Shelley S. Tworoger
Department of Epidemiology, Harvard School of Public Health, Boston, Massachusetts, United States of America
Channing Division of Network Medicine, Department of Medicine, Brigham and Women's Hospital and Harvard Medical School, Boston, Massachusetts, United States of America

Linda J. Titus
Department of Community & Family Medicine, Department of Pediatrics, Dartmouth-Hitchcock Medical Center Lebanon, New Hampshire, United States of America

Øystein Helland and Line Bjørge
Department of Obstetrics and Gynecology, Haukeland University Hospital, Bergen, Norway
Department of Clinical Science, University of Bergen, Bergen, Norway

Mihaela Popa
KinN Therapeutics, Bergen, Norway

Olav K. Vintermyr and Anders Molven
The Gade Laboratory for Pathology, Department of Clinical Medicine, University of Bergen, Bergen, Norway
Department of Pathology, Haukeland University Hospital, Bergen, Norway

Bjørn Tore Gjertsen and Emmet McCormack
Department of Clinical Science, University of Bergen, Bergen, Norway
Department of Medicine, Hematology Section, Haukeland University Hospital, Bergen, Norway

Krista M. Pettee, Kaitlyn M. Dvorak and Kathryn M. Eisenmann
Department of Biochemistry and Cancer Biology, University of Toledo Health Science Campus, Toledo, Ohio, United States of America

Andrea L. Nestor-Kalinoski
Department of Surgery, University of Toledo Health Science Campus, Toledo, Ohio, United States of America

Index